# Basic and Bedside
# Electrocardiography

# Basic and Bedside
# Electrocardiography

### Romulo F. Baltazar, MD, FACC

*Director, Noninvasive Cardiology*
*Sinai Hospital of Baltimore*
*Assistant Professor, Medicine*
*Johns Hopkins University*
*Baltimore, Maryland*

Wolters Kluwer | Lippincott Williams & Wilkins
Health
Philadelphia · Baltimore · New York · London
Buenos Aires · Hong Kong · Sydney · Tokyo

*Acquisitions Editor:* Frances Destefano
*Managing Editor:* Leanne McMillan
*Marketing Manager:* Kimberly Schonberger
*Production Editor:* Beth Martz
*Design Coordinator:* Stephen Druding
*Compositor:* Aptara, Inc.

351 West Camden Street          530 Walnut Street
Baltimore, MD 21201              Philadelphia, PA 19106

Printed in the United Staes of America

9  8

**Library of Congress Cataloging-in-Publication Data**

Baltazar, Romulo F.
   Basic and bedside electrocardiography / Romulo F. Baltazar.
       p. ; cm.
   Includes index.
   ISBN-13: 978-0-7817-8804-5
   ISBN-10: 0-7817-8804-8
  1.   Electrocardiography.   I. Title.
   [DNLM: 1.   Electrocardiography. 2.   Heart Diseases—diagnosis. 3.   Heart
Diseases—therapy.   WG 140 B197b 2009]
   RC683.5.E5B283 2009
   616.1′207547—dc22

                                        2008056135

DISCLAIMER

Care has been taken to confirm the accuracy of the information present and to describe generally accepted practices. However, the authors, editors, and publisher are not responsible for errors or omissions or for any consequences from application of the information in this book and make no warranty, expressed or implied, with respect to the currency, completeness, or accuracy of the contents of the publication. Application of this information in a particular situation remains the professional responsibility of the practitioner; the clinical treatments described and recommended may not be considered absolute and universal recommendations.

The authors, editors, and publisher have exerted every effort to ensure that drug selection and dosage set forth in this text are in accordance with the current recommendations and practice at the time of publication. However, in view of ongoing research, changes in government regulations, and the constant flow of information relating to drug therapy and drug reactions, the reader is urged to check the package insert for each drug for any change in indications and dosage and for added warnings and precautions. This is particularly important when the recommended agent is a new or infrequently employed drug.

Some drugs and medical devices presented in this publication have Food and Drug Administration (FDA) clearance for limited use in restricted research settings. It is the responsibility of the health care provider to ascertain the FDA status of each drug or device planned for use in their clinical practice.

To purchase additional copies of this book, call our customer service department at **(800) 638-3030** or fax orders to **(301) 223-2320**. International customers should call **(301) 223-2300**.

Visit Lippincott Williams & Wilkins on the Internet: http://www.lww.com. Lippincott Williams & Wilkins customer service representatives are available from 8:30 am to 6:00 pm, EST.

*This book is dedicated to my wife, Ophelia,
for her inspiration, support and encouragement in
the preparation of this book.*

# Preface

More than 100 years since its introduction, electrocardiography continues to provide invaluable clinical information. Even with the development of modern and more expensive technologies, its significance has not declined. To the contrary, its clinical application continues to expand, and presently, it is the most utilized diagnostic modality in the whole practice of medicine. In the hospital setting, it is routinely used to monitor both cardiac and noncardiac patients, especially in acute care units and during the performance of various cardiac and noncardiac procedures. Thus, the information provided by the electrocardiogram should be standard knowledge for every medical and paramedical professional who is involved with patient care.

This book is purposely written in a format that will assist the beginner, including medical students, nurses, and paramedical professionals, in understanding basic electrocardiography. It is also intended for interns, residents, physician assistants, fellows, anesthesiologists, and clinical cardiologists by including standard of care treatment of patients with electrocardiographic abnormalities based on the most recent practice guidelines when guidelines are available. Thus, the book is a combination of both basic and bedside electrocardiography.

The book integrates the comments and suggestions of many interns, residents, and attending physicians to whom I owe a great deal of gratitude. I would like to thank Drs. Miruais Hamed, Paul Aoun, Eileen Zingman, Olga Szalasny, Katja Vassiliades, Manish Arora, Onyi Onuoha, Brandon Togioka, Darshana Purohit, Ranjani Ramanathan, Binu Matthew, Paolo Caimi, Mulugeta Fissha, Hany Bashandy, Cindy Huang, Suzan Fattohy, Rachel Hartman, Kevin Hayes, Khawaja Farook, Jason Javillo, Jennifer Morales, Ubadullah Sharief, Ledys de Marsico, Celian Valero, Samarina Ahmad, Kweku Hayford, Haritha Pendli, Maya Morrison, and many others. I am also grateful to Kittane Vishnupriya for his very helpful comments and for the ECG that he painstakingly obtained to illustrate the significance of the posterior leads in the diagnosis of posterolateral myocardial infarction when he was a coronary care resident. I am also grateful to Drs. Gabriela Szabo, Ameena Etherington, and Soma Sengupta for reviewing chapters in the book, and Laura Baldwin, our superb cardiology technician, who has taught me how to retrieve and record electrocardiograms from our archives.

I am also grateful to Dr. Morton Mower who has been my mentor since I was a resident. His suggestions for improving the book are greatly appreciated. I would also like to express my deep appreciation to Dr. Steven Gambert, Chief of the Department of Medicine, Johns Hopkins University/Sinai Hospital Program in Internal Medicine, for his support and encouragement and for his enthusiasm in having this book published.

Finally, I am grateful to my daughter, Cristina, who is instrumental in teaching me how to use the computer in the preparation of this book and my son Romulo, Jr who decided on Radiology as his specialty, for his comments and suggestions for simplifying some of the chapters, especially those dealing with Basic Electrocardiography.

*Romulo F. Baltazar, MD, FACC*
*Director, Noninvasive Cardiology, Department of Medicine*
*Johns Hopkins University/Sinai Hospital Program in*
*Internal Medicine*

# Contents

# Basic Anatomy and Electrophysiology

## Basic Anatomy of the Heart

- **The cardiac chambers:** The heart is the center of the circulatory system and is the organ that pumps blood to the different parts of the body. It consists of two upper receiving chambers—the right atrium and left atrium—and two lower pumping muscular chambers—the right ventricle and left ventricle (Fig. 1.1).
  - **Right atrium:** The right atrium receives venous blood from the different parts of the body through the superior and inferior vena cavae and directs the blood to the right ventricle.
  - **Right ventricle:** The right ventricle pumps blood to the pulmonary artery for delivery to the lungs.
  - **Left atrium:** The left atrium receives oxygenated blood from the lungs through four separate pulmonary veins and delivers blood to the left ventricle.
  - **Left ventricle:** The left ventricle pumps oxygenated blood to the aorta for delivery to the different parts of the body.

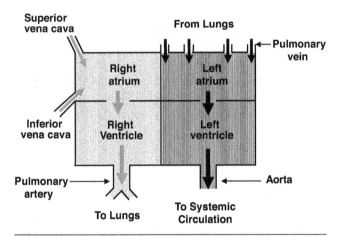

**Figure 1.1: Anatomy of the Heart.** Diagrammatic representation of the heart showing two upper receiving chambers—the right and left atria—and two lower muscular pumping chambers—the right and left ventricles. Arrows point to the direction of blood flow.

## The Sinus Node and Intraventricular Conduction System

- **The sinus node and conduction system:** The heart has a generator that gives rise to an electrical impulse and an electrical circuit; this allows the cardiac impulse to propagate from atria to ventricles in an orderly sequence. The generator of the heart is the sinus node and the electrical circuit is the intraventricular conduction system (Fig. 1.2A, B).
- **Intraventricular conduction system:** The bundle of His, right and left bundle branches, the fascicular branches of the left bundle branch, and Purkinje fibers constitute the intraventricular conduction system. Their cells are specialized for rapid and orderly conduction of the electrical impulse and may be regarded as the electrical circuit of the heart.

## Basic Anatomy of the Heart

- **Sinus node:** The sinus node is the origin of the cardiac impulse and is the pacemaker of the heart. It is located high within the right atrium near the entrance of the superior vena cava.
- **Atria:** The atria consist of a thin layer of muscle cells that conduct the sinus impulse directly to the atrioventricular (AV) node. The atria also contracts upon arrival of the impulse from the sinus node. With contraction of the atria, additional blood is pumped to the ventricles.
- **AV node:** The AV node is the only pathway through which the sinus impulse can reach the ventricles. It is located at the floor of the right atrium, adjacent to the ventricular septum. The AV node slows down the conduction of the sinus impulse to the ventricles so that contraction of the atria and ventricles does not occur simultaneously. This results in a better cardiac output.

**Figure 1.2:** **The Sinus Node and the Intraventricular Conduction System of the Heart.** **(A)** Diagrammatic representation of the sinus node, atria, AV node, and the intraventricular conduction system of the heart. **(B)** Diagram showing the sequence of conduction of the cardiac impulse from sinus node to the ventricles. AV, atrioventricular; BB, bundle branch; LA, left atrium; LV, left ventricle; RA, right atrium; RV, right ventricle.

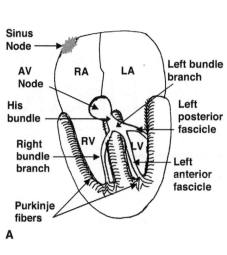

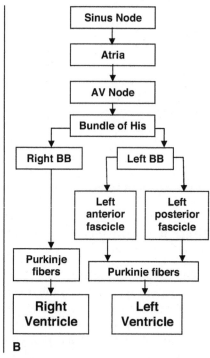

- **Bundle of His:** The AV node continues into the bundle of His, a short structure that immediately divides into two main branches: the left and right bundle branches.
- **Right bundle branch:** The right bundle branch is a long and thin branch of the His bundle that courses to the right side of the ventricular septum. It terminates into a network of Purkinje fibers in the endocardium of the right ventricle.
- **Left bundle branch:** The left bundle branch is a short branch of the His bundle that spreads to the left side of the ventricular septum in a fanlike fashion forming three distinct fascicles.
  - **Left anterior fascicle:** This fascicle courses to the anterior and superior walls of the left ventricle.
  - **Midseptal fascicle:** This fascicle branches to the ventricular septum and is intricately connected with the anterior and posterior fascicles.
  - **Left posterior fascicle:** This fascicle courses to the posterior and inferior walls before terminating in a network of Purkinje fibers.

- **Purkinje system:** The Purkinje system is the terminal portion of the conduction system consisting of a network of fibers within the endocardium of both ventricles. It spreads the impulse directly to the myocardium, causing both ventricles to contract in synchrony.
- **Ventricles:** The ventricles are the main pumping chambers of the heart. Because the muscles of the ventricles are the thickest structure in the heart, they generate the largest deflection in the electrocardiogram (ECG).

## Basic Electrophysiology

- **Basic electrophysiology:** The heart consists of three special types of cells with different electrophysiologic properties (Fig. 1.3). These cells include:
  - **Muscle cells:** Muscle cells are specialized for contraction and are present in the atria and ventricles.

**Figure 1.3:**    **Action Potential of a Muscle Cell, Conducting Cell and Pacemaking Cell.** The action potential of a ventricular muscle cell specialized for contraction **(A)**, His-Purkinje cell specialized for impulse conduction **(B)**, and sinus node cell with special properties of automaticity **(C)**.

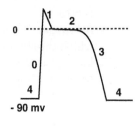

A: Muscle Cell

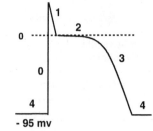

B: Conducting Cell

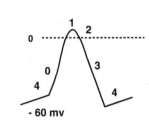

C: Pacemaking Cell

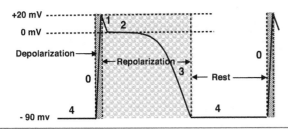

**Figure 1.4:    Action Potential of a Ventricular Muscle Cell.** The action potential of a ventricular muscle cell is shown. Phase 4 corresponds to the resting potential, which is approximately −90 mV. When the cell is depolarized, the potential abruptly changes from −90 mV to +20 mV and is represented by a rapid upstroke or phase 0. Phase 1 returns the overshoot to neutral. Phase 2 corresponds to the plateau phase in which the potential is maintained at 0 mV for a constant duration. Phase 3 returns the potential rapidly to resting baseline of −90 mV.

- **Conducting cells:** Conducting cells are specialized for rapid conduction of the electrical impulse and are present within the entire His-Purkinje system.
- **Pacemaking cells:** Pacemaking cells have properties of automaticity and are capable of generating electrical impulses. These cells are present in the sinus node and throughout the His-Purkinje system.
- All myocardial cells are electrically polarized with the inside of the cell more electrically negative than the outside. This negative potential is due to the difference in concentration of electrolytes inside the cell compared with outside. Because the cells are polarized, they are capable of being discharged. When the cells are discharged, an action potential is generated. Recordings of action potentials of a ventricular muscle cell, conducting cell from the His-Purkinje system and a pacemaking cell from the sinus node are shown in Figure 1.3.
- **Action potential of a ventricular muscle cell:** When a ventricular muscle cell discharges, an action potential is generated. A recorded action potential is shown in Figure 1.4. The action potential can be divided into five separate phases: 0, 1, 2, 3, and 4. Taken together, the five phases of the action potential represent a complete electrical cycle with phase 0 representing depolarization, phases 1 to 3 representing repolarization, and phase 4 representing rest or quiescence.
  - **Phase 4:** A ventricular muscle cell has a resting potential of approximately −90 mV, meaning the cell is more negative inside than outside by about 90 mV. This is primarily because of the higher concentration of potassium inside the cell than outside. This resting state corresponds to phase 4 of the action potential.
  - **Phase 0:** Depolarization of the cell corresponds to phase 0 of the action potential. During phase 0, the

polarity of the cell changes rapidly from −90 mV to 0 mV, transiently overshooting the point of equilibrium by +20 mV. This rapid depolarization is due to the transit of positively charged sodium from outside the cell to inside and is represented by the rapid upstroke of the action potential.
  - **Phase 1:** This corresponds to the return of the overshoot to 0 mV.
  - **Phase 2:** This corresponds to the plateau phase of the action potential, which is maintained at approximately 0 mV.
  - **Phase 3:** This is due to rapid repolarization returning the polarity of the cell immediately to its resting potential of −90 mV.
- **Action potential of sinus node cell:** The action potential of a sinus node cell, which is a pacemaker cell, is different from a muscle cell. The features of a pacemaker cell that make it different from a nonpacemaking cell are summarized in the diagram (Fig. 1.5).
  - **Spontaneous depolarization:** The most important difference between a pacemaker and a non-pacemaker cell is that during phase 4, cells with pacemaking properties exhibit slow spontaneous diastolic depolarization, which is characterized by a slowly rising upward slope of the resting potential. This is due to slowly decreasing negativity of the cell caused by the slow entry of sodium ions into the cell. Because sodium carries positive charges, the cell becomes less and less negative until it reaches a certain threshold (threshold potential), above which the cell automatically discharges. This property is not present in non-pacemaking cells because non-pacemaking cells have flat or very slow rising diastolic slopes during phase 4, which never reach threshold potential.
  - **Resting potential:** The resting potential of a sinus node cell is approximately −60 mV and therefore is less negative than the resting potential of a ventricular muscle cell, which is approximately −90 mV. This causes phase 0 to rise slowly resulting only in a small overshoot of 0 to 10 mV (see Fig. 1.5) as compared with that seen in the non-pacemaker cell.
- **Repolarization:** After the cells are depolarized, they have to recover before the arrival of the next impulse. This process of recovery is called repolarization. Repolarization is a longer process than depolarization and includes phases 1, 2, and 3 of the action potential. During repolarization, the cell may not be able to respond to another stimulus. The likelihood of response depends on the electrical status of the cell (Fig. 1.6).
  - **Absolute refractory period:** The cell is unable to respond to any kind of stimulus during this period. It includes phases 1 and 2.

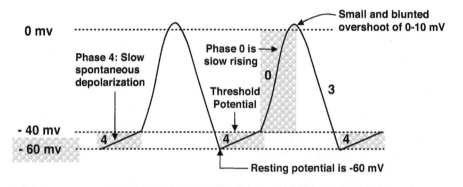

**Figure 1.5:   Action Potential of a Sinus Node Cell.** The action potential of a sinus node cell is shown. The resting potential is approximately −60 mV and is less negative than the resting potential of a ventricular muscle cell, which is approximately −90 mV. Slow spontaneous depolarization is present during phase 4. Phase 0 is slow rising with only a small overshoot. These features differentiate a pacemaking cell from a non-pacemaking cell and are highlighted.

■ **Effective refractory period:** The cell is able to generate a potential; however, it is too weak to be propagated. This includes a small portion of phase 3.

■ **Relative refractory period:** The cell is partially repolarized and may be able to respond to a stimulus if the stimulus is stronger than usual. This period includes a portion of phase 3 extending to threshold potential, which is about −70 mV.

■ **Supernormal phase:** The cell may respond to a less than normal stimulus. This period includes the end of phase 3 when repolarization is almost complete and has reached a potential that is more negative than the threshold potential of −70 mV.

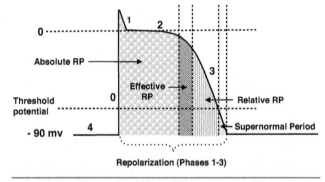

**Figure 1.6:   Repolarization and Refractory Periods.** Repolarization includes phases 1 to 3 of the action potential. The absolute refractory period includes phases 1 and 2 in which the cell cannot be stimulated by any impulse. The effective refractory period includes a small portion of phase 3 in which a stimulus can elicit a local response but not strong enough to be propagated. Relative refractory period is that portion of phase 3 that extends to threshold potential. The cell will respond to a stimulus that is stronger than normal. The supernormal phase starts just below threshold potential where the cell can respond to a stimulus that is less than normal. RP, refractory period.

# Basic Anatomy and Electrophysiology

## Basic Anatomy

■ **The sinus node:** The sinus node is located in the superior and lateral border of the right atrium. The most cranial portion starts from the epicardium at the junction of the superior vena cava and right atrium. Its most caudal portion is located subendocardially. The sinus node contains pacemaker cells that are widely distributed throughout its entire length. These cells have properties of automaticity and are capable of discharging spontaneously. Although there are other cells in the heart that are also capable of discharging spontaneously, the cells in the sinus node have the fastest rate of discharge. The sinus node therefore is the pacemaker of the heart. The sinus node is supplied by the sinus node artery that originates from the right coronary artery 60% to 65% of the time. The rest of the vascular supply originates from the left circumflex coronary artery.

■ **Internodal tracts:** There are three internodal tracts connecting the sinus node to the AV node namely the anterior, posterior, and middle internodal tracts. The significance of these internodal tracts is uncertain because the sinus impulse is conducted to the AV node through the atria.

■ **The AV node:** The AV node is smaller than the sinus node and is located in the lower right atrium just above the insertion of the septal leaflet of the tricuspid valve and anterior to the entrance of the coronary sinus to the lower right atrium. The AV node consists of three areas with distinct properties: the upper, middle, and lower portions. The upper portion also called AN (atrionodal) region connects the atria to the middle portion, which is called N (nodal) region. The lower portion, also called NH (nodo-His) region, connects with the bundle of His. The middle region is primarily responsible for delaying AV conduction. It is also where acetylcholine is released. It has no automatic properties in contrast to the upper and lower regions, which contain cells with properties of automaticity. In 90% of patients, the AV node is supplied by the AV nodal artery, which is a branch of the right coronary artery. In the remaining 10%, the AV node artery comes from the left circumflex coronary artery.

- **The His-Purkinje system:** The AV node continues as the His bundle, which immediately divides into the right and the left bundle branches. The right bundle branch is a direct continuation of the bundle of His and continues down the right side of the interventricular septum toward the right ventricular apex and base of the anterior papillary muscle. The left bundle branch fans into several branches. These branches can be grouped into three main subdivisions or fascicles: the anterior, midseptal, and posterior fascicles. These fascicles are interconnected with each other. The significance of the midseptal fascicle is uncertain, although it is probably responsible for the initial depolarization of the ventricular septum. The right bundle branch and the fascicles end into a network of Purkinje fibers over the endocardial surface of both ventricles. Conduction across the His-Purkinje system is not significantly affected by sympathetic and parasympathetic influences. The blood supply of the His bundle comes from both anterior and posterior descending coronary arteries through their septal branches.

## Basic Electrophysiology

- There are three special types of cells in the heart, each with its own distinctive electrophysiologic property. They include muscle cells such as those of the atria and ventricles, conducting cells such as those of the His-Purkinje system, and pacemaking cells such as those of the sinus node.
- All cells are polarized with the inside of the cell more negative than the outside. This difference in the electrical charge is due to the different concentration of electrolytes inside the cell compared with outside. The major electrolytes that determine the difference in gradient between the inside and outside the cell are:
  - **Potassium**—the concentration of $K^+$ is 30 to 50 times higher inside than outside the cell.
  - **Sodium**—the concentration of $Na^+$ is reversed from that of potassium and is almost 10 times higher outside than inside the cell.
  - **Calcium**—the concentration of $Ca^{2+}$ is higher outside than inside the cell.
- The cell membrane is relatively impermeable to electrolytes. The movement of ions into and out of the cell membrane is controlled by channels that are specific to certain ions. $Na^+$ channels are present that are specific only for sodium ions. $K^+$ and $Ca^{2+}$ channels are also present that are specific only

for potassium and calcium ions, respectively. These ions, however, cannot enter into and out of the cell any time. The channels open and close only at given moment. In other words, they are gated. The voltage of the cell membrane controls the gates; thus, opening and closing of these channels are voltage sensitive. Channels that are specific only for sodium ions, called fast sodium channels, are closed when the potential or voltage of the cell is –90 mV (resting potential). The fast sodium channels will open only when the cell is depolarized, resulting in rapid entry of sodium ions into the cell. This corresponds to the rapid upstroke (phase 0) of the action potential.

## The Action Potential of Muscle Cells in the Atria and Ventricles

- **The sodium pump:** The resting potential of muscle cells in the ventricles is approximately –90 mV. It is slightly less in the atria. During the resting state, the cell membrane is impermeable to sodium. A higher concentration of sodium is maintained outside the cell compared with inside the cell, because of the presence of a $Na^+/K^+$ pump located in the cell membrane. The $Na^+/K^+$ pump exchanges three $Na^+$ ions from inside the cell for two $K^+$ ions outside the cell. This exchange process requires energy, which is derived from the hydrolysis of adenosine triphosphate by the enzyme sodium-potassium adenosine triphosphatase (ATPase). Because there are three ions of $Na^+$ exchanged for two ions of $K^+$, a positive ion is lost during the exchange making the inside of the cell more negative.

  - The increasing negativity of the cell when $Na^+$ is exchanged for $K^+$ is due to the presence of large negatively charged proteins inside the cell. These large proteins are unable to diffuse out of the cell because of their size. Thus, when three ions of $Na^+$ exit the cell in exchange for two ions of $K^+$ entering the cell, the large proteins will have one negative charge that is not neutralized, making the inside of the cell more negative until a potential of –90 mV is reached.

  - **Mechanism of action of digitalis:** If the $Na^+/K^+$ ATPase pump is inhibited, sodium is removed through the $Na^+/Ca^{2+}$ exchange mechanism. Sodium inside the cell is exchanged for calcium, which causes calcium to accumulate within the cell. This increase in intracellular calcium through inhibition of the Na/K ATPase pump is the mechanism by which digitalis exerts its inotropic effect. In the presence of digitalis toxicity, this exchange can continue even after the cell has completed its repolarization (beyond phase 3). This may cause the potential of the cell to become transiently less negative, resulting in delayed afterdepolarization. Such afterdepolarizations do not always reach threshold potential. In the case when threshold potential is reached, it may result in repeated oscillations of the cell membrane and can cause tachycardia due to triggered activity.

■ An action potential has five phases—phases 0, 1, 2, 3, and 4. A complete electrical cardiac cycle includes depolarization (which corresponds to phase 0), repolarization (phases 1, 2, and 3), and a period of rest or quiescence (corresponding to phase 4 of the action potential).

■ **Phase 0:** Phase 0 corresponds to the very rapid upstroke of the action potential.

□ Phase 0 starts when the muscle cell is depolarized by the sinus impulse, which is propagated from one cell to the next adjacent cell. When the cell is depolarized, the fast $Na^+$ channels in the cell membrane are activated, allowing sodium ions to enter the cell. Because sodium ions are positively charged, they neutralize the negative ions making the potential inside the cell less negative. After the threshold potential of approximately −70 mV is reached, all fast sodium channels open, allowing sodium, which is approximately 10 to 15 times higher outside than inside the cell, to enter rapidly. The explosive entry of $Na^+$ into the cell is the cause of the rapid upstroke of the action potential where the polarity of the cell not only becomes neutral (0 mV) but will result in an overshoot of approximately +20 to +30 mV.

□ The entry of $Na^+$ into the cell occurs only over a fraction of a second, because the fast sodium channel closes immediately when the membrane potential becomes neutral. After the fast sodium channel closes, it cannot be reactivated again and will not reopen until the potential of the cell is restored to its original resting potential of −90 mV.

□ Depolarization or phase 0 of the action potential is equivalent to the R wave (or QRS complex) of a single myocardial cell. Because there are millions of myocardial cells within the ventricles that are simultaneously depolarizing, it will take approximately 0.06 to 0.10 seconds to depolarize all the myocardial cells in both ventricles. This period corresponds to the total duration of the QRS complex in the surface ECG. Thus, when there is left ventricular hypertrophy or when there is bundle branch block, the duration of the QRS complex becomes wider because it will take longer to activate the entire ventricle.

□ After depolarization, the cell has to repolarize so that it can prepare itself for the next wave of excitation. Repolarization includes phases 1 to 3 of the action potential.

■ **Phase 1:** Early rapid repolarization starts immediately after phase 0, with the return of the polarity of the cell from approximately +20 to +30 mV to almost neutral (0 mV).

□ The decrease in potential from +20 to +30 mV to 0 mV is due to the abrupt closure of fast sodium channels and transient activation of the potassium channels causing outward movement of $K^+$. This transient outward movement of potassium is more prominent in the epicardium compared with endocardium, which may explain the shorter action potential dura-

tion of epicardial cells compared with endocardial cells. This difference in action potential duration is clinically important because this can favor reentry (see Brugada syndrome, Chapter 23, Acute Coronary Syndrome—ST Elevation Myocardial Infarction).

□ In the surface ECG, phase 1 and early phase 2 coincides with the J point, which marks the end of the QRS complex and beginning of the ST segment.

■ **Phase 2:** Phase 2 represents the plateau phase in which the potential of the cell remains unchanged at approximately 0 mV for a sustained duration.

□ The opening of the fast sodium channels during phase 0 of the action potential is also accompanied by the opening of the calcium channels when the voltage of the cell has reached approximately −40 mV. Unlike the fast sodium channel that opens and closes transiently, the flow of calcium into the cell is slower but is more sustained. Because the cell membrane is much more permeable to potassium ions than to other ions and because there is a much higher concentration of potassium inside than outside the cell, potassium leaks out of the cell (loss of positive ions), counterbalancing the entry of calcium into the cell (gain of positive ions). These two opposing forces maintain the polarity of the cell in equilibrium at approximately 0 mV for a sustained duration that corresponds to the plateau of the action potential.

□ The entry of calcium into the cell also triggers the release of more calcium from storage sites in the sarcoplasmic reticulum. This "calcium-triggered calcium release" mechanism is responsible for initiating contraction of the muscle cell. Throughout the duration of phase 2, the cells in the ventricles remain in a sustained state of contraction. During this period, the cells remain absolutely refractory and cannot be depolarized by an external stimulus.

□ **Phase 2** corresponds to the ST segment in the ECG, which normally remains isoelectric throughout its duration.

■ **Phase 3:** Phase 3 represents rapid ventricular repolarization. During phase 3, the polarity of the cell becomes more negative until it reaches its original resting potential of −90 mV.

□ The increasing negativity of the cell during phase 3 is due to inactivation of the calcium channels with decreased entry of calcium into the cell. However, the efflux of potassium out of the cell continues, making the potential of the cell more negative until it reaches −90 mV. After the resting potential of −90 mV is reached, repolarization of the cell is complete, and the cell is again ready to be depolarized.

□ **Phase 3**, or rapid ventricular repolarization, corresponds to the T wave in the ECG. The end of the repolarization period corresponds to the end of the T wave and marks the beginning of phase 4.

- **Phase 4:** Phase 4 represents the resting or quiescent state of the myocardial cell. The polarity of the cell when repolarization is completed is approximately −90 mV.

  □ During the resting state, the $K^+$ channels in the cell membrane are open while the channels of other ions remain closed. Because of the much higher concentration of $K^+$ inside than outside the cell, outward flow of $K^+$ continues. The loss of $K^+$ ions increases the negativity inside the cell. As the potential of the cell becomes more negative, an electrical force is created that attracts the positively charged potassium ions back into the cell against its concentration gradient. Thus, during phase 4, two forces acting in opposite directions cause the $K^+$ ions either to migrate in (because of electrical force) or migrate out (because of difference in $K^+$ concentration across the cell membrane) until a steady state is reached where migration of the $K^+$ into and out of the cell reaches an equilibrium. This corresponds to the final resting potential of a ventricular muscle cell, which is approximately −90 mV. This resting electrical potential can be predicted for potassium using the Nernst equation, where the resting potential of the cell is influenced by the difference in concentration of $K^+$ across the cell membrane and by the electrical forces attracting $K^+$ back into the cell.

  □ In ventricular muscle cells, phase 4 is maintained constantly at approximately −90 mV, making the slope relatively flat. The muscle cell can be discharged only by an outside stimulus, which is the arrival of the propagated sinus impulse.

  □ **Phase 4** corresponds to the T-Q interval in the ECG. This interval is isoelectric until it is interrupted by the next wave of depolarization.

## Conducting Cells of the His-Purkinje System

- The His-Purkinje system is specialized for rapid conduction. The action potential of the His-Purkinje cells is very similar to that of atrial and ventricular muscle cells except that the resting potential is less negative at approximately −95 mV. The more negative the action potential, the faster is the rate of rise of phase 0 of the action potential. This results in a more rapid (steeper) slope of phase 0, a higher overshoot and a more prolonged duration of the action potential. This explains why conduction of impulses across the His-Purkinje fibers is approximately five times faster than ordinary muscle cells.

## Pacemaker Cells in the Sinus Node

- Pacemaker cells in the sinus node and AV junction have properties of automaticity. These cells can discharge spontaneously independent of an outside stimulus. Muscle cells in the atria and ventricles, in contrast, do not possess the property of automaticity. However, they may develop this property if they are injured or become ischemic.

- The action potentials of automatic cells of the sinus node and AV node differ from those of non-pacemaker cells. Most importantly, they demonstrate a slow spontaneous diastolic depolarization during phase 4 of the action potential. These differences are discussed next.

- **Phase 4:**

  □ During phase 4, the resting potential of the automatic cells exhibit spontaneous depolarization. The potential of the pacemaker cell becomes less and less negative until it reaches threshold potential. This decreasing negativity of the resting potential is called slow spontaneous diastolic depolarization. This is the most important property that differentiates a pacemaking cell from a non-pacemaking cell. The non-pacemaking cell has a flat diastolic slope during phase 4 and does not exhibit slow spontaneous depolarization. Thus, the potential of the non-pacemaking cell never reaches threshold.

  □ The presence of spontaneous diastolic depolarization is due to the presence of sodium channels that are open during diastole. These sodium channels are not the same as the fast sodium channels that are responsible for phase 0 of the action potential. They are activated immediately after the cell reaches its most negative potential, causing sodium ions to enter the cell slowly. This slow entry of sodium into the cell is called pacemaker or funny current. This renders the polarity of the cell during phase 4 less and less negative until the threshold potential is reached.

  □ Also during phase 4, the resting potential of pacemaking cells of the sinus node measures approximately −50 to −60 mV and is therefore less negative than the resting potential of atrial and ventricular muscle cells, which measures approximately −90 mV. This less negative potential of no more than −50 to −60 mV causes the fast sodium channel to be inactivated permanently. The resting potential of the cell has to be restored to −90 mV before the fast sodium channels can be activated. Thus, phase 0 of the action potential of the sinus node and pacemaking cells of the AV junction is not due to the entry of sodium through fast sodium channels, but is mediated by the entry of calcium into the cell. After phase 4 reaches threshold potential, which is approximately −40 mV, the calcium channels open, resulting in the entry of calcium into the cell, which causes phase 0 of the action potential.

  □ Among all cells of the heart with pacemaking properties, the cells in the sinus node have the fastest rate of rise during phase 4 of the action potential. This accounts for why the sinus node has the fastest cyclical rate per minute and is the pacemaker of the heart. Other cells with automatic properties can be found in parts of the atria, AV junction, His-Purkinje system, and muscle cells of the mitral and tricuspid valves. Although these cells also exhibit slow diastolic depolarization, the rate of rise of the diastolic slope of phase 4 of these cells is much slower. Thus, these cells will be discharged by the propagated sinus impulse before their potential can reach threshold potential.

☐ There is an hierarchical order in the AV conduction system in which cells that are closest to the AV node have the fastest rate of rise during phase 4 of the action potential compared with cells that are located more distally. Thus, when the sinus node fails as the pacemaker of the heart, cells in the AV node at its junction with the bundle of His usually come to the rescue because these automatic cells have the fastest rate compared with other potential pacemakers of the heart.

▪ **Phase 0:**

☐ As previously mentioned, the fast sodium channels do not play any role in triggering phase 0 of the action potential in the pacemaker cells of the sinus node and AV junction since the resting potential of these cells are not capable of reaching –90 mV. Thus, the fast sodium channels remain closed and do not contribute to phase 0 of the action potential.

☐ Depolarization of the cell occurs through calcium channels that open when the resting potential of the cell spontaneously reaches –40 mV.

☐ Because the resting potential is less negative at –60 mV and phase 0 is mediated by calcium ions, the rate of rise of phase 0 is slower. This results in a slope that is less steep with a lower overshoot than that of muscle cells of the atria and ventricles.

## Refractory Periods

▪ The myocardial cell needs to repolarize before the arrival of the next impulse. If complete repolarization has not been achieved, the cell may or may not respond to a stimulus, depending on the intensity of the stimulus and the extent to which the cell has recovered at the time the stimulus is delivered. Not surprisingly, refractory periods are defined according to the phase of the action potential at which the impulse arrives.

▪ **Absolute refractory period:** The absolute refractory period is the period in the action potential during which the cell cannot respond to any stimulus. This period includes phase 1 and phase 2 of the action potential.

▪ **Effective refractory period:** The effective refractory period is the period during which the cell can be stimulated; however, the action potential that is generated is not strong enough to propagate to other cells. This period includes a short interval of phase 3 (approximately –25 mV).

▪ **Relative refractory period:** The relative refractory period starts from the end of the effective refractory period and extends to a potential slightly less negative than –70 mV, which is the threshold potential. Not all of the fast sodium channels are fully recovered at this time. Thus, the potential generated has a lower amplitude and a slower rate of rise of phase 0 of the action potential. The impulse will still be propagated but conduction velocity is slower.

▪ **Supernormal period:** The cell may respond to less than ordinary stimuli if the cell is stimulated at a potential that is slightly below (more negative than) its threshold potential of –70 mV. The potential of the cell would therefore be only a few millivolts from becoming threshold potential. Thus, a smaller than normal stimulus is sufficient to excite the cell. This short interval corresponds to the supernormal period of repolarization.

## Suggested Readings

Conover MB. Normal electrical activation of the heart. In: *Understanding Electrocardiography.* 8th ed. St. Louis: Mosby; 2003:8–22.

Dunn MI, Lipman BS. Basic physiologic principles. In: *Lipman-Massie Clinical Electrocardiography.* 8th ed. Chicago: Yearbook Medical Publishers Inc; 1989:24–50.

Greineder K, Strichartz GR, Lilly LS. Basic cardiac structure and function. In: Lilly LS, ed. *Pathophysiology of Heart Disease.* 2nd ed. Baltimore: Lippincott Williams & Wilkins; 1993: 1– 23.

Shih H-T. Anatomy of the action potential in the heart. *Texas Heart J.* 1994;21:30–41.

# Basic Electrocardiography

## The Normal Sinus Impulse

- The sinus node is the origin of the normal electrical impulse. Although there are other cells in the heart that can also discharge spontaneously, the sinus node has the fastest rate of discharge and is the pacemaker of the heart.
- **Normal Sinus Rhythm:** Any impulse originating from the sinus node is called normal sinus rhythm. The sinus node discharges at a rate of 60 to 100 beats per minute (bpm), although the rate could vary depending on the metabolic needs of the body.
  - **Sinus bradycardia:** When the rate of the sinus node is <60 bpm, the rhythm is called sinus bradycardia.
  - **Sinus tachycardia:** When the rate is >100 bpm, the rhythm is called sinus tachycardia.
  - **Sinus arrhythmia:** When the sinus impulse is irregular, the rhythm is called sinus arrhythmia.
- The electrical impulse that is generated from the sinus node spreads from the atria to the ventricles in an orderly sequence. In this manner, contraction of the atria and ventricles is closely synchronized to maximize the efficiency of the heart as a pump (Fig. 2.1).

## Activation of the Atria—The P Wave

- **The Sinus Impulse:** When the sinus node discharges, no deflection is recorded because the impulse from the sinus node is not strong enough to generate an electrical signal. The first deflection that is recorded after the sinus node discharges is the P wave.
- **P Wave:** The P wave is the first deflection in the electrocardiogram (ECG) and is due to activation of the atria.
  - **Configuration:** The configuration of the normal sinus P wave is smooth and well rounded. Because the sinus node is located at the upper border of the right atrium, the sinus impulse has to travel from the right atrium to the left atrium on its way to the ventricles. The first half of the P wave therefore is due to activation of the right atrium (Fig. 2.2A). The second half is due to activation of the left atrium (Fig. 2.2B).
  - **Duration:** The width or duration of the normal sinus P wave measures ≤2.5 small blocks (≤0.10 seconds). This is the length of time it takes to activate both atria.
  - **Amplitude:** The height or amplitude of the normal sinus P wave also measures ≤2.5 small blocks (≤0.25 mV).

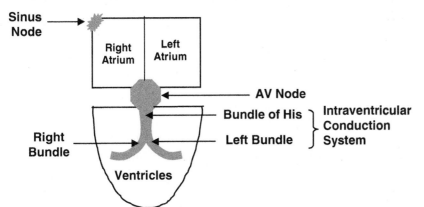

**Figure 2.1: Diagrammatic Representation of the Sinus Node and Conduction System.** The sinus node is the origin of the normal electrical impulse and is the pacemaker of the heart. The sinus impulse spreads to the atria before it is propagated to the ventricles through the atrioventricular node and special conduction system.

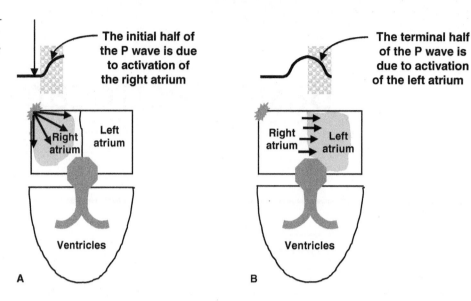

**Figure 2.2:    Atrial Activation— the P Wave.** When the sinus node discharges, no electrical activity is recorded in the electrocardiogram. The first deflection is the P wave, which represents activation of the atria. The initial half of the P wave represents activation of the right atrium and the terminal half represents activation of the left atrium.

## Activation of the Atrioventricular Node

- After depolarization of the atria, the only pathway by which the sinus impulse can reach the ventricles is through the atrioventricular (AV) node and intraventricular conduction system.

- **The AV node:** The AV node consists of a network of special cells that normally delay conduction of the atrial impulse to the ventricles. As the impulse traverses the AV node on its way to the ventricles, it does not generate any electrical activity in the ECG. Therefore, an isoelectric or flat line is recorded immediately after the P wave (Fig. 2.3).

### Intraventricular Conduction System

After the impulse emerges from the AV node, it is conducted rapidly through the His bundle, bundle branches,

and fascicles, which constitute the intraventricular conduction system, before terminating in a branching network of Purkinje fibers. The spread of the electrical impulse in the His-Purkinje system also does not cause any deflection in the ECG, similar to that of the AV node. This is represented as a continuation of the isoelectric or flat line after the P wave.

## Activation of the Ventricles— The QRS Complex

- **QRS Complex:** The QRS complex represents activation of the ventricles. The QRS complex generates the largest deflection in the ECG because the ventricles contain the largest mass of muscle cells in the heart, collectively referred to as the myocardium (Fig. 2.4).

**Figure 2.3:    Activation of the Atrioventricular Node and His-Purkinje System.** Propagation of the impulse at the atrioventricular node and His-Purkinje system will not cause any deflection in the electrocardiogram and is represented as an isoelectric or flat line after the P wave.

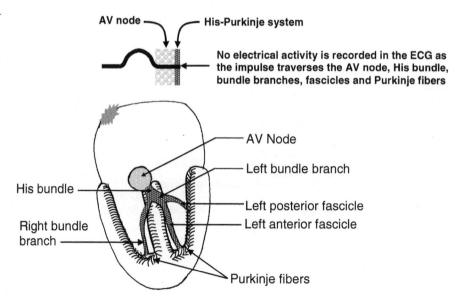

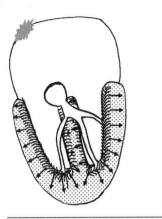
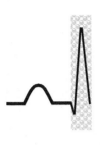

The QRS complex represents simultaneous activation of both ventricles

**Figure 2.4:    Activation of the Ventricles—the QRS Complex.** Activation of the ventricles is represented as a QRS complex in the electrocardiogram. Because the Purkinje fibers are located in the endocardium, the endocardium is the first to be activated. The impulse spreads from endocardium to epicardium in an outward direction. Arrows point to the direction of activation.

- The spread of the sinus impulse through the His-Purkinje system is very rapid and efficient, but is electrically silent with no impulse recorded in the ECG. The QRS complex is recorded only when the impulse has spread from the Purkinje fibers to the myocardium.

- The myocardium can be arbitrarily divided into three layers: the endocardium, which is the inner layer, the mid-myocardium, and the epicardium, which is the outer layer of the myocardium.

- The Purkinje fibers are located in the endocardium of both ventricles. Because the electrical impulse arrives first at the Purkinje fibers, the ventricles are activated from endocardium to epicardium in an outward direction.

- The QRS complex corresponds to phase 0 of the action potential of all individual myocardial cells of both ventricles. Because the ventricles consist of a thick layer of myocardial cells, not all cells are depolarized at the same time. Depolarization of the whole myocardium can vary from 0.06 to 0.10 seconds or longer. This duration corresponds to the width of the QRS complex in the ECG.

## The QRS Complex

- **QRS Complex:** The QRS complex has various waves that go up and down from baseline. These waves are identified as follows: Q, R, S, R′, and S′. If additional waves are present, R″ or S″ designations may be added. Regardless of the size of the deflections, capital and small letters are used empirically mainly for convenience, although, generally, capital letters designate large waves and small letters, small waves (Fig. 2.5).

  - **Q wave:** The Q wave is defined as the first wave of the QRS complex below the baseline. If only a deep Q wave is present (no R wave), the QRS complex is described as a QS complex.

  - **R wave:** The R wave is defined as the first positive (upward) deflection of the QRS complex. If only an R wave is present (no Q wave or S wave), the QRS complex is described as an R wave.

  - **S wave:** The S wave is the negative deflection after the R wave.

  - **R′:** The R′ (R prime) is the next positive wave after the S wave.

  - **S′:** The S′ (S prime) is the next negative deflection after the R′.

  - **R″ or S″:** These waves are rarely used, however if additional waves are needed to describe the QRS complex, the letter R″ (R double prime) is used for the next positive wave and S″ (S double prime) for the next negative wave.

- **QRS complex:** The QRS complex is identified as a QRS complex regardless of the number of waves present. Thus, a tall R wave without a Q wave or S wave is still identified as a QRS complex.

## The J Point, ST Segment, and T Wave

- The QRS complex is followed by a flat line called the ST segment. The end of the QRS complex and beginning of the ST segment is called the J point. The flat ST segment is followed immediately by another positive deflection called the T wave.

**Figure 2.5:    QRS Nomenclature.** Diagram shows how the waves are identified in the QRS complex.

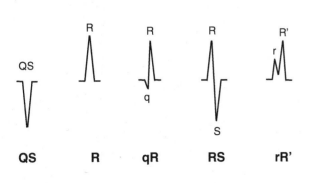
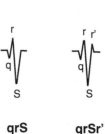

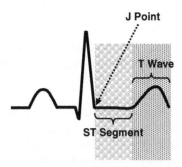

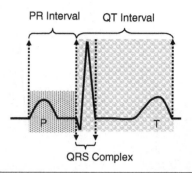

**Figure 2.6: Repolarization of the Ventricles.** Ventricular repolarization begins immediately after depolarization and starts at the J point, which marks the end of the QRS complex, and extends to the end of the T wave. This corresponds to phases 1, 2, and 3 of the action potential. Ventricular repolarization allows the ventricles to recover completely and prepares the myocardial cells for the next wave of depolarization.

**Figure 2.7: The PR Interval, QRS Complex, and QT Interval.** The PR interval is measured from the beginning of the P wave to the beginning of the QRS complex. The QRS complex is measured from the beginning of the first deflection to the end of the last deflection and the QT interval is measured from the beginning of the QRS complex to the end of the T wave.

- **J point:** The J point, also called the J junction, marks the end of the QRS complex and beginning of the ST segment (Fig. 2.6).
- **ST segment:** The ST segment starts from the J point to the beginning of the T wave. The ST segment is flat or isoelectric and corresponds to phase 2 (plateau phase) of the action potential of the ventricular myocardial cells. It represents the time when all cells have just been depolarized and the muscle cells are in a state of sustained contraction. The ventricular muscle cells are completely refractory during this period and cannot be excited by an outside stimulus.
- **T wave:** The T wave represents rapid ventricular repolarization. This segment of ventricular repolarization corresponds to phase 3 of the transmembrane action potential. During phase 3, the action potential abruptly returns to its resting potential of −90 mV.
- The J point, ST segment, and T wave represent the whole process of ventricular repolarization corresponding to phases 1, 2, and 3 of the transmembrane action potential. Repolarization returns the polarity of the myocardial cells to resting potential and prepares the ventricles for the next wave of depolarization.

## The PR Interval, QRS Complex, and QT Interval

- The duration of the PR interval, QRS complex, and QT interval are routinely measured in the standard 12-lead ECG. These intervals are shown in Figure 2.7.
  - **PR interval:** The PR interval is measured from the beginning of the P wave to the beginning of the QRS

complex. If the QRS complex starts with a Q wave, the PR interval is measured from the beginning of the P wave to the beginning of the Q wave (P-Q interval), but is nevertheless called PR interval. The normal PR interval measures 0.12 to 0.20 seconds in the adult. It includes the time it takes for the sinus impulse to travel from atria to ventricles. The PR interval is prolonged when there is delay in conduction of the sinus impulse to the ventricles and is shortened when there is an extra pathway connecting the atrium directly to the ventricle.
  - **QRS complex:** The QRS complex is measured from the beginning of the first deflection, whether it starts with a Q wave or an R wave, and extends to the end of the last deflection. The normal QRS duration varies from 0.06 to 0.10 seconds. The QRS duration is increased when there is ventricular hypertrophy, bundle branch block, or when there is premature excitation of the ventricles because of the presence of an accessory pathway.

## The QT Interval

- **QT Interval:** The QT interval includes the QRS complex, ST segment, and T wave corresponding to phases 0 to 3 of the action potential. It is measured from the beginning of the QRS complex to the end of the T wave. Note that the presence of a U wave is not included in the measurement. In assessing the duration of the QT interval, multiple leads should be selected and the QT interval is the longest QT that can be measured in the whole 12-lead ECG recording.
- **QTc:** The QT interval is affected by heart rate. It becomes longer when the heart rate is slower and shorter

$$QTc = \frac{QT \text{ interval (in seconds)}}{\sqrt{R\text{-}R \text{ interval (in seconds)}}}$$

**Figure 2.8:   The QT Interval.** The QT interval is measured from the beginning of the QRS complex to the end of the T wave. When the heart rate is >70 bpm, one can "eyeball" that the QTc is normal if the QT interval is equal to or less than half the R-R interval. When this occurs, no calculation is necessary. If the QT interval is more than half the R-R interval, the QTc may not be normal and should be calculated (see example in Fig. 2.9).

when the heart rate is faster. The QT interval therefore should always be corrected for heart rate. The corrected QT interval is the QTc.

- The simplest and most commonly used formula for correcting the QT interval for heart rate is the Bazett formula shown here.

- The normal QTc should not exceed 0.42 seconds in men and 0.44 seconds in women. The QTc is prolonged when it measures >0.44 seconds in men and >0.46 seconds in women and children.

- An easy rule to remember in calculating the QTc when the heart rate is >70 bpm is that the QTc is normal (<0.46 seconds) if the QT interval is equal to or less than half the R-R interval (Fig. 2.8).

- **Calculating the QTc:** Table 2.1 is useful in calculating the QTc when a calculator is not available. In the example in Figure 2.9, the short technique of visually inspecting the QT interval can be used because the heart rate is >70 bpm. The QT interval (10 small blocks) is more than half the preceding R-R interval (14 small blocks). Thus, the QTc may not be normal and needs to be calculated.

  - **First: Measure the QT interval:** The QT interval measures 10 small blocks. This is equivalent to 0.40 seconds (Table 2.1, column 1, QT interval in small block).

  - **Second: Measure the R-R interval:** The R-R interval measures 14 small blocks, which is equivalent to 0.56 seconds. The square root of 0.56 seconds is 0.75 seconds (see Table 2.1).

  - **Finally: Calculate the QTc:** Using the Bazett formula as shown below: QTc = 0.40 ÷ 0.75 = 0.53 seconds. The QTc is prolonged.

- Rapid calculation of the QTc using the Bazett formula is shown below.

- **The Normal U Wave:** The end of the T wave completes the normal cardiac cycle, which includes the P wave, the QRS complex, and the T wave. The T wave, however, may often be followed by a small positive deflection called the U wave. The U wave is not always present, but it may be the last complex in the ECG to be recorded (Fig. 2.10).

  - The size of the normal U wave is small, measuring approximately one-tenth of the size of the T wave.

  - U waves are best recorded in the anterior precordial leads $V_2$ and $V_3$ because these chest leads are closest to the ventricular myocardium.

  - U waves are usually visible when the heart rate is slow (<65 bpm) and rarely visible with faster heart rates (>95 bpm).

$$QTc = \frac{QT \text{ interval (in seconds)}}{\sqrt{R\text{-}R \text{ interval (in seconds)}}} = \frac{0.40}{0.75} = 0.53 \text{ sec}$$

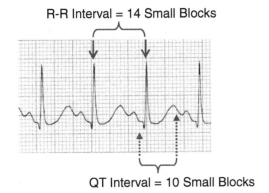

R-R Interval = 14 Small Blocks

QT Interval = 10 Small Blocks

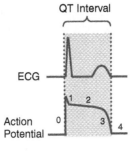

QT Interval

ECG

Action Potential

**Figure 2.9:   Calculating the QTc.** If a calculator is not available, the QTc can be calculated by using Table 2.1. The preceding R-R interval is measured because the QT interval is dependent on the previous R-R interval. In this figure, the QT interval (10 small blocks) is more than half the preceding R-R interval (14 small blocks), thus the QTc may not be normal and should be calculated as shown in the text. The right panel is a reminder that the QT interval is equivalent to the total duration of the action potential (phases 0 to 3).

## TABLE 2.1

### Calculating the QTc

$$QTc\,(sec) = \frac{QT\ interval\,(sec)}{\sqrt{RR\ interval\,(sec)}}$$

| QT Interval | | R-R Interval (Small Blocks) | Heart Rate (Beats per Minute) | R-R Interval (sec) | Square Root of R-R Interval (sec) |
|---|---|---|---|---|---|
| QT (Small Blocks) | QT (sec) | | | | |
| 45 | 1.80 | 45 | 33 | 1.80 | 1.34 |
| 44 | 1.76 | 44 | 34 | 1.76 | 1.33 |
| 43 | 1.72 | 43 | 35 | 1.72 | 1.31 |
| 42 | 1.68 | 42 | 36 | 1.68 | 1.30 |
| 41 | 1.64 | 41 | 37 | 1.64 | 1.28 |
| 40 | 1.60 | 40 | 38 | 1.60 | 1.26 |
| 39 | 1.56 | 39 | 39 | 1.56 | 1.25 |
| 38 | 1.52 | 38 | 39 | 1.52 | 1.23 |
| 37 | 1.48 | 37 | 41 | 1.48 | 1.22 |
| 36 | 1.44 | 36 | 42 | 1.44 | 1.20 |
| 35 | 1.40 | 35 | 43 | 1.40 | 1.18 |
| 34 | 1.36 | 34 | 44 | 1.36 | 1.17 |
| 33 | 1.32 | 33 | 45 | 1.32 | 1.15 |
| 32 | 1.28 | 32 | 47 | 1.28 | 1.13 |
| 31 | 1.24 | 31 | 48 | 1.24 | 1.11 |
| 30 | 1.20 | 30 | 50 | 1.20 | 1.10 |
| 29 | 1.16 | 29 | 52 | 1.16 | 1.08 |
| 28 | 1.12 | 28 | 54 | 1.12 | 1.06 |
| 27 | 1.08 | 27 | 56 | 1.08 | 1.04 |
| 26 | 1.04 | 26 | 58 | 1.04 | 1.02 |
| 25 | 1.00 | 25 | 60 | 1.00 | 1.00 |
| 24 | 0.96 | 24 | 63 | 0.96 | 0.98 |
| 23 | 0.92 | 23 | 65 | 0.92 | 0.96 |
| 22 | 0.88 | 22 | 68 | 0.88 | 0.94 |
| 21 | 0.84 | 21 | 71 | 0.84 | 0.92 |
| 20 | 0.80 | 20 | 75 | 0.80 | 0.89 |
| 19 | 0.76 | 19 | 79 | 0.76 | 0.87 |
| 18 | 0.75 | 18 | 83 | 0.75 | 0.87 |
| 17 | 0.68 | 17 | 88 | 0.68 | 0.82 |
| 16 | 0.64 | 16 | 94 | 0.64 | 0.80 |
| 15 | 0.60 | 15 | 100 | 0.60 | 0.77 |
| 14 | 0.56 | 14 | 107 | 0.56 | 0.75 |
| 13 | 0.52 | 13 | 115 | 0.52 | 0.72 |
| 12 | 0.48 | 12 | 125 | 0.48 | 0.69 |
| 11 | 0.44 | 11 | 136 | 0.44 | 0.66 |
| 10 | 0.40 | 10 | 150 | 0.40 | 0.63 |
| 9 | 0.36 | 9 | 167 | 0.36 | 0.60 |
| 8 | 0.32 | 8 | 188 | 0.32 | 0.57 |
| 7 | 0.28 | 7 | 214 | 0.28 | 0.53 |

Column 2 converts the measured QT interval to seconds; the last column converts the measured R-R interval to its square root.

- A normal U wave is upright in all leads except aVR because the axis of the U wave follows that of the T wave.
- The origin of the normal U wave is uncertain, although it is believed to be due to repolarization of the His-Purkinje system.
- **Abnormal U Wave:** U waves are often seen in normal individuals, but can be abnormal when they are inverted or when they equal or exceed the size of the T wave. This occurs in the setting of hypokalemia.
- **T-Q Segment:** The T-Q segment is measured from the end of the T wave of the previous complex to the Q wave of the next QRS complex. It represents electrical diastole corresponding to phase 4 of the action potential.

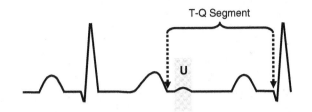

**Figure 2.10: The U Wave and T-Q Segment.** The U wave is the last deflection in the electrocardiogram and is best recorded in leads V$_2$ and V$_3$ because of the close proximity of these leads to the ventricular myocardium. The cause of the U wave is most likely the repolarization of the His-Purkinje system. U waves are abnormal when they are inverted or become unduly prominent, as may be seen in the setting of hypokalemia. The T-Q segment corresponds to phase 4 of the action potential. It marks the end of the previous action potential and the beginning of the next potential.

## Summary of ECG Deflections

See Figure 2.11.

- **P wave:** The P wave represents activation of the atria.
- **PR interval:** The PR interval starts from the beginning of the P wave to the beginning of the QRS complex and represents the time required for the sinus impulse to travel from the atria to the ventricles.
- **PR segment:** The PR segment starts at the end of the P wave to the beginning of the QRS complex and corresponds to the time it takes for the impulse to travel from AV node to ventricles.
- **QRS complex:** This represents activation of all the muscle cells in the ventricles and corresponds to phase 0 of the action potential.
- **J point:** The J point marks the end of the QRS complex and beginning of the ST segment. It corresponds to phase 1 of the action potential.

- **ST segment:** The ST segment is the isoelectric portion between the J point and the beginning of the T wave. It corresponds to phase 2 (plateau) of the action potential.
- **T wave:** The T wave represents rapid repolarization of the ventricles and corresponds to phase 3 of the action potential.
- **QT:** The QT interval is measured from the beginning of the QRS complex to the end of the T wave and corresponds to electrical systole.
- **TQ:** The TQ segment starts from the end of the T wave to the beginning of the next QRS complex. This represents phase 4 of the action potential and corresponds to electrical diastole.
- **U wave:** The U wave, if present, is the last positive deflection in the ECG. It is likely due to repolarization of the His-Purkinje system.

## Abnormal Waves in the ECG

- There are other waves in the ECG that have been described. These waves are not normally present but should be recognized because they are pathologic and diagnostic of a clinical entity when present.
  - **Delta wave:** The delta wave is a slow and slurred upstroke of the initial portion of the QRS complex and is usually seen in conjunction with a short PR interval (Fig. 2.12A). Its presence is diagnostic of the Wolff-Parkinson-White syndrome. Delta waves are caused by an accessory pathway that connects the atrium directly to the ventricles across the atrioventricular groove resulting in pre-excitation of the ventricles (see Chapter 20, Wolff-Parkinson-White Syndrome).
  - **Osborn wave:** The Osborn wave, also called a J wave, is a markedly exaggerated elevation of the J point that results in an H shape configuration of

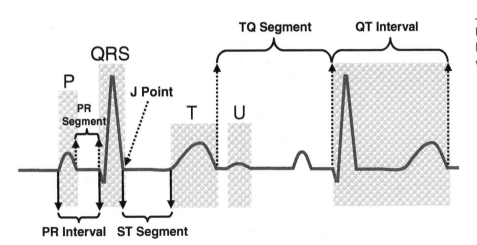

**Figure 2.11: Summary of the Electrocardiogram Waves, Intervals, and Segments.**

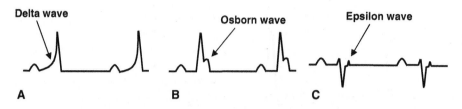

Figure 2.12:   **Abnormal Waves in the electrocardiogram.** **(A)** Delta waves characterized by slowly rising upstroke of the QRS complex from preexcitation (Wolff-Parkinson-White syndrome). **(B)** Osborn waves, which resemble an "h" because of hypothermia and hypercalcemia. **(C)** Epsilon waves seen as extra notch after the QRS in $V_1$, $V_2$, or $V_3$ diagnostic of arrhythmogenic right ventricular dysplasia.

the QRS complex. The presence of the Osborn wave is associated with hypothermia or hypercalcemia (Fig. 2.12B).

■ **Epsilon wave:** The epsilon wave is an extra notch at the end of the QRS or early portion of the ST segment most commonly seen in $V_1$ to $V_3$. This extra notch represents delayed activation of the outflow tract of the right ventricle and is diagnostic of arrhythmogenic right ventricular dysplasia, also called arrhythmogenic right ventricular cardiomyopathy (Fig. 2.12C). Arrhythmogenic right ventricular dysplasia is an inherited form of cardiomyopathy characterized by the presence of fibro-fatty infiltrates within the myocardium of the right ventricle that can result in ventricular arrhythmias. It is a common cause of sudden cardiac death in young individuals.

# Transmembrane Action Potential and the Surface ECG

■ The diagram (Fig. 2.13) shows the relationship between the action potential of a single ventricular myocardial cell and the surface ECG. A complete cardiac cycle can be divided into two phases: systole and diastole.

■ **Systole:** Systole corresponds to the QT interval and includes:

☐ **Depolarization:** Depolarization is phase 0 of the action potential. This is equivalent to the QRS complex in the ECG.

☐ **Repolarization:** Repolarization includes phases 1, 2, and 3, which correspond to the J point, ST segment, and T wave in the ECG.

Figure 2.13:   **The Transmembrane Action Potential and the Surface Electrocardiogram.** Transmembrane action potential of a ventricular myocardial cell **(A)** and the corresponding surface electrocardiogram **(B)**. Phase 0 of the action potential is equivalent to the QRS complex, phase 1 the J point, phase 2 the ST segment, phase 3 the T wave, and phase 4 the TQ segment. Note that repolarization and depolarization of the myocardium occur during systole, which corresponds to the QT interval. Diastole, which is phase 4, the rest period, corresponds to the TQ interval.

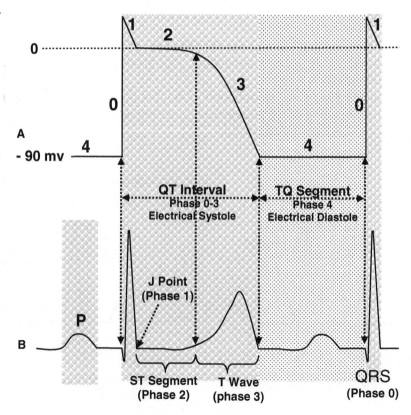

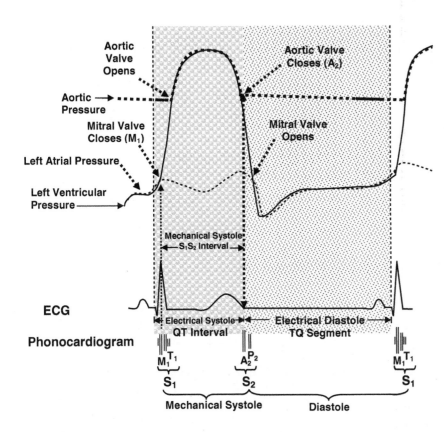

**Figure 2.14:    Electrical and Mechanical Systole and Diastole.** The electrocardiogram (ECG), left ventricular, left atrial, and aortic root pressure tracings are shown. Electrical systole corresponds to the QT interval in the ECG. Mechanical systole starts from $S_1$ (first heart sound) because of closure of the mitral ($M_1$) and tricuspid ($T_1$) valves, and extends to $S_2$ (second heart sound) because of closure of the aortic ($A_2$) and pulmonic ($P_2$) valves. There is a slight electromechanical delay from the onset of the QRS complex to the onset of $S_1$. Electrical diastole is equivalent to the TQ segment in the ECG. This is equivalent to mechanical diastole, which starts from $S_2$ and extends to $S_1$.

- **Diastole:** Diastole occurs during phase 4, or the resting period of the cell. This corresponds to the TQ segment in the ECG.

## Timing of Systole and Diastole

- It is important to recognize that the ECG represents electrical events and that a time lag occurs before mechanical contraction and relaxation.
  - **Systole:** In the ECG, electrical systole starts with the QRS complex and ends with the T wave corresponding to the QT interval. At bedside, mechanical sys-

tole begins with the first heart sound or $S_1$ and ends with the second sound or $S_2$ (Fig. 2.14).
  - **Diastole:** In the ECG, diastole starts at the end of the T wave to the next Q wave (TQ). At bedside, diastole extends from $S_2$ to $S_1$.

## The 12-Lead ECG

- Shown here are examples of complete 12-lead ECGs. A continuous lead II rhythm strip is recorded at the bottom of each tracing. The first ECG (Fig. 2.15) is a normal ECG. The second ECG (Fig. 2.16) shows prominent U waves in an otherwise normal ECG.

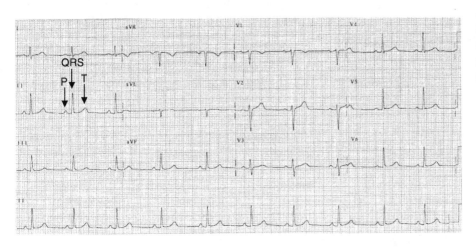

**Figure 2.15:    Normal Electrocardiogram.** The rhythm is normal sinus with a rate of 62 beats per minute.

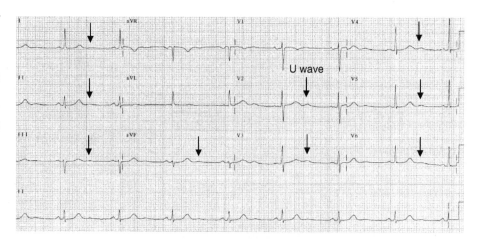

**Figure 2.16:   Prominent U Waves.** Twelve-lead electrocardiogram showing U waves in almost all leads. U waves are usually seen when the heart rate is slow and are most prominent in the anterior precordial leads because these leads are closest to the ventricles. The U waves are marked by the arrows.

## The Normal Electrocardiogram

### The ECG Deflections

1. The P wave represents activation of the atria.
2. The QRS complex represents activation of the ventricles.
3. The T wave represents rapid repolarization of the ventricles.
4. U wave represents repolarization of the His-Purkinje system.

### Segments and Intervals

1. PR interval represents the time it takes for the sinus impulse to travel from the atria to the ventricles.
2. QT interval represents electrical systole and extends from the onset of the QRS complex to end of the T wave.
3. The J point marks the end of the QRS complex and beginning of the ST segment.
4. JT interval is the QT interval without the QRS complex.
5. The ST segment begins immediately after the QRS complex and extends to the onset of the T wave.
6. TQ interval represents electrical diastole and extends from the end of the T wave to the beginning of the next QRS complex.

### The ECG Deflections, Segments, and Intervals and their Clinical Implications

- **The P wave:** The sinus node does not leave any imprint when it discharges. The P wave is the first deflection in the ECG and indicates that the sinus impulse has spread to the atria. The P wave therefore represents activation of the atria and is the only ECG evidence that the sinus node has discharged.

- **The sinus P wave**
  - Because the sinus impulse is not represented in the ECG when the sinus node discharges, the configuration of the

P wave is the main criterion in identifying that the impulse is sinus or non-sinus in origin. The sinus node is located at the right upper border of the right atrium close to the entrance of the superior vena cava. Because of its anatomic location, the sinus impulse has to travel from right atrium to left atrium in a leftward and downward (inferior) direction. This is represented in the ECG as an upright P wave in leads I, II, and aVF, as well as in $V_3$ to $V_6$. Lead II usually records the most upright P wave deflection and is the most important lead in recognizing that the rhythm is normal sinus. If the P wave is inverted in lead II, the impulse is unlikely to be of sinus node origin.

- The sinus impulse follows the same pathway every time it activates the atria; thus, every sinus impulse has the same P wave configuration.

- The P wave duration should not exceed 2.5 small blocks (≤0.10 seconds or 100 milliseconds). The height of the P wave also should not exceed 2.5 small blocks (≤2.5 mm) and is measured vertically from the top of the baseline to the top of the P wave. The duration of the P wave represents activation of the left and right atria. According to the American College of Cardiology/American Heart Association/Heart Rhythm Society, the P wave duration should be measured in at least three leads that are recorded simultaneously—preferably leads I, II, and $V_1$—from the beginning of the P wave to the end of the P wave. The P wave is abnormal when there is increased amplitude or duration, when the shape of the wave is peaked, notched, or bifid, or when it is inverted or absent in lead II.

  - ☐ **Increased duration of the P wave:** A prolonged P wave suggests enlargement of the left atrium or intra-atrial block.

  - ☐ **Increased amplitude of the P wave:** Increased P wave amplitude suggests enlargement of the right atrium.

- Activation of the atria is immediately followed by atrial contraction. The mechanical contraction of the atria is not audible. However, when the ventricles are stiff or noncompliant, as occurs when there is left ventricular hypertrophy, a fourth heart sound ($S_4$) may be audible because of vibrations caused by blood hitting the ventricular walls during atrial contraction. A fourth heart sound may not be present when there are no P waves; for instance, when the rhythm is junctional or when there is atrial fibrillation.

- **Ta wave:** The P wave may be followed by a repolarization wave called the Ta wave. The Ta wave is the T wave of the P wave. The Ta wave is small and is usually not visible because it becomes obscured by the coinciding QRS complex. The direction of the Ta wave in the ECG is opposite that of the P wave. Thus, when the P wave is upright, the Ta wave is inverted.

- **The PR interval:** The PR interval represents the time required for the sinus impulse to reach the ventricles. It includes the time it takes for the sinus impulse to travel through the atria, AV node, bundle of His, bundle branches, fascicles of the left bundle branch, and the Purkinje network of fibers until the ventricles are activated.

  - The normal PR interval measures 0.12 to 0.20 seconds in the adult. The PR interval is measured from the beginning of the P wave to the beginning of the QRS complex. The longest as well as the shortest PR interval in the 12-lead ECG tracing should be measured so that delay in the conduction of the sinus impulse to the ventricles and premature excitation of the ventricles are not overlooked.

    - **Prolonged PR interval:** The PR interval is prolonged when it measures >0.20 seconds (200 milliseconds). This delay in the conduction of the sinus impulse from atria to ventricles is usually at the level of the AV node. The whole 12-lead ECG is measured for the longest PR interval preferably leads I, II, and $V_1$.

    - **Short PR interval:** The PR interval is short when conduction of the impulse from atria to ventricles is shorter than normal (<0.12 seconds or 120 milliseconds). This usually occurs when an accessory pathway or bypass tract is present connecting the atrium directly to the ventricle or when conduction of the impulse across the AV node is enhanced because of a small AV node or from pharmacologic agents that speed AV nodal conduction. This will also occur when there is an ectopic impulse, meaning that the P wave originates from the atria or AV junction and not from the sinus node.

- **PR segment:** The PR segment is the isoelectric or flat line between the P wave and the QRS complex and is measured from the end of the P wave to the beginning of the QRS complex. It represents the spread of the impulse at the AV node and His-Purkinje system, with most of the delay occurring at the level of the AV node. This delay is important so that atrial and ventricular contraction is coordinated and does not occur simultaneously. Because the PR segment is isoelectric, it is used as baseline for measuring the various deflections in the ECG.

- **QRS complex:** The QRS complex is the next deflection after the P wave. It represents activation of both ventricles. It is the largest complex in the ECG because the ventricles contain the largest mass of working myocardium in the heart. This is in contrast to the thinner muscles in the atria, which corresponds to a smaller P wave. The first portion of the ventricle to be activated is the middle third of the ventricular septum because the left bundle branch is shorter than the right bundle branch.

- **Waves of the QRS complex:** The QRS complex consists of the following waves or deflections: Q, R, S, R′, S′, R″, and S″. The use of capital and small letters in identifying the waves of the QRS complex is arbitrary.

- **Duration of the QRS complex:** The QRS complex is measured from the beginning of the first deflection, which may be a Q wave or R wave, to the end of the last deflection. The width or duration of the QRS complex normally varies from 0.06 to 0.10 seconds in the adult but may be less in infants and children. The QRS complex corresponds to phase 0 of the transmembrane action potential of a single muscle cell. Because there are millions of muscle cells in the ventricles that are activated, the total duration of the QRS complex will depend on how efficiently the whole ventricle is depolarized. Thus, when there is increased muscle mass due to hypertrophy of the left ventricle or when there is delay in the spread of the electrical impulse because of bundle branch block or the impulse originates directly from the ventricles or from a ventricular pacemaker, the duration of the QRS complex becomes prolonged.

- **Amplitude:** The height of the QRS complex in the limb leads should measure ≥5 mm in at least one lead. This includes the total amplitude above and below the baseline. In the chest lead, it should measure ≥10 mm in at least one lead.

  - **Low voltage:** Low voltage is present when the tallest QRS complex in any limb lead is <5 mm or the tallest complex in any chest lead is <10 mm. Low voltage may be confined only to the limb leads or only to the chest leads or it may be generalized involving both limb and chest leads. Low voltage can occur when transmission of the cardiac impulse to the recording electrode is diminished because of peripheral edema, ascites, anasarca, chronic obstructive pulmonary disease (especially emphysema), obesity, pericardial, or pleural effusion. Low voltage can also occur if the recording electrode is distant from the origin of the impulse.

  - **Increased voltage:** The voltage of the QRS complex may be increased when there is hypertrophy of the ventricles. It may be a normal finding in young adults.

- **Electrical versus mechanical systole:** The onset of the QRS complex marks the beginning of **electrical** systole, which is hemodynamically silent. After the ventricles are depolarized, there is a brief delay before the ventricles contract causing both mitral and tricuspid valves to close during systole. Closure of both mitral and tricuspid valves is audible as the first heart sound ($S_1$), which marks the beginning of **mechanical** systole.

- **QT interval:** The QT interval is measured from the beginning of the QRS complex to the end of the T wave. The American College of Cardiology/American Heart Association/Heart Rhythm Society recommend that the QT interval should be measured using at least three different leads and should be the longest QT interval that can be measured in the 12-lead ECG.

  - The QT interval is measured from the earliest onset of the QRS complex to the latest termination of the T wave.

  - The duration of the QT interval is affected by heart rate. Thus, the QT interval corrected for heart rate is the QTc. The QTc is calculated using the Bazett formula: QTc (in seconds) = QT interval (in seconds) ÷ square root of the preceding R-R interval (in seconds).

  - The normal QTc is longer in women than in men. The QTc interval should not exceed 0.44 seconds (440 milliseconds) in women and 0.42 seconds (420 milliseconds) in men. A prolonged QT interval is defined as a QTc >0.44 seconds (440 milliseconds) in men and >0.46 seconds (460 milliseconds) in women and children. If bundle branch block or intraventricular conduction defect of >0.12 seconds is present, the QTc is prolonged if it measures >0.50 seconds (500 milliseconds).

  - A prolonged QTc interval can be acquired or inherited. It predisposes to the occurrence of a ventricular arrhythmia called torsades de pointes. A prolonged QTc, either acquired or inherited, should always be identified because this subtle abnormality can be lethal.

  - The difference between the longest and shortest QT interval, when the QT intervals are measured in all leads in a 12-lead ECG, is called QT dispersion. Wide QT dispersion of >100 milliseconds predicts a patient who is prone to ventricular arrhythmias.

- **J Point:** The end of the QRS complex and the beginning of the ST segment is called the J point. The J point marks the end of depolarization and the beginning of repolarization of the transmembrane action potential.

  - **J point elevation:** J point elevation is frequently seen in normal patients and can be attributed to the difference in repolarization between the endocardial and epicardial cells. The ventricular epicardium exhibits a spike and dome configuration during phases 1 and 2 of the action potential that is not present in the endocardium. This difference in potential during early repolarization causes current to flow between the endocardium and epicardium. This current is recorded as elevation of the J point in the surface ECG. The difference in repolarization becomes even more pronounced in the setting of hypothermia or hypercalcemia. When the J point becomes very prominent, it is often called a J wave or Osborn wave.

- **ST segment:** The ST segment is the interval between the end of the QRS complex and the beginning of the T wave. This corresponds to the plateau (phase 2) of the transmembrane

action potential. During phase 2, the transmembrane potential of the ventricular myocardial cells remains constant at 0 mV for a relatively long period. Thus, the ST segment remains isoelectric and at the same baseline level as the PR and TP segments. An ST segment is considered abnormal when it deviates above or below this baseline by 1 mm. The ST segment is also abnormal when there is a change in its morphology such as when it becomes concave or convex or has an upsloping or downsloping configuration. Contraction of the ventricular myocardium is sustained due to entry of calcium into the cell, which triggers the release of more calcium from intracellular storage sites, namely the sarcoplasmic reticulum. During this period, the ventricles are absolutely refractory to any stimuli.

- **ST elevation in normal individuals:** Elevation of the ST segment is often seen in normal healthy individuals especially in men. In one study, 91% of 6014 normal healthy men in the US Air Force aged 16 to 58 had 1 to 3 mm of ST segment elevation. ST elevation therefore is an expected normal finding in men.

  - The ST elevation in normal healthy males is commonly seen in a younger age group especially among African American men. The prevalence declines gradually with age. In one study, ST elevation of at least 1 mm was present in 93% of men aged 17 to 24 years, but in only 30% by age 76 years. In contrast, women less commonly demonstrate ST elevation, and its presence is not age related. In the same study, approximately 20% of women had ST elevation of at least 1 mm and there was no age predilection.

  - ST segment elevation in normal healthy individuals was most often seen in precordial leads $V_1$ to $V_4$ and was most marked in $V_2$. The morphology of the normal ST elevation is concave.

  - The ST segment elevation in men is much more pronounced than that noted in women with most of the men having ST elevation of $\geq 1$ mm. Most women have ST elevation measuring <1 mm. Thus, ST elevation of <1 mm has been designated as a female pattern and ST elevation of at least 1 mm associated with a sharp take-off of the ST segment of at least 20° from baseline, has been designated as a male pattern. The pattern is indeterminate if ST elevation of at least 1 mm is present but the takeoff of the ST segment from baseline is <20°. The male and female patterns can be visually recognized without making any measurements in most normal ECGs.

  - Another pattern of ST segment elevation seen in normal healthy individuals is one associated with early repolarization. This type of ST elevation is often accompanied by a J wave at the terminal end of the QRS complex. The ST elevation is most frequently seen in $V_4$ and is frequently accompanied by tall and peaked T waves (see Chapter 23, Acute Coronary Syndrome: ST Elevation Myocardial Infarction).

☐ Another ST elevation considered normal variant is the presence of ST elevation accompanied by inversion of the T wave in precordial leads $V_3$ to $V_5$.

- **Abnormal ST elevation:** Abnormal causes of ST elevation include acute myocardial infarction, coronary vasospasm, acute pericarditis, ventricular aneurysm, left ventricular hypertrophy, hyperkalemia, left bundle branch block, and the Brugada syndrome. This is further discussed in Chapter 23, Acute Coronary Syndrome: ST Elevation Myocardial Infarction.

- **T wave:** The T wave corresponds to phase 3 of the transmembrane action potential and represents rapid repolarization. The different layers of the myocardium exhibit different repolarization characteristics.

  - Repolarization of the myocardium normally starts from epicardium to endocardium because the action potential duration of epicardial cells is shorter than the other cells in the myocardium. Thus, the onset of the T wave represents the beginning of repolarization of the epicardium and the top of the T wave corresponds to the complete repolarization of the epicardium.

  - Repolarization of the endocardium takes longer than repolarization of the epicardium. Therefore, the repolarization of the endocardium is completed slightly later at the downslope of the T wave.

  - In addition to the endocardial and epicardial cells, there is also a population of M cells constituting 30% to 40% of the mid-myocardium. The M cells have different electrophysiologic properties with repolarization taking even longer than that seen in epicardial and endocardial cells. M cell repolarization consequently corresponds to the end of the T wave.

  - The duration and amplitude of the T wave is variable, although, generally, the direction (axis) of the T wave in the 12-lead ECG follows the direction of the QRS complex. Thus, when the R wave is tall, the T wave is upright, and when the R wave is smaller than the size of the S wave, the T wave is inverted.

  - The shape of the normal T wave is rounded and smooth and slightly asymmetric with the upstroke inscribed slowly and the downslope more steeply. The T wave is considered abnormal if the shape becomes peaked, notched, or distorted or if the amplitude is increased to more than 5 mm in the limb leads and >10 mm in the precordial leads. It is also abnormal when the T wave becomes symmetrical or inverted. This is further discussed in Chapter 24 (Acute Coronary Syndrome: Non-ST Elevation Myocardial Infarction and Unstable Angina).

  - At bedside, the end of the T wave coincides with the closure of the aortic and pulmonic valves. This is audible as $S_2$ during auscultation. The aortic second heart sound therefore can be used for timing purposes to identify the end of left ventricular systole and beginning of diastole. Any event before the onset of $S_2$ is systolic and any event occurring after $S_2$ (but before the next $S_1$) is diastolic.

- **TQ interval:** The TQ interval is measured from the end of the T wave to the onset of the next QRS complex. It corresponds to phase 4 of the transmembrane action potential. The T-P or TQ segment is used as the isoelectric baseline for measuring deviations of the J point or ST segment (elevation or depression) because the transmembrane action potential is at baseline and there is no ongoing electrical activity at this time. Thus, the TQ segment is not affected by other waves. However, if there is sinus tachycardia and the PR interval is markedly prolonged and the P wave is inscribed at the end of the T wave, then the long PR segment is used as an alternate baseline for measuring deviations of the J point or ST segment.

  - **T-P segment:** The T-P segment is a subportion of the TQ interval, which represents the interval between the end of ventricular repolarization (end of T wave) and the onset of the next sinus impulse (P wave). It marks the end of the previous cycle and the start of the next cardiac cycle beginning with the sinus impulse. This segment usually serves as baseline for measuring deviations of the J point or ST segment.

- At bedside, diastole starts with the closure of the aortic and pulmonic valves (audible as the second heart sound $S_2$) and continues until the closure of the mitral and tricuspid valves (audible as the first heart sound $S_1$). This closely corresponds to the TQ interval in the ECG.

- **The U wave:** Although a U wave may be seen as another deflection after the T wave, this is not consistently present. U waves are commonly visible when the heart rate is slow (usually <65 bpm) and are rarely recorded with heart rates above 95 bpm. U waves are best recorded in the anterior precordial leads due to the proximity of these leads to the ventricular myocardium. Repolarization of the His-Purkinje system coincides with the inscription of the U wave in the ECG and is more delayed than the repolarization of the M cells. The U wave therefore is most probably because of repolarization of the His-Purkinje system.

  - The U wave follows the direction of the T wave and QRS complex. Thus, the U wave is upright when the T wave is upright. When the U wave is inverted or prominent, it is considered pathologic.

  - An abnormal U wave indicates the presence of myocardial disease or electrolyte abnormality. Prominent U waves may be due to hypokalemia or drugs such as quinidine. Inversion of the U wave is always pathologic and is most commonly due to myocardial ischemia, hypertension, or valvular regurgitation. Its presence may be transient or it may be more persistent.

- **Abnormal waves:** The delta wave, epsilon wave, and Osborn wave are other waves in the ECG that should be recognized because these waves are pathologic. J. Willis Hurst traced the historical origin of these waves as follows:

  - **Delta wave:** The slow, slurred upstroke of the QRS complex, associated with the Wolff-Parkinson-White syndrome, is due to premature excitation of the ventricle because of the presence of an accessory pathway connecting the atrium directly to the ventricle. This early deflection of the QRS complex is called the delta wave because it resembles the shape of a triangle ($\Delta$) which is the symbol of the Greek capital letter delta. (Note that the slow slurred upslope of the initial QRS complex resembles the left side of the triangle.)

- **Epsilon wave:** The epsilon wave is associated with right ventricular dysplasia and represents late activation of the right ventricular free wall. This is represented as a small deflection at the end of the QRS complex and is best recorded in leads $V_1$ to $V_3$. Epsilon comes next to the Greek letter delta. The delta wave occurs at the beginning of the QRS complex (because of early activation of the ventricle and is a preexcitation wave), whereas the epsilon wave occurs at the end of the QRS complex (because of late activation of the free wall of the right ventricle and is a postexcitation wave).

- **Osborn wave:** When the J point is exaggerated, it is called J wave. The wave is named after Osborn, who described the association of this wave to hypothermia.

## Suggested Readings

Antzelevitch C. The M Cell. *J Cardiovasc Pharmacol Ther.* 1997;2:73–76.

Ariyarajah V, Frisella ME, Spodick DH. Reevaluation of the criterion for interatrial block. *Am J Cardiol.* 2006;98:936–937.

Buxton AE, Calkins H, Callans DJ, et al. ACC/AHA/HRS 2006 key data elements and definitions for electrophysiology studies and procedures: a report of the American College of Cardiology/American Heart Association Task Force on Clinical Data Standards (ACC/AHA/HRS Writing Committee to Develop Data Standards on Electrophysiology). *J Am Coll Cardiol.* 2006;48:2360–2396.

Correale E, Battista R, Ricciardiello V, et al. The negative U wave: a pathogenetic enigma but a useful often overlooked bedside diagnostic and prognostic clue in ischemic heart disease. *Clin Cardiol.* 2004;27:674–677.

Dunn MI, Lipman BS. Basic physiologic principles. In: *Lipman-Massie Clinical Electrocardiography.* 8th ed. Chicago: Yearbook Medical Publishers, Inc; 1989:24–50.

Hurst JW. Naming of the waves in the ECG, with a brief account of their genesis. *Circulation.* 1998;98:1937–1942.

Marriott HJL. Complexes and intervals. In: *Practical Electrocardiography.* 5th ed. Baltimore: Williams and Wilkins; 1972: 16–33.

Moss AJ. Long QT syndrome. *JAMA.* 2003;289:2041–2044.

Phoon CKL. Mathematic validation of a shorthand rule for calculating QTc. *Am J Cardiol.* 1998;82:400–402.

Sgarbossa EB, Wagner GS. Electrocardiography. In: *Textbook of Cardiovascular Medicine.* 2nd ed. Editor is Topol EJ Philadelphia: Lippincott-Williams and Wilkins; 2002:1330–1383.

Surawicz B. U waves: facts, hypothesis, misconceptions and misnomers. *J Cardiovasc Electrophysiol.* 1998;9:1117–1128.

Surawicz B, Parikh SR. Prevalence of male and female patterns of early ventricular repolarization in the normal ECG of males and females from childhood to old age. *J Am Coll Cardiol.* 2002;40:1870–1876.

Yan GX, Antzelevitch C. Cellular basis for the normal T wave and the electrocardiographic manifestations of the long-QT syndrome. *Circulation.* 1998;98:1928–1936.

Yan GX, Lankipalli RS, Burke JF, et al. Ventricular repolarization components of the electrocardiogram, cellular basis and clinical significance. *J Am Coll Cardiol.* 2003;42:401–409.

Yan GX, Shimizu W, Antzelevitch C. Characteristics and distribution of M cells in arterially perfused canine left ventricular wedge preparations. *Circulation.* 1998;98:1921–1927.

# The Lead System

## Basic Principles

- The electrical impulses originating from the heart can be transmitted to the body surface because the body contains fluids and chemicals that can conduct electricity. These electrical impulses can be recorded by placing electrodes to the different areas of the body. Thus, if a left arm electrode is connected to the positive pole of a galvanometer and a right arm electrode is connected to the negative pole, the magnitude as well as the direction of the electrical impulse can be measured.
  - Any flow of current directed toward the positive (left arm) electrode is conventionally recorded as an upright deflection (Fig. 3.1A).
  - Any flow of current away from the positive electrode is recorded as a downward deflection (Fig. 3.1B).
  - The height of the electrocardiogram (ECG) deflection represents the difference in potential between the two electrodes.

## Bipolar Leads I, II, and III

- **Bipolar Leads:** An imaginary line connecting any two electrodes is called a lead. A lead is bipolar when both positive and negative electrodes contribute to the deflection in the ECG. The positive and negative electrodes are placed at an equal distance away from the heart and the resulting ECG deflection is the sum of the electrical forces going in opposite directions. Leads I, II, and III are examples of bipolar leads.
  - **Lead I:** Lead I is conventionally constructed such that the left arm electrode is attached to the positive pole of the galvanometer and the right arm to the negative pole (Fig. 3.2A). If the direction of the impulse is toward the left arm, an upward or positive deflection is recorded. If the direction of the impulse is toward the right arm, a negative or downward deflection is recorded.

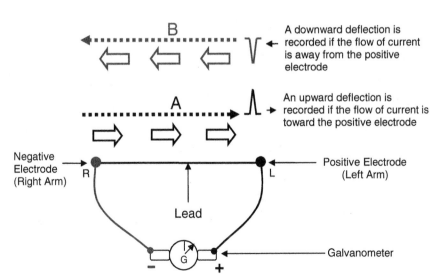

A downward deflection is recorded if the flow of current is away from the positive electrode

An upward deflection is recorded if the flow of current is toward the positive electrode

Negative Electrode (Right Arm)

Positive Electrode (Left Arm)

Lead

Galvanometer

**Figure 3.1: Lead.** The direction and magnitude of the electrical impulse can be measured with a galvanometer (G). The left arm electrode is conventionally attached to the positive pole of the galvanometer and the right arm electrode to the negative pole. An imaginary line connecting the two electrodes is called a lead. Any flow of current directed toward the positive electrode will be recorded as an upright deflection **(A)**. Any current moving away from the positive electrode is recorded as a downward deflection **(B)**.

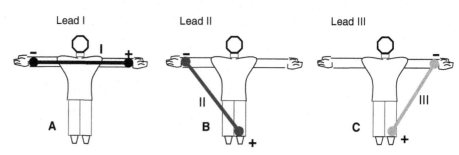

**Figure 3.2: Bipolar Leads I, II, and III. A–C** represent the location of the electrodes for leads I, II, and III, respectively. Any flow of current toward the positive electrode will record a positive deflection. The imaginary line connecting the two electrodes is the ECG lead.

■ **Lead II:** The left leg is attached to the positive pole and the right arm to the negative pole (Fig. 3.2B). When the direction of the impulse is toward the left leg, a positive deflection is recorded. When the direction of the impulse is toward the right arm, a downward deflection is recorded.

■ **Lead III:** The left leg is attached to the positive pole and the left arm to the negative pole (Fig. 3.2C). When the direction of the impulse is toward the left leg, an upward deflection is recorded. When the direction of the impulse is toward the left arm, a downward deflection is recorded.

■ Lead I transects an imaginary line from one shoulder to the other shoulder and represents an axis of 0° to 180° (Fig. 3.3A).

■ Lead II transects an imaginary line between the left leg and right arm and represents an axis of +60° to –120° (Fig. 3.3B).

■ Lead III transects an imaginary line between the left leg and the left arm and represents an axis of +120° and –60° (Fig. 3.3C).

■ Leads I, II, and III can be arranged to form the Einthoven triangle (Fig. 3.3D, E) as shown. The leads can also be superimposed on each other by combining all three leads at their mid-points to form a triaxial

reference system representing the frontal plane of the body (Fig. 3.3F).

■ **Unipolar Leads:** When one electrode is capable of detecting an electrical potential (exploring electrode) and the other electrode is placed at a distant location so that it will not be affected by the electrical field (indifferent electrode), the lead that is created is a unipolar lead. A unipolar lead therefore has only one electrode that contributes to the deflection in the ECG. The other electrode serves as a ground electrode and is theoretically neutral.

■ **The exploring electrode:** Only the exploring electrode is capable of measuring the flow of current. This electrode is connected to the positive pole of the galvanometer. If the flow of current is directed toward the exploring electrode, an upward deflection is recorded. If the flow of current is away from the exploring electrode, a downward deflection is recorded. The exploring electrodes of the three unipolar limb leads are conventionally placed in the right arm, left arm and left foot and were originally called VR, VL, and VF respectively.

■ **The ground electrode:** The ground electrode is constructed by placing a resistance of 5,000 ohms to each of the three limb electrodes and connecting them together to form a central terminal (Fig. 3.4).

**Figure 3.3: Bipolar Leads I, II, and III. A, B,** and **C** represent leads I, II, and III, respectively. The leads form an Einthoven triangle **(D, E)**, which can be rearranged to form a triaxial reference system by combining all three leads at each midpoint as shown **(F)**.

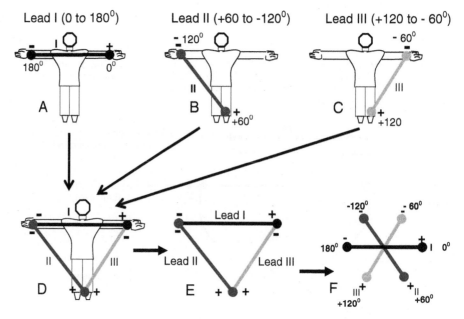

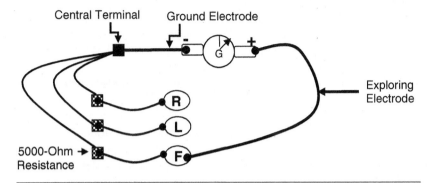

**Figure 3.4:    Unipolar Leads VR, VL, and VF.** Diagram shows the original construction of the unipolar limb leads VR, VL, and VF. Each limb lead is connected to a resistance of 5,000 ohms to form a central terminal. The central terminal serves as the ground electrode and is connected to the negative pole of the galvanometer. The exploring electrode, which in this example is in the left foot, is connected to the positive pole. R, right arm; L, left arm; F, left foot.

The central terminal is connected to the negative pole of the galvanometer. This serves as the ground electrode, which has a potential of zero or near zero.

## Augmented Unipolar Leads AVR, AVL, and AVF

■ **Augmented unipolar leads aVR, aVL, and aVF:** When the exploring electrode was disconnected from

the central terminal, the size of the ECG deflection increased by 50%. Thus, the augmented unipolar leads VR, VL, and VF were renamed aVR, aVL, and aVF and became the standard unipolar limb leads.

■ **Lead aVR:** The unipolar electrode is positioned over the right arm and is capable of detecting the flow of electrical impulse directed toward the right shoulder. The location of aVR is –150° (Fig. 3.5A).

■ **Lead aVL:** The unipolar electrode is positioned over the left arm and is capable of detecting potentials

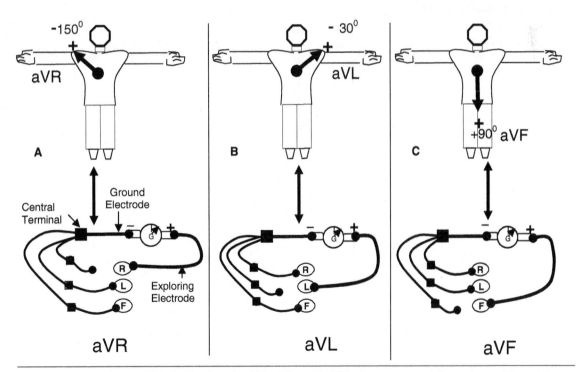

**Figure 3.5:    Augmented Unipolar Leads aVR, aVL, and aVF.** The upper panel shows the position of the exploring electrode for leads aVR, aVL, and aVF. The lower panel shows the connection of the exploring electrode and the central terminal. R, right arm; L, left arm; F, left foot.

directed toward the left shoulder. The location of aVL is −30° (Fig. 3.5B).

- **Lead aVF:** The unipolar electrode is positioned over the left leg and is capable of detecting potentials directed toward the left groin. The location of aVF is +90° (Fig. 3.5C).

## Unipolar Leads AVR, AVL, and AVF

- The three augmented unipolar leads aVR, aVL, and aVF (Fig. 3.6A), and the three standard bipolar leads I, II, and III (Fig. 3.6B) complete the six leads representing the frontal plane of the body. These six leads can be rearranged to form a hexaxial reference system as shown (Fig. 3.6C). All unipolar leads are identified with a letter V.
- The location of each lead as well as the position of the positive and negative terminals of each lead is crucial in understanding the 12-lead ECG.

## The Precordial Leads

- **Precordial leads:** Six precordial leads were later added to the six frontal leads to complete the 12-lead ECG. All

six precordial leads are unipolar and are identified with a letter V. When the lead is unipolar, only the exploring electrode contributes to the generation of the electrical complex.

- **Exploring electrode:** The location of the exploring electrodes in the chest is universally standardized. The electrodes are labeled $V_1$ to $V_6$. The standard universal position of $V_1$ to $V_6$ are as follows:
  - $V_1$ is located at the 4th intercostal space immediately to the right of the sternum.
  - $V_2$ is located at the 4th intercostal space immediately to the left of the sternum.
  - $V_3$ is located between $V_2$ and $V_4$.
  - $V_4$ is located at the 5th intercostal space, left midclavicular line.
  - $V_5$ is located at the same horizontal level as $V_4$, left anterior axillary line.
  - $V_6$ is located at the same level as $V_5$, left mid axillary line.
- **Ground electrode:** The ground electrode is the central terminal similar to Figure 3.4 and is constructed by placing a resistance of 5,000 ohms to each of the three limb electrodes (Fig. 3.7). The central terminal is connected to the negative pole of the galvanometer and serves as the ground electrode, which has a potential of zero.

**Figure 3.6: Hexaxial Reference System Representing the Frontal Plane.** The standard bipolar leads I, II, and III and the augmented unipolar limb leads aVR, aVL, and aVF make up the hexaxial reference system representing the frontal plane. **(A)** The location of these leads in relation to the body. **(B, C)** How these six leads are related to each other.

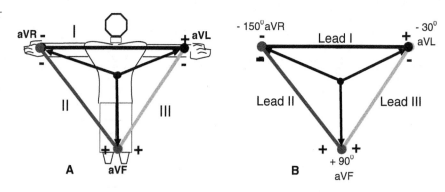

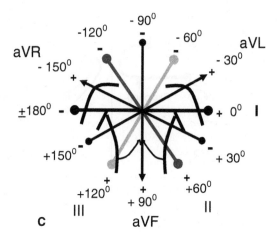

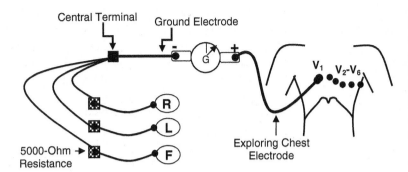

**Figure 3.7:   The Precordial Leads.** The construction of the unipolar chest leads is shown diagrammatically. The precordial electrode is the exploring electrode. Six exploring electrodes are positioned in $V_1$ to $V_6$. The ground electrode consists of three limb electrodes individually attached to a 5,000-ohm resistance and connected together to form a central terminal. R, right arm; L, left arm; F, left foot.

## The 12-Lead ECG

■ The six frontal or limb leads and the six horizontal or precordial leads complete the 12-lead ECG (Fig. 3.8A, B).

## ⬜ Standard and Special Leads

■ **Standard 12-lead ECG:** The 12-lead ECG is recorded with the patient supine and a pillow supporting the head.

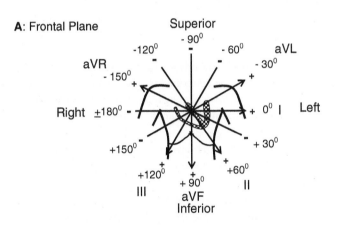

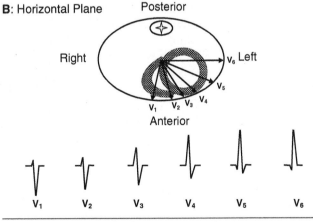

**Figure 3.8:   The 12-Lead Electrocardiogram. (A)** The position of the six limb leads in the frontal plane. **(B)** The six precordial leads in the horizontal plane.

The latest recommendations of the American Heart Association regarding the ECG include the following:

■ Until further studies are available, the extremity electrodes are placed distal to the shoulders and hips and not necessarily at the wrists or ankles. This reduces motion artifacts and ECG voltage and duration are less affected than if the leads are placed more distally.

■ All leads in the standard 12-lead ECG are effectively bipolar. This is based on the principle that all leads consist of an electrode that is paired to another electrode. This includes the standard limb leads as well as the leads where the exploring electrode is paired with an indifferent electrode consisting of the central terminal or its modification. Thus, standard leads I, II, and III; augmented limb leads aVR, aVL, and aVF; and the six precordial leads $V_1$ to $V_6$ are all effectively bipolar and the use of bipolar and unipolar to describe these leads is discouraged.

■ Misplacement of the precordial leads is a common cause of variability in the ECG, especially when serial tracings are being interpreted. The position of $V_4$ should be followed horizontally; thus, $V_5$ and $V_6$ should be in the same horizontal position as $V_4$ rather than at a lower position if the course of the 5th intercostal space is followed laterally. In women, it is recommended that the precordial electrodes should be placed under rather than over the breast, thus allowing $V_5$ and $V_6$ to follow the horizontal position of $V_4$. If the anterior axillary line is not well defined, $V_5$ is positioned midway between $V_4$ and $V_6$. The position of $V_1$ and $V_2$ is at the 4th intercostal space at the right and left sternal borders respectively. When $V_1$ and $V_2$ are erroneously placed higher at the 2nd intercostal space, the following changes may occur:

⬜ A smaller r wave is recorded from $V_1$ to $V_3$. The R wave reduction is approximately 1 mm per interspace, causing poor R wave progression, which can be mistaken for anterior myocardial infarction (MI).

⬜ Terminal r′ waves with T wave inversion resulting in rSr′ pattern in $V_1$ and $V_2$ are recorded similar to the configuration in lead aVR.

⬜ If the diaphragm is displaced downward and the heart becomes vertically oriented, as when there is chronic obstructive lung disease, the normal location of $V_3$ and $V_4$ will place these leads in a relatively higher position than the ventricles; thus, deep S waves will be recorded in these leads, which can be mistaken for anterior MI.

■ Finally, when the extremity leads are modified so that the leads are placed in the torso rather than the extremities, the ECG is not considered equivalent to the standard ECG. Similarly, tracings obtained in the sitting or upright position is not equivalent to the standard ECG, which is recorded supine.

■ It has also been observed that when $V_1$ and $V_2$ are placed higher than their normal location, small q waves may be recorded in $V_2$ and $V_3$, especially in the presence of left anterior fascicular block.

■ **Special Electrodes:** In addition to the 12 standard ECG leads, special leads can be created by repositioning some electrodes to the different areas on the chest.

■ **Special leads $V_7$, $V_8$, and $V_9$:** $V_7$ is located at the left posterior axillary line at the same level as $V_6$. $V_8$ is located just below the angle of the left scapula at the same level as $V_7$ and $V_9$ just lateral to the spine at the same level as $V_8$. These leads supplement the 12-lead ECG in the diagnosis of posterolateral ST elevation MI and should be recorded when reciprocal ST segment depression is present in $V_1$ to $V_3$.

■ **Right sided precordial leads $V_3R$, $V_4R$, $V_5R$, and $V_6R$:** After recording the usual standard 12-lead ECG, special leads $V_3R$, $V_4R$, $V_5R$, and $V_6R$ can be added by moving precordial leads $V_3$, $V_4$, $V_5$, and $V_6$ to the right side of the chest corresponding to the same location as that on the left. These leads are very useful in the diagnosis of right ventricular MI, dextrocardia, and right ventricular hypertrophy. These leads should be recorded routinely when there is acute coronary syndrome with ST elevation MI involving the inferior wall (leads II, III, and aVF).

■ **Other lead placement used for detection of arrhythmias:**

  □ **CF, CL, and CR leads:** Bipolar leads have electrodes positioned in the arms or leg, which are equidistant from the heart. When one electrode is moved to the precordium and the other electrode is retained in its original position in the arm or leg, the chest electrode will contribute more to the recording than the remote electrode.

  □ Thus, a CL lead is created if one electrode is placed on the chest and the more remote electrode is retained in its original position in the left arm. If the chest electrode is placed in $V_1$ and the remote electrode is at the left arm, the lead is identified as $CL_1$.

  □ CR lead is created when the remote electrode is retained in the right arm. If the chest electrode is placed in $V_1$ and the remote electrode is at the right arm, the lead is identified as $CR_1$.

  □ CF lead is created when the remote electrode is retained in the left foot. If the chest electrode is placed in $V_1$ and the remote electrode is at the left foot, the lead is identified as $CF_1$.

  □ **Modified $CL_1$ or $MCL_1$:** $MCL_1$ is a lead that resembles $V_1$. The lead is bipolar and is a modified $CL_1$ lead. The positive electrode is placed at $V_1$ and the negative electrode is placed close to the left shoulder. A ground electrode is placed at the other shoulder. It is frequently used for detecting arrhythmias during continuous monitoring of patients admitted to the coronary care unit.

  □ **Lewis lead:** When the P wave is difficult to recognize, the right arm electrode is moved to the 2nd right intercostal space just beside the sternum and the left arm electrode to the 4th right intercostal space also beside the sternum. Lead I is used for recording.

  □ **Fontaine lead:** The Fontaine leads are special leads for recording epsilon waves in patients with arrhythmogenic right ventricular dysplasia. The epsilon waves are usually difficult to record using only the standard 12 leads. The right arm electrode is placed at the manubrium and the left arm electrode at the xiphoid. Additionally, the left foot electrode may be moved to position $V_4$. Leads I, II, and III are used for recording.

  □ **Other modifications:** Other special leads can be created if the P waves cannot be visualized by placing the right arm electrode at $V_1$ position and the left arm electrode anywhere to the left of the sternum or more posteriorly at $V_7$ position. Lead I is recorded.

  □ **Esophageal and intracardiac electrodes:** These electrodes can be connected to any precordial or V lead, usually $V_1$, for recording atrial activity (P waves) if the P wave cannot be visualized in the surface ECG.

    □ A pill electrode can be swallowed and positioned behind the left atrium in the esophagus and connected to a precordial lead usually $V_1$. The ECG is recorded in $V_1$.

    □ An electrode can also be inserted transvenously and positioned into the right atrium. The electrode is connected to a precordial lead and recorded as above.

    □ A central venous catheter, which is often already in place for intravenous administration of medications, is filled with saline. A syringe needle is inserted to the injecting port of the central line and attached with an alligator clamp to a precordial lead, usually $V_1$. The ECG is recorded in $V_1$. This special lead is for recording atrial activity if the P waves are not visible in the surface ECG.

## Suggested Readings

Burch GE, Winsor T. Principles of electrocardiography. In: *A Primer of Electrocardiography*, 5th ed. Philadelphia: Lea and Febiger; 1966;17–66.

Burch GE, Winsor T. Precordial leads. In: *A Primer of Electrocardiography*, 5th ed. Philadelphia: Lea and Febiger; 1966;146–184.

Dunn MI, Lippman BS. Basic ECG principles. In: *Lippman-Massie Clinical Electrocardiography*, 8th ed. Chicago: Yearbook Medical Publishers; 1989:51–62.

Hurst JW. Naming of the waves in the ECG, with a brief account of their genesis. *Circulation*. 1998;1937–1942.

Kligfield P, Gettes LS, Bailey JJ, et al. Recommendations for the standardization and interpretation of the electrocardiogram: part I: the electrocardiogram and its technology: a scientific statement from the American Heart Association Electrocardiography and Arrhythmias Committee, Council on Clinical Cardiology; the American College of Cardiology Foundation; and the Heart Rhythm Society. *J Am Coll Cardiol*. 2007;49:1109–1127.

Madias JE, Narayan V, Attari M. Detection of P waves via a "saline-filled central venous catheter electrocardiographic lead" in patients with low electrocardiographic voltage due to anasarca. *Am J Cardiol*. 2003;91:910–914.

Marriott HJL. Chapter 4. Electrical Axis. In: *Practical Electrocardiography*, 5th ed. Baltimore: Willliams & Wilkins; 1972:34–43.

Wagner GS. Cardiac electrical activity and recording the electrocardiogram. In: *Marriott's Practical Electrocardiography*, 10th ed. Philadelphia: Lippincott Williams and Wilkins; 2001;2–41.

# 4

# The Electrical Axis and Cardiac Rotation

## The Frontal and Horizontal Planes

- Figuring the direction or axis of the QRS complex (or any wave in the electrocardiogram [ECG]) requires a thorough understanding of the location of each of the different leads in the 12-lead ECG. This knowledge is crucial and provides the basic foundation for understanding electrocardiography. Before attempting to read this chapter, a review of the previous chapter is mandatory.
- The ECG mirrors both frontal and horizontal planes of the body and is thus tridimensional.
    - **Frontal plane:** The frontal plane is represented by leads I, II, III, aVR, aVL, and aVF. It includes the left/right and superior/inferior orientation of the body (Fig. 4.1A). The electrical position of the heart in the frontal plane is described as axis deviation. Thus, the axis of the QRS complex may be normal or it may be deviated to the left, to the right or to the northwest quadrant.
    - **Horizontal plane:** The horizontal plane is represented by leads $V_1$ to $V_6$ (Fig. 4.1B). It includes left/right and anteroposterior orientation of the body. The position of the heart in the horizontal plane is described as rotation. Thus, the rotation of

the heart may be normal or it may be rotated clockwise or counterclockwise.

## The Frontal Plane

- **Frontal plane:** Using the hexaxial reference system (Fig. 4.2), the frontal plane can be divided into four quadrants.
    - **Normal quadrant:** The left lower quadrant between 0° and +90° represents normal quadrant.
    - **Left upper quadrant:** The left upper quadrant between 0° and −90° represents left axis deviation.
    - **Right lower quadrant:** The right lower quadrant between +90° and +180° represents right axis deviation.
    - **Right upper quadrant:** The quadrant between −90° and ±180° is either extreme right or extreme left axis deviation. Often, it is not possible to differentiate whether the axis has deviated extremely to the right or extremely to the left; thus, this axis is often called northwest axis.
- **Normal axis:** The normal QRS axis depends on the age of the patient.

**Figure 4.1:  The 12-Lead Electrocardiogram.** The location of the different leads in the frontal **(A)** and horizontal **(B)** planes is shown.

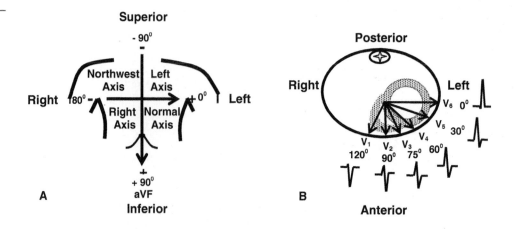

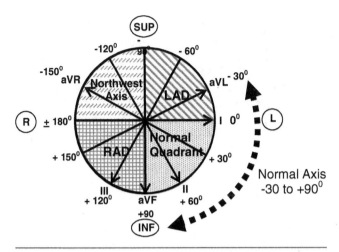

**Figure 4.2:   The Frontal Plane and the Hexaxial Reference System.** The frontal plane is represented by the six limb leads. The position of the limb leads and the location of the different quadrants in the frontal plane are shown. Note that the leads are 30° apart. The normal axis in the adult extends from −30° to +90°, thus −1° to −30° is considered normal axis. LAD, left axis deviation; RAD, right axis deviation; L, left; R, right; SUP, superior; INF, inferior.

- In newborns up to 6 months of age, the normal QRS axis is >+90° (vertical axis). With increasing age, the axis moves horizontally leftward toward 0°. It is rare in children to have a horizontal axis.

- In adults, the normal axis extends horizontally from +90° to −30°. The axis −1° to −30° is located in the left upper quadrant and is left axis deviation. How-

ever, because the normal axis extends up to −30°, an axis of −1° to −30° is considered part of the normal axis (Fig. 4.2).

## Figuring Out the Electrical Axis

- **Basic considerations:** Before attempting to determine the axis of any deflection in the ECG, the location of all the six leads in the frontal plane as well as the location of the positive and negative terminals of each lead should be mastered. The ECG deflection is maximally upright if the flow of current is directed toward the positive side of the lead and is maximally inverted if the flow of current is directed toward the negative side. Thus, if the flow of current is parallel to lead I (0° to 180°), lead I will record the tallest deflection if the flow of current is directed toward 0° and the deepest deflection if the flow of current is directed toward 180° (Fig. 4.3A, B).

- The lead perpendicular to lead I will record an isoelectric complex. Isoelectric or equiphasic implies that the deflection above and below the baseline are about equal. Since lead aVF is perpendicular to lead I, lead aVF will record an isoelectric deflection (Fig. 4.3C, D).

- **Determining the electrical axis:** The electrical axis or direction of the QRS complex (or any wave in the ECG) can be determined by several methods. Although the area under the QRS complex provides a more accurate electrical axis, the area is not readily measurable. For convenience, the amplitude of the QRS complex is measured instead.

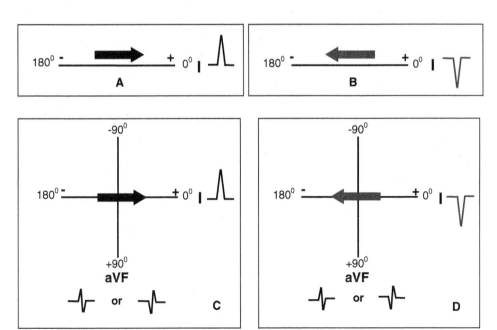

**Figure 4.3:   Leads I and aVF.** Lead I and aVF are perpendicular to each other. The electrocardiogram deflection in lead I will register the tallest deflection if the current is directed toward the positive electrode (0°) as shown in **A**. It will record the deepest deflection if the current is directed toward 180° or the negative electrode as shown in **B**. The lead perpendicular to lead I will record an isoelectric deflection. Because aVF is perpendicular to lead I, aVF will record an isoelectric complex **(C, D)**.

**Figure 4.4: Perpendicular Leads.** In the frontal plane, the following leads are perpendicular to each other: Leads I and aVF (**A**), Leads II and aVL (**B**) and lead III and aVR (**C**).

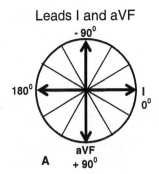

Leads I and aVF

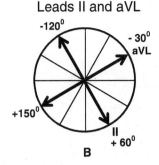

Leads II and aVL

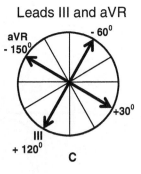

Leads III and aVR

- **Method 1: Look for an isoelectric complex:** When an isoelectric QRS complex is present in any lead in the frontal plane, the axis of the QRS complex is perpendicular to the lead with the isoelectric complex. The following leads in the frontal plane are perpendicular to each other.
  - **Lead I is perpendicular to lead aVF** (Fig. 4.4A).
    - □ When an equiphasic QRS complex is recorded in lead I (0°), the axis of the QRS complex is +90° or −90°.
    - □ Similarly, when an equiphasic QRS complex is recorded in lead aVF (+90°), the axis of the QRS complex is 0° or 180°.
  - **Lead II is perpendicular to lead aVL** (Fig. 4.4B).
    - □ When an equiphasic QRS complex is recorded in lead II (+60°), the axis of the QRS complex is −30° or +150°.
    - □ Similarly, when an equiphasic QRS complex is recorded in lead aVL (−30°), the axis of the QRS complex is +60° or −120°.
  - **Lead III is perpendicular to lead aVR** (Fig. 4.4C).
    - □ When an equiphasic QRS complex is recorded in lead III (+120°), the axis of the QRS complex is −150° or +30°.
    - □ Similarly, when an equiphasic QRS complex is recorded in lead aVR (−150°), the axis of the QRS complex is +120° or −60°.

## Figuring Out the Electrical Axis when an Equiphasic Complex is Present

- **Lead I is equiphasic:** If the QRS complex in lead I (0°) is equiphasic, the flow of current is toward lead aVF, because lead aVF is perpendicular to lead I. If the flow of current is toward +90°, which is the positive side of aVF, the tallest deflection will be recorded in aVF (Fig. 4.5A). If the flow of current is toward −90° away from the positive side of aVF, lead aVF will record the deepest deflection (Fig. 4.5B).

- Figures 4.5C and D summarize the possible deflections of the other leads in the frontal plane if lead I is equiphasic.

- **Lead II is equiphasic:** If lead II (+60°) is equiphasic, the flow of current is in the direction of lead aVL, because lead aVL is perpendicular to lead II. If the electrical current is directed toward −30°, the tallest deflection will be recorded in lead aVL (Fig. 4.6A) because this is the positive side of lead aVL. On the other hand, if the flow of current is toward +150°, lead aVL will record the deepest deflection, because this is away from the positive side of lead aVL (Fig. 4.6B).

- Figures 4.6C and D summarize the possible deflections of the different leads in the frontal plane of the ECG if lead II is equiphasic.

- **Lead III is equiphasic:** If the QRS complex in lead III (+120°) is equiphasic, the flow of current is in the direction of lead aVR, because lead aVR is perpendicular to lead III. If the electrical current is directed toward −150°, the tallest deflection will be recorded in lead aVR (Fig. 4.7A) because this is the positive side of lead aVR. On the other hand, if the flow of current is toward +30°, lead aVR will record the deepest deflection because this is the negative side of lead aVR (Fig. 4.7B).

- Figures 4.7C and D summarize the possible deflections of the different leads in the frontal plane if lead III is equiphasic.

## Figuring Out the Axis of the QRS Complex; Summary and Practice Tracings

- When an isoelectric deflection is recorded in any lead in the frontal plane, the mean axis of the QRS complex can be easily calculated (Figs. 4.8–4.13).

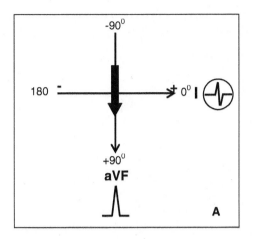

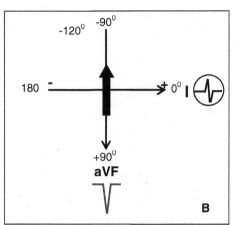

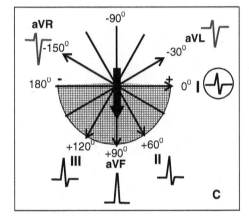

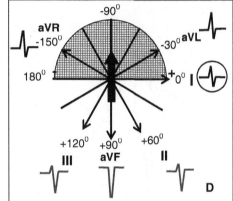

**Figure 4.5:   Lead I is Equiphasic.** If the QRS complex in lead I is equiphasic **(A, B)**, lead aVF will register the tallest deflection if the current is directed toward the positive side of aVF at +90° **(A)** and the deepest deflection if the current is directed toward –90°, away from the positive side of aVF **(B)**. The electrocardiogram configuration of the other leads if lead I is equiphasic is summarized in **C** and **D**.

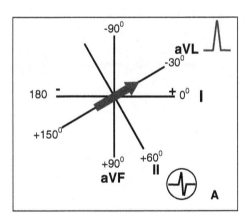

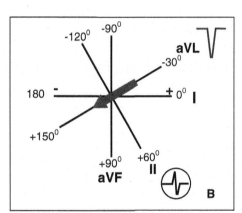

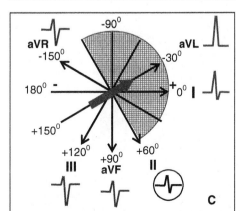

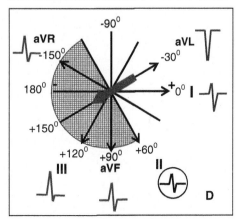

**Figure 4.6:   Lead II is Equiphasic.** If the QRS complex in lead II is equiphasic **(A, B)**, lead aVL will register the tallest deflection if the current is moving toward –30°, which is the positive side of aVL **(A)**. If the electrical current is moving away from the positive side of lead aVL or toward +150°, lead aVL will record the most negative deflection **(B)**. The configuration of the electrocardiogram in the other leads is summarized in **C** and **D**.

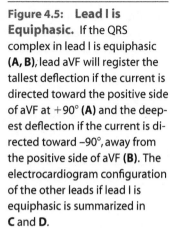

**Figure 4.7:    Lead III is Equiphasic.** If the QRS complex in lead III is equiphasic **(A, B)**, lead aVR will register the tallest deflection if the current is moving toward −150°, which is the positive side of aVR **(A)**. If the current is moving away from the positive side of lead aVR toward +30°, lead aVR will record the most negative deflection **(B)**. The configuration of the electrocardiogram in the other leads when lead III is equiphasic is summarized in **C** and **D**.

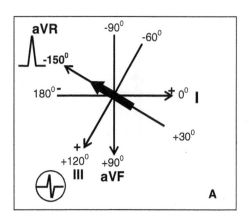

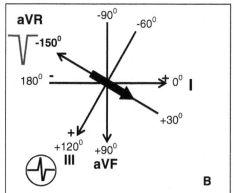

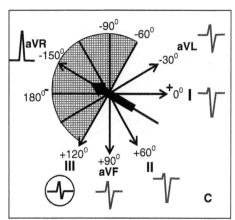

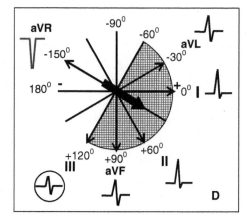

**Figure 4.8:    Isoelectric Deflection in Lead I.** Lead I is isoelectric. Because lead I is perpendicular to aVF, and lead aVF has a tall complex, the axis is +90°.

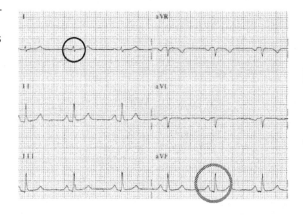

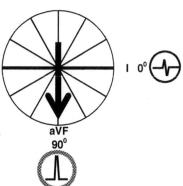

**Figure 4.9:    Isoelectric Deflection in aVL.** Lead aVL is isoelectric. Because lead aVL is perpendicular to lead II, and lead II shows the tallest deflection, the axis is +60°.

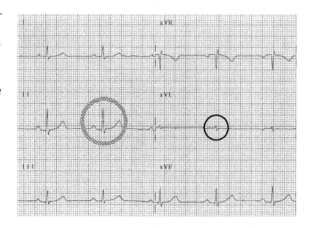

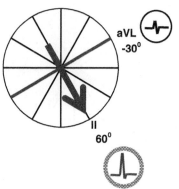

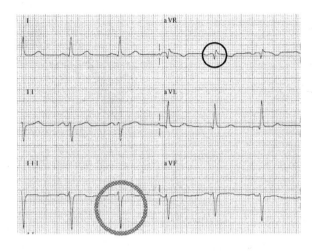

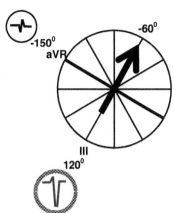

**Figure 4.10: Isoelectric Deflection in aVR.** Lead aVR is isoelectric. Because aVR is perpendicular to lead III, and lead III has the deepest complex, the axis is −60°. Note that tall R waves are present in aVL (−30°), which is beside the negative side of lead III.

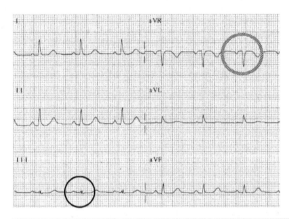

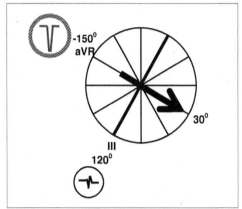

**Figure 4.11: Isoelectric Deflection in III.** Lead III is isoelectric. Because III is perpendicular to lead aVR, and lead aVR has a negative complex, the axis is away from the positive side of aVR or +30°. This is substantiated by the presence of tall R waves in leads I and lead II. These leads flank the negative side of lead aVR.

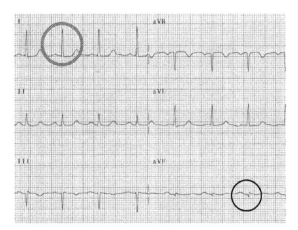

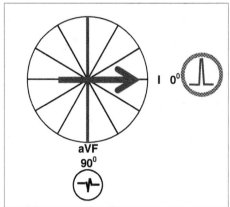

**Figure 4.12: Isoelectric Deflection in aVF.** Lead aVF is isoelectric. Because aVF is perpendicular to lead I, and lead I has the tallest complex, the axis is 0°.

**Figure 4.13:**
**Isoelectric Deflection in aVR.** Lead aVR is iso-electric. Because aVR is perpendicular to lead III, and lead III has the tallest complex, the axis is +120°.

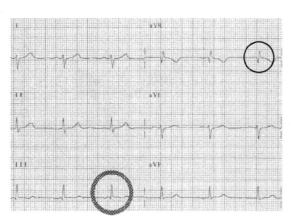

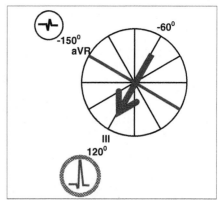

- The diagrams in Figure 4.14 summarize how to rapidly assess the axis of the QRS complex when an equiphasic complex is present.

## Method 2

As shown in the previous examples, the axis of the QRS complex can be calculated rapidly using the "eyeball" technique when an isoelectric complex is present in any lead in the frontal plane. Not all ECGs, however, will have an isoelectric complex. If an isoelectric complex is not present, the mean QRS axis can be estimated just as rapidly by the following method.

- **Select the smallest QRS complex:** The axis is obtained using the same method as calculating the axis when an isoelectric complex is present.

  □ Thus, in Figure 4.15, lead aVL is selected because the complex is the smallest and is almost isoelectric. Lead aVL is perpendicular to lead II. Because lead II shows the tallest complex, the axis is approximately 60°. Adjustment has to be made to correct for the actual axis because the complex in lead aVL is not actually isoelectric.

  □ Because aVL is negative (R < S), the axis is adjusted further away from 60°, thus the axis is approximately 70° rather than 60°.

  □ Had aVL been positive (R > S), the axis is adjusted closer to 50° rather than 70°.

## Method 3: Plotting the Amplitude of the QRS Complex using Two Perpendicular Leads

If there are no isoelectric complexes in the frontal plane, a simple way of calculating the axis is to select any pair of leads that are perpendicular to each other like leads I and aVF. The ECG in Figure 4.15 does not show any isoelectric QRS complex and will be used for calculation. The QRS complexes in leads I and aVF are shown in Figure 4.16.

- **Step 1:** The total amplitude of the QRS complex in lead I is +4 units. This is measured by subtracting any upright deflection from any downward deflection (R +5 units, S −1 unit; total +4 units).

- **Step 2:** The total amplitude of the QRS complex in lead aVF is +9 units.

- **Step 3:** Perpendicular lines are dropped for 4 units from the positive side of lead I and for 9 units from the positive side of lead aVF until these two lines intersect (Fig. 4.16). The point of intersection is marked by an arrowhead and connected to the center of the hexaxial reference system. The line drawn represents a vector, which has both direction and magnitude. The direction of the vector is indicated by the arrowhead. Thus, the mean electrical axis of the QRS complex is +70°.

- The diagram in Fig. 4.17 summarizes the different ECG deflections that will be recorded if several unipolar recording electrodes are placed along the path of an electrical impulse traveling from left to right toward 0°:

  - The electrode at 0° will record the most positive deflection.

  - The electrode at 180° will show the most negative deflection.

  - The electrode perpendicular to the direction of the impulse (+90° and −90°) will record an equiphasic or isoelectric complex.

  - Any recording electrode that is located within 90° of the direction of the electrical current (checkered area) will record a positive deflection (R > S wave).

  - Any electrode that is further away and is >90° of the direction of the electrical impulse will show a negative deflection (R < S wave).

- The diagrams in Fig. 4.18 summarize the location of the QRS axis when an equiphasic QRS complex is not present in the frontal plane (Fig. 4.18).

## The Precordial Leads

- **Horizontal plane:** The six precordial leads $V_1$ to $V_6$ are also called horizontal or transverse leads since they represent the horizontal or transverse plane of the

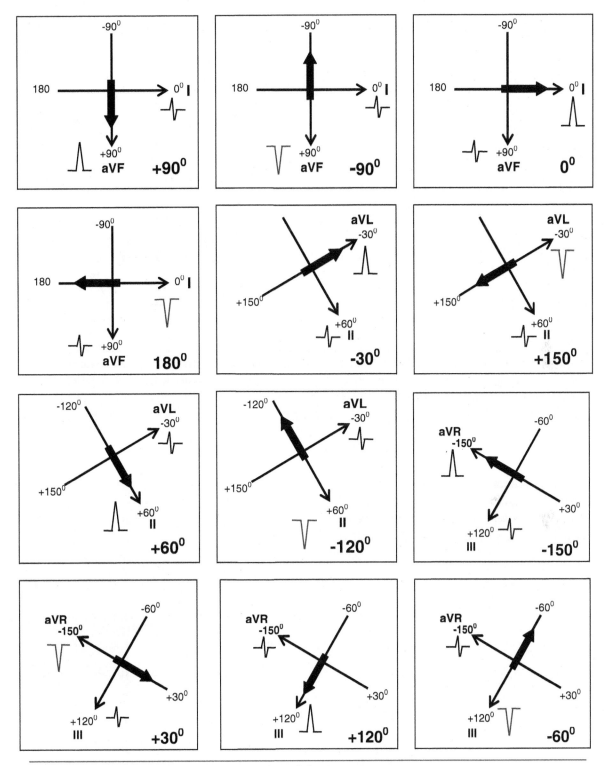

**Figure 4.14:    Diagrams Showing the Location of the QRS.** Bold arrows point to the QRS axis when an equiphasic complex is present.

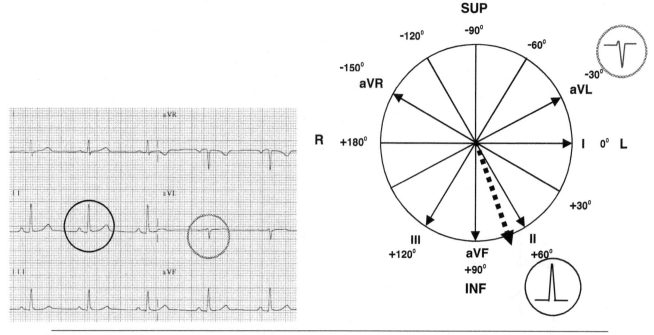

**Figure 4.15:    Figuring Out the Axis when no Isoelectric Complex is Present.** Lead aVL is selected because the complex is the smallest and almost isoelectric. Lead aVL is perpendicular to lead II. Because lead II shows the tallest complex, the axis is close to 60°. Lead aVL, however, is not actually isoelectric but is negative (r < S); thus, the axis of the QRS complex is adjusted further away and is closer to 70° (*dotted arrow*) than 60°.

chest. The horizontal plane includes the left/right as well as the anteroposterior sides of the chest (Fig. 4.19).

- **Leads V₁ and V₂:** Leads $V_1$ and $V_2$ are right-sided precordial leads and are positioned directly over the right ventricle. The QRS complexes in $V_1$ and $V_2$ represent electrical forces generated from the right

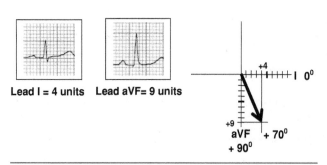

Lead I = 4 units    Lead aVF= 9 units

**Figure 4.16:    Figuring the QRS Axis.** The electrocardiogram showing leads I and aVF. The total amplitude of the QRS complex of +4 units is identified on the positive side of lead I. The total amplitude of +9 units is also identified on the positive side of lead aVF. Lines are dropped perpendicularly from leads I and aVF until the line intersects. The lines intersect at +70°, which mark the axis of the QRS complex.

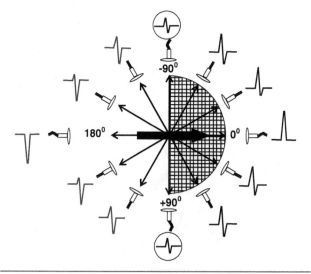

**Figure 4.17:    The Electrocardiogram Configurations of an Electrical Impulse Traveling Toward 0°.** The diagram summarizes the different electrocardiogram configurations of an impulse traveling at 0° if several electrodes are placed along its path. Any lead within 90° of the direction of the electrical impulse (checkered area) will record a positive deflection. Any lead that is further away (>90°) will record a negative deflection. The most positive or tallest deflection is recorded by the electrode positioned at 0° and the most negative by the electrode at 180°.

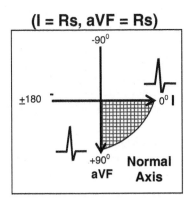

(I = Rs, aVF = Rs)

-90°
±180
0° I
+90°
aVF
**Normal Axis**

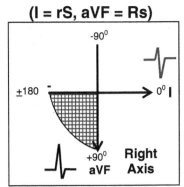

(I = rS, aVF = Rs)

-90°
±180
0° I
+90°
aVF
**Right Axis**

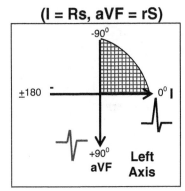

(I = Rs, aVF = rS)

-90°
±180
0° I
+90°
aVF
**Left Axis**

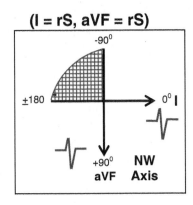

(I = rS, aVF = rS)

-90°
±180
0° I
+90°
aVF
**NW Axis**

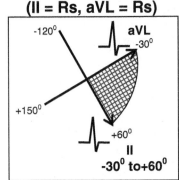

(II = Rs, aVL = Rs)

-120°
aVL
-30°
+150°
+60°
**II**
**-30° to +60°**

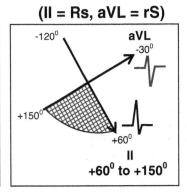

(II = Rs, aVL = rS)

-120°
aVL
-30°
+150°
+60°
**II**
**+60° to +150°**

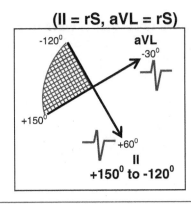

(II = rS, aVL = rS)

-120°
aVL
-30°
+150°
+60°
**II**
**+150° to -120°**

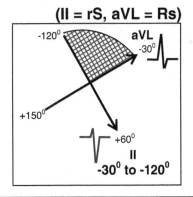

(II = rS, aVL = Rs)

-120°
aVL
-30°
+150°
+60°
**II**
**-30° to -120°**

**Figure 4.18: Checkered Area shows the Location of the QRS Axis when an Equiphasic QRS Complex is Not Present.** NW, northwest.

ventricle and generally show small r and deep S waves.

- **Leads V$_5$ and V$_6$:** Leads V$_5$ and V$_6$ are left-sided precordial leads that directly overlie the left ventricle. The QRS complexes represent electrical forces generated from the left ventricle, which show small q waves followed by tall R waves.

- **Leads V$_3$ and V$_4$:** The QRS complexes are equiphasic in leads V$_3$ and V$_4$ because these leads represent the septal area and is the transition zone between

the deep S waves in V$_1$ and V$_2$ and the tall R waves in V$_5$ and V$_6$ (Fig. 4.19).

## Cardiac Rotation

- **Cardiac rotation:** In the horizontal plane, a change in the electrical position of the heart is described as rotation. The heart may rotate clockwise or counterclock-

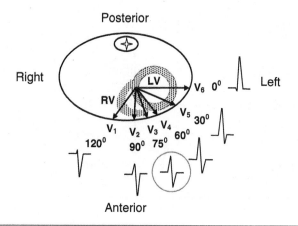

**Figure 4.19: Precordial Leads V₁ to V₆.** The location of the precordial leads and the expected normal configuration of the QRS complexes from V₁ to V₆ are shown. The QRS complex is equiphasic in V₃, which is circled. V₃ and V₄ represent the transition zone between the deep S waves in V₁ and V₂ and the tall R waves in V₅ and V₆. LV, left ventricle; RV, right ventricle.

wise (Fig. 4.20), resulting in a shift of the transition zone to the left or to the right of V₃ or V₄.

■ **Clockwise rotation or delayed transition:** When the heart rotates clockwise, the transition zone, which is usually in V₃ or V₄, moves to the left toward V₅ or V₆. This is called clockwise rotation, delayed transition, or late transition. When the apex of the heart is viewed from under the diaphragm, the front of the heart moves to the left, causing the right ventricle to move more anteriorly (Fig. 4.20A).

■ **Counterclockwise rotation or early transition:** When the heart rotates counterclockwise, the transition zone moves earlier, toward V₁ or V₂. This is called counterclockwise rotation or early transition. When the apex of the heart is viewed from under the diaphragm, the front of the heart moves to the right causing the left ventricle to move more anteriorly (Fig. 4.20C).

■ In cardiac rotation, it is important to recognize that the heart is being visualized from under the diaphragm looking up. This is opposite from the way the precordial electrodes are conventionally visualized, which is from the top looking down. Thus, in cardiac rotation, the anterior and posterior orientation of the body and the direction of cardiac rotation is reversed (compare Fig. 4.19 and 4.20).

■ Rotation of the heart is determined by identifying the transition zone where the QRS complex is equiphasic (Fig. 4.21). Rotation is normal if the transition zone is located in V₃ or V₄ (Fig. 21A, B). Figures 4.21C and D show counterclockwise rotation or early transition, and Figures 4.21E and F show late transition or clockwise rotation. The transition zones are circled (Figs. 4.22–4.24).

## Tall R Waves in V₁

■ **R wave taller than S wave in V₁:** In children, the R wave may be taller than the S wave in V₁. This is unusual in adults (Figs. 4.25A and 4.26, normal ECG).

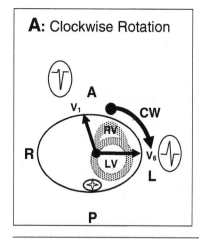
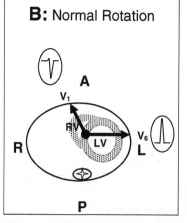
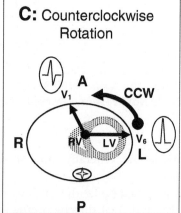

**Figure 4.20: Clockwise and Counterclockwise Rotation.** Rotation of the heart is viewed from under the diaphragm. **(A)** Clockwise rotation. The front of the heart moves to the left as shown by the arrow causing the right ventricle to move more anteriorly. **(B)** Normal rotation. **(C)** Counterclockwise rotation. The front of the heart moves to the right causing the left ventricle to move more anteriorly. A, anterior; CCW, counterclockwise rotation; CW, clockwise rotation; L, left; LV, left ventricle; P, posterior; R, right; RV, right ventricle.

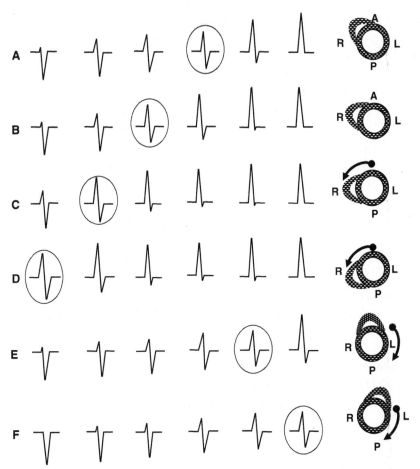

**Figure 4.21: Transition Zones. (A, B)** Normal transition where the R and S waves are equiphasic in $V_3$ or $V_4$. **(C, D)** Early transition or counterclockwise rotation with the transition zone in $V_1$ or $V_2$. **(E, F)** Late transition or clockwise rotation with the equiphasic QRS complex in $V_5$ or $V_6$. The transition zones are circled. A, anterior; P, posterior; R, right; L, left.

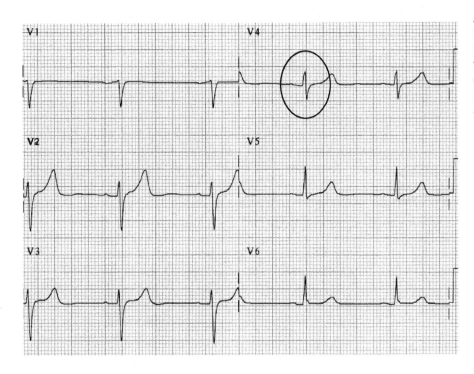

**Figure 4.22: Normal Rotation.** Precordial leads $V_1$ to $V_6$ are shown. There is gradual progression of the R waves from $V_1$ to $V_6$. $V_4$ is equiphasic (*circled*), representing the normal transition zone.

**Figure 4.23:    Counterclockwise Rotation or Early Transition.** There is early transition of the QRS complexes with the equiphasic zone in $V_1$. This represents counterclockwise rotation or early transition.

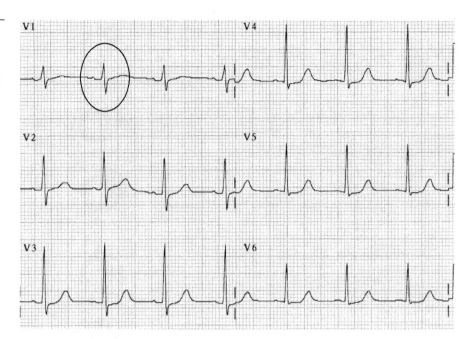

When R wave is taller than the S wave in $V_1$, the following should be excluded before this finding is considered a normal variant.

- Right bundle branch block (RBBB)
- Right ventricular hypertrophy
- Pre-excitation or Wolff Parkinson White (WPW) ECG
- Straight posterior myocardial infarction (MI)

- Pacemaker rhythm
- Ventricular ectopic impulses
- **RBBB:** In RBBB, the QRS complexes are wide measuring ≥0.12 seconds (Figs. 4.25B and 4.27). This is the most important feature distinguishing RBBB from the other entities with tall R waves in $V_1$. Terminal R′ waves are also present in $V_1$ and wide S waves are present in $V_5$ and $V_6$ or lead I (see Chapter 10, Intraventricular Conduction Defect: Bundle Branch Block).

**Figure 4.24:    Clockwise Rotation or Late Transition.** There is gradual progression of the R wave from $V_1$ to $V_6$ until the QRS complex becomes equiphasic in $V_6$. This represents clockwise rotation or late transition.

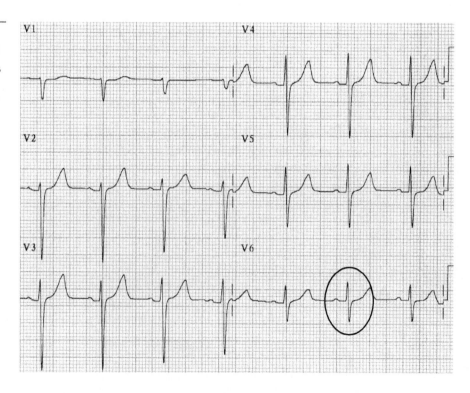

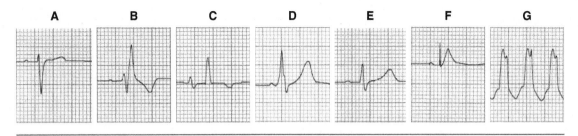

**Figure 4.25:** **Tall R Wave in V$_1$.** **(A)** Normal electrocardiogram. The R wave is smaller than the S wave. **(B)** Right bundle branch block. **(C)** Right ventricular hypertrophy. **(D)** Pre-excitation. **(E)** Straight posterior myocardial infarction. **(F)** Pacemaker-induced ventricular complex. **(G)** Ectopic ventricular complexes from the left ventricle.

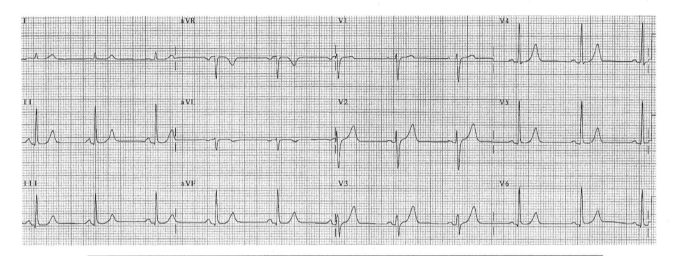

**Figure 4.26:** **Normal Electrocardiogram.** Note that the R waves are smaller than the S waves in V$_1$.

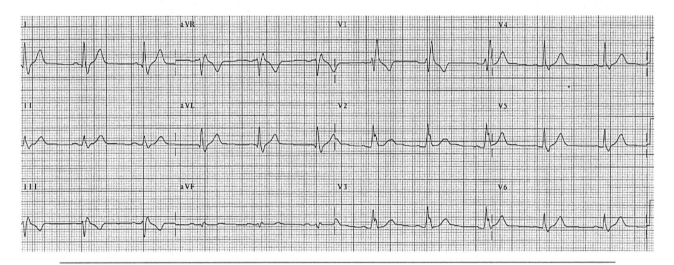

**Figure 4.27:** **Right Bundle Branch Block.** The QRS complexes are wide and tall terminal R waves are present in V$_1$.

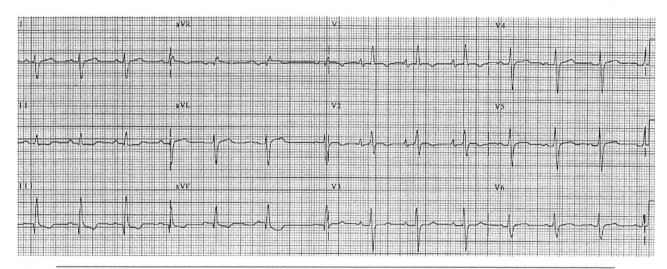

**Figure 4.28:    Right Ventricular Hypertrophy.** When right ventricular hypertrophy is the cause of the tall R waves in V$_1$, right axis deviation of ≥90° is almost always present. The diagnosis of right ventricular hypertrophy is unlikely if the axis is not shifted to the right.

■ **Right ventricular hypertrophy:** In right ventricular hypertrophy, a tall R wave in V$_1$ is almost always associated with right axis deviation of approximately ≥90° (Figs. 4.25C and 4.28). The diagnosis of RVH is uncertain unless there is right axis deviation in the frontal leads.

■ **Pre-excitation or WPW ECG:** In WPW syndrome, evidence of pre-excitation is present in the baseline ECG with short P-R interval and presence of a delta wave. The R waves are tall in V$_1$ when the bypass tract is left-sided (Figs. 4.25D and 4.29).

■ **Posterior MI:** Straight posterior MI is usually seen in older patients, not in children or young adults. It is often associated with inferior MI with pathologic q waves in leads II, III, and aVF (Figs. 4.25E and 4.30) or history of previous MI.

■ **Pacemaker rhythm:** When the rhythm is induced by an artificial pacemaker, a pacemaker artifact always precedes the QRS complex. Generally, a pacemaker-induced QRS complex has a QS or rS configuration in V$_1$ because the right ventricle is usually the chamber paced. However, when the R wave is tall in V$_1$ and is more prominent than the S wave (R or Rs complex), left ventricular or biventricular pacing should be considered as shown in Figures 4.25F and 4.31 (see Chapter 26, The ECG of Cardiac Pacemakers).

■ **Ventricular ectopic impulses:** Ventricular ectopic impulses may show tall R waves in V$_1$. This can occur when the ectopic impulses originate from the left ventricle (Figs. 4.25G and 4.32).

■ **Normal variant:** The ECG is shown (Fig. 4.33).

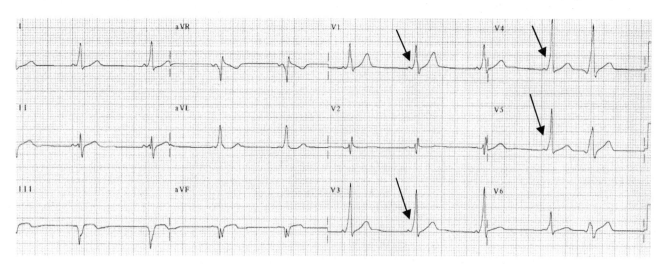

**Figure 4.29:    Pre-excitation (Wolff Parkinson White Electrocardiogram).** A short P-R interval with delta wave (*arrows*) from pre-excitation is noted. In pre-excitation, the R waves are tall in V$_1$ when the bypass tract is left-sided.

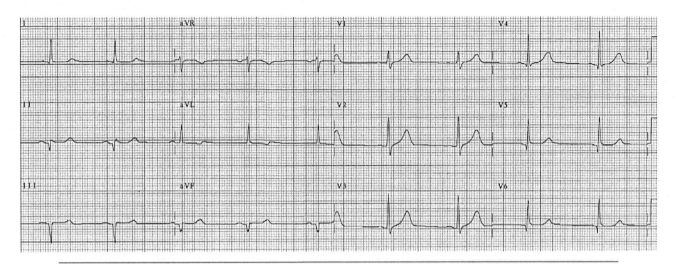

**Figure 4.30: Posterior Myocardial Infarction.** In posterior myocardial infarction (MI), tall R waves in $V_1$ is usually associated with inferior MI. Note the presence of pathologic q waves in leads II, III, and aVF.

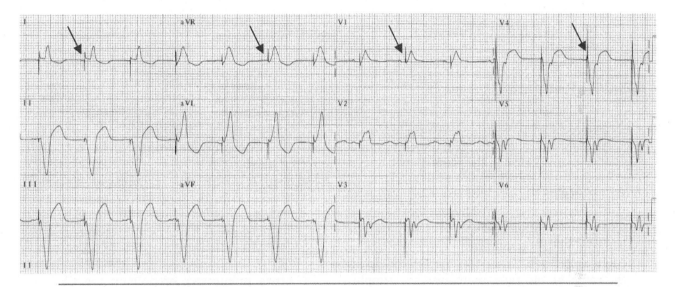

**Figure 4.31: Pacemaker-induced QRS Complexes.** Tall R waves in $V_1$ from pacemaker-induced rhythm. Arrows point to the pacemaker artifacts.

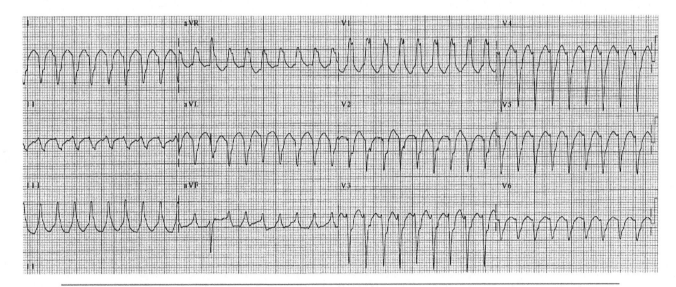

**Figure 4.32: Wide Complex Tachycardia with Tall R Waves in $V_1$.** Tall R waves in $V_1$ may be due to ectopic impulses originating from the left ventricle.

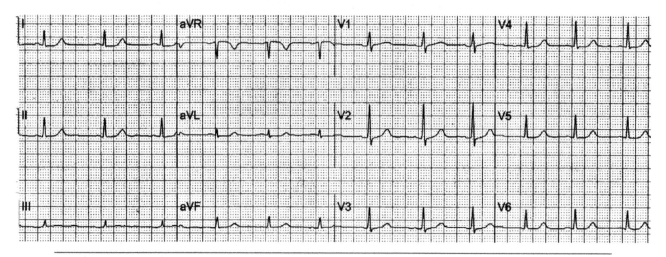

**Figure 4.33:    Normal Variant.** The electrocardiogram shows tall R waves in $V_1$ and $V_2$ in a patient with completely normal cardiac findings. Before considering tall R waves in $V_1$ and $V_2$ as normal variant, other causes should be excluded.

## Clockwise Rotation

- **Clockwise rotation:** In clockwise rotation or late transition, the transition zone of the QRS complexes in the precordial leads is shifted to the left of $V_4$ resulting in deep S waves from $V_1$ to $V_5$ or often up to $V_6$ (Fig. 4.34). Clockwise rotation is usually the result of the following:
  - **Left ventricular hypertrophy:** This can be due to several causes, including dilated cardiomyopathy or left-sided valvular insufficiency.
  - **Right ventricular hypertrophy:** Depending on the cause of the right ventricular hypertrophy, clockwise rotation may be present instead of a tall R in $V_1$. This often occurs when there is mitral stenosis, pulmonary hypertension and chronic obstructive pulmonary disease (see Chapter 7, Chamber Enlargement and Hypertrophy).

- **Biventricular hypertrophy:** Both ventricles are enlarged.

- **Chronic obstructive pulmonary disease:** In chronic obstructive pulmonary disease such as emphysema or chronic bronchitis, the diaphragm is displaced downward causing the heart to rotate clockwise and become vertically oriented (Fig. 4.34).

- **Acute pulmonary embolism:** See Chapter 7, Chamber Enlargement and Hypertrophy.

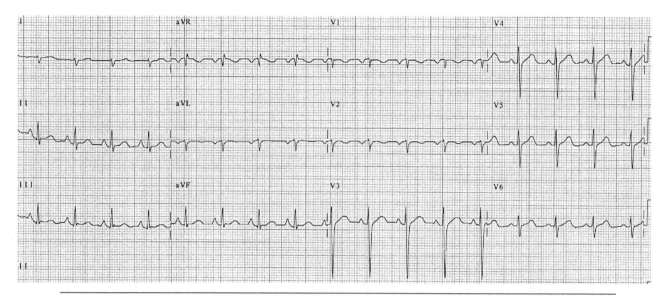

**Figure 4.34:    Clockwise Rotation.** In clockwise rotation, the transition zone is shifted to the left, resulting in deep S waves from $V_1$ to $V_6$. Note that the R waves are smaller than the S wave in $V_5$ and in $V_6$ because of a shift in the transition zone to the left of $V_6$. The electrocardiogram also shows right axis deviation; peaked P waves in II, III, and aVF; and low voltage in lead I. The cardiac rotation is due to chronic obstructive pulmonary disease.

- **Left anterior fascicular block:** See Chapter 9, Intraventricular Conduction Defect: Fascicular Block.
- **Other causes:** Cardiac rotation resulting from shift in mediastinum or thoracic deformities including pectus excavatum.

## Suggested Readings

Burch GE, Winsor T. Principles of electrocardiography. In: *A Primer of Electrocardiography*, 5th ed. Philadelphia: Lea and Febiger; 1966:17–66.

Burch GE, Winsor T. Precordial leads. In: *A Primer of Electrocardiography*, 5th ed. Philadelphia: Lea and Febiger; 1966: 146–184.

Dunn MI, Lippman BS. Basic ECG principles. In: *Lippman-Massie Clinical Electrocardiography*, 8th ed. Chicago: Yearbook Medical Publishers; 1989:51–62.

Marriott HJL. Electrical axis. In: *Practical Electrocardiography*, 5th ed. Baltimore: Willliams & Wilkins; 1972:34–43.

Wagner GS. Cardiac electrical activity. In: *Marriott's Practical Electrocardiography*, 10th ed. Philadelphia: Lippincott Williams & Wilkins; 2001;2–19.

Wagner GS. Recording the electrocardiogram. In: *Marriott's Practical Electrocardiography*, 10th ed. Philadelphia: Lippincott Williams & Wilkins; 2001;26–41.

# Heart Rate and Voltage

## The ECG Paper

- The standard electrocardiogram (ECG) is recorded at a paper speed of 25 mm per second. The voltage is calibrated so that 1 mV gives a vertical deflection of 10 mm.
- **ECG paper:** The ECG paper consists of parallel vertical and horizontal lines forming small squares 1 mm wide and 1 mm high. Every fifth line is highlighted and is darker than the other lines, thus defining a larger square of five small squares vertically and horizontally. An example of an ECG is shown in Figure 5.1.
  - **Width:** The width of the ECG paper represents time. Every millimeter or one small block is equivalent to 0.04 seconds, because the ECG records with a paper speed of 25 mm/second. Every highlighted line containing five small squares is equivalent to 0.20 seconds.

- **Height:** The height represents voltage. Because the height is standardized to give a deflection of 10 mm per mV, every small square is equivalent to 0.10 mV. The calibration marker is routinely recorded at the beginning or end of a 12-lead tracing (Fig. 5.1).

## Calculating the Heart Rate

- There are several methods of calculating the heart rate from the ECG.
  - **Using the large boxes:** The heart rate, expressed in beats per minute (bpm), can be calculated by counting the number of large boxes between two R waves (Fig. 5.2).
- **Using the small boxes:** Another method of calculating the heart rate is by counting the number of small

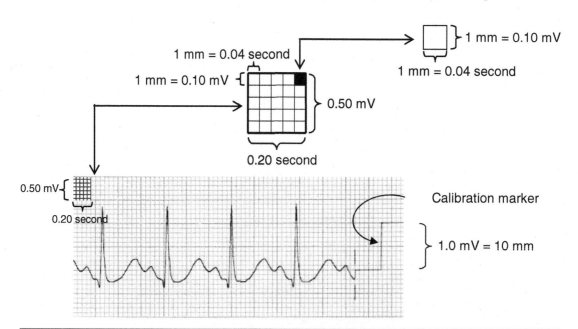

**Figure 5.1: The Electrocardiogram (ECG) Paper.** The ECG paper is divided into small squares. The width of the smallest square is 1 mm, which is equivalent to 0.04 seconds. The height of the smallest square is 1 mm, which is equivalent to 0.10 mV. When a 12-lead ECG is obtained, a calibration signal is routinely recorded such that 1.0 mV gives a deflection of 10 mm.

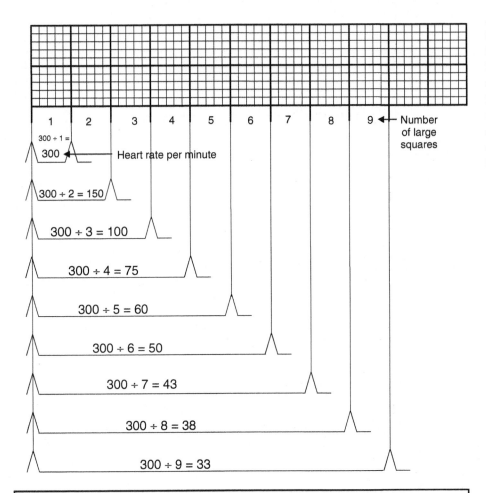

**Figure 5.2: Calculating the Heart Rate Using the Large Squares.** The heart rate can be calculated by the formula 300 ÷ the number of large squares between two R waves. Thus, if there are 5 large squares between 2 QRS complexes, the heart rate is 60 beats per minute (300 ÷ 5 = 60).

**Heart rate per minute = 300 ÷ Number of large squares**

boxes between two R waves. This is the most accurate method when the heart rate is regular and fast (Fig. 5.3).

- **Using 3-second time markers:** A third method of calculating the heart rate is by using the 3-second time markers, which are printed at the top margin of the ECG paper. The distance between the time markers is 3 seconds. The heart rate is calculated by counting the number of QRS complexes within 3 seconds and multiplied by 20. The first complex is the reference point and is not counted (Fig. 5.4).

- **Using 6-second time markers:** If the heart rate is irregular or very slow (Fig. 5.5), a longer time interval such as 6-second time marker or even 12-second time marker is chosen. The heart rate is calculated by counting the number of QRS complexes within 6 seconds and multiplied by 10. If 12 seconds are used, the number of complexes is multiplied by 5, to obtain the heart rate per minute.

- Not all ECG papers have 3-second time lines. A 3-second time line, however, can be created by counting 15 large blocks in the ECG paper. Similarly, a

6-second time line can be created by counting 30 large blocks.

- **Using commercially available heart rate sticks:** Several commercially available heart rate meters can be used to calculate heart rates. The meter is placed on the ECG rhythm strip and the heart rate is read directly from the meter stick as shown (Figs. 5.6 and 5.7). Using a heart rate meter stick is a very convenient way of measuring heart rates. Unfortunately, they are not always available when needed.

- **Using a heart rate table:** When the heart rate is regular, a heart rate table can be used for calculating heart rates. When calculating heart rates, it is more convenient to use the larger boxes for slower heart rates and the smaller boxes for fast heart rates if the heart rate is regular. Note that the same heart rate can be obtained by using the formula 300 divided by the number of big boxes or 1,500 divided by the number of small boxes, as explained earlier. If the heart rate is irregular as in patients with atrial fibrillation, a 6- or 12-second rhythm strip is more accurate (Fig. 5.8).

**Figure 5.3: Calculating the Heart Rate Using the Small Squares.** Using the small squares, the heart rate can be calculated by the formula 1,500 ÷ the number of small boxes between two R waves. Thus, if there are 5 small squares between 2 QRS complexes, the heart rate is 300 beats per minute (1,500 ÷ 5 = 300).

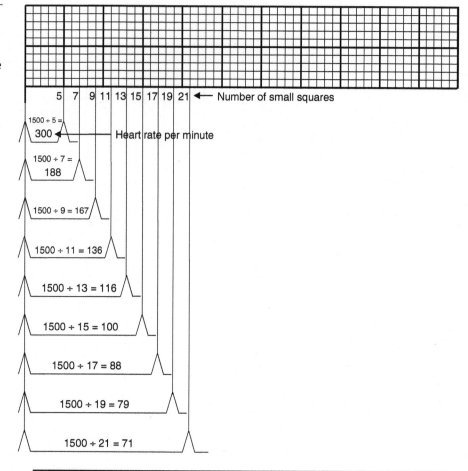

**Heart rate per minute = 1500 ÷ Number of small squares**

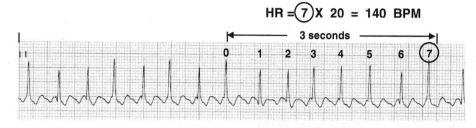

**Figure 5.4: Calculating the Heart Rate Using the 3-Second Time Markers.** There are seven complexes within the 3-second time line. The heart rate is 7 × 20 = 140 beats per minute. Note that the first QRS complex is the reference point and is not counted.

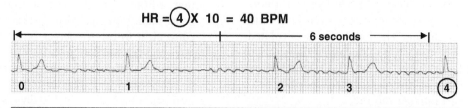

**Figure 5.5: Calculating the Heart Rate Using the Time Markers.** Because the heart rate is very slow, a longer interval is measured and two 3-second markers (6 seconds) are used. There are four complexes within the 6-second time line. Thus, the heart rate is 4 × 10 = 40 beats per minute.

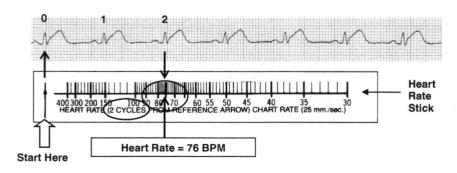

**Figure 5.6: Heart Rate Meter Stick Using Two Cardiac Cycles.** An example of a heart rate meter stick is shown. This heart rate stick uses two cardiac cycles to measure the heart rate. Two QRS complexes are measured starting from the reference point, which is identified by an arrow on the left side of the meter stick. The heart rate is read directly from the meter stick and is 76 beats per minute.

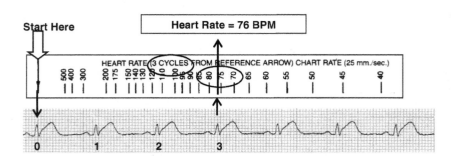

**Figure 5.7: Heart Rate Meter Stick Using Three Cardiac Cycles.** This particular meter stick uses three cardiac cycles to calculate the heart rate. Three cardiac cycles are counted starting from the reference point, which is at the left side of the meter stick. The heart rate is read directly from the meter stick and is 76 beats per minute.

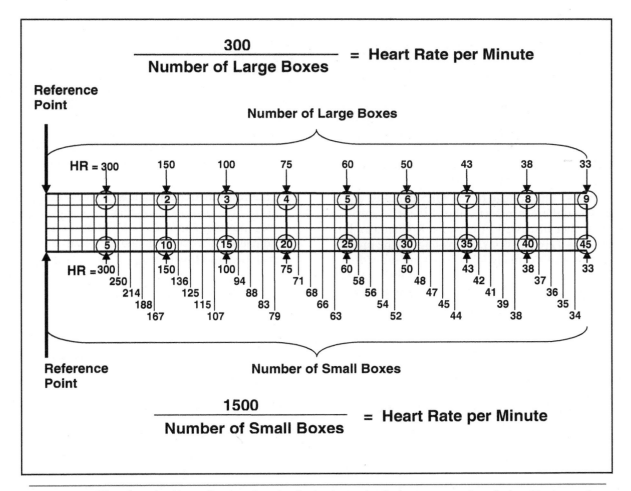

**Figure 5.8: Figuring the Heart Rate.** When the rhythm is regular, the heart rate can be calculated by measuring the distance between two QRS complexes using the large boxes (*upper portion of the diagram*) or the small boxes (*lower portion of the diagram*). The larger boxes are more convenient to use when the heart rate is <100 beats per minute, whereas the smaller boxes are more accurate to use when the heart rate is faster and >100 beats per minute.

**Figure 5.9:  Tall Voltage.** Two sets of electrocardiograms (ECGs) were obtained from the same patient representing the precordial leads and a lead II rhythm strip. **(A)** The ECG was recorded at normal calibration. Note that the amplitude of the QRS complexes is very tall with the calibration set at normal standard voltage (10 mm = 1.0 mV). **(B)** The ECG was recorded at half standard voltage (5 mm = 1.0 mV). Note that the amplitude of the QRS complexes is smaller, the ECG is less cluttered, and the height of the QRS complexes is easier to measure. The calibration signals are recorded at the end of each tracing and are marked by the arrows.

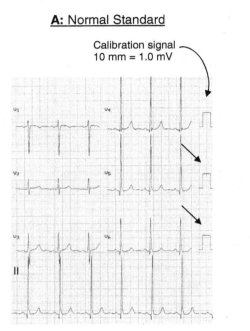
**A: Normal Standard**

Calibration signal
10 mm = 1.0 mV

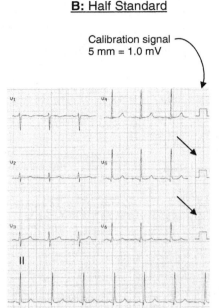
**B: Half Standard**

Calibration signal
5 mm = 1.0 mV

## ECG Voltage

- **Voltage:** The height or amplitude in the ECG paper represents voltage. The calibration signal is routinely printed at the beginning or end of the 12-lead recording (Fig. 5.9) and is standardized so that 1 mV gives a deflection of 10 mm. If the QRS complexes are too small (low voltage) or too tall (tall voltage), the standardization can be doubled or halved accordingly by flipping a switch in the ECG machine.

- **Tall voltage:** The voltage of the QRS complex is increased when there is hypertrophy of the left ventricle. This is further discussed in Chapter 7, Chamber Enlargement and Hypertrophy. The voltage in the precordial leads is also normally taller in young individuals, especially African American males, in patients who are thin or emaciated, and in patients with mastectomy, especially of the left breast.

- **Low voltage:** Excess fat, fluid, or air does not conduct impulses well and will attenuate the size of the complexes. The distance between the heart and the recording electrode will also influence the voltage in the ECG. Thus, the complexes in the limb leads are smaller than the complexes in the precordial leads because the location of the limb electrodes is farther from the heart. Fluid around the heart, lungs, abdomen, body, or extremities as well as obesity will also attenuate the size of the complexes. The low voltage may be generalized or it may be confined to the limb or frontal leads.

  - **Low voltage in the limb leads:** Low voltage confined to the limb leads indicates that not a single QRS complex measures 5 mm (0.5 mV) in any of the frontal or limb leads. The voltage in the chest leads is normal.

  - **Generalized low voltage:** Generalized low voltage indicates that not a single QRS complex measures 5 mm (0.5 mV) in the limb leads and 10 mm (1.0 mV) in the chest leads (Fig. 5.10).

**Figure 5.10:  Low Voltage with Electrical Alternans.** Twelve-lead electrocardiogram showing generalize low voltage. Note that not a single QRS complex measures 5 mm in the limb leads or 10 mm in the precordial leads. In addition, there is also beat-to-beat variation in the size of the QRS complexes because of electrical alternans *(arrows)*. The presence of a large pericardial effusion was verified by an echocardiogram.

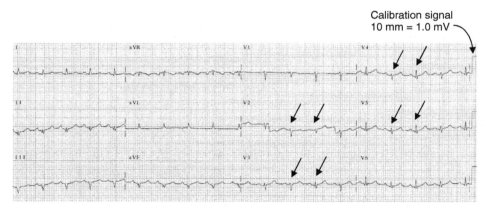

Calibration signal
10 mm = 1.0 mV

## Electrical Alternans

In electrical alternans, there is a beat-to-beat variation in the size of the QRS complexes usually by >1 mm. An example of alternating voltage of the QRS complex resulting from significant pericardial effusion is shown in Figure 5.10.

## ⬚ Calculating the Heart Rate and Measuring the Voltage

### ECG Findings

- **Heart rate:** The number of heartbeats per minute can be counted accurately using the ECG.
- **Voltage:** The voltage of any wave in the ECG can also be measured by its amplitude.

### Mechanism

- **Heart rate:** The QRS complex represents activation of the ventricles, which causes the heart to pump blood to the different parts of the body. The heart beat per minute can be counted by palpating the radial pulse or more accurately by counting the number of QRS complexes in the ECG.
- **Voltage:** The height of the different complexes in the ECG depends on a number of factors, which can either increase or decrease their amplitude. Increased ventricular mass and close proximity of the recording electrode to the origin of the impulse will enhance the voltage. On the other hand, the presence of fat, fluid, or air and a longer distance between the origin of the impulse and the recording electrode will attenuate the voltage in the ECG.

### Clinical Implications

- **Heart rate:** Included as one of the vital signs in the evaluation of any patient is the heart rate. When the patient is on a cardiac monitor, the heart rate is displayed together with the ECG rhythm. The heat rate can also be obtained very accurately in a recorded ECG. This can be done rapidly by measuring the distance between two R waves when the heart rate is regular. If the heart rate is irregular, a longer rhythm strip is needed for a more precise reading. Note that the heart rate obtained by ECG is more accurate than the pulse rate obtained at bedside because not all the impulses recorded in the ECG may be strong enough to generate a cardiac output that is palpable as a pulse, especially in sick patients who are hypotensive or in heart failure or when the patient has an irregular rhythm. In these patients, the pulse rate is not always equal to the heart rate.
  - **Regular heart rate:** When the rate is <100 bpm, the larger boxes are more convenient to use. When the rate is >100 bpm, the smaller boxes are more convenient and more accurate to use. The distance between two QRS complexes in large or small boxes is used for counting the ventricular rate and the distance between two P waves for counting the atrial rate.
    - **Large boxes:** The heart rate per minute can be calculated using the formula: 300 ÷ number of large boxes between two R waves. The formula is based on the following information.
    - Standard ECG paper speed = 25 mm per second or 1,500 mm per minute. Because one large box = 5 mm, ECG paper speed is 1,500 ÷ 5, or 300 large boxes per minute.
    - Heart rate per minute = 300 ÷ number of large boxes between two QRS complexes.
    - **Small boxes:** The heart rate per minute is obtained by dividing 1,500 by the number of small boxes between two R waves. The formula is derived from the following information:
    - Standard ECG paper speed = 25 mm per second or 1,500 mm per minute.
    - Heart rate per minute = 1,500 ÷ number of small boxes between two QRS complexes.
  - **Irregular heart rate:** When the heart rate is irregular (atrial flutter or atrial fibrillation), a longer interval should be measured to provide a more precise rate. A 3-second time line can be created if it is not marked in the rhythm strip. A 3-second interval is equal to 15 large boxes.
    - If a 3-second time interval is used, multiply the number of QRS complexes by 20.
    - If a 6-second time interval is used, multiply the number of complexes by 10.
    - If a 12-second time interval is used, multiply the number of complexes by 5.
    - Note that the first QRS complex is used as a reference point and is not counted.
- **Voltage:** Tall voltage in the ECG suggests that there is increased mass of the right or left ventricle. This is further discussed in Chapter 7, Chamber Enlargement and Hypertrophy. Decreased voltage of the QRS complex occur when transmission of the cardiac impulse to the recording electrode is diminished and are frequently seen in patients who are obese or patients with chronic pulmonary disease, pleural or pericardial effusions, generalized edema, hypothyroidism, or when there is infiltrative cardiomyopathy, such as in amyloidosis, causing reduction in the number of myocytes in the ventricles and atria.
- **Electrical alternans:** Alternating voltage of the QRS complex can occur when there is significant pericardial effusion, which allows the heart to swing in a pendular fashion within the pericardial cavity. When the heart moves closer to the chest wall, the QRS complex becomes taller. When it is pushed further away from the chest wall by the next beat, the QRS complex becomes smaller. The alternating size of the QRS complex is best recorded in the precordial electrodes especially $V_2$ to $V_5$ because these leads are closest to the heart. Electrical alternans because

of pericardial effusion can occur only if the pericardial effusion is large enough to allow the heart to swing within the pericardial cavity. Alternation of the QRS complex because of pericardial effusion is a sign of cardiac tamponade. Electrical alternans can also occur even in the absence of pericardial effusion when there is abnormal conduction of the electrical impulse in the ventricles alternating with normal conduction. It can also occur during supraventricular tachycardia or when there is severe myocardial ischemia. Electrical alternans can involve any wave of the ECG including P waves, QRS complexes, and T waves.

## Suggested Readings

Marriot HJL. Rhythm and rate. In: *Practical Electrocardiography*. 5th ed. Baltimore: Williams & Wilkins; 1972;11–15.

Surawicz B, Fisch C. Cardiac alternans: diverse mechanisms and clinical manifestations. *J Am Coll Cardiol*. 1992;20:483–499.

# Depolarization and Repolarization

## Single Muscle Cell

- Deflections in the electrocardiogram (ECG) including the P waves, QRS complexes, and T waves are due to depolarization and repolarization of the atria and ventricles. The following discussion will provide a basic understanding of how these ECG deflections are generated.

- Every heartbeat is preceded by an electrical impulse that originates from the sinus node. This impulse is propagated from one cell to the next adjacent cell until the whole myocardium is depolarized. After it is discharged, the muscle cell immediately undergoes a process of repolarization that permits the cell to again depolarize at the arrival of the next impulse.

- **Single muscle cell:** The resting potential of a single muscle cell is approximately −90 mV with the inside of the cell more negative than the outside (Fig. 6.1A). This difference in potential makes the cell capable of being discharged. When the myocardial cell is depolarized, the polarity reverses with the inside of the cell becoming more positive than the outside (Fig. 6.1B).

## Depolarization of a Single Muscle Cell

- **Depolarization:** During depolarization, the activation wave travels from one end of the myocardial cell to the other end (Fig. 6.2A).

- **Positive deflection:** If a recording electrode is placed in front of the traveling impulse (at position 1, Fig. 6.2B), a positive deflection is recorded.

- **Negative deflection:** If a recording electrode is placed behind the moving impulse (at position 2), a negative deflection is recorded.

- **Moving dipole:** A positive deflection is recorded when the activation wave is advancing toward the recording electrode because the activation wave is traveling with the positive charge in front, which is facing the recording electrode. When the activation wave is moving away from a recording electrode, a negative deflection is recorded because the activation wave has a negative charge behind, which is facing the recording electrode. The activation wave in essence is a moving vector with opposite charges, one positive and the other negative. This moving vector with opposite charges is called a dipole (Fig. 6.2B). During depolarization, the dipole always travels with the positive charge in front and the negative charge behind.

## Repolarization of a Single Muscle Cell

- **Repolarization:** Repolarization restores the polarity of the cell to its original potential of −90 mV and is recorded as a T wave in the ECG. In a single myocardial cell, repolarization starts in the same area where the cell was first depolarized, because this part of the cell has had the most time to recover. The repolarization wave

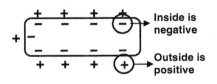

**A. Resting Myocardial Cell**

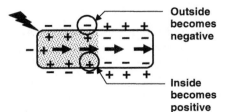

**B. During Depolarization**

**Figure 6.1: Muscle Cell at Rest and During Depolarization. (A)** The resting myocardial cell is negative inside the cell relative to the outside. **(B)** During depolarization, the activation wave travels from one end to the other end, changing the polarity inside the cell from negative to positive. Arrows point to the direction of depolarization.

**Figure 6.2: Depolarization. (A)** The arrows indicate the direction of the activation wave, which is a zone of advancing positive charges. The front of the activation wave is circled. **(B)** The wave of depolarization is represented as a moving dipole with the positive charge traveling in front and the negative charge behind. A recording electrode at position 1 will record a positive deflection because the dipole is traveling with the positive charge facing the electrode. A recording electrode at position 2 will record a negative deflection since the electrode is facing the negative charge of the moving dipole.

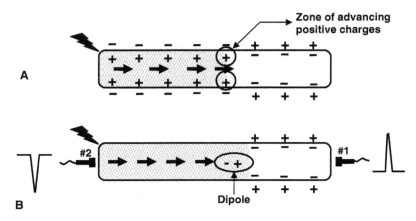

moves in the same direction as the wave of depolarization, only this time, the repolarization wave is a zone of advancing negative charges (Fig. 6.3A). Thus, the dipole is traveling with the negative charge in front and the positive charge behind (Fig. 6.3B).

■ **Inverted T wave:** During repolarization, the recording electrode positioned in front of the repolarization wave (position 1, Fig. 6.3B) will record an inverted T wave. This is because the electrode is facing the negative charge of the advancing dipole.

■ **Upright T wave:** The recording electrode placed behind the repolarization wave (position 2) will record an upright T wave because the electrode is facing the positive charge of the moving dipole.

■ **Depolarization and repolarization of a muscle cell:** Depolarization and repolarization of a single muscle cell travel in the same direction. Thus, the R wave and the T wave are inscribed in opposite directions.

## Depolarization and Repolarization of the Atria

■ **Atrial depolarization and repolarization:** The atrial impulse originates from the sinus node and spreads within the thin atrial wall in a circumferential fashion until both atria are depolarized. Atrial depolarization and repolarization parallels that of a single muscle cell (Fig. 6.4).

■ **Depolarization—P wave:** Depolarization of the atria occurs longitudinally with the impulse spreading from one cell to the next adjacent cell. It is recorded as a P wave in the ECG. Any electrode in front of the advancing wave will record a positive deflection. Any electrode behind the advancing wave will record a negative deflection.

■ **Repolarization—Ta wave:** Repolarization of the atria is also represented by a T wave, but is more

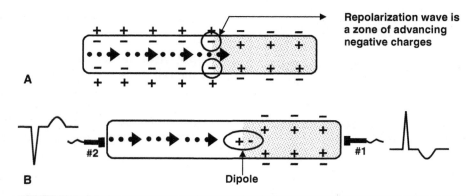

**Figure 6.3: Repolarization of a Single Muscle Cell. (A)** The front of the repolarization wave is circled and is a zone of advancing negative charges. The direction of the repolarization wave is shown by the arrows. **(B)** A recording electrode in front of the repolarization wave at position 1 will record an inverted T wave because the electrode is facing the negative charge of the moving dipole. A recording electrode behind the repolarization wave at position 2 will record a positive or upright T wave because the electrode is facing the positive charge of the moving dipole.

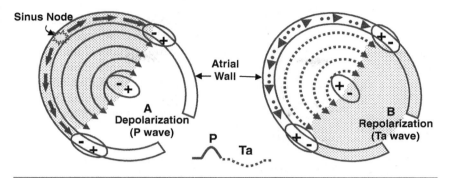

**Figure 6.4:   Atrial Depolarization and Repolarization. (A)** Depolarization of the atria is represented as a P wave in the electrocardiogram. The impulse follows the length of the thin atrial muscle and spreads circumferentially. **(B)** Repolarization is represented as a Ta wave and follows the same direction as depolarization. Thus, the P wave and the Ta wave are inscribed in opposite directions. Arrows represent the direction of the spread of the electrical impulse.

specifically called a Ta wave to differentiate it from the T wave of ventricular repolarization. Repolarization is similar to a single muscle cell and starts from the area that was first depolarized because these cells have had the longest time to recover. Any electrode in front of the repolarization wave will record a negative deflection. The Ta wave is usually not visible because the wave is too small to be recorded. When present, it usually coincides with the QRS complex in the ECG and is therefore obscured.

■ **Depolarization and repolarization of the atria:** Similar to a single muscle cell, depolarization and repolarization of the atria follow the same direction. Thus, the P wave and Ta wave are inscribed in opposite directions.

## Depolarization and Repolarization of the Ventricles

■ **Ventricular depolarization:** The ventricles consist of a thick layer of cells called the myocardium. The myocardium can be divided arbitrarily into three layers—the endocardium, which is the inner layer; the midmyocardium or middle layer; and epicardium or outer layer. Unlike the atria, the ventricles are depolarized by special conduction pathways called the intraventricular conduction system consisting of the bundle of His, bundle branches, and fascicles. The intraventricular conduction system terminates in a network of Purkinje fibers, which are subendocardial in location. Depolarization of both ventricles is synchronous and occurs from endocardium to epicardium because the Purkinje fibers are located subendocardially (Fig. 6.5). When the ventricles are depolarized, a QRS complex is recorded. If a recording electrode is placed on the chest wall

immediately adjacent to the epicardium, an upright deflection (tall R wave) will be recorded.

## Intrinsicoid Deflection

■ **Intrinsic deflection:** If a recording electrode is experimentally placed directly over the epicardium of the left ventricle, an R wave will be recorded because the ventricles are activated from endocardium to epicardium. The abrupt turnaround from the peak of the R wave toward baseline is called the intrinsic deflection. It indicates that the impulse has arrived at the site of the recording electrode.

### Depolarization

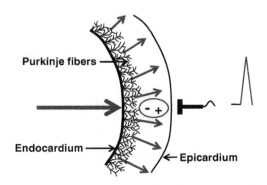

**Figure 6.5:   Depolarization of the Ventricles.** Depolarization of the free wall of the ventricles starts from the endocardium and spreads outward toward the epicardium (*arrows*) because the Purkinje fibers are located subendocardially. A precordial lead such as V₅ will record a positive deflection because the electrode is facing the positive end of the moving dipole.

A

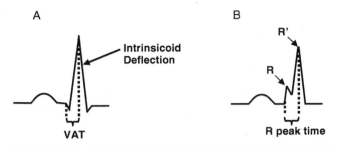

B

**Figure 6.6:   Intrinsicoid Deflection. (A)** The ventricular activation time (VAT) starts from the onset of the QRS complex to the peak of the R wave. The intrinsicoid deflection is the downward deflection that immediately follows the peak of the R wave. **(B)** When there is bundle branch block, the *R peak time* is the preferred terminology to identify the onset of the intrinsicoid deflection and is measured from the onset of the QRS complex to the peak of the R′ wave.

■ **Intrinsicoid deflection:** Clinically, the recording electrode is normally placed on the chest wall and not directly over the epicardium. What is recorded is not the intrinsic deflection, but its equivalent, the intrinsicoid deflection. The time it takes for the impulse to arrive at the recording electrode is the ventricular activation time and is measured from the onset of the QRS complex to the top of the R wave. The abrupt downward deflection of the R wave that immediately follows is the intrinsicoid deflection (Fig. 6.6). When there is right ventricular hypertrophy, the onset of the intrinsicoid deflection is delayed in right-sided precordial leads $V_1$ or $V_2$ (normal, ≤0.03 seconds). When there is left ventricular hypertrophy, the onset of the intrinsicoid deflection is delayed in left sided precordial leads $V_5$ or $V_6$ (normal, ≤0.05 seconds).

■ **R peak time:** When there is intraventricular conduction delay, the working group of the World Health Organization/International Society and Federation for Cardiology prefers to use the term *R peak time* to indicate the onset of the intrinsicoid deflection and is measured from the onset of the QRS complex to the peak of the R or R′ wave.

## The Normal Sequence of Ventricular Activation

■ **The normal QRS complex:** When the conduction system is intact, the sequence of ventricular activation occurs in a predictable fashion that can be broken down into three stages; vector 1 depolarization of the ventricular septum, vector 2 depolarization of the free walls of both ventricles, and vector 3 depolarization of the posterobasal wall of the left ventricle and posterobasal septum.

■ **Vector 1—depolarization of the ventricular septum:** When the sinus impulse finally arrives at the ventricles, the first portion of the ventricle to be activated is the middle third of the left side of the ventricular septum. This is because the left bundle branch is shorter than right bundle branch. The septum is activated from left to right as represented by the arrows in Figure 6.7A. Any electrode located to the right of the ventricular septum (such as $V_1$) will record a positive deflection (small r wave) because the impulse is traveling toward the positive side of the electrode. Any electrode located to the left of the septum (such as precordial leads $V_5$, $V_6$, and limb leads I and aVL) will record a negative deflection (small q wave) because the impulse is traveling away from the positive side of these electrodes. This small

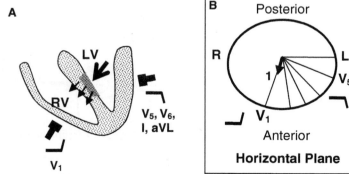

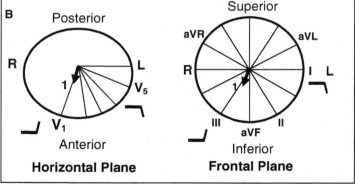

**Figure 6.7:   Vector 1—Initial Activation of the Ventricles. (A)** The earliest portion of the ventricles to be activated is the left side of the ventricular septum (*arrow*) at its mid-portion. The initial electrocardiogram for $V_1$ and for $V_{5-6}$ or leads I and aVL are shown. **(B)** In the horizontal and frontal planes, the direction of the initial vector is represented by the arrows indicated by the number 1. This initial impulse is directed to the right, anteriorly and inferiorly. LV, left ventricle; RV, right ventricle; R, right; L, left.

q wave is often called septal q wave to indicate that the initial vector of the QRS complex is due to septal activation. The total duration of the normal septal q wave should not exceed 0.03 seconds.

■ **Vector 2—depolarization of both ventricles:** Depolarization of the free wall of both ventricles occurs simultaneously, beginning within the endocardium adjacent to the subendocardial Purkinje fibers and spreading outward toward the epicardium. Activation of the remaining ventricular septum occurs on both sides of the septum simultaneously, which cancels each other. Activation of the free wall of both ventricles also occurs in opposite directions, and similarly neutralizes one another. Because the right ventricle is thinner than the left ventricle, a certain portion of the forces generated by the thicker left ventricle will remain unopposed. Additionally, apical depolarization forces are not neutralized because the area opposite the apex is occupied by the non-muscular mitral and tricuspid valves. Taken together, these two forces manifest in a vector 2 that is directed to the left and slightly posteriorly, either inferiorly or superiorly, and corresponds to the mean axis of the QRS complex. A downward deflection (deep S) is recorded in $V_1$ and an upward deflection (tall R) is recorded in $V_5$–$V_6$ (Fig. 6.8).

■ **Vector 3—terminal portion of the QRS complex:** Depolarization of the ventricles occurs in an apex to base direction. Thus, the last portion of the ventricles to become depolarized includes the posterobasal wall of the left ventricle and posterobasal portion of the ventricular septum. These structures are located superiorly in relation to the other structures of the heart. Thus, the late forces are directed superiorly and posteriorly (Fig. 6.9).

■ Vectors one through three are oversimplifications of the complex process of ventricular depolarization and are summarized in Figure 6.10. These vectors differ both spatially and temporally and produce a unique QRS complex that is contingent on the location of the recording electrode.

## Ventricular Repolarization

■ **Repolarization:** Unlike the situation in the single muscle cell or the atria where depolarization and repolarization travel in the same direction, depolarization and repolarization of the ventricular myocardium occur in opposite directions. Thus, depolarization starts from endocardium to epicardium (Fig. 6.11A) and repolarization is reverse, occurring from epicardium to endocardium (Fig. 6.11B). This causes the QRS complex and T wave to be inscribed in the same direction. Thus, precordial electrodes $V_5$ and $V_6$ will record a positive deflection (tall R wave) during depolarization and also a positive deflection during repolarization (upright T wave) because these precordial electrodes are facing the positive end of the moving dipole.

■ Several explanations have been offered as to why the epicardial cells recover earlier than the endocardial cells even if they are the last to be depolarized. More recently, it has been shown that the action potential duration of endocardial cells is longer when compared

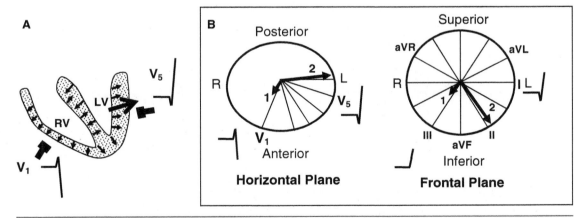

**Figure 6.8:  Vector 2 or Depolarization of the Free Walls of Both Ventricles. (A)** Both ventricles are depolarized from endocardium to epicardium in an outward direction (*small arrows*). The mean direction of vector 2 is represented by the large arrow, which is toward the left, posteriorly and superiorly or inferiorly. **(B)** The mean direction of vector 2 is shown in the horizontal and frontal planes. Vector 2 corresponds to the mean axis of the QRS complex, which is −30° to +90° in the frontal plane. In the above example, the frontal plane vector is close to +60° and is inferior. RV, right ventricle; LV, left ventricle; R, right; L, left.

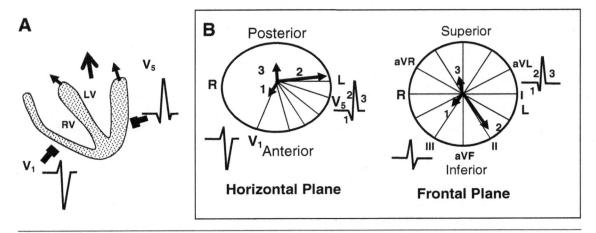

**Figure 6.9: Vector 3—Terminal Portion of the QRS Complex. (A)** The posterobasal portion of the septum and left ventricle are the last segments to be depolarized. The terminal vector is directed superiorly and posteriorly. **(B)** The direction of vector 3 in the horizontal and frontal planes is shown. L, left; R, right; LV, left ventricle; RV, right ventricle.

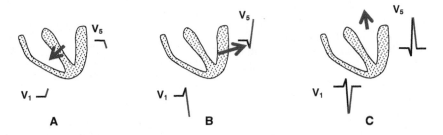

**Figure 6.10: Summary of the Sequence of Ventricular Activation.** The initial vector **(A)** represents depolarization of the left side of the ventricular septum at its mid-portion, which is directed to the right, anteriorly and inferiorly. **(B)** Vector 2 is directed to the left, posteriorly and superiorly or inferiorly corresponding to the mean axis of the QRS complex. **(C)** Vector 3 is directed superiorly and posteriorly.

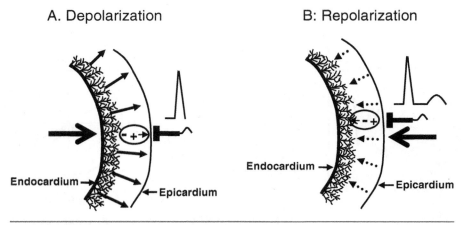

**Figure 6.11: Ventricular Repolarization. (A)** Diagram showing depolarization of the ventricular myocardium, which starts from endocardium to epicardium. This causes the QRS complex to be upright since the depolarization wave is advancing toward the recording electrode. Arrows point to the direction of depolarization. **(B)** Repolarization of the ventricular myocardium is from epicardium to endocardium. Because the repolarization wave is moving away from the recording electrode, the recording electrode is facing the positive side of the moving dipole. Thus, a positive deflection (upright T wave) is recorded. Arrows point to the direction of repolarization.

with epicardial cells. This is most probably the main reason why the epicardial cells recover earlier than endocardial cells causing repolarization to start from epicardium to endocardium.

## Depolarization and Repolarization of the Atria and Ventricles

### Depolarization and Repolarization

- **Single muscle cell:** In a single muscle cell, depolarization and repolarization travel in the same direction. Thus, the R wave and the T wave are normally inscribed in opposite directions. If the QRS complex is upright or positive, then the T wave is normally inverted, and if the QRS is negative or inscribed downward, then the T wave is normally upright.

- **Atria:** The direction of depolarization and repolarization of the atria is similar to that of a single muscle cell. The sinus impulse spreads longitudinally from right atrium to left atrium. Repolarization occurs in the same direction. Thus, if an electrode records an upright P wave, the repolarization or Ta wave is inverted and if the electrode records an inverted P wave, the Ta wave is upright.

- **Ventricles:** Depolarization and repolarization of the ventricles occur in opposite directions. Thus, if the QRS complex is upright or positive, then the T wave is also upright. If the QRS complex is negative, then the T wave is inverted.

### Mechanism

- **Single muscle cell:** In a single muscle cell, depolarization and repolarization occur in the same direction because the area that is first depolarized has had a longer time to recover.

- **Atria:** The atria consist of a thin layer of cells. Unlike the ventricles, the atria do not have a special conducting system. Thus, the impulse is spread from one muscle cell to the next muscle cell longitudinally until both atria are depolarized. Depolarization and repolarization is similar to a single muscle cell and occur in the same direction.

- **Ventricles:** The ventricles consist of a thick layer of muscle cells and are depolarized from endocardium to epicardium because the Purkinje fibers are located subendocardially. Unlike the atria and the single muscle cell where depolarization and repolarization occur in the same direction, depolarization and repolarization of the ventricles occur in opposite directions. The reason as to why the epicardial cells recover earlier than the endocardial cells despite being the last to be depolarized may be due to the following reasons.

- The endocardial cells have longer action potential duration compared with epicardial cells.

- Myocardial perfusion occurs mainly during diastole when the ventricles are relaxed and the pressures within the cavities are lowest. Because repolarization (T wave) occurs during systole when the myocardium is mechanically contracting, there is no significant myocardial perfusion within the subendocardial layer because it is subjected to a much higher tension than the epicardium.

- The endocardium has a higher rate of metabolism as compared with the epicardium and thus requires more oxygen than the epicardium.

- The subendocardial layer is the deepest part of the myocardium. Because the coronary arteries are anatomically epicardial in location, the subendocardial areas are the farthest from the coronary circulation, making the endocardium relatively ischemic as compared with the epicardium.

## Suggested Readings

Burch GE, Winsor T. Principles of electrocardiography. In: *A Primer of Electrocardiography.* 5th ed. Philadelphia: Lea & Febiger; 1966;1–66.

Dunn MI, Lipman BS. Basic physiologic principles. In: *Lipman-Massie Clinical Electrocardiography.* 8th ed. Chicago: Yearbook Medical Publishers; 1989;24–50.

Marriott HJL. Genesis of the precordial pattern. In: *Practical Electrocardiography.* 5th ed. Baltimore: Williams & Wilkins Co.; 1972;44–55.

Sgarbossa EB, Wagner GS. Electrocardiography. In: Topol EJ ed. *Textbook of Cardiovascular Medicine.* 2nd ed. Philadelphia: Lippincott Williams & Wilkins; 2002:1330–1383.

Willems JL, Robles de Medina EO, Bernard R, et al. Criteria for intraventricular conduction disturbances and pre-excitation. *J Am Coll Cardiol.* 1985;1261–1275.

# Chamber Enlargement and Hypertrophy

## The Normal P Wave

- **Normal sinus rhythm:** The sinus node is the origin of the normal impulse. The normal sinus P wave has the following features.
  - **Frontal plane:**
    - □ **Axis:** The axis of the normal P wave is approximately 45° to 60°. Thus, the P wave is upright in lead II. This is the most important lead in recognizing that the rhythm is normal sinus. If the P wave is not upright in lead II, the P wave is probably ectopic (not of sinus node origin).
    - □ **Contour:** The normal P wave is smooth and well rounded and should not be peaked or notched.
    - □ **Amplitude:** The normal P wave is ≤2.5 mm in height.
    - □ **Duration:** The normal P wave is ≤2.5 mm wide or ≤100 milliseconds in duration.
  - **Horizontal plane:**
    - □ Sinus P waves are normally upright in $V_3$ to $V_6$. In $V_1$ and often in $V_2$, the contour of the normal P wave may be upright, inverted or biphasic. Biphasic means that the initial portion of the P wave is upright and the terminal portion is inverted (Fig. 7.1).

The inverted portion should measure <1 mm in duration and <1 mm in depth.

## Right Atrial Enlargement

- **Right atrial enlargement:** The following changes occur when there is right atrial enlargement.
  - **Frontal plane:**
    - □ **Axis:** The axis of the P wave is shifted to the right of +60°. Thus, the P waves are tall in leads II, III, and aVF. The P waves in lead III are usually taller than in lead I ($P_3 > P_1$).
    - □ **Contour:** The contour of the P wave is peaked and pointed. These changes are often described as "P-pulmonale" because right atrial enlargement is frequently caused by pulmonary disease.
    - □ **Amplitude:** The height or amplitude of the P wave increases to >2.5 mm. These P wave changes are best seen in leads II, III, and aVF (Fig. 7.2).
    - □ **Duration:** The total duration of the P wave is not prolonged unless the left atrium is also enlarged. Because the right atrium is activated earlier than

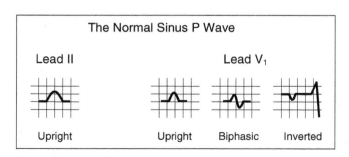

**Figure 7.1: The Normal P Wave.** The sinus P wave is well rounded and smooth and is upright in leads I, II, and aVF measuring ≤2.5 mm in height and ≤2.5 mm in width. In $V_1$, a normal P wave can be upright, biphasic, or inverted

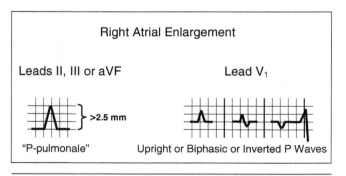

**Figure 7.2: Right Atrial Enlargement.** In right atrial enlargement, the P waves are peaked and tall with an amplitude >2.5 mm in leads II, III, or aVF. Changes in $V_1$ are less obvious, although the upward deflection is often peaked. The duration of the P wave is not widened.

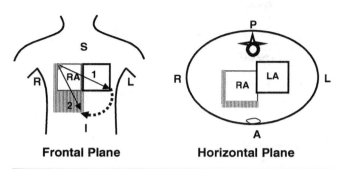

**Figure 7.3:    Right Atrial Enlargement.** In the frontal plane, the right atrium enlarges downward and to the right causing a shift in the P wave axis to the right (*from arrow 1 to arrow 2*). In the horizontal plane, the enlargement of the right atrium is slightly anterior, which may cause slight peaking of the P waves in lead $V_1$. The shaded portion indicates the changes that occur when the right atrium enlarges. S, superior; I, inferior; R, right; L, left; A, anterior; P, posterior; RA, right atrium; LA, left atrium.

the left atrium, any delay in the propagation of the impulse from enlargement of the right atrium will coincide with the activation of the left atrium.

■ **Horizontal plane:** In $V_1$, there may not be any significant P wave changes. The P wave remains normally upright, biphasic, or inverted. The initial upright portion may be slightly peaked or pointed or it might be slightly taller than normal.

■ When there is right atrial enlargement, the right atrium enlarges downward and to the right, thus the axis of the P wave is shifted vertically to the right of $+60°$ (Fig. 7.3). This causes the P wave in lead III to be taller than the P wave in lead I.

## Electrocardiogram of Right Atrial Enlargement

1. The P waves are tall and peaked measuring $>2.5$ mm in leads II, III, or aVF (Fig. 7.4).

2. The duration of the P wave is not increased unless the left atrium is also enlarged.

## Mechanism

■ **Normal sinus P waves:** The sinus node is located at the right upper border of the right atrium near the entrance of the superior vena cava. The sinus impulse has to spread from right atrium to left atrium downward in a right-to-left direction. The initial portion of the P wave represents right atrial activation and the terminal portion, left atrial activation. In the frontal plane, the normal P wave axis is approximately $+45°$ to $+60°$ and is upright in leads I, II, and aVF. The tallest P wave is usually recorded in lead II and the amplitude of the normal P wave is $\leq 2.5$ blocks. In $V_1$, the normal sinus P wave can be upright, biphasic, or inverted. The normal cutoff for the total duration varies among different authors. The World Health Organization/International Society and Federation of Cardiology Task Force define the normal duration as $\leq 110$ milliseconds, which is not easy to measure in the electrocardiogram (ECG). A width of $\leq 2.5$ small blocks ($\leq 100$ milliseconds) will be used as the normal P wave duration in this text.

■ **Right atrial enlargement:** The right atrium enlarges downward and to the right causing the direction of the sinus impulse to slightly shift to the right of $+60°$. This causes the P waves to be taller and more peaked in leads II, III, and aVF. Thus the P wave in lead III is usually taller than the P wave in lead I ($P_3 > P_1$). In $V_1$ and $V_2$, the initial portion of the P wave may increase in amplitude, although the terminal

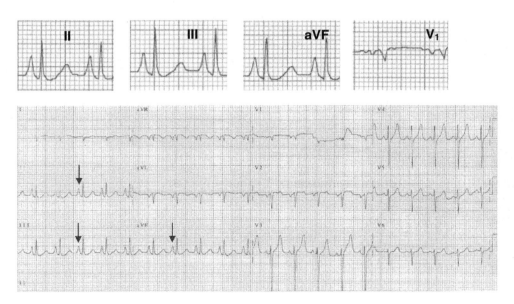

**Figure 7.4:    Right Atrial Enlargement.** Twelve-lead electrocardiogram showing right atrial enlargement. Tall and peaked P waves, also called "P-pulmonale," are seen in leads II, III, and aVF (*arrows*). Note that the P waves are taller in lead III than in lead I. Leads II, III, aVF, and $V_1$ are magnified to show the abnormal P wave contour. The patient has chronic obstructive pulmonary disease.

portion representing left atrial activation is not affected. Because the right atrium is activated earlier than the left atrium, any delay in activation of the atria due to enlargement of the right atrium will coincide with activation of the left atrium. Thus, the duration of the P wave is not prolonged.

## Clinical Implications

■ Enlargement of the right or left atrium occurring independently is rare. It is usually associated with disease of the valvular structures or the ventricles. The most common cause of right atrial enlargement without left atrial enlargement in the adult population is pulmonary disease. Thus, the tall, narrow, and peaked P wave of right atrial enlargement is often described as "P-pulmonale." Right atrial enlargement can be due to tricuspid or pulmonary valve disease, pulmonary hypertension, acute pulmonary embolism, and right ventricular failure or hypertrophy from varied causes.

■ Enlargement of either atria predisposes to atrial arrhythmias, especially atrial flutter or atrial fibrillation. It is uncommon for atrial flutter or fibrillation to become sustained and self-perpetuating unless the atria are enlarged or diseased.

■ When the lungs are hyperinflated because of emphysema, the diaphragm is pushed downward. The right atrium may also be displaced downward. When this occurs, the P wave in $V_1$ may become totally inverted because the diaphragm and the heart are pushed vertically downward while the standard location of the $V_1$ electrode remains unchanged at the 4th intercostal space to the right of the sternum. The inverted P wave may be mistaken for an enlarged left atrium.

■ Right atrial enlargement is due to volume or pressure overload within the right atria. This causes the right atrial size to increase. Right atrial enlargement is recognized at bedside by the presence of distended neck veins. When the patient is semirecumbent at an angle of 45°, and the neck veins are distended above the clavicle, the pressure in the right atrium is elevated.

## Treatment and Prognosis

■ The treatment and prognosis of right atrial enlargement will depend on the etiology of the right atrial enlargement.

## Left Atrial Enlargement

■ **Left atrial enlargement:** The ECG changes of left atrial enlargement are best reflected in the terminal half of the P wave because the right atrium is activated earlier than the left atrium. The ECG features of left atrial enlargement are summarized in Figure 7.5.

■ **Frontal plane:**

□ **Axis:** The axis of the P wave is shifted to the left, thus the P waves are taller in lead I than in lead III ($P_1 > P_3$).

□ **Contour:** The contour of the P wave is bifid or "M" shaped. The first hump represents activation of the right atrium and the second hump represents activation of the left atrium. These two humps are separated by at least one small block and are best seen in leads I, II, aVF, $V_5$, and $V_6$. This type of P wave is often called "P-mitrale," indicating that at some time in the past, mitral

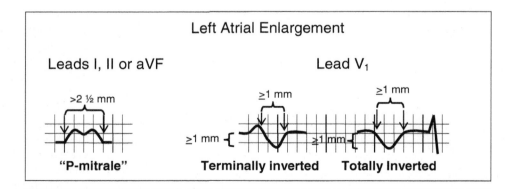

**Figure 7.5: Left Atrial Enlargement.** The duration of the P wave is prolonged measuring >2.5 mm in leads I, II, or aVF, with a bifid or M-shaped configuration. This type of P wave is called "P-mitrale." In lead $V_1$, the P wave may be totally inverted or it may be biphasic. The inverted portion is broad and deep measuring ≥1 mm wide and ≥1 mm deep.

stenosis is the most common cause of left atrial enlargement.

□ **Amplitude:** The height or amplitude of the P wave is not significantly increased.

□ **Duration:** The duration or width of the P wave is increased and should measure >2.5 mm (>100 milliseconds).

■ **Horizontal plane:**

□ In lead $V_1$, the P wave is biphasic or inverted. The inverted portion measures ≥1 mm in depth and ≥1 mm (0.04 seconds) in duration.

The left atrium enlarges to the left and posteriorly shifting the P wave axis to the left of +45°. The P wave abnormalities are best seen in leads I, II, aVF and $V_1$ (Figs. 7.6 and 7.7).

## Bi-Atrial Enlargement

■ **Bi-atrial enlargement:** When both atria are enlarged, the criteria for right atrial and left atrial enlargement are both present because the atria are activated separately (Fig. 7.8).

■ **Frontal plane:** In the frontal plane, the P waves are tall measuring >2.5 mm because of right atrial

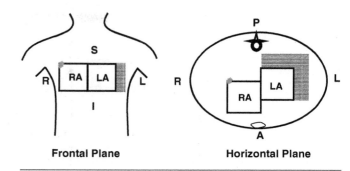

**Frontal Plane**          **Horizontal Plane**

**Figure 7.6:   Left Atrial Enlargement.** The left atrium enlarges to the left and posteriorly. Because activation of the atria is sequential, starting from right atrium to left atrium, the duration of the P wave is prolonged. The P waves are not only wide but are notched in leads I, II, and aVF. The terminal portion is inverted in lead $V_1$. S, superior; I, inferior; R, right; L, left; A, anterior; P, posterior; RA, right atrium; LA, left atrium.

enlargement. At the same time, the P waves are broad, notched, or M-shaped measuring >2.5 mm wide from left atrial enlargement. These changes are best seen in leads I, II, and aVF (Fig. 7.9).

■ **Horizontal plane:** In the horizontal plane, the P wave in $V_1$ is biphasic or inverted. The initial positive portion is usually peaked due to right atrial enlargement

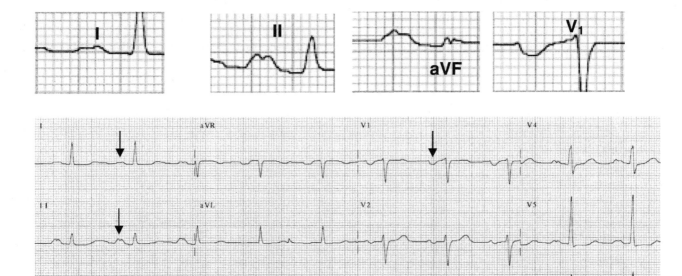

**Figure 7.7:   Left Atrial Enlargement.** The P waves are wide in leads I, II, III, and aVF as well as several other leads. The configuration of the P wave is M-shaped (P-mitrale). The P wave is negative in $V_1$. The negative deflection measures at least 1 × 1 (1 mm wide and 1 mm deep).

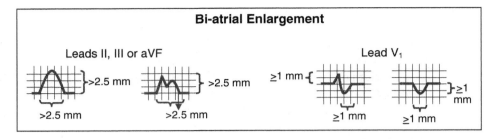

**Bi-atrial Enlargement**

**Figure 7.8:    Bi-atrial Enlargement.** Bi-atrial enlargement is characterized by tall and broad P waves measuring >2.5 mm in height and >2.5 mm in duration. In V$_1$, the P wave is biphasic or inverted. The initial portion may be peaked due to right atrial enlargement. The inverted portion is broad and deep measuring ≥1 mm wide and ≥1 mm deep because of left atrial enlargement.

and the terminal negative portion is ≥1 mm wide and ≥1 mm deep from left atrial enlargement.

## Intra-Atrial Block

- **Intra-atrial block:** According to an ad hoc working group organized by the World Health Organization and International Society and Federation in Cardiology, the P wave duration should not exceed 0.11 seconds in the adult. The normal cutoff for the P wave duration, however, varies among authors. Increased duration of the P wave implies that there is intra-atrial block that may be due to left atrial en-

largement but can also be caused by scarring or fibrosis of the atria.

- **Left atrial enlargement:** In left atrial enlargement, the P wave duration is always prolonged because of intra-atrial block or prolonged atrial conduction. Increased left atrial pressure or volume is not always present. Thus, left atrial abnormality may be a better terminology to describe the P wave changes associated with left atrial enlargement.

- A 12-lead ECG is shown in Figure 7.10. The P waves are notched with an M-shape configuration in lead II. The P wave measures >2.5 mm wide with both peaks separated by one small block. The configuration of the P wave is consistent with "P-mitrale." The P wave in V$_1$ is not deep or wide. Although there is intra-atrial block, not all the P wave changes satisfy the criteria for left atrial enlargement.

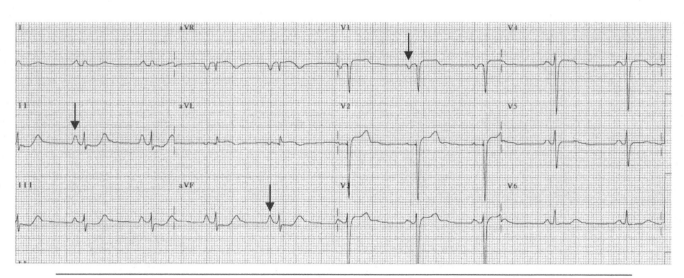

**Figure 7.9:    Electrocardiogram of Bi-atrial Enlargement.** The P waves are peaked and wide. In leads II and aVF, the P waves are >2.5 mm tall and >2.5 mm wide (>100 milliseconds in duration). In V$_1$, the P waves are terminally negative and are 1 mm wide and 1 mm deep.

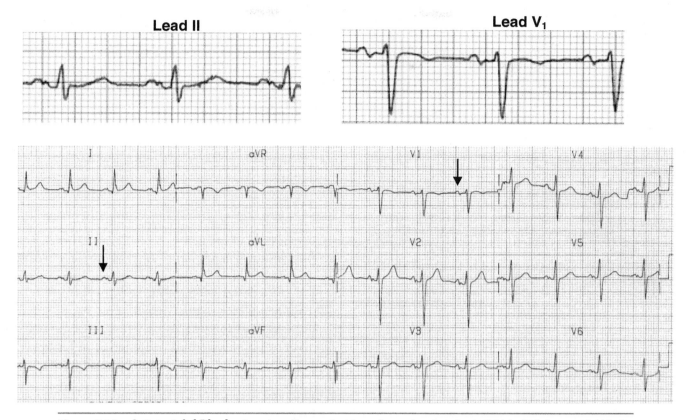

**Figure 7.10:    Intra-atrial Block.**  Any sinus P wave that is prolonged, measuring >2.5 blocks is intra-atrial block. This could be due to left atrial enlargement, but could also be due to other causes. Leads II and V₁ are enlarged so that the P waves are better visualized.

## ■ Left Atrial Enlargement

### ECG of Left Atrial Enlargement

1. The duration of the P wave is increased in leads I, II, or aVF. The P waves are often notched with M shape pattern measuring >2.5 mm in width or >100 milliseconds in duration.
2. Terminally inverted P waves in $V_1$ measuring ≥1 mm in depth and ≥1 mm in duration.

### Mechanism

■ When there is left atrial enlargement, the initial portion of the P wave representing right atrial activation is not altered. The terminal portion representing left atrial activation becomes longer, resulting in a broader P wave. Thus, the total duration of the P wave is prolonged. The general direction of the P wave is slightly altered becoming more horizontal at 20° to 40°. Thus, the P wave in lead I is taller than the P wave in lead III ($P_1$ > $P_3$). The P wave abnormalities are best seen in lead II and often in leads I and aVF and precordial leads $V_5$ and $V_6$. The P wave is frequently bifid with two separate humps, at least 0.04 seconds apart. The first hump represents right atrial activation and the second hump represents activation of the enlarged left atrium. Because mitral valve disease is a common cause of left atrial enlargement, the notched and M-shaped P wave of left atrial enlargement is described as "P-mitrale."

■ Because the left atrium is oriented to the left and posterior to that of the right atrium, an enlarged left atrium will cause the terminal forces of the P wave to be directed to the left and posteriorly. In $V_1$, the terminal portion, which represents left atrial activation, will be oriented more posteriorly than normal, causing the P wave to be broad and deep measuring at least 1 mm wide and 1 mm deep equivalent to one small box.

### Clinical Significance

■ Primary disease involving the left atrium alone is rare. Enlargement of the left atrium, therefore, is secondary to abnormalities involving the mitral valve or the left ventricle including mitral stenosis or insufficiency, left ventricular systolic, or diastolic dysfunction from several causes such as hypertension, coronary artery disease, cardiomyopathy, and aortic valve disease.

■ Left atrial enlargement is a common finding in patients with left ventricular hypertrophy (LVH). The presence of left atrial enlargement is one of the criteria for the ECG diagnosis of LVH.

■ Because the atria are activated circumferentially, and the electrical impulse travels through the length of the atrial wall, "enlargement" is preferred over "hypertrophy" when describing the presence of atrial enlargement. The P wave changes in the ECG do not reflect thickening or hypertrophy of the atrial wall, but rather, increase in the dimension of the atrial cavity or prolonged conduction in the atria from intra-atrial block. Additionally, when pulmonary hypertension occurs from pulmonary embolism or heart failure, the P wave changes can occur acutely. It can also regress acutely when the pulmonary pressure resolves, which is unlikely if the changes are due to atrial hypertrophy. This is in contrast to the ventricles, where electrical activation is from endocardium to epicardium. The changes in the QRS complex represent increased left ventricular mass or thickness. Thus, either "enlargement" or "hypertrophy" is appropriate in describing the increased ventricular mass, whereas atrial enlargement or atrial abnormality is more appropriate in describing the changes in the atria.

## Treatment and Prognosis

■ Left atrial enlargement is most often associated with abnormalities of either the mitral valve or left ventricle. The treatment and prognosis will depend on the underlying cause of the left atrial enlargement.

## Left Ventricular Hypertrophy

■ **LVH:** The sensitivity of the ECG in detecting LVH is limited; thus, several criteria have been proposed. Most of these ECG abnormalities are based on increased voltage of the QRS complex from increased mass of the

left ventricle when there is LVH. These changes include the following (see Figs. 7.11 and 7.12).

■ **Abnormalities in the QRS complex**
  □ Deep S waves in $V_1$ or $V_2$ measuring >30 mm
  □ Tall R waves in $V_5$ or $V_6$ measuring >30 mm
  □ S in $V_1$ + R in $V_5$ or $V_6$ >35 mm
  □ Tall R waves in aVL measuring >11 mm
  □ Tall R or deep S in any limb lead >20 mm
  □ R in aVL + S in $V_3$ >28 mm (men) and >20 mm (women)
  □ The total amplitude of the QRS complex exceeds 175 mm in all 12 leads
  □ Onset of intrinsicoid deflection >0.05 seconds in $V_5$ or $V_6$
  □ Increased duration of the QRS complex >0.09 seconds
  □ Left axis deviation $\geq-30°$

■ **Abnormalities in the P wave**
  □ Left atrial abnormality

■ **Abnormalities in the ST segment and T wave**
  □ ST depression and T inversion in leads with tall R waves (left ventricular strain)

■ **Increased voltage of the QRS complex:** The voltage of the QRS complex is increased when there is LVH. Unfortunately, the amplitude of the QRS complex may not be a reliable marker of LVH because it can be altered by several factors other than increased thickness of the left ventricular wall.

■ **LVH without increased voltage:** Patients with LVH may not exhibit any increase in QRS voltage because of obesity, peripheral edema, anasarca,

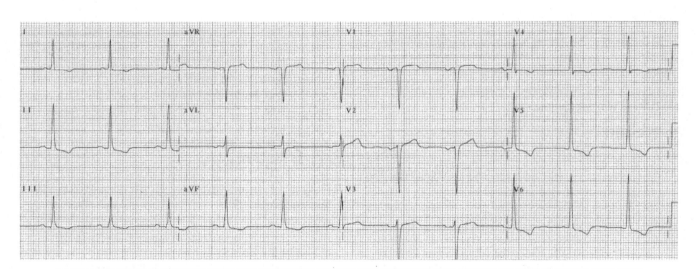

**Figure 7.11: Left Ventricular Hypertrophy.** Twelve-lead electrocardiogram showing left ventricular hypertrophy. The P wave in $V_1$ is 1 mm wide and 1 mm deep because of left atrial enlargement. The voltage of the QRS complex is increased with deep S waves in $V_1$ and tall R waves in $V_5$ and $V_6$. ST depression with T wave inversion is present in leads with tall R waves (LV strain).

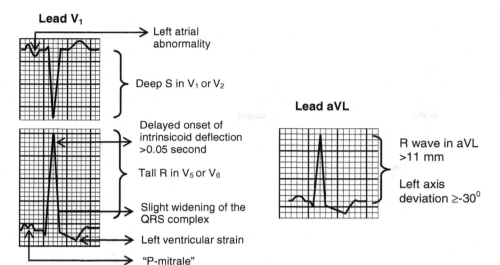

**Figure 7.12:** **Left Ventricular Hypertrophy.** Diagrammatic representation of the different electrocardiogram changes in left ventricular hypertrophy.

increased diameter of the chest, lung disease especially emphysema, large breasts, biventricular hypertrophy, amyloidosis, pericardial effusion, pleural effusion, and hypothyroidism.

- **Increased voltage not resulting from LVH:** Conversely, increased voltage of the QRS complex may be present even in the absence of LVH in adolescent boys, anemia, left mastectomy, and in thin individuals.

■ **Left atrial abnormality:** Enlargement of the left atrium is included as one of the diagnostic hallmarks of LVH. During diastole when the mitral valve is open, the left atrium and left ventricle behave as a common chamber. Thus, changes in pressure and volume in the left ventricle are also reflected in the left atrium.

■ **Ventricular activation time:** Ventricular activation time represents the time it takes for the ventricular impulse to arrive at the recording electrode and is measured from the onset of the QRS complex to the top of the R or R' wave (Fig. 7.13A, B). The thicker the myocardium, the longer it takes for the impulse to travel from endocardium to epicardium. Thus, when there is LVH, the ventricular activation time of leads overlying the left ventricle ($V_5$ or $V_6$) is prolonged (>0.05 seconds).

■ **Intrinsicoid deflection:** The intrinsicoid deflection corresponds to the time that the depolarization wave has arrived at the recording electrode and is represented by the sudden downward deflection of the R wave toward baseline. If there is LVH, the onset of the

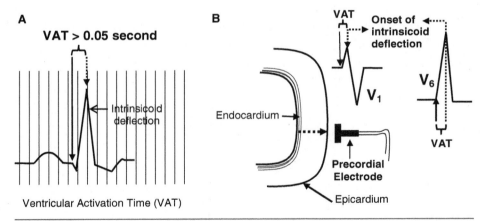

**Figure 7.13:** **Intrinsicoid Deflection.** The ventricular activation time (VAT) is measured from the onset of the QRS complex to the top of the R wave. The intrinsicoid deflection is represented by the immediate downward deflection of the R wave toward baseline (**A**). When there is left ventricular hypertrophy, the onset of the intrinsicoid deflection (dotted lines in **A** and **B**) is delayed in $V_5$ or $V_6$. When there is right ventricular hypertrophy, the onset of the intrinsicoid deflection is delayed in $V_1$ or $V_2$.

intrinsicoid deflection in leads $V_5$ or $V_6$ is delayed (Fig. 7.13B).

- **Abnormalities in the ST segment and T wave:** Because depolarization of the left ventricle is abnormal, repolarization is also abnormal resulting in ST segment depression and T wave inversion in leads with tall R waves. Left ventricular strain is frequently used to describe this pattern of ST depression and T wave inversion (Fig. 7.12).

- LVH is a compensatory mechanism in response to both pressure and volume overload.
    - **Pressure overload:** LVH from pressure overload is usually due to systemic hypertension, aortic stenosis, coarctation of the aorta, or hypertrophic obstructive cardiomyopathy. When there is pressure or systolic overload, the left ventricle becomes concentrically hypertrophied. The walls of the left ventricle are thickened although the size of the left ventricular cavity remains normal. The ECG shows tall R waves in $V_5$ and $V_6$ associated with depression of the ST segment and inversion of the T wave. These ST-T changes are often described as due to left ventricular "strain" (Figs. 7.11 and 7.12).
    - **Volume overload:** This type of LVH is due to increased volume of the left ventricle as would occur when there is mitral regurgitation, aortic regurgitation, ventricular septal defect, peripheral arteriovenous shunts, anemia, and thyrotoxicosis. When there is volume or diastolic overload, the left ventricle becomes eccentrically hypertrophied. The left ventricular cavity becomes dilated. There is also increased left ventricular mass. The ECG shows prominent Q waves, tall R waves, and tall and upright T waves in $V_5$ and $V_6$ (Fig. 7.14).

- LVH associated with left ventricular strain is more common than LVH from volume overload because hypertension is the most common cause of LVH.

## The ECG of LVH

- Several ECG criteria have been used in the diagnosis of LVH. These include:
    - **Increased amplitude or voltage of the QRS complex**
        - Limb leads
            - R wave in any limb lead measuring $\geq 20$ mm
            - S wave in any limb lead measuring $\geq 20$ mm
            - R wave in aVL $> 11$ mm
            - R in lead I + S in III $> 25$ mm
        - Precordial leads
            - S wave in $V_1$ or $V_2$ $\geq 30$ mm
            - R wave in $V_5$ or $V_6$ $\geq 30$ mm
            - R wave in $V_5$ or $V_6$ $> 26$ mm
            - S wave in $V_1$, $V_2$ or $V_3$ $\geq 25$ mm
            - R wave in $V_4$, $V_5$ or $V_6$ $\geq 25$ mm
            - $SV_1$ + $RV_5$ or $V_6$ $> 35$ mm
            - Tallest S + tallest R in $V_1$ to $V_6$ $> 45$ mm
            - R wave in $V_6$ > R wave in $V_5$
        - Limb + Precordial leads
            - R wave in aVL + S wave in $V_3$ $> 20$ mm in females
            - R wave in aVL + S wave in $V_3$ $> 28$ mm in males
            - Total QRS voltage from all 12 ECG leads $> 175$ mm
    - **Increased duration of the QRS complex**
        - Delayed onset of intrinsicoid deflection $\geq 0.05$ seconds in $V_5$ or $V_6$
        - Increased duration of the QRS complex $\geq 0.09$ seconds

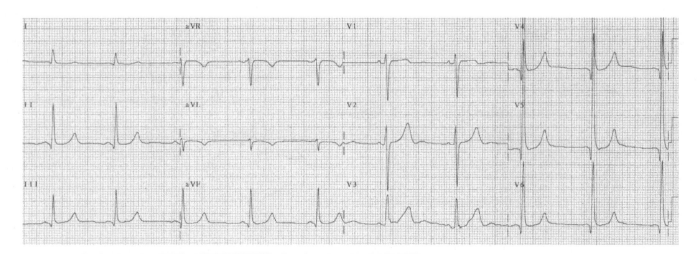

**Figure 7.14: Left Ventricular Hypertrophy from Volume Overload.** Twelve-lead electrocardiogram (ECG) showing tall voltage measuring >45 mm in $V_5$ and >25 mm in $V_6$ combined with prominent Q waves and tall T waves. This pattern of LVH is usually due to volume overload. This ECG is from a 55-year-old man with sickle cell anemia with gross cardiomegaly by chest x-ray.

- **Left atrial abnormality**
  - ☐ Terminal negativity of the P wave in $V_1$ measuring 1 mm × 1 mm
- **Left axis deviation**
  - ☐ ≥−30°
  - ☐ ≥−15°
- **ST-T abnormalities indicating left ventricular strain in $V_5$ or $V_6$**
  - ☐ ST segment depression
  - ☐ T wave inversion

The following are the criteria that are frequently used in the diagnosis of LVH.

- **Sokolow-Lyon Index:** This is the most commonly used criteria for the diagnosis of LVH.
  - R in $V_5$ or $V_6$ + S in $V_1$ = >35 mm
  - R in aVL >11 mm
- **Romhilt and Estes:**
  - 3 points each
    - ☐ P wave from left atrial abnormality
    - ☐ Any increase in voltage of the QRS complex
      - ☐ R or S in limb lead = ≥20 mm
      - ☐ S in $V_1$ or $V_2$ = ≥30 mm
      - ☐ R in $V_5$ or $V_6$ = ≥30 mm
    - ☐ ST-T abnormalities
      - ☐ Any shift in the ST segment (without digitalis) = 3
  - 2 points
    - ☐ Left axis deviation of ≥−30°
  - 1 point each
    - ☐ Slight widening of the QRS complex of ≥0.09 seconds
    - ☐ Intrinsicoid deflection in $V_5$ or $V_6$ of ≥0.05 seconds
    - ☐ ST-T abnormalities with digitalis

**Score of ≥5 points = LVH; score of 4 points = probable LVH**

- **Cornell voltage criteria:**
  - R in aVL + S in $V_3$ = >28 mm in men and >20 mm in women.
- **Cornell product:**
  - Cornell voltage multiplied by the QRS duration in milliseconds = >2,440 milliseconds. (In women, 6 mm is added to Cornell voltage.)
- **Total QRS voltage:**
  - Total QRS voltage or total amplitude of the QRS complex obtained from all 12 leads. The normal voltage averages 129 mm (range, 80 to 185 mm) with 175 mm as the upper limits of normal.

## Mechanism

- **Increased voltage of the QRS complex:** Increased voltage of the QRS complex is frequently used as one of the criteria for LVH. When the ventricles are activated, the free walls of both ventricles (vector 2) are activated simultaneously from

endocardium to epicardium. These forces occur in opposite directions and cancel out. Because the left ventricle is normally thicker than the right ventricle, the left ventricle continues to undergo electrical activation even after activation of the right ventricle is completed. Therefore, activation of the left ventricle continues unopposed. This vector corresponds to the main axis of the QRS complex and is oriented to the left and posteriorly. Tall R waves are normally recorded in leads $V_{5-6}$ and deep S waves are recorded in lead $V_1$ and often in $V_2$. When there is left ventricular hypertrophy, these findings become exaggerated. The R waves become taller in left sided leads $V_5$, $V_6$, and aVL. Right-sided chest leads such as $V_1$ and $V_2$, will record deep S waves. When there is respiratory variation, the largest deflection is selected to represent the magnitude of the QRS complex.

- **Pressure overload:** LVH from increased systolic pressure can occur when there is aortic or subaortic obstruction or when there is systemic hypertension. This type of LVH is often called pressure overload or systolic overload and is usually characterized by the presence of a thick left ventricle with normal cavity dimension. R waves are tall in the left sided chest leads $V_5$ or $V_6$ and deep S waves are present in right-sided chest leads $V_1$ or $V_2$. The ST segments are depressed and T waves are inverted in leads with tall R waves. These ST-T abnormalities are frequently described as left ventricular strain. This type of LVH is associated with a high systolic pressure.

- **Volume overload:** LVH can also be due to volume overload such as valvular regurgitation, ventricular septal defect, patent ductus arteriosus, and other extracardiac left-to-right shunts. This type of LVH is often called volume overload or diastolic overload and is usually characterized by the presence of a dilated left ventricular cavity. Prominent Q waves are present in leads with tall R waves such as $V_5$ and $V_6$ accompanied by tall rather then inverted T waves.

- **Left atrial abnormality:** LVH is frequently associated with enlargement of the left atrium. When there is LVH, there is increased left ventricular end diastolic pressure or volume. This will also increase left atrial pressure or volume because the left atrium and left ventricle behave as common chamber when the mitral valve is open during diastole.

- **Prolonged ventricular activation time:** The ventricular activation time represents the time it takes for the impulse to activate the myocardium below the recording electrode. The thicker the myocardium, the longer it takes for the electrical impulse to travel from endocardium to epicardium. This is measured from the onset of the QRS complex to the top of the R wave. Thus, the electrodes overlying the left ventricle, such as leads $V_5$ or $V_6$, will record a longer ventricular activation time of >0.05 seconds when there is LVH.

- **Delayed onset of the intrinsicoid deflection:** The intrinsicoid deflection represents that moment in time that the impulse has reached the epicardium and is represented as a downward deflection of the R wave toward baseline. The onset of the intrinsicoid deflection signals that the whole myocardium below the recording electrode has been fully activated. Because the ventricular activation time is prolonged when there is LVH, the onset of the intrinsicoid deflection in $V_5$ or $V_6$ is also delayed.

■ **Increased duration of the QRS complex:** When there is LVH, left ventricular mass is increased; thus, activation of the left ventricle will take longer. When LVH is present, the duration of the QRS complex is increased. The QRS is widened not only because of the increased muscle mass or increased ventricular activation time but intraventricular conduction delay may be present.

■ **Left axis deviation ≥−30°:** Left axis deviation may occur when there is LVH because of increased muscle mass resulting in a more horizontal axis of the QRS complex. Additionally, LVH is frequently associated with left anterior fascicular block or incomplete left bundle branch block, which can shift the QRS axis more markedly to the left.

■ **ST and T wave abnormalities:** The ST segment and T wave represent ventricular repolarization corresponding to phases 2 and 3 of the transmembrane action potential, respectively. Normally, when the ventricles are activated, repolarization begins immediately. During phase 2, corresponding to the ST segment, the electrical potential is normally maintained at almost 0 potential for a sustained duration; thus, there is no deflection recorded in the ECG. The T wave is inscribed only when sufficient potential is generated during repolarization corresponding to the down slope or phase 3 of the transmembrane action potential.

■ **ST depression:** When there is LVH, ventricular activation is prolonged. Repolarization begins in some areas of the ventricle even before the whole myocardium is completely depolarized. This allows repolarization to occur relatively earlier than usual, which can reach sufficient magnitude to cause downward deviation of the ST segment in leads with tall R waves.

■ **T wave inversion:** The T wave in LVH is inverted and is opposite in direction to that of the QRS complex. This implies that depolarization and repolarization of the myocardium occur in the same direction, which is the opposite of normal. The prolonged activation time of the thickened left ventricle allows the endocardium to recover earlier even before the whole thickness of the myocardium is completely depolarized. Thus, repolarization proceeds from endocardium to epicardium, resulting in depression of the ST segment and inversion of the T waves in leads with tall R waves. Additionally, when the left ventricle is thickened, the myocardium may outstrip its normal blood supply even in the absence of occlusive coronary disease. Thus, the whole thickness of the left ventricle becomes relatively ischemic. The endocardium, which is the first to be depolarized, will recover earlier because it had a longer time to recover.

## Clinical Significance

■ Although LVH is a physiologic response to pressure or volume overload, it is a marker of increased cardiovascular morbidity and is a known risk factor for sudden cardiovascular death. The presence of LVH may be a predictor of LV dysfunction within 5 years after its detection.

■ Hypertension is the most common cause of LVH. In hypertensive patients, LVH occurs as a compensatory adaptation from pressure overload. LVH due to hypertension can regress with antihypertensive medications. All antihypertensive medications are generally effective in regressing LVH except hydralazine and minoxidil. There is clinical evidence to show that regression of LVH in patients with hypertension reduces cardiovascular events. A baseline ECG therefore is standard examination in patients initially diagnosed with hypertension.

■ The several ECG criteria proposed for the diagnosis of LVH suggest that none of these criteria is optimal. The sensitivity of the ECG in diagnosing LVH is relatively poor and is <50%. However, when LVH is diagnosed by ECG, the specificity is high and is approximately ≥90%. The diagnosis of LVH in the ECG is primarily dependent on the presence of increased voltage. Unfortunately, voltage can be affected by many conditions other than LVH. The echocardiogram is more sensitive and more specific than the ECG for the detection of LVH, but is less readily available and much more expensive. The ECG remains the procedure of choice and is the most important modality in detecting LVH in patients with hypertension.

■ When there is LVH, physical examination will show the following findings:

■ **Normal apical impulse:** The apex of the heart is normally occupied by the left ventricle. The apex impulse, which is the lowest and most lateral cardiac impulse in the precordium, is due to left ventricular contraction and normally occupies <2 cm (the size of a quarter) and confined to only one intercostal space. In some patients, the apex impulse may not be palpable.

■ **Concentric LVH:** When the left ventricle is concentrically hypertrophied, the left ventricular cavity is not enlarged and the apex impulse is not displaced. The area occupied by the apex impulse, however, becomes wider measuring about 2 to 3 cm or more in diameter, thus occupying an area that may involve two intercostal spaces. Furthermore, the apex impulse becomes more sustained and longer in duration compared with the short precordial tap that is normally expected when the left ventricle is not hypertrophied. A prominent 4th heart sound is usually audible if the patient is in normal sinus rhythm, which may be palpable as a prominent outward pulsation at the apex before systole. This is better appreciated when the patient is lying in lateral decubitus position.

■ **Eccentric LVH:** When there is eccentric LVH, the left ventricular cavity is dilated. The apex impulse is displaced laterally and downward and may reach the 6th or 7th intercostal space at the left anterior axillary line. The precordial impulse becomes more diffuse involving a wider area in the precordium.

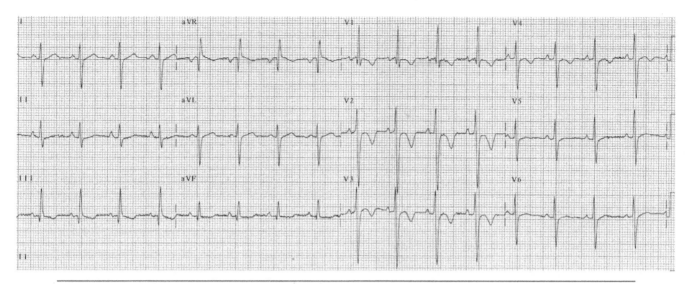

**Figure 7.15:  Right Ventricular Hypertrophy.** There is right axis deviation, the QRS complexes are tall in $V_1$ and P waves are peaked in II and aVF. This pattern of right ventricular hypertrophy is described as type A and is frequently seen in severe right ventricular hypertrophy often associated with congenital heart disease or severe mitral stenosis.

## Treatment and Prognosis

- LVH detected by ECG is a risk factor for increased cardiovascular death. When ECG changes of LVH occur, the risk for cardiovascular morbidity and mortality increases, and the risk is even higher when ST and T wave abnormalities are also present. The treatment and prognosis of patients with LVH will depend on the etiology of the LVH. In patients with hypertension, regression of LVH with antihypertensive agents is possible. There are clinical data to show that regression of LVH in patients with hypertension decreases mortality and morbidity from cardiovascular death.

## Right Ventricular Hypertrophy

- **Right ventricular hypertrophy:** Right ventricular hypertrophy (RVH) is recognized in the ECG by the following findings (Fig. 7.15).
  - **Abnormalities in the QRS complex**
    - □ Right axis deviation of approximately ≥90°. This should always be present before the diagnosis of RVH is considered.
    - □ qR complex in $V_1$
    - □ R wave measuring ≥7 mm in $V_1$
    - □ R wave taller than the S wave in $V_1$ (R/S ratio ≥1)
    - □ Delayed onset of the intrinsicoid deflection in $V_1$ >0.03 seconds
    - □ rS complex from $V_1$ to $V_6$ with right axis deviation
    - □ $S_1 S_2 S_3$ pattern in adults
  - **Abnormalities in the P wave**
    - □ Right atrial abnormality (P-pulmonale)

- **Abnormalities in the ST segment and T wave**
  - □ ST segment depression and T wave inversion in anterior precordial leads ($V_1$ and $V_2$)
- In adult patients, the thickness of the right ventricle seldom exceeds that of the left ventricle even when RVH is present. Because both ventricles are activated simultaneously, the forces generated by the right ventricle are masked by the forces generated by the left ventricle. Thus, the diagnosis of RVH by ECG may be difficult unless the right ventricle is severely hypertrophied.
- **Types of RVH:** The ECG manifestations of RVH may be different. Three different types have been described: types A, B, and C (Fig. 7.16).

### Other Patterns of RVH

- **Chronic pulmonary disease:** When there is chronic obstructive pulmonary disease such as emphysema or chronic bronchitis, the overinflated lungs push the diaphragm downward, causing the heart to become vertically oriented. When this occurs, the axes of the P wave, QRS complex, and T wave are all shifted rightward and inferiorly toward lead aVF (90°), resulting in the so called "lead I sign." Because lead I (0°) is perpendicular to lead aVF, lead I and often $V_6$ will conspicuously show small deflections (Fig. 7.17) because the P, QRS, and T waves become isoelectric in these leads. The ventricles also rotate in a clockwise fashion, causing poor R wave progression and delay in the transition zone. Other signs of type C RVH like right axis deviation and P-pulmonale are usually present.
- **$S_1 S_2 S_3$ pattern:** $S_1 S_2 S_3$ pattern implies that S waves are present in leads I, II, and III. When the $S_1 S_2 S_3$ pattern is present, the direction of the mean QRS axis is superior

**Figure 7.16:    Right Ventricular Hypertrophy.** Three types of right ventricular hypertrophy (RVH) are shown. **(A)** Type A RVH. **(B)** Type B RVH. **(C)** An example of type C RVH.

A. Type A RVH

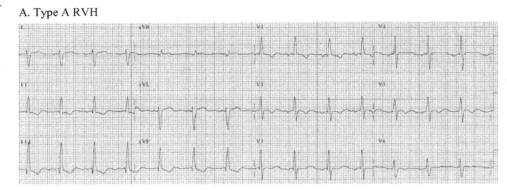

B. Type B RVH

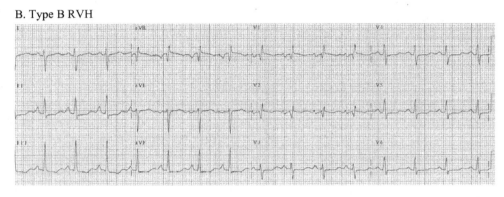

C. Type C RVH

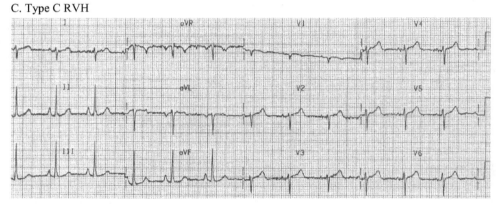

and to the right, away from leads II and aVF. This brings the main axis of the QRS complex to the northwest quadrant, as shown in the ECG in Figure 7.18. $S_1 S_2 S_3$ pattern is not specific for RVH because it can occur normally in young children without any evidence of RVH or cardiac disease. In older individuals, this pattern is suggestive of RVH, especially when other signs of RVH such as right atrial enlargement (P-pulmonale) or prominent R waves are present in $V_1$. Additionally, the size of the S waves in leads I, II, and III are usually deeper than the size of the R waves.

## Acute Pulmonary Embolism

■ **Acute pulmonary embolism:** Acute pulmonary embolism may also result in acute right heart strain

(Fig. 7.19). Most patients with acute pulmonary embolism are usually ill and restless and are therefore tachypneic and tachycardic. Sinus tachycardia and incomplete right bundle branch block are the most frequent ECG findings. The following are the ECG changes of acute pulmonary embolism.

■ **Rhythm:**
   □ Sinus tachycardia, atrial flutter, or atrial fibrillation
■ **Changes in the QRS complex:**
   □ Right axis deviation of approximately $\geq 90°$
   □ $S_1 Q_3 T_3$ pattern (S wave in lead I, Q with inverted T wave in III)
   □ rSR′ pattern in $V_1$ usually of acute onset
   □ $V_1$ may also show QS, qR, or R > S pattern
   □ Clockwise rotation with persistent S in $V_6$ similar to type C RVH

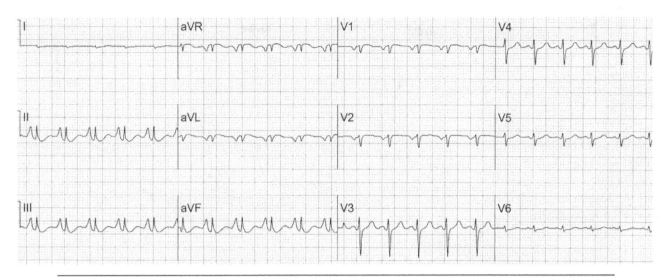

**Figure 7.17:  Chronic Obstructive Pulmonary Disease.**  In chronic obstructive pulmonary disease, the heart is vertically oriented because of the hyperinflated lungs pushing the diaphragm downward. This causes the P, QRS, and T deflections to be oriented vertically toward 90° resulting in the so called "lead I sign," where all the deflections in lead I become conspicuous by their diminutive appearance. This could also occur in $V_6$, because $V_6$ is also perpendicular in relation to lead aVF. In addition, the heart is rotated clockwise with peak P-pulmonale in II, III, and aVF. These changes are consistent with type C RVH.

■ **Changes in the P wave:**
  □ P-pulmonale with peaking of the P waves in leads II, III, and aVF
  □ Ta waves become exaggerated in leads II, III, and aVF, causing 1 mm of ST depression in the inferior leads
■ **Changes in the ST segment and T waves**
  □ ST elevation in $V_1$
  □ Inverted T waves in $V_1$ to $V_3$ or up to $V_6$

## Combined Ventricular Hypertrophy

■ **Biventricular hypertrophy:** When both the right and left ventricles are hypertrophied, there is cancellation of the forces generated by both ventricles. Thus, the ECG may remain unchanged, and the diagnosis of biventricular hypertrophy is often difficult. Occasionally, the following ECG changes may be present as shown in Fig. 7.20.
  ■ **Tall biphasic complexes in mid-precordial leads:** The transition leads $V_3$ or $V_4$ may show increased

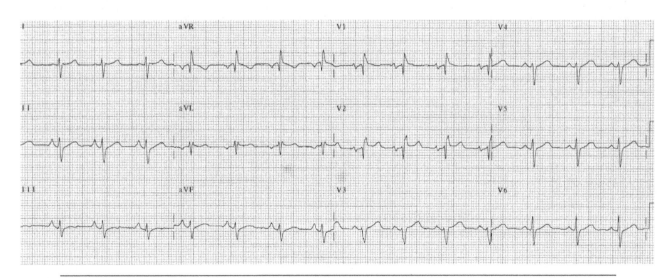

**Figure 7.18:  $S_1 S_2 S_3$ Pattern.**  This pattern simply implies that an S wave is present in leads I, II, and III. The direction of the impulse is away from these leads and is usually at the northwest quadrant causing a tall R wave in aVR. $S_1$ $S_2 S_3$ may suggest right ventricular hypertrophy in older individuals, especially when the P waves are peaked in lead II because of right atrial enlargement, when R waves are tall in $V_1$, or the size of the S waves is deeper than the size of the R waves in all three leads.

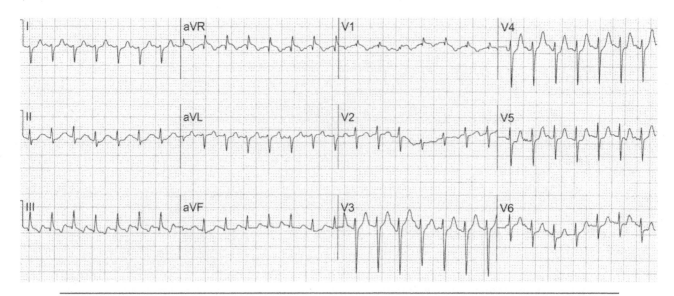

**Figure 7.19: Acute Pulmonary Embolism.** The electrocardiogram shows sinus tachycardia, right axis deviation $\leq 90°$, $S_1 Q_3 T_3$ pattern, rR' pattern in $V_1$, and persistent S in the precordial leads extending to $V_6$. These findings are usually acute in onset due to acute right heart strain.

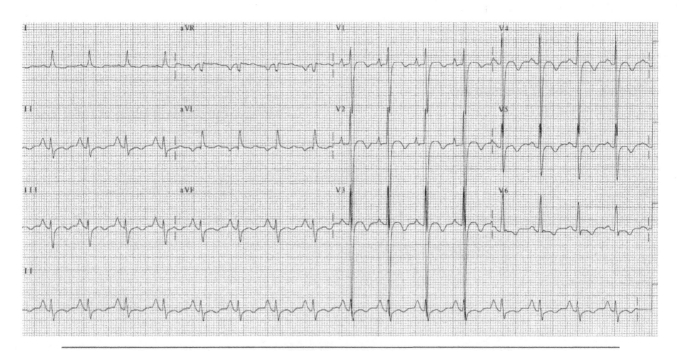

**Figure 7.20: Combined Ventricular Hypertrophy.** When both ventricles are hypertrophied, the electrocardiogram changes of right and left ventricular hypertrophy cancel each other and may be difficult to diagnose. In this example, there is increased voltage of the QRS complex, especially over the transition zones $V_3$ and $V_4$, which shows tall R waves and deep S waves. There is also evidence of left ventricular hypertrophy and right atrial enlargement. Note also that there is voltage discordance, in that the precordial leads show tall voltages, whereas the limb leads that are bipolar leads have lower voltage.

amplitude of the QRS complex with increased R waves combined with deep S waves (Katz-Wachtel phenomenon).

- **Right atrial enlargement combined with LVH:** LVH by any standard criteria combined with P pulmonale as shown in Fig. 7.20.
- **Voltage discordance:** Biventricular hypertrophy may also manifest as voltage discordance between the limb and precordial leads. Precordial leads are unipolar leads and are closer to the heart than the limb leads. Thus, tall QRS complexes are recorded in the precordial leads, whereas the limb leads, which are further away especially bipolar leads I, II, and III, will record low voltages.

## ECG Findings in RVH

## Abnormalities in the QRS complexes

- Right axis deviation of approximately $\geq 90°$. This should always be present before the diagnosis of RVH is considered.
- qR in $V_1$
- R wave in $V_1 \geq 7$ mm
- Tall R waves in $V_1$ or $V_2$ (R/S ratio $\geq 1$)
- Delayed intrinsicoid deflection in $V_1$ or $V_2 > 0.03$ seconds.
- rS complex from $V_1$ to $V_6$ (clockwise rotation) with right axis deviation
- $S_1 S_2 S_3$ pattern in adult patients
- rSR' or RBBB in $V_1$ with right axis deviation

## Abnormalities in the P waves

- Peaked P waves in leads II, III and aVF (P-pulmonale)

## Abnormalities in the ST segment and T waves

- ST depression and T wave inversion in right sided precordial leads ($V_1$)
- T wave inversion in $V_2$ to $V_6$

## Mechanism

- Because of its thinner wall and smaller mass, the right ventricle does not contribute significantly to the generation of the QRS complex. Thus, when the ventricles are synchronously activated, the forces generated from the right ventricle are masked by those generated from the left ventricle. When there is RVH, the right ventricular wall becomes thickened and the right ventricular mass is increased, resulting in a larger contribution of the right ventricle in generating the QRS complex. In adults, the thickness of the right ventricle does not exceed that of the left ventricle even when RVH is present, thus the ECG changes of RVH continue to be masked by the forces generated by the thicker

left ventricle. In certain types of congenital heart diseases, however, the RV wall is much thicker than the LV wall, such as in tetralogy of Fallot or in congenital pulmonary stenosis. When this occurs, the ECG findings of RVH become more obvious.

- **Changes in the frontal or limb leads:** RVH is better appreciated in the precordial leads than the limb leads because the precordial leads overlie the ventricles directly. Nevertheless, there are certain changes in the limb leads that may suggest RVH.
  - **Right axis deviation:** Right axis deviation is one of the most reliable signs in the diagnosis of RVH. Because the right ventricle is anterior and to the right of the left ventricle, increase in right ventricular mass will shift the QRS axis to the right and anteriorly. Thus, the axis of the QRS complex is shifted toward 80° to 120° or further to the right when RVH is present. RVH is the most common cause of right axis deviation in the adult. The diagnosis of RVH is unlikely unless the axis of the QRS complex is shifted to the right.
  - **$S_1 S_2 S_3$ pattern:** This pattern simply means that there is an S wave in lead I, lead II, and lead III. The presence of S waves in these leads is due to the terminal forces of the QRS complex being oriented rightward and superiorly toward the northwest quadrant. This is due to activation of the posterobasal portion of the right ventricle terminally. The presence of $S_1 S_2 S_3$, however, is not always diagnostic of RVH because it is also seen in normal healthy individuals, especially the younger age group. When there is $S_1 S_2 S_3$ pattern, RVH may be present when other changes in the QRS complex are present, such as tall R waves in $V_1$, P-pulmonale, or when the S waves are deeper than the size of the R waves in all three leads.
  - **Abnormalities of the P wave:** Right atrial enlargement is a frequent accompaniment of right ventricular enlargement. Thus, the presence of peaked P waves with increased amplitude (P-pulmonale), best recorded in leads II, III, and aVF suggest RVH unless the P wave changes are due to tricuspid stenosis, which is rare in adults.
- **Changes in the precordial leads:** Because the precordial leads are directly on top of the ventricles, more information is provided by these leads when compared with the more distal limb leads.
  - **Tall R waves in $V_1$ or $V_2$ with R/S ratio $\geq 1$:** Increased voltage in the right-sided precordial leads occur when there is increased thickness of the right ventricular wall. This will be recorded as tall R waves in $V_1$ or $V_2$ with R/S ratio $\geq 1$. R/S ratio $\geq 1$ means that the height of the R wave in $V_1$ is equal to or higher in amplitude than the S wave, which is the reverse of normal in the adult population.
  - **rS complex from $V_1$ to $V_6$ with right axis deviation:** This is also called clockwise rotation or delayed transition. Deep S waves or rS complex from $V_1$ to $V_6$ may be

due to RVH or LVH. For RVH to be present there should also be right axis deviation. When RVH is present, the right ventricle rotates anteriorly, causing the left ventricle to rotate in a more posterior orientation. If the ventricles are viewed from below looking upward, the rotation of both ventricles will be clockwise when there is right ventricular enlargement. Because the precordial leads are recorded in their standard location from $V_1$ to $V_6$, the transition zone is not crossed unless the electrodes are moved to the left and more posteriorly. This type of RVH is frequently associated with chronic lung disease (type C RVH).

■ **Prolonged ventricular activation time with delayed onset of the intrinsicoid deflection in $V_1$ or $V_2$.** When the ventricular activation time is prolonged, the onset of the intrinsicoid deflection is delayed. The ventricular activation time of the right ventricle is measured in $V_1$ from the onset of the QRS complex to the peak of the R or R′ wave and represents the time required for the impulse to activate the right ventricular wall. The ventricular activation time of the right ventricle normally measures $\leq 0.03$ seconds and is increased to $\geq 0.04$ seconds when there is right ventricular hypertrophy. The onset of the intrinsicoid deflection, measured in $V_1$ or $V_2$, represents the time when the electrical impulse has reached the right ventricular epicardium and generally coincides with the peak of the R wave or immediately thereafter, when the R wave is deflected downward toward baseline.

## Clinical Significance

■ In adults, RVH can result from many different causes. RVH may be due to pressure overload such as pulmonic stenosis or primary pulmonary hypertension. This type of RVH predominantly results in increased thickness of the right ventricle. It may also be due to volume overload such as atrial septal defect and tricuspid or pulmonic regurgitations, resulting in volume overload with dilatation of the right ventricular cavity. RVH can also result from the presence of lung disease, which may distort the anatomical relationship between the heart and the chest wall. Or it may be due to left heart failure where an increase in left ventricular mass is associated with an increase in right ventricular mass. These changes may develop insidiously or abruptly, as when pulmonary hypertension occurs in the setting of acute pulmonary embolism. The ECG presentations of RVH, therefore, in these different clinical settings are not necessarily similar. Different patterns of RVH have been described which includes types A, B, and C based on the morphology of the QRS complex in the precordial leads. Types A and B are easy to recognize as RVH because the size of the R wave is taller than the S wave in $V_1$, whereas in type C the size of the R wave is smaller than the S wave in $V_1$ and may not be recognized as RVH. In all three types, the axis of the QRS complex is shifted to the right.

■ **Type A RVH:** This is the most recognizable type of RVH. The R waves are tall in $V_1$, often in $V_2$ and $V_3$. The R wave is usually monophasic (no S wave) in $V_1$. If an S wave is present, the R wave is always taller than the height of the S wave with an R/S ratio $>1$. $V_5$ and $V_6$ may show deeper S waves than R waves. In type A RVH, the thickness of the right ventricle is greater than the thickness of the left ventricle, and the right ventricle is the dominant ventricle. This type of RVH is the most commonly recognized and is seen in severe pulmonic stenosis, primary pulmonary hypertension, or mitral stenosis with severe pulmonary hypertension. The axis of the QRS complex is significantly deviated to the right at approximately $+120°$.

■ **Type B RVH:** The R wave in $V_1$ is slightly taller than the S wave or the ratio between the R wave and S wave is $\geq 1$. $V_1$ may also exhibit an rsr′ pattern. The QRS complex in $V_5$ and $V_6$ is not different from normal. This type of RVH is usually due to atrial septal defect or mitral stenosis with mild to moderate pulmonary hypertension. The frontal axis is vertical at approximately $90°$.

■ **Type C RVH:** This type of RVH is difficult to recognize and is frequently missed because the R wave in $V_1$ is not tall and is smaller than the S wave. Instead, a deep S wave is present in $V_1$ and in $V_2$ that extends up to $V_6$. Thus, $V_1$ to $V_6$ will show rS complexes. In $V_6$, the R wave continues to be smaller in amplitude than the S wave. The axis of the QRS complex is approximately $90°$ or less. This type of RVH is usually due to chronic obstructive lung disease but could also occur acutely as a manifestation of acute pulmonary embolism.

■ Prolongation of the QRS complex usually does not occur when there is RVH because the thickness of the right ventricle wall usually does not exceed that of the left ventricle, even when RVH is present. Thus, the forces generated by the right ventricle are cancelled by the forces from the left ventricle. When widening of the QRS complex is present, there may be associated right bundle branch block because the right bundle branch is very susceptible to injury when there is increased right ventricular pressure.

■ The right ventricle is to the right and anterior to that of the left ventricle. Pulsations from the right ventricle are not normally visible or palpable. However, when the right ventricle is enlarged or hypertrophied, a sustained systolic precordial impulse is palpable along the left parasternal area. Prominent "a" waves are seen in the neck veins. Very often, tricuspid regurgitation is also present causing a "cv" wave in the jugular neck veins accompanied by prominent pulsations of the liver or the ear lobes bilaterally. Third and fourth gallop sounds may also be audible along the lower left sternal border. Their right ventricular origin can be verified by increase in intensity of these gallop sounds with inspiration.

## Treatment and Prognosis

■ When RVH is present, the underlying cause should be evaluated. The treatment and prognosis will depend on the etiology of the RVH.

## Suggested Readings

Ariyarajah V, Frisella ME, Spodick DH. Reevaluation of the criterion for interatrial block. *Am J Cardiol.* 2006;98:936–937.

Buxton AE, Calkins H, Callans DJ, et al. ACC/AHA/HRS 2006 key data elements and definitions for electrophysiological studies and procedures: a report of the American College of Cardiology/American Heart Association Task Force on clinical data standards (ACC/AHA/HRS writing committee to develop data standards on electrophysiology. *J Am Coll Cardiol.* 2006;48:2360–2396.

Casale PN, Devereux RB, Alonso DR, et al. Improved sex-specific criteria of left ventricular hypertrophy for clinical and computer interpretation of electrocardiograms: validation with autopsy findings. *Circulation.* 1987;75:565–572.

Chow TC, Helm RA, Kaplan S. *Right Ventricular Hypertrophy in Clinical Vectorcardiography.* 2nd ed. New York: Grune and Stratton; 1974.

Conover MB. Chamber hypertrophy and enlargement. In: *Understanding Electrocardiography.* 8th ed. St. Louis: Mosby; 2003:407–419.

Devereux RB, Wachtell K, Gerdts E, et al. Prognostic significance of left ventricular mass change during treatment of hypertension. *JAMA* 2004;292:2350–2356.

Dunn MI, Lipman BS. *Lipman-Massie Clinical Electrocardiography.* Chicago: Yearbook Medical Publishers, Inc.; 1989.

Gardin JM, Lauer MS. Left ventricular hypertrophy: the next treatable silent killer. *JAMA.* 2004;292:2396–2398.

Haider AW, Larson MG, Benjamin EJ, et al. Increased left ventricular mass and hypertrophy are associated with increased risk for sudden death. *J Am Coll Cardiol.* 1998;32:1454–1459.

Josephson ME, Kastor JA, Morganroth J. Electrocardiographic left atrial enlargement. Electrophysiologic, echocardiographic and hemodynamic correlates. *J Am Coll Cardiol.* 1977;39:967–971.

Kligfield P, Gettes LS, Bailey JJ, et al. Recommendations for the standardization and interpretation of the electrocardiogram. *J Am Coll Cardiol.* 2007;49:1109–1127.

Marriott HJL. Chamber enlargement. In: *Practical Electrocardiography.* 5th ed. Baltimore: The William and Wilkins Company; 1972:56–66.

Mirvis DM, Goldberger AL. Electrocardiography. In: Zipes DP, Libby P, Bonow RO, et al., eds. *Braunwald's Heart Disease, a Textbook of Cardiovascular Medicine.* 7th ed. Philadelphia: Elsevier Saunders; 2005:118–125.

Nicholas WJ, Liebson PR. ECG changes in COPD: what do they mean? *J Respir Dis.* 1987;8:103–120.

Odom II H, Davis L, Dinh HA, et al. QRS voltage measurements in autopsied men free of cardiopulmonary disease: a basis for evaluating total QRS voltage as an index of left ventricular hypertrophy. *Am J Cardiol.* 1986;58:801–804.

Okin PM, Roman MU, Devereux RB, et al. Time-voltage QRS area of the 12-lead electrocardiogram: detection of left ventricular hypertrophy. *Hypertension.* 1998:31:937–942.

Okin PM, Devereux RB, Jern S, et al. Regression of electrocardiographic left ventricular hypertrophy during antihypertensive treatment and the prediction of major cardiovascular events. *JAMA.* 2004;292:2343–2349.

Romhilt DW, Estes EH Jr. A point-score system for the ECG diagnosis of left ventricular hypertrophy. *Am Heart J.* 1968;75:752.

Sokolow M, Lyon TP. The ventricular complex in left ventricular hypertrophy as obtained by unipolar precordial and limb leads. *Am Heart J.* 1949;37:161–186.

Willems JL, Robles de Medina EO, Bernard R, et al. Criteria for intraventricular conduction disturbances and pre-excitation. *J Am Coll Cardiol.* 1985;5:1261–1275.

# Atrioventricular Block

## Types of AV Block

- The atria and ventricles are contiguous structures separated by a dense mass of fibrous tissues that are electrically inert. This prevents the direct spread of electrical impulses between the atria and ventricles. The only pathway by which the sinus impulse can reach the ventricles is through the normal atrioventricular (AV) conduction system (Fig. 8.1).

- The normal AV conduction system consists of the AV node, bundle of His, bundle branches, and fascicular branches of the left bundle branch. The sinus impulse can be delayed or interrupted anywhere along this conduction pathway, resulting in varying degrees of AV block.

- There are three types of AV block based on the severity of the conduction abnormality:
  - **First-degree AV block**
  - **Second-degree AV block**
    - ☐ Mobitz type I or AV Wenckebach
    - ☐ Mobitz type II
    - ☐ Advanced or high grade
  - **Third-degree or complete AV block**

## First-Degree AV Block

- **Normal AV conduction:** The normal PR interval measures 0.12 to 0.20 seconds in the adult (Fig. 8.2). It represents the time required for the sinus impulse to travel from atria to ventricles.

- **First-degree AV block:** First-degree AV block simply means that the PR interval is prolonged and measures >0.20 seconds (Fig. 8.3). It indicates delay in the conduction of the sinus impulse from atria to ventricles with most of the delay occurring at the level of the AV node.

- Although the PR interval is prolonged in first-degree AV block, all P waves are conducted to the ventricles and are always followed by QRS complexes (Fig. 8.4). First-degree AV block therefore is a conduction delay rather than actual block. This conduction delay can occur anywhere between the atria and the ventricles.

- First-degree AV block is usually a conduction delay at the AV node. This can be due to a variety of causes including enhanced vagal tone; use of pharmacologic agents that prolong AV conduction such as beta blockers, calcium channel blockers, and digitalis; or it might indicate disease of the AV conduction system.

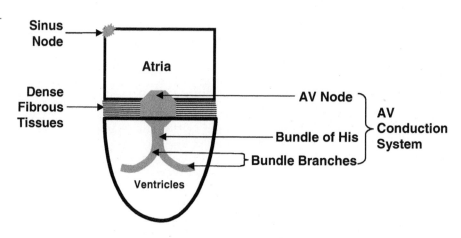

**Figure 8.1: Diagrammatic Representation of the Atrioventricular (AV) Conduction System.** The atria and ventricles are separated by a dense mass of fibrous tissues. This prevents the spread of atrial impulses directly to the ventricles. The only pathway by which the atrial impulse can propagate to the ventricles is through the AV conduction system.

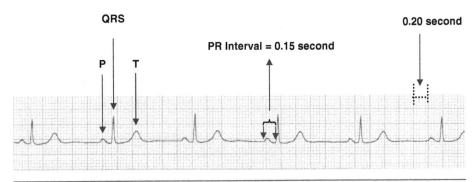

**Figure 8.2:   Normal Atrioventricular (AV) Conduction.** Rhythm strip showing normal PR interval measuring 0.15 seconds. The PR interval is measured from the beginning of the P wave to the beginning of the QRS complex and normally varies from 0.12 to 0.20 seconds. If a Q wave is present, the PR interval is measured from the beginning of the P wave to the beginning of the Q wave (P-Q interval). The PR interval represents the time required for the sinus impulse to travel from atria to ventricles.

- Once a sinus P wave is not conducted to the ventricles, the AV block has advanced to second degree (Fig. 8.5).

## Common Mistakes in First-Degree AV Block

- The diagnosis of first-degree AV block is usually straightforward but can be very confusing if the PR interval is unusually prolonged. The P wave may be hidden within the T wave or it can be mistaken for a T wave of the previous complex (Figs. 8.6C and 8.7).

- First-degree AV block does not cause symptoms. However, when the P wave falls within the Q-T interval of the previous cardiac cycle, which corresponds to ventricular systole, simultaneous contraction of both atria and ventricles may cause symptoms of low cardiac output (Figs. 8.6C and 8.7).

## ▣ First-Degree AV Block

### Electrocardiogram Findings

1. The PR interval is prolonged and measures >0.20 seconds.
2. Every P wave is followed by a QRS complex.

### Mechanism

- The PR interval represents the time required for the sinus impulse to travel from atria to ventricles. There are several structures involved in the propagation of the sinus impulse to the ventricles. These include the atria, AV node, His bundle, bundle branches, and fascicles. The sinus impulse can be delayed anywhere between the atria and ventricles although the prolongation of the PR interval is almost always due to slowing of conduction within the AV node. Less commonly, first-degree AV block can occur in the His-Purkinje system or within the atria.

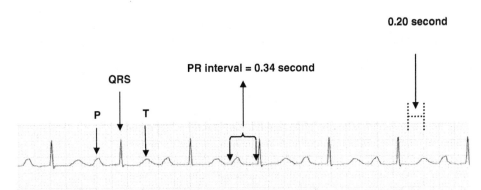

**Figure 8.3:   First-Degree Atrioventricular (AV) Block.** Rhythm strip showing PR interval of 0.34 seconds. Any PR interval measuring >0.20 seconds is first-degree AV block and indicates that there is a delay in the conduction of the sinus impulse from atria to ventricles.

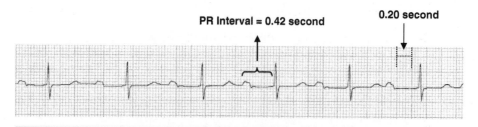

Figure 8.4: **First-Degree Atrioventricular (AV) Block.** The PR interval measures 0.42 seconds and is unusually prolonged. Regardless of the duration of the PR interval as long as every P wave is followed by a QRS complex, the conduction abnormality is first-degree AV block.

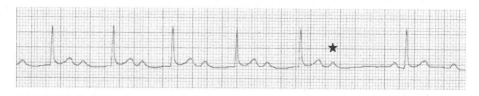

Figure 8.5: **Second-Degree Atrioventricular (AV) Block.** When a sinus P wave is not conducted to the ventricles and is not followed by a QRS complex (*star*), the conduction abnormality is no longer first-degree but has advanced to second-degree AV block.

Lead II Rhythm Strips

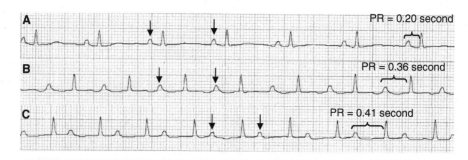

Figure 8.6: **First-Degree Atrioventricular (AV) Block.** When the PR interval is unusually prolonged, the P wave may be mistaken for a T wave. Rhythm strips **(A, B, C)** are from the same patient taken on separate occasions. **(A)** Top normal PR interval of 0.20 seconds. Arrows identify the P waves. The PR interval is longer in **(B)** (0.36 seconds) and is even much longer in **(C)** (0.41 seconds). In **(C)**, the PR interval is unusually prolonged such that the P waves can be mistaken for T waves of the previous complex.

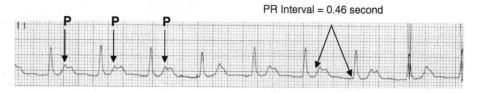

Figure 8.7: **First-Degree Atrioventricular (AV) Block with Unusually Prolonged PR Interval.** The PR interval measures 0.46 seconds and is unusually prolonged. The P wave is difficult to recognize (*arrows*) because it is superimposed on the T wave of the previous complex. This can result in synchronous contraction of both atria and ventricles, which may cause symptoms of low cardiac output.

## Clinical Significance

■ First-degree AV block is the mildest form of AV conduction abnormality characterized by delay in conduction of the sinus impulse from atria to ventricles. All P waves conduct to the ventricles, thus first-degree AV block is a misnomer because the impulse is only delayed. There is no actual block.

■ First-degree AV block may not be appreciated if the PR interval is markedly prolonged or the P wave is buried within the T wave of the previous complex. In both instances, the P wave may be difficult to identify.

■ First-degree AV block can be the result of enhanced vagal tone; administration of pharmacologic agents that can block the AV node such as beta blockers, calcium blockers, digitalis; and other antiarrhythmic agents. It can be caused by hypothyroidism, rheumatic fever, or intrinsic disease of the AV node and conducting system from ischemia, inflammation, infiltration, and fibrosis.

■ The first heart sound is usually diminished in intensity when there is first-degree AV block. If the PR interval is prolonged, the AV valves slowly drift back to a semiclosed position before the ventricles contract, resulting in a soft first heart sound. When the PR interval is unusually prolonged and the P wave is inscribed at the T wave or ST segment of the preceding complex, cannon A waves may be seen in the jugular neck veins because atrial contraction occurs simultaneously with ventricular systole, which may result in diminished cardiac output.

## Treatment

■ First-degree AV block is benign and does not require any treatment. The etiology of the AV block should be recognized and corrected.

■ First-degree AV block may compromise left ventricular filling if the PR interval is >0.30 seconds because atrial contraction may occur during ventricular systole. This may elevate atrial and pulmonary venous pressures and reduce ventricular filling and cardiac output resulting in symptoms of congestion and low output very similar to the symptoms associated with the pacemaker syndrome (see Chapter 26, The ECG of Cardiac Pacemakers). If the long PR interval is not reversible and temporary AV pacing can improve the symptoms related to low cardiac output, the American College of Cardiology (ACC), American Heart Association (AHA), and Heart Rhythm Society (HRS) guidelines for permanent pacemaker implantation consider this type of first-degree AV block as a class IIa indication for permanent pacing (meaning that the weight of evidence is in favor of usefulness or efficacy of the procedure).

## Prognosis

■ Prognosis is generally good and favorable especially if the cause is reversible. If the cause is due to structural cardiac abnormalities, first-degree AV block may progress to higher grades of AV block. The prognosis therefore depends on the associated cardiac abnormalities rather than the presence of first-degree AV block.

## Second-Degree AV Block

■ **Second-degree AV block:** There are three types of second-degree AV block.
  ■ Mobitz type I also called AV Wenckebach
  ■ Mobitz type II
  ■ Advanced, also called high-grade second-degree AV block

■ **Type I and type II second-degree AV block:** In type I and type II second-degree AV block, two or more consecutive P waves are conducted to the ventricles and only single P waves are blocked (Fig. 8.8).

■ **Advanced second-degree AV block:** The AV block is advanced when the second-degree block cannot be classified as type I or type II. An example of advanced second-degree AV block is when two or more consecutive P waves are blocked as in 3:1, 4:1, or 5:1 AV block (Fig. 8.9). Another example is when only a single P wave is followed by a QRS complex as in 2:1 AV block (Fig. 8.10).

### Type I Second-Degree AV Block

■ **Type I second-degree AV block:** Type I second-degree AV block is also called AV Wenckebach. The following features characterize type I second-degree AV block (Figs. 8.11 and 8.12):
  ■ Two or more consecutive P waves are conducted.
  ■ Only single P waves are blocked.

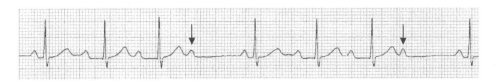

**Figure 8.8:   Type I Second-Degree Atrioventricular (AV) Block.** The rhythm strip shows type I second-degree AV block. Three P waves are conducted with gradual prolongation of the PR interval. Only one P wave (marked by the arrows) is not followed by a QRS complex.

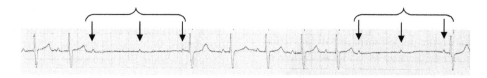

**Figure 8.9:    Advanced 3:1 Second-Degree Atrioventricular (AV) Block.** The rhythm strip shows intermittent 3:1 AV block (*brackets*). The first two P waves are not conducted. When two or more consecutive P waves are not conducted, the rhythm is advanced second-degree block. Arrows point to the P waves.

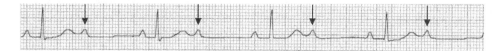

**Figure 8.10:    Advanced 2:1 Second-Degree Atrioventricular (AV) Block.** In 2:1 AV block, the first P wave is conducted and the next P wave is blocked (*arrows*). A common error is to classify 2:1 AV block as a type II second-degree AV block. Because only one P wave is followed by a QRS complex, the AV block cannot be classified as type I or II.

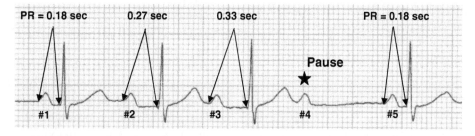

**Figure 8.11:    Type I Second-Degree Atrioventricular (AV) Block.** The rhythm strip shows 4:3 AV Wenckebach with four P waves (labeled 1 to 4) conducting only three QRS complexes. The PR interval gradually prolongs before a ventricular complex is dropped (*star*). The long pause allows the conduction system to rest and recover so that the next P wave (5) is conducted more efficiently, resulting in a PR interval that measures the shortest. The QRS complexes are narrow and only a single P wave is not conducted (4).

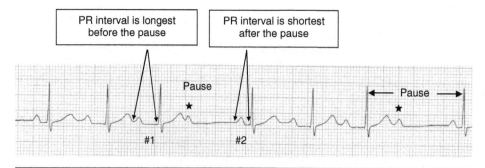

**Figure 8.12:    Type I Second-Degree Atrioventricular (AV) Block.** Instead of measuring for gradual prolongation of the PR interval, one can simply compare the PR interval before (1) and after (2) the pause. If the PR interval shortens after the pause, type I AV block is present. The stars identify single P waves that are not conducted.

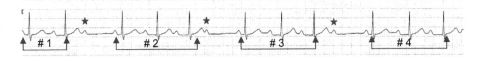

**Figure 8.13:** **Group Beating.** Group beating simply means that if you "eyeball" the tracing from left to right, one gets the impression that the beats (the QRS complexes) are grouped together because of the spaces created by P waves without QRS complexes (*stars*). Four such groups can be identified in the above tracing (groups 1 to 4). Group beating is frequently seen in type I atrioventricular (AV) block because AV Wenckebach has a tendency to be repetitive. The above is an example of 4:3 AV Wenckebach meaning that there are four P waves for every three QRS complexes.

- There is gradual prolongation of the PR interval before a ventricular complex is dropped.
- The PR interval always shortens immediately after the pause.
- The QRS complexes may be narrow or wide but are typically narrow.

## Type I Second-Degree AV Block

- There are additional features commonly seen in classical type I second-degree AV block:
  - Group beating is present (Fig. 8.13)
  - The R-R intervals (distance between two R waves) are variable (Fig. 8.14). The R-R interval straddling a blocked P wave is less than the R-R interval straddling a conducted sinus impulse.
- **Conduction ratio:** The conduction ratio refers to the total number of P waves to the total number of QRS complexes that are conducted. Thus, a 4:3 AV Wenckebach implies that of four consecutive P waves, only three are conducted; a 5:4 AV Wenckebach means that of five consecutive P waves, only four are conducted.

- Shortening of the PR interval after a pause is much easier to recognize than gradual prolongation of the PR interval, as shown in Figure 8.15. This always favors second-degree type I AV block.
- Type I second-degree AV block may have narrow or wide QRS complexes.
- **Localizing the AV block:** Type I second-degree AV block is almost always localized at the level of the AV node, although it can also occur below the AV node (infranodal) at the level of the His-Purkinje system. The presence of bundle branch block (Fig. 8.16) or myocardial infarction (Fig. 8.17) may be helpful in localizing whether the block is nodal or infranodal.
  - **Narrow QRS complexes:** When the QRS complexes are narrow, the block is almost always confined to the AV node (Fig. 8.18). A block occurring at the bundle of His (intra-His block) is possible, but is rare.
  - **Wide QRS complexes:** When the QRS complexes are wide because of the presence of bundle branch block, the block may be AV nodal although an infranodal block at the level of the bundle branches is more likely (Fig. 8.16).

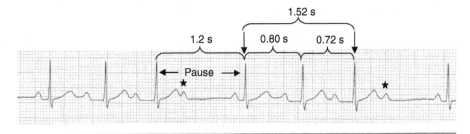

**Figure 8.14:** **Varying R-R Interval in Type I Second-Degree Atrioventricular (AV) Block.** Type I can be differentiated from type II second-degree AV block by the R-R intervals. In type I AV block, the R-R intervals are variable because the PR intervals are also variable. Note that the R-R interval straddling a blocked P wave (1.2 seconds) is less than the R-R interval straddling a conducted sinus impulse (1.52 seconds). This is in contrast to type II block, where the R-R intervals are fixed because the PR intervals are also fixed (see Fig. 8.20). The longest R-R interval occurs immediately after the pause (0.80 seconds) with gradual shortening of the next R-R interval (0.72 seconds). The stars mark the P waves that are not conducted.

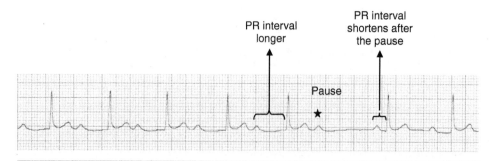

**Figure 8.15: Type I Second-Degree Atrioventricular (AV) Block.** The PR interval looks fixed but suddenly shortens after the pause. The shortening of the PR interval is characteristic of type I second-degree AV block. The star identifies a P wave without a QRS complex. Note that gradual lengthening of the PR interval is not obvious before the pause.

■ **Acute myocardial infarction (MI):**

　□ **Acute inferior MI:** When AV block occurs in the setting of an acute inferior MI, the location of the AV block is at the AV node (Fig. 8.17, see also Figs. 8.30 and 8.39). The QRS complexes are narrow.

　□ **Acute anterior MI:** When AV block occurs in the setting of an acute anterior MI, the AV block is below the AV node (infranodal block). The QRS complexes are usually wide (See section on Complete AV Block).

## ECG Findings of Type I AV Block

1. Two or more consecutive P waves are conducted.
2. Only single P waves are blocked.
3. There is gradual prolongation of the PR interval before a ventricular complex is dropped.
4. The PR interval always shortens immediately after the pause.
5. The QRS complexes are usually narrow.
6. Group beating is present.
7. The R-R intervals are variable. The longest R-R interval is noted immediately after the pause and shortening of the R-R interval occurs successively thereafter.

## Mechanism

■ Type I second-degree AV block or AV Wenckebach is usually a block at the level of the AV node although it can occur

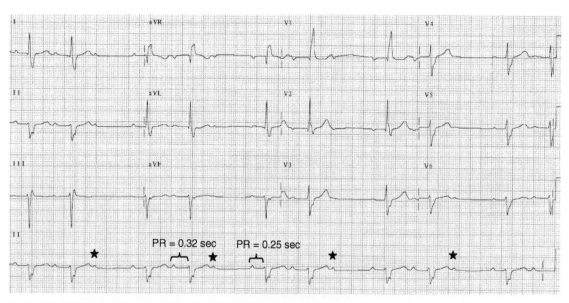

**Figure 8.16: Second-Degree Atrioventricular (AV) Block with Wide QRS Complexes.** The QRS complexes in AV Wenckebach are usually narrow. In this example, the QRS complexes are wide because of the presence of right bundle branch block and left anterior fascicular block. The rhythm strip at the bottom of the tracing shows 3:2 AV Wenckebach. Note that the PR interval is longer before the pause (0.32 seconds) and shortens immediately after the pause (0.25 seconds). Shortening of the PR interval after the pause is consistent with type I second-degree AV block. The P waves that are not conducted are identified by the stars.

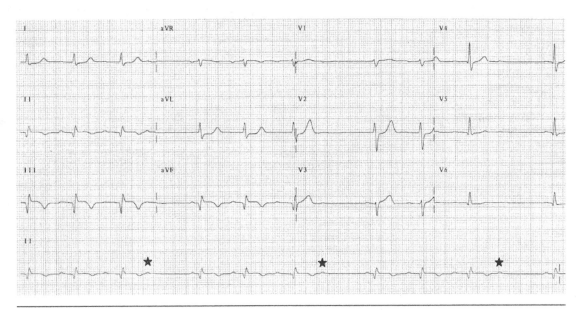

**Figure 8.17:  Atrioventricular (AV) Block and Acute Inferior Myocardial Infarction (MI).** When type I block occurs in the setting of acute inferior MI as shown, the block is AV nodal. The stars identify the blocked P waves.

anywhere in the AV conduction system. When the QRS complexes are narrow, the block is almost always AV nodal. A block in the distal His-Purkinje system is suspected when there is bundle branch block (a sign of distal conduction system disease) or when the AV block occurs in the setting of an acute anterior MI.

■ Because the sinus impulses constantly bombard the AV node, conduction through the AV node becomes progressively delayed until a sinus impulse can no longer be conducted, resulting in a P wave without a QRS complex. The pause allows the AV node to rest and recover, allowing the next impulse to be conducted more efficiently resulting in a shorter PR interval.

## Clinical Significance

■ Type I AV block may be a normal finding in healthy individuals, especially during sleep, because of enhanced vagal tone. It may be caused by intense vagal stimulation such as vomiting or coughing. The arrhythmia may be caused by agents that block the AV node, such as calcium blockers, beta blockers, or digitalis. These examples of AV block are the result of extrinsic causes and are reversible. AV block can also be due to structural cardiac disease such as degenerative and calcific disease of the conduction system, ischemia, infarction or inflammation of the AV node, or intraventricular conduction system including acute myocarditis, rheumatic fever, and Lyme disease. These examples of AV block are due to intrinsic disease of the AV node and conduction system and may not be reversible.

■ Type I AV block is usually confined to the AV node. The QRS complexes are narrow. Type I AV block with wide QRS complexes may be AV nodal but is more frequently infranodal. When the block is infranodal, the cause of the AV block is usually due to structural cardiac disease.

■ **AV nodal block:** AV block at the level of the AV node is generally benign with a good prognosis. Even when type I block progresses to complete AV block, the AV block is usually reversible. Furthermore, the rhythm that comes to the rescue (escape rhythm), is from the AV junction.

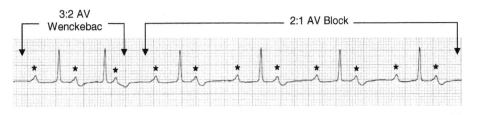

**Figure 8.18:  Two to One Atrioventricular (AV) Block.** The initial portion of the tracing shows a classical 3:2 AV Wenckebach with gradual prolongation of the PR interval. This is followed by 2:1 AV block. The presence of 2:1 block associated with classical AV Wenckebach with narrow QRS complexes suggests that the 2:1 AV block is AV nodal. The stars identify the P waves.

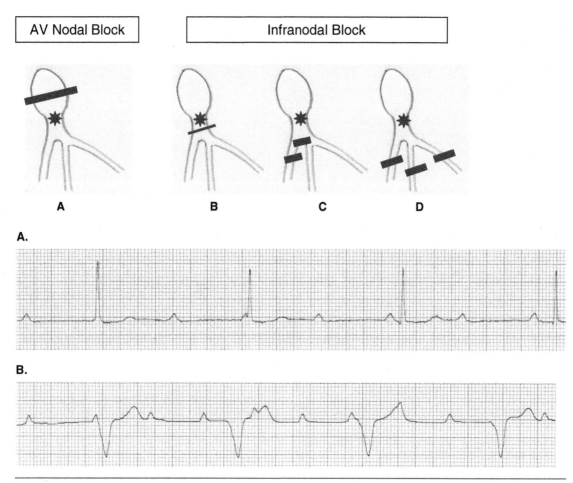

**Figure 8.19:    Complete Atrioventricular (AV) block and Junctional Escape Rhythm.** Complete AV block can occur anywhere in the conduction system. In the upper column, complete AV block is at the AV node **(A)**; in **(B)**, at the bundle of His; in **(C)**, both bundle branches; and in **(D)**, right bundle branch and both fascicles of the left bundle. If the block is AV nodal **(A)**, the escape rhythm will be AV junctional (star) and will have narrow QRS complexes (electrocardiogram **A**). However, if the block is infranodal (diagrams **B, C,** and **D**), AV junctional rhythm is not possible and the escape rhythm will be ventricular with wide QRS complex (electrocardiogram **B**).

AV junctional rhythm is more stable and more physiologic than a ventricular escape rhythm and has a relatively fast rate that can be further enhanced with atropine.

■ **Infranodal block:** Type I block with wide QRS complexes may be nodal or infranodal. Infranodal AV block may occur at the level of the bundle of His, bundle branches, or distal fascicles. Infranodal AV block is almost always associated with bundle branch block and the immediate prognosis is more ominous when compared with that occurring at the AV node (Fig. 8.19).

■ Type I AV block is a common complication of acute inferior MI and is usually reversible since the block is at the level of the AV node.

## Treatment

■ **Symptomatic patients:**

■ For symptomatic patients with type I second-degree AV block that does not resolve, especially in patients with left

ventricular systolic dysfunction, the ACC/AHA/HRS guidelines recommend the insertion of a permanent pacemaker as a Class I indication regardless of the location of the AV block. (Class I means there is evidence or general agreement that the procedure is beneficial, useful, and effective.)

■ Patients with second-degree AV block with symptoms similar to those of the pacemaker syndrome; insertion of a permanent pacemaker is a Class IIa recommendation.

■ Patients with neuromuscular disease with second-degree AV block with or without symptoms; insertion of a permanent pacemaker is a Class IIb recommendation.

■ **Asymptomatic patients:** Type I second-degree AV nodal block is usually reversible and generally does not require any therapy. The cause of the AV block should be identified and corrected. The following are the ACC/AHA/HRS recommendations regarding insertion of permanent pacemakers in completely asymptomatic patients with type I second-degree AV block.

- **AV nodal block:**
  - ☐ If the block is AV nodal and the patient is hemodynamically stable and asymptomatic, with a heart rate >50 beats per minute (bpm), insertion of a permanent pacemaker is a Class III recommendation. Class III means that there is evidence or general agreement that the procedure is not useful and in some cases may be harmful.
  - ☐ If the block is AV nodal and is expected to resolve and unlikely to recur (such as effect of drugs, Lyme disease, hypoxia from sleep apnea), permanent pacing is also a Class III recommendation.
- **Infranodal block:**
  - ☐ If the AV block is infranodal, at the level of the bundle of His (intra-His) or bundle branches (infra-His), insertion of a permanent pacemaker is a Class IIa indication. This includes asymptomatic patients with infranodal block diagnosed during an electrophysiologic study for other indications.
- **Any level:** Some patients with second-degree AV block at any level may be completely asymptomatic, but may need permanent pacing for the following conditions:
  - ☐ Patients who develop second of third-degree AV block during exercise in the absence of myocardial ischemia. This is a Class I recommendation.
  - ☐ Myotonic muscular dystrophy, Erb dystrophy, and peroneal muscular dystrophy with any degree of AV block (including first-degree AV block) with or without symptoms because of unpredictable progression of AV conduction disease. This is a class IIb recommendation.
- Emergency treatment of symptomatic patients with bradycardia includes atropine (see Treatment of Complete AV Block in this Chapter) and if not effective, a temporary transvenous or transcutaneous pacemaker may be necessary before a permanent pacemaker can be implanted.
- Other pharmacologic agents that can be tried for treatment of the bradycardia before a pacemaker can be inserted include adrenergic agents such as isoproterenol, epinephrine, or dobutamine. These are further discussed under treatment of complete heart block in this chapter.

## Prognosis

- Type I AV block most often occurs at the level of the AV node and is usually reversible with a good prognosis. The AV block is often seen in normal healthy athletic individuals, especially during sleep.
- If the AV block occurs more distally at the level of the His-Purkinje system, structural cardiac disease is usually present. The overall prognosis in these patients will depend on the underlying cardiac abnormality. If the underlying cause is degenerative disease confined to the conduction system, the prognosis is similar to a patient without the conduction abnormality after a permanent pacemaker is implanted.

## Type II Second-Degree AV Block

- **Mobitz type II second-degree AV block:** Mobitz type II second-degree AV block is characterized by the following features:
  - Two or more consecutive P waves are conducted.
  - Only single P waves are blocked.
  - All PR intervals measure the same throughout. The PR interval is fixed and does not prolong before or shorten after a pause (Figs. 8.20 and 8.21).
  - The QRS complexes are usually wide (Figs. 8.20 and 8.21) because of the presence of bundle branch block.
  - The R-R intervals (distance between R waves) are constant and measure the same throughout as long as the sinus rhythm is stable—that is, the heart rate or P-P intervals are regular (Fig. 8.22).
- **Type II block with wide QRS complexes:** Mobitz type II second-degree AV block is always an infranodal block and occurs exclusively at the level of the

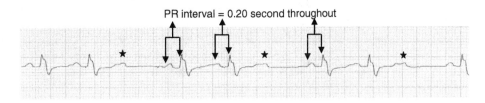

PR interval = 0.20 second throughout

**Figure 8.20:    Type II Second-Degree Atrioventricular (AV) Block.** In Mobitz type II AV block, the PR intervals are fixed and measure the same throughout. It does not lengthen before nor shorten after a QRS complex is dropped. Note that only single P waves are blocked (*stars*) and that the QRS complexes are wide because of the presence of a bundle branch block.

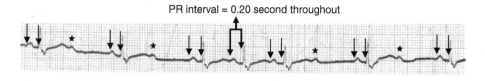

**Figure 8.21:**    **Type II Second-Degree Atrioventricular (AV) Block.** The PR intervals are fixed (distances between paired arrows measure 0.20 seconds throughout). The QRS complexes are wide and only single P waves are not conducted (*stars*).

His-Purkinje system (Fig. 8.23). Type II block is unlikely unless there is evidence of infranodal disease such as bundle branch block or anterior MI.

- **Type II block with narrow QRS complexes:** Type II block with narrow QRS complexes is possible, although rare. The block involves the His bundle (intra-His block) rather than the bundle branches. If the PR interval looks fixed, but the QRS complexes are narrow and no evidence of anterior MI is present, the block may be AV nodal rather than infranodal. More often, the PR interval looks fixed because there is only minimal prolongation in the surface electrocardiogram (ECG), which is difficult to demonstrate unless the PR interval is measured carefully (Fig. 8.24).

- **Treatment:** Even in completely asymptomatic patients, a permanent pacemaker should be considered when the diagnosis is type II second-degree AV block.

  - **Type II AV block with wide QRS complexes:** Insertion of a permanent pacemaker is a Class I indication for patients with type II second-degree AV block associated with wide QRS complexes.

  - **Type II AV block with narrow QRS complexes:** If the QRS complexes are narrow and type II second-degree AV block is present, insertion of a permanent pacemaker is a Class IIa indication. If the level of the AV block is uncertain, an electrophysiologic study should be performed before a permanent pacemaker is implanted.

- **Prognosis:** Because type II second-degree AV block is an infranodal disease, the immediate prognosis is more ominous than type I AV block, where the block is usually AV nodal (Fig. 8.25). Infranodal disease is associ-

ated with structural heart disease and is progressive and usually not reversible. When complete AV block occurs, it is usually sudden without warning.

## ECG Findings of Type II Second-degree AV Block

1. Two or more consecutive P waves are conducted.
2. Only single P waves are blocked.
3. The PR intervals are fixed and do not vary. The PR interval does not prolong before or shorten after the pause.
4. The QRS complexes are wide due to the presence of bundle branch block.
5. If the sinus rate is stable, the R-R intervals are fixed. The R-R interval between three successively conducted sinus complexes is equal to the R-R interval straddling the pause.

## Mechanism

- In Mobitz type II second-degree AV block, one bundle branch has a fixed block and the other bundle branch is intermittently blocked, resulting in P waves that are not conducted. The PR interval remains constant throughout. The PR interval immediately after the pause should not shorten and should measure the same as the PR interval before the pause.

- Mobitz type II second-degree AV block occurs exclusively at the His-Purkinje system, usually at the level of the bundle branches. Although the block can occur within the His bundle, an intra-His block is rare. Before the diagnosis of type II block is secured, there should be evidence of infranodal disease in the form of left bundle branch block or right bundle

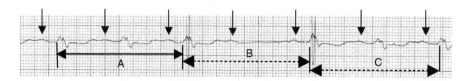

**Figure 8.22:**    **Constant R-R Intervals.** In type II second-degree atrioventricular (AV) block, the R-R intervals are constant because the PR intervals are also constant. Distance **A** and **C** with three consecutive complexes measure the same as distance **B** with a dropped QRS complex. Thus, the RR interval straddling a pause (distance **B**) measures the same as the R-R interval straddling a conducted sinus impulse (**A** or **C**). The P waves are marked by the arrows.

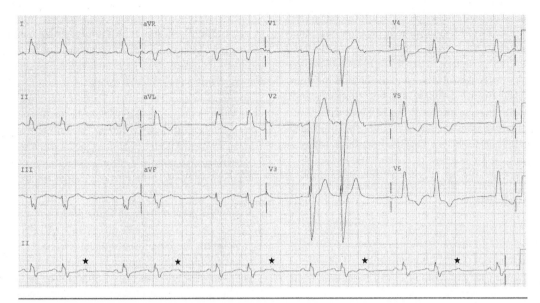

**Figure 8.23:    Mobitz Type II Second-Degree Atrioventricular (AV) Block.** The 12-lead electro-cardiogram shows all the findings of type II second-degree AV block. The PR interval is fixed, only single P waves are blocked (*stars*), two consecutive P waves are conducted, and there is left bundle branch block.

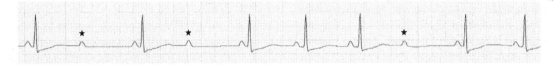

**Figure 8.24:    Fixed PR Interval with Narrow QRS Complexes.** The PR interval looks fixed and the QRS complexes are narrow. However, if the PR interval is measured carefully, there is subtle shortening imme-diately after the pause. Shortening of the PR interval after a pause suggests type I second-degree atrioventric-ular block. The stars identify the nonconducted P waves.

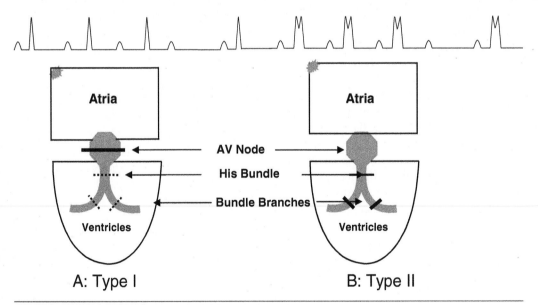

**Figure 8.25:    Location of Atrioventricular (AV) Block.** In type I second-degree AV block or AV Wenckebach **(A)**, the AV block is almost always at the AV node although it can also occur anywhere in the His-Purkinje system. In type II second-degree AV block **(B)**, the AV block occurs exclusively at the bundle of His, bundle branches, and distal conduction system. The lines transecting the AV conduction system indi-cate the potential sites of AV block.

branch block with or without fascicular block. When one bundle branch is blocked, intermittent block of the other bundle causes the QRS complex to be dropped intermittently. If the QRS complex is narrow and the PR interval looks fixed, the possibility of a block at the level of the bundle of His is likely (intra-His block), although this is rare and, more commonly, may be due to AV nodal block with minimal prolongation of the PR interval that may be difficult to appreciate in the surface ECG unless the PR interval is measured carefully.

## Clinical Significance

■ Type II block is an infranodal disease involving the bundle of His, and, more commonly, the bundle branches and fascicles. Type II block does not occur at the level of the AV node.

■ It is a common mistake to include 2:1 AV block as Mobitz type II block. It is not possible to distinguish type I from type II block when there is 2:1 AV block because prolongation of the PR interval cannot be observed when only one P wave is conducted. In 2:1 AV block, the PR interval looks fixed because only a single P wave is conducted.

■ When an acute infarct is complicated by type II second-degree AV block, the location of the infarct is anterior. Even with insertion of a pacemaker, mortality remains high because an anterior infarct with second-degree AV block is usually an extensive infarct.

■ If there is difficulty in differentiating type I (usually AV nodal) from type II (always infranodal) block, sympathetic and parasympathetic manipulation may be tried. Both sinus node and AV node are influenced by sympathetic and parasympathetic stimulation, whereas the intraventricular conduction system below the AV node is affected mainly by sympathetic but not by parasympathetic stimuli. Sympathetic stimulation such as exercise increases the rate of the sinus node and enhances conduction across the AV node. Atropine and adrenergic agents can cause the same effect. Thus, exercise, atropine, or adrenergic agents will increase the sinus rate and will also improve AV nodal block, but will not improve and may even worsen type II or infranodal block. On the other hand, parasympathetic stimulation such as carotid sinus compression can improve infranodal block by slowing the sinus rate and prolonging AV conduction, thus allowing the distal conduction system and infranodal block more time to recover.

■ Type II block is usually caused by structural cardiac disease such as sclerosis or calcification of the conducting system resulting from aging. It can also be due to ischemia, infarction, and infiltrative diseases including sarcoid, amyloid, and neuromuscular dystrophy. It can occur postoperatively after cardiac surgery or ablation procedures.

## Treatment

■ Because type II block is an infranodal disease, a permanent pacemaker should be inserted even in asymptomatic pa-

tients. If type II AV block is associated with wide QRS complexes, this is a Class I indication for permanent pacing, according to the ACC/AHA/HRS guidelines. If the QRS complexes are narrow, the recommendation becomes Class IIa.

■ Patients with type II block can develop complete heart block suddenly without warning. Thus, a transcutaneous pacemaker or a temporary pacemaker should be available even if the patient is not bradycardic. If the patient suddenly develops complete AV block before a pacemaker can be inserted, adrenergic agents such as isoproterenol or epinephrine may be given to increase the intrinsic rate of the escape rhythm. Infranodal block will not respond to atropine (see Treatment of Complete AV Block in this Chapter).

■ When the QRS complexes are narrow and the PR intervals look fixed, the diagnosis of Mobitz type II block may be questionable. If the diagnosis of type II block is uncertain, an electrophysiologic study may be necessary to ascertain that the block is infranodal before a permanent pacemaker is implanted, especially in asymptomatic patients with second-degree AV block.

## Prognosis

■ Because type II block is an infranodal disease, the immediate prognosis is more ominous than type I second-degree AV block. When complete AV block occurs, the escape rhythm has to originate below the level of the block. Thus, only a ventricular escape rhythm can come to the rescue. Unlike type I block, type II block is commonly associated with structural heart disease; therefore, the conduction abnormality is usually not reversible and progression to complete AV block may be sudden without warning (see complete AV block).

■ The overall prognosis of type II block depends on the presence or absence of associated cardiac abnormalities.

■ If the AV block is confined to the conduction system and no evidence of structural cardiac disease is present, insertion of a permanent pacemaker to correct the conduction abnormality will result in the same natural history as a patient without the conduction abnormality.

■ If the conduction abnormality is associated with structural cardiac disease, such as ischemic heart disease or cardiomyopathy, the prognosis will depend on the etiology of the cardiac abnormality.

## Advanced 2:1 Second-Degree AV Block

■ **Advanced second-degree AV block:** 2:1 AV block is an example of advanced second-degree AV block.

■ In 2:1 block, every other P wave is conducted alternating with every other P wave that is blocked (Figs. 8.26 and 8.27).

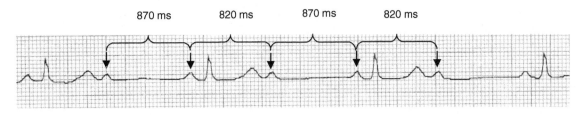

**Figure 8.26: 2:1 Second-Degree Atrioventricular (AV) Block with Narrow QRS Complexes.** Every other P wave is conducted alternating with every other P wave that is blocked (*arrows*) consistent with 2:1 AV block. Two to one AV block is not a type II block because only a single P wave is conducted. Note that the QRS complexes are narrow, thus an infranodal block is unlikely. Because there is no evidence of distal conduction system disease, the 2:1 AV block is most likely at the level of the AV node. Note also that the P-P interval with a QRS complex is shorter (820 milliseconds) than the P-P interval without a QRS complex (870 milliseconds) because of ventriculophasic sinus arrhythmia.

- The QRS complexes may be narrow or wide (Figs. 8.26 and 8.27).

- A common error is to include 2:1 AV block as a type II block because the PR interval is fixed. Two to one AV block is neither type I nor type II second-degree block. The PR interval looks fixed because only a single P wave is conducted, thus only one PR interval can be measured. To differentiate type I from type II block, at least two consecutive P waves should be conducted so that the lengthening of the PR interval can be observed.

- **Ventriculophasic sinus arrhythmia:** During 2:1 AV block, sinus arrhythmia may be present. The sinus arrhythmia is ventriculophasic if the P-P interval with a QRS complex is shorter than the P-P interval without a QRS complex (Fig. 8.26).

- 2:1 AV block may be nodal or infranodal. To differentiate one from the other, continuous monitoring should be performed until conduction improves and more than one consecutive P wave is conducted (3:2 or better). When this occurs, the level of the AV block may be localized.
  - When conduction improves and 2:1 block is seen in association with type I block, the block is AV nodal (Fig. 8.28).
  - When conduction improves and 2:1 block is seen in association with type II block (fixed PR intervals and wide QRS complexes), the block is infranodal (Fig. 8.29).

- **Acute MI and AV block:** When 2:1 block complicates acute MI, the location of the infarct is helpful in identifying the level of the AV block. If the infarct is inferior and the QRS complexes are narrow, the AV block is at the level of the AV node (Fig. 8.30).

## Advanced Second-Degree AV Block: 3:1 and Higher

- **Advanced second-degree AV block:** When the AV block is 2:1, 3:1, 4:1, or higher, the AV block cannot be classified as type I or type II because only a single P wave is conducted (2:1 block) or two or more consecutive P waves are blocked (3:1 AV block or higher). These are examples of advanced second-degree AV block (Figs. 8.31–8.33).

- The conduction ratio refers to the number of P waves that are blocked before a P wave is conducted. Thus, a 3:1 conduction ratio implies that of three consecutive P waves, only one is conducted.

- Advanced AV block with narrow QRS complexes may be nodal or infranodal (Figs. 8.31 and 8.32). When the QRS complexes are wide, the block is almost always infranodal (Fig. 8.33).

## ECG Findings of Advanced Second-Degree AV Block

1. Advanced or high-grade AV block is a form of second-degree block where two or more consecutive P waves are not

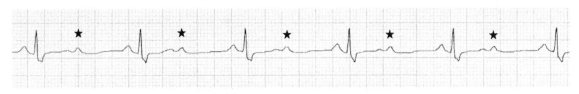

**Figure 8.27: 2:1 Second-Degree Atrioventricular (AV) Block with Wide QRS Complexes.** The rhythm is 2:1 AV block similar to Figure 8.26. In this example, the QRS complexes are wide because of right bundle branch block, a sign of distal conduction system disease. This type of 2:1 block can be infranodal occurring at the level of the bundle branches although AV nodal block is also possible. The stars point to the nonconducted P waves.

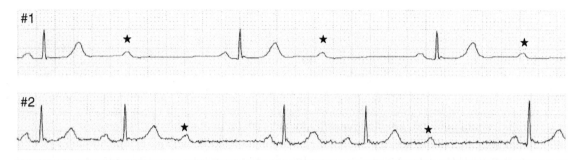

**Figure 8.28: 2:1 Second-Degree Atrioventricular (AV) Block Occurring with AV Wenckebach.**
Rhythm strip 1 shows 2:1 AV block. Rhythm strip 2 is from the same patient taken several minutes later showing 3:2 AV Wenckebach. Because 2:1 AV block is seen in association with classical AV Wenckebach with narrow complexes, the 2:1 block is at the level of the AV node. The stars identify the blocked P waves.

conducted as in 3:1, 4:1, or 5:1 AV block. A 2:1 AV block is also included as a form of advanced second-degree AV block because only a single P wave is conducted.

2. The QRS complexes may be narrow or wide.
3. The long pauses are often terminated by escape beats.

## Mechanism

- Advanced second-degree AV block can occur at the level of the AV node (AV nodal block). It can also occur more distally at the level of the His-Purkinje system (infranodal block).
  - **AV nodal block:** Advanced second-degree AV block occurring at the AV node may have narrow or wide QRS complexes, although typically the QRS complexes are narrow.
  - **Infranodal block:** Advanced second-degree AV block can occur at the level of the bundle of His or more distally at the level of the bundle branches. The QRS complexes may be narrow or wide, although typically the QRS complexes are wide.

☐ **Bundle of His:** Advanced second-degree block can occur at the level of the bundle of His, but this type of AV block (intra-His block) is uncommon. The QRS complexes are narrow.

☐ **Bundle branches:** When the block is at the level of the bundle branches, the baseline ECG will show wide QRS complexes because of right or left bundle branch block.

- Ventriculophasic sinus arrhythmia may occur when there is 2:1 AV block. The P-P interval with a QRS complex is shorter than the P-P interval without a QRS complex. The P-P interval with a QRS complex has stroke volume that can stretch the carotid baroreceptors, causing vagal inhibition that is most pronounced in the next cardiac cycle. This results in a longer P-P interval in the cardiac cycle without a QRS complex.

## Clinical Significance

- It is a common mistake to classify 2:1 AV block always as a type II block because the PR interval is fixed. Because there is

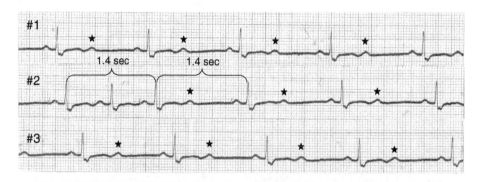

**Figure 8.29: 2:1 Second-Degree Atrioventricular (AV) Block with Wide QRS Complexes.** The rhythm strips labeled 1, 2, and 3 are continuous. Rhythm strip 1 shows 2:1 AV block; rhythm strip 2 shows three consecutively conducted P waves with a classical Mobitz type II pattern. The PR interval is fixed and the R-R interval is also fixed. In rhythm strip 3, 2:1 AV block is again present. The transient occurrence of Mobitz type II AV block, which is an infranodal block, suggests that the 2:1 block is infranodal, occurring at the level of the bundle branches. The stars identify the blocked P waves.

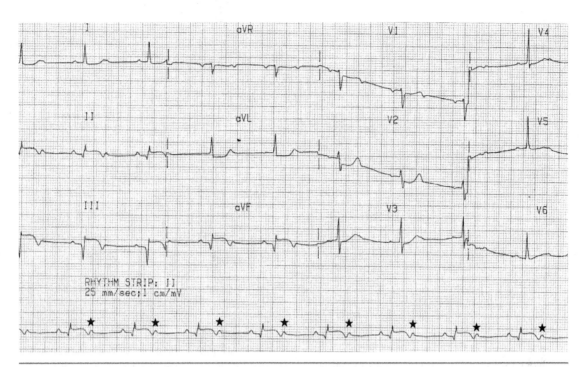

**Figure 8.30: Two to One Atrioventricular (AV) Block and Acute Inferior Myocardial Infarction (MI).** Twelve-lead electrocardiogram showing 2:1 AV block with narrow QRS complexes occurring as a complication of acute inferior MI. The stars identify the P waves that are not conducted. The presence of acute inferior MI with narrow QRS complexes localizes the AV block at the level of the AV node.

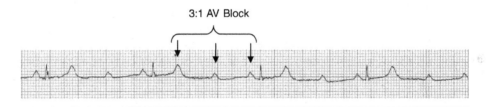

**Figure 8.31: Advanced Second-Degree Atrioventricular (AV) Block.** The rhythm is normal sinus with 3:1 AV block (*bracket*). The QRS complexes are narrow. When the QRS complexes are narrow, the block may be nodal or infranodal, but is usually nodal. The P waves are marked by the arrows.

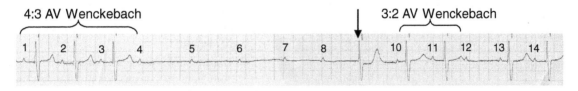

**Figure 8.32: Advanced Second-Degree Atrioventricular (AV) Block.** There are five consecutive P waves (labeled 4 to 8) that are not conducted. The pause is terminated by a junctional escape complex (*arrow*). Beats 1 to 4 and 10 to 12 show classical AV Wenckebach with gradual lengthening of the PR interval followed by a P wave that is not conducted (beats 4 and 12). The PR interval shortens immediately after the pause (beat 13). The presence of classical AV Wenckebach with narrow complexes indicates that the advanced AV block is at the level of the AV node. The presence of an AV junctional escape complex also indicates that the block is AV nodal.

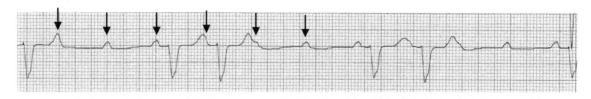

**Figure 8.33:   Advanced (3:1) Second-Degree Atrioventricular (AV) Block.** When advanced second-degree AV block has wide QRS complexes, the block is almost always infranodal. In this example, one bundle branch has a fixed blocked and the other bundle branch is intermittently blocked, resulting in nonconducted P waves. The arrows identify the P waves.

only a single conducted P wave and the next P wave is blocked, there is only one PR interval that can be measured. Thus, it is not possible to classify 2:1 block as type I or type II. At least two consecutive P waves should be conducted to differentiate type I from type II block. A 2:1 AV block is an example of advanced AV block. It is preferable to leave the diagnosis of 2:1 block simply as 2:1 second-degree AV block without specifying that the AV block is type I or type II.

■ Infranodal block implies a more serious conduction abnormality than AV nodal block. The location of the conduction abnormality can be identified as nodal or infranodal by the following features.

  ■ When 2:1 AV block or a higher conduction ratio, such as 3:1 or 4:1 AV block is associated with AV Wenckebach with narrow QRS complexes, the block is at the level of the AV node.

  ■ When 2:1 AV block or a higher conduction ratio is associated with type II block with a fixed PR interval and wide QRS complexes, the block is below the AV node.

  ■ When advanced AV block is associated with the use of pharmacologic agents that can block the AV node (beta blockers, calcium blockers, or digitalis), the block is AV nodal.

  ■ When advanced AV block occurs in the setting of an acute infarction:

    □ If the infarct is inferior, the block is AV nodal. The QRS complexes are narrow.

    □ If the infarct is anterior, the block is infranodal. This is usually associated with wide QRS complexes.

  ■ If the AV block is infranodal, evidence of infranodal disease, such as right or left bundle branch block, should be present. In general, advanced AV block with wide QRS complexes with a conduction ratio of 3:1 or higher commonly involves the His-Purkinje system.

  ■ If an escape beat is present, the origin of the escape complex may be helpful in localizing the level of the AV block.

    □ If the escape beat has a narrow QRS complex, the block is AV nodal. A block within the bundle of His (intra-His) is possible but uncommon.

    □ If the escape complex is wide, the AV block is usually infranodal.

  □ The causes of advanced second-degree AV block are identical to those of types I and II AV block.

## Treatment

■ Advanced AV block, including 2:1 AV block at the level of the AV node, is usually transient with a good prognosis. Therapy is not required if the patient is asymptomatic and the heart rate exceeds 50 bpm. However, if symptoms related to bradycardia occur, atropine is the drug of choice (see Treatment of Complete AV Block in this Chapter). Atropine is not effective if the AV block is infranodal. An intravenous adrenergic agent such as isoproterenol, 2 to 10 mcg/minute or epinephrine 2 to 20 mcg/minute, may be given emergently as a continuous infusion until a transvenous (or transcutaneous) pacemaker becomes available. The dose is titrated according to the desired heart rate (see Treatment of Complete AV Block in this Chapter).

■ In patients where the AV block is not reversible, a permanent pacemaker is indicated. The following are indications for insertion of permanent pacemaker in advanced second-degree AV block according to the ACC/AHA/HRS guidelines.

  ■ **Symptomatic patients:** For patients with advanced second-degree AV block who have symptoms or ventricular arrhythmias related to the bradycardia, insertion of a permanent pacemaker is a Class I recommendation regardless of the anatomic level of the AV block.

  ■ **Asymptomatic patients:** In asymptomatic patients with advanced second-degree AV block, permanent pacing is a Class I indication in the following conditions regardless of the site of the AV block.

    □ Patients with arrhythmias and other medical conditions that require drugs that can cause symptomatic bradycardia.

    □ Documented asystole ≥3.0 seconds or any escape rate <40 bpm in patients with sinus rhythm who are awake and asymptomatic.

    □ In patients with atrial fibrillation with ≥1 pauses of ≥5 seconds.

    □ After catheter ablation of the AV junction.

    □ Postcardiac surgery AV block that is not expected to resolve.

    □ Neuromuscular diseases including myotonic muscular dystrophy, Kearns-Sayre syndrome, Erb dystrophy, and peroneal muscular atrophy with or without symptoms.

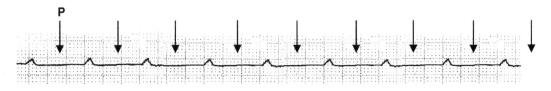

**Figure 8.34:** **Third-Degree or Complete Atrioventricular (AV) Block.** In complete AV block, it is not possible for any atrial impulse to propagate to the ventricles, therefore only P waves (and no QRS complexes) will be present. Unless the ventricles are activated by another impulse originating below the level of the block, the ventricles will remain asystolic, resulting in syncope or sudden death.

☐ During exercise in the absence of myocardial ischemia.

☐ Asymptomatic patients with advanced AV block at the infranodal level diagnosed during electrophysiologic study for other indications. This is a Class IIa recommendation.

☐ AV block that is expected to resolve or unlikely to recur such as those resulting from drug toxicity, Lyme disease, or during hypoxia related to sleep apnea in the absence of symptoms is a Class III recommendation.

## Prognosis

■ The prognosis of high-grade AV block depends on the etiology of the AV block. Patients with isolated advanced AV block resulting from degenerative disease of the conduction system may have the same prognosis as those without advanced AV block after a permanent pacemaker is implanted.

## Third-Degree or Complete AV Block

■ **Complete or third-degree AV block:** In complete or third-degree AV block, there is complete failure of all atrial impulses to conduct to the ventricles; therefore,

only P waves will be present (Fig. 8.34). These P waves are unable to reach the ventricles because they are blocked or interrupted somewhere in the AV conduction system (Fig. 8.35). Unless an escape rhythm comes to the rescue, the ventricles will remain asystolic and the patient will develop syncope or die suddenly.

■ The origin of the escape rhythm will depend on the location of the AV block. These escape complexes are completely independent from the sinus P waves, resulting in complete dissociation between the P waves and the QRS complexes.

## Localizing the AV Block

■ Complete AV block may occur at the level of the AV node or it may be infranodal, occurring below the AV node anywhere in the His bundle, bundle branches, and more distal conduction system.

■ **AV nodal block:** If complete AV block occurs at the level of the AV node, a junctional escape rhythm usually comes to the rescue.

■ **AV junctional escape rhythm:** The AV junction includes the AV node all the way down to the bifurca-

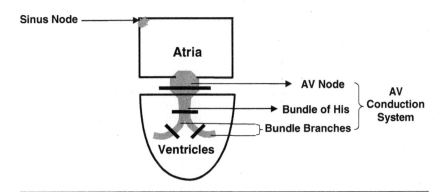

**Figure 8.35:** **Complete Atrioventricular (AV) Block.** Complete AV block can occur anywhere along the AV conduction system. It can occur at the AV node or bundle of His. It can involve both bundle branches simultaneously or the right bundle plus both fascicles of the left bundle branch. When complete AV block is present, the location of the conduction abnormality should always be identified because prognosis will depend on the location of the AV block.

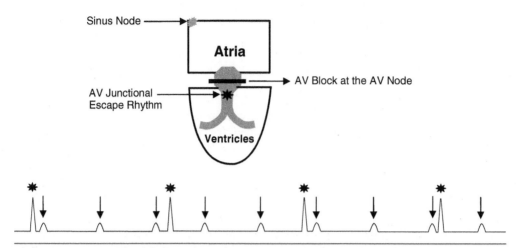

**Figure 8.36:    Complete Atrioventricular (AV) block with Narrow QRS Complexes.** If complete AV block occurs at the level of the AV node, a junctional escape rhythm (*star*) comes to the rescue. The QRS complexes are narrow because the impulse originates above the bifurcation of the bundle of His and can activate both ventricles simultaneously. Arrows point to sinus P waves, which are completely dissociated from the QRS complexes.

tion of the bundle of His. The escape rhythm usually originates below the AV node at its junction with the bundle of His. Any impulse originating above the bifurcation of the bundle of His such as a junctional rhythm can activate both ventricles simultaneously, resulting in a narrow QRS complex (Fig. 8.36). The presence of AV junctional rhythm indicates that the block is at the level of the AV node. If the AV junction is suppressed or inhibited or is structurally abnormal, a ventricular escape rhythm may come to the rescue.

- **Ventricular escape rhythm:** A ventricular escape rhythm has wide QRS complexes because it originates below the bifurcation of the bundle of His (Fig. 8.37). The presence of a ventricular escape rhythm usually indicates that the block is infranodal, although the AV block may occasionally occur at the level of the AV node.

- **Infranodal block:** When the block is infranodal, it usually occurs at the level of the bundle branches or fascicles. It can also occur at the level of the bundle of His, although a block at the level of the bundle of His (intra-His block) is rare. When the block is infranodal, only a ventricular escape rhythm with wide QRS complexes can come to the rescue. The QRS complexes are wide because the impulse originates below the bifurcation of the bundle of His; thus, the ventricles are not activated simultaneously. Conduction of the impulse is delayed and is transmitted from one ventricle to the other by muscle cell to muscle cell conduction. A junctional escape rhythm cannot come to the rescue because it will not be able to continue down the conducting system and will not be able to reach the ventricles.

- The origin of the escape rhythm is helpful in localizing the level of the AV block as shown in Figure 8.19.

- The presence of an acute MI is useful in localizing the AV block.

  - **Acute anterior MI:** When complete AV block occurs in the setting of an acute anterior MI, the AV block is infranodal. The AV block is frequently preceded by left or right bundle branch block and the escape rhythm is ventricular (Fig. 8.38).

  - **Acute inferior MI:** When complete AV block occurs in the setting of an acute inferior MI, the AV block is at the AV node (Fig. 8.39).

- Figure 8.39 shows acute inferior MI with complete AV dissociation. The presence of acute inferior MI with junctional rhythm (narrow QRS complexes) suggests that the AV block is at the level of the AV node.

- Although a junctional escape rhythm points to the AV node as the site of the AV block, a ventricular escape rhythm does not indicate that the AV block is always infranodal. In Figure 8.40, the first three escape complexes are ventricular, suggesting an infranodal location of the AV block. The last three escape complexes, however, are narrow and are junctional in origin. This makes an infranodal block highly unlikely. The presence of junctional escape complexes therefore suggests that the AV block is AV nodal.

- The surface ECG is an excellent diagnostic tool in localizing the level of AV block, making electrophysiologic testing rarely necessary. However, when the level of AV block remains uncertain, intracardiac ECG may be used to verify the exact location of the AV conduction abnormality.

- Intracardiac ECG can be obtained by inserting an electrode catheter into a vein and advancing it to the right ventricle at the area of the bundle of His.

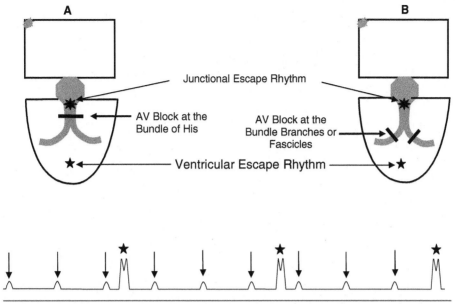

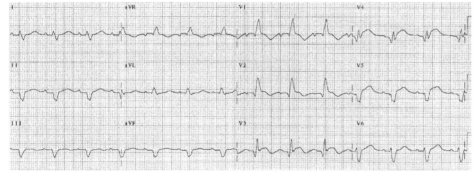

**Figure 8.37: Complete Atrioventricular (AV) Block with Wide QRS Complexes.** The atrial impulses, identified by the arrows, cannot conduct to the ventricles because of complete AV block, which can occur at the level of the bundle of His **(A)** or bundle branches and fascicles **(B)**. A block at the level of the bundle of His is possible but is rare. When there is infranodal block, the QRS complexes are wide because the escape rhythm originates from the ventricles (*star*). It is not possible for a junctional escape rhythm (*asterisk*) to come to the rescue because the origin of the impulse is proximal to the block and will not be able to propagate to the ventricles.

A: Acute anteroseptal MI:

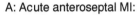

**Figure 8.38: Atrioventricular (AV) Block Complicating Acute Anterior Myocardial Infarction (MI).** Electrocardiogram (ECG) **A** shows acute anteroseptal MI complicated by first-degree AV block, right bundle branch block, and left anterior fascicular block. ECG **B** shows complete AV dissociation. The P waves are marked by the arrows.

B: Complete AV dissociation:

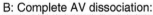

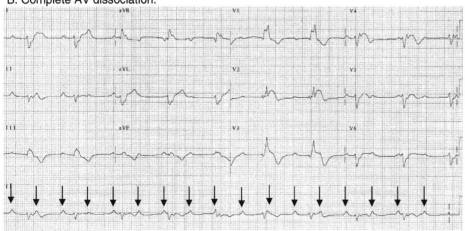

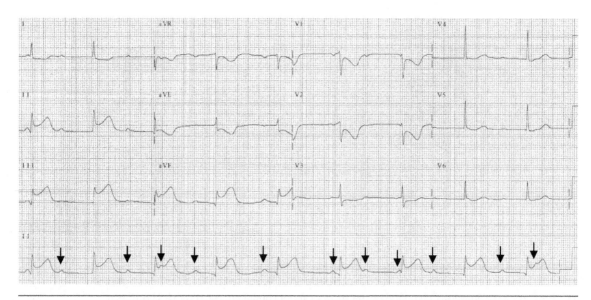

**Figure 8.39:    Acute Inferior Myocardial Infarction (MI) with Complete Atrioventricular (AV) Dissociation.** When acute inferior MI is accompanied by AV dissociation, the AV block is at the level of the AV node. The arrows identify the P waves. Note also that the escape rhythm is AV junctional with narrow QRS complexes.

- **Surface ECG:** When the atria and ventricles are activated by the sinus impulse, the surface ECG records a P wave, which corresponds to atrial activation and a QRS complex, which corresponds to ventricular activation (Fig. 8.41A).

- **Intracardiac ECG:** The intracardiac ECG will be able to record not only atrial (A) and ventricular (V) activation, which corresponds to the P wave and QRS complex in the surface ECG, but can also record activation of the His bundle (H), which is represented as a deflection between the P wave and the QRS complex (Fig. 8.41B).

## Intracardiac ECG or His Bundle Recording

- The His deflection allows the PR or A-V interval to be divided into two components:
  - **A-H interval:** This represents conduction between atria and His bundle corresponding to the transmission of the impulse across the AV node.

- **H-V interval:** This represents conduction between the His bundle and ventricles corresponding to the transmission of impulse in the bundle branches and distal conduction system.

- When an atrial impulse is blocked and is not followed by a QRS complex, the intracardiac recording can localize the AV block.
  - **AV nodal:** If the atrial impulse is not followed by His deflection (and ventricular complex), the AV block is AV nodal (Fig. 8.42A).
  - **Infranodal:** If the atrial impulse is followed by His spike but not a ventricular complex, the AV block is infranodal (Fig. 8.42B).
  - **Intra-His:** The atrial impulse can be blocked at the level of the bundle of His (intra-His block), although this is rare.

- In complete AV block, the ventricular rate should always be slower than the atrial rate and not the other way around. The ventricles and AV conduction system should be given enough time to recover so that the atrial

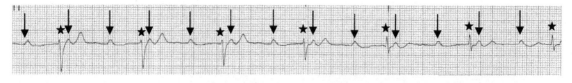

**Figure 8.40:    Complete Atrioventricular (AV) Block.** The presence of ventricular escape rhythm does not indicate that the block is always infranodal. The rhythm strip shows complete AV block. The QRS complexes are marked by the stars. The first three complexes are wide and represent ventricular escape complexes suggesting that the AV block is infranodal. The last three complexes, however, are narrow, representing junctional rhythm that makes an infranodal block unlikely.

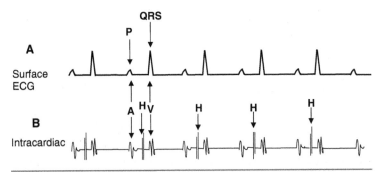

**Figure 8.41:   The Surface Electrocardiogram (ECG) and Intracardiac Recording.** The surface ECG is capable of recording only the P wave and the QRS complex, whereas an intracardiac study is capable of recording not only atrial (A) and ventricular (V) activation but also that of the His (H) bundle. The presence of the His deflection allows the PR interval to be divided into two main components: the A-H interval (atrium to His interval), which represents conduction through the AV node (normal 60 to 125 milliseconds) and H-V interval, which represents conduction through the distal conduction system between the His bundle and ventricles (normal, 35 to 55 milliseconds).

impulse will not find the ventricles refractory. Thus, the ventricular rate should not only be slower than the atrial rate but should be <50 bpm, usually in the low to mid-40s before the AV block is considered complete.

■ Complete AV block can occur regardless of the atrial rhythm, which could be normal sinus (Fig. 8.43), atrial flutter (Fig. 8.44), or atrial fibrillation (Fig. 8.45).

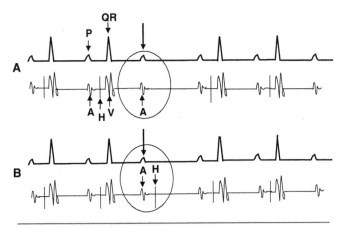

**Figure 8.42:   Intracardiac Electrocardiogram (ECG).** **(A)** Atrioventricular (AV) block at the level of the AV node. The surface ECG shows a P wave that is not conducted (arrow). The intracardiac ECG shows an atrial deflection **(A)** that is not followed by a His deflection thus the AV block is AV nodal. **(B)** AV block involving the distal conduction system. The surface ECG shows a P wave that is not conducted (*arrow*). Intracardiac ECG shows an atrial deflection followed by a His deflection but not a ventricular deflection suggesting that the AV block is distal to the His bundle at the bundle branches and distal conduction system. A, atrial complex; H, His spike; V, ventricular complex.

## Common Mistakes in AV Block

■ **Sinus arrest:** When only QRS complexes are present and atrial activity is absent (no P waves), the rhythm is sinus arrest and not complete AV block (Figs. 8.46 and 8.47).

■ **Complete AV block versus advanced second-degree AV block:** In complete AV block, there should be complete dissociation between the P waves and the QRS complexes. If a single P wave captures a QRS complex, the AV block is no longer complete (Fig. 8.48).

■ **Blocked Premature Atrial Complexes (PACs):** Blocked premature atrial complexes may be mistaken for nonconducted sinus P waves and mistaken for second-degree AV block (Fig. 8.49).

■ **Concealed conduction:** Concealed conduction is commonly mistaken for AV block. Concealed conduction indicates that a previous impulse had infiltrated the conduction system. This will have an effect on the next impulse. Figure 8.50 shows a sinus P wave (star) that is not followed by a QRS complex. This can be mistaken for second-degree AV block. Although a nonconducted sinus P wave is obvious, there is a premature ventricular impulse preceding the P wave. This premature impulse depolarized not only the ventricles, but also the AV conduction system retrogradely, rendering the AV node refractory. The effect of the premature impulse on the conduction system is not apparent until the arrival of the next sinus impulse, which is unable to conduct to the ventricles because the AV node is still refractory. This is an example of concealed conduction and not second-degree AV block. Figure 8.51 is a similar example of concealed conduction showing sinus P waves that are not conducted (arrows). The blocked P waves are preceded by premature ventricular complexes.

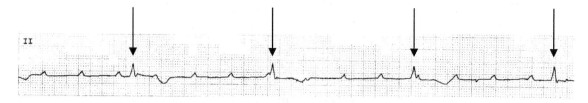

**Figure 8.43: Complete Atrioventricular (AV) Block.** The rhythm is normal sinus with a rate of 96 beats per minute. The ventricular rate is 26 beats per minute (*arrows*). Note that the P waves are completely dissociated and have no relation to the QRS complexes because complete AV block. Note also that the atrial rate is faster than the ventricular rate.

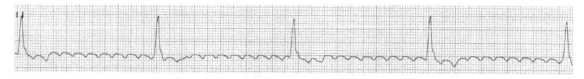

**Figure 8.44: Complete Atrioventricular (AV) Block.** The rhythm is atrial flutter. The ventricular rate is slow and regular and is <30 beats per minute because of complete AV block. The presence of wide QRS complexes indicates that the escape rhythm is ventricular in origin and suggests that the block is infranodal.

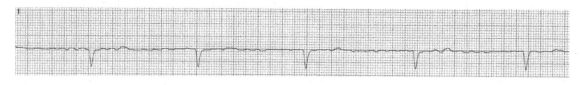

**Figure 8.45: Complete Atrioventricular (AV) Block.** The rhythm is atrial fibrillation with complete AV block with a slow ventricular rate of approximately 33 beats per minute. The QRS complexes are wide and regular, suggesting that the escape rhythm is ventricular in origin. This favors an infranodal block. In atrial fibrillation, the R-R intervals are irregularly irregular. When the R-R intervals suddenly become regular, complete AV block should always be considered.

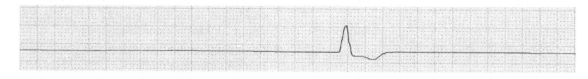

**Figure 8.46: This is Not Complete Atrioventricular (AV) Block.** Because there is no atrial activity, atrioventricular block is not present. The underlying mechanism is due to complete absence of sinus node activity (sinus arrest) because of sick sinus syndrome. The sinus arrest is terminated by a ventricular escape complex.

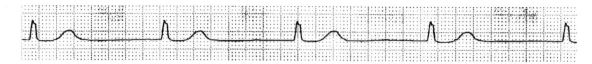

**Figure 8.47: Sinus Node Dysfunction Mistaken for Complete Atrioventricular Block.** Again, there is no evidence of atrial activity; therefore, atrioventricular (AV) block is not present. The rhythm is AV junctional with a slow ventricular rate of 39 beats per minute because of sick sinus syndrome.

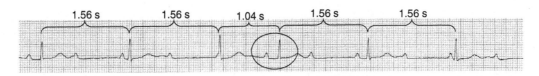

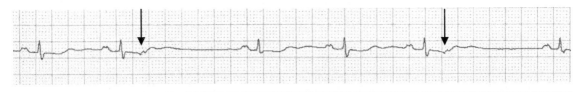

**Figure 8.48:    Advanced Atrioventricular Block (AV) Mistaken for Complete AV Block.**  The P wave with a circle captures a QRS complex resulting in sudden shortening of the R-R interval to 1.04 seconds. If one P wave is able to capture the ventricles as shown, the atrioventricular (AV) block is not complete. This is an example of advanced but not complete AV block.

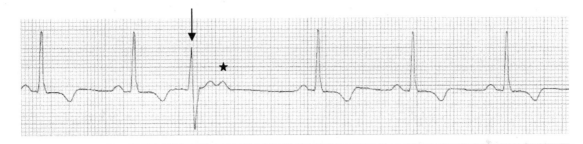

**Figure 8.49:    Blocked Premature Atrial Complexes (PACs) Resembling Second-Degree Atrioventricular (AV) Block.**  The blocked PACs are marked by the arrows. Note that the P waves are premature and are followed by pauses. These nonconducted premature atrial complexes may be mistaken for sinus P waves and the rhythm can be mistaken for second-degree AV block.

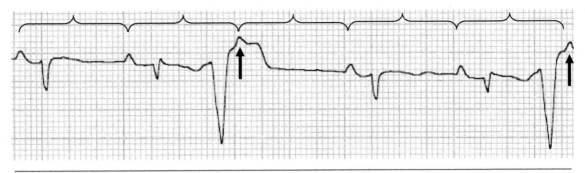

**Figure 8.50:    Concealed Conduction.**  The rhythm strip shows a sinus P wave without a QRS complex (*star*), which can be mistaken for second-degree atrioventricular (AV) block. Preceding the sinus P wave is a premature ventricular complex (*arrow*) that retrogradely penetrated the AV conduction system, making the AV node refractory. Thus, the next sinus impulse was not conducted. This is an example of concealed conduction and not second-degree AV block.

**Figure 8.51:    Concealed Conduction.**  Sinus P waves without QRS complexes (*arrows*) are noted only after every ventricular ectopic impulse. This is an example of concealed conduction and not second-degree atrioventricular block.

## TABLE 8.1

### Indications for Insertion of Permanent Cardiac Pacemakers in Patients with Acquired AV Block in Adults

| Third-degree and advanced second-degree AV block at any anatomic level | **Symptomatic individuals:** Bradycardia causes symptoms (including heart failure) or ventricular arrhythmias presumed to be due to AV block.<br>**Asymptomatic individuals:**<br>• Arrhythmias and other medical conditions that require drug therapy that results in symptomatic bradycardia.<br>• Documented asystole of ≥3.0 seconds or escape rate is <40 beats per minute in awake or asymptomatic patients in sinus rhythm.<br>• Atrial fibrillation and bradycardia of ≥1 or more episodes of ≥5 seconds duration.<br>• Heart rate >40 beats per minute when awake but with persistent third-degree AV block with cardiomegaly or left ventricular dysfunction.<br>• Second or third-degree AV block during exercise in the absence of myocardial ischemia.<br>**After cardiac procedures:**<br>• Postablation of the AV junction<br>• AV block occurring after cardiac surgery that is not expected to resolve<br>**AV block Associated with neuromuscular diseases:[a]**<br>• The patient may be symptomatic or asymptomatic |
|---|---|
| Type II second-degree AV block | **Symptomatic patients:**<br>• Symptomatic patients because of bradycardia.<br>**Asymptomatic patients:**<br>• Type II second-degree AV block with wide QRS complexes.<br>• Type II second-degree AV block with narrow QRS complexes (Class IIa). |
| Type I second-degree AV block | **Symptomatic individuals:**<br>• Symptoms of low output and hypotension because of bradycardia regardless of the level of AV block.<br>• Patient may not be bradycardic but symptoms are similar to pacemaker syndrome (Class IIa).<br>**Asymptomatic individuals:**<br>• AV block at or below the level of the bundle of His usually diagnosed during electrophysiological study performed for other indications (Class IIa).<br>**Patients with neuromuscular disease:[a]**<br>• Patients may be symptomatic or asymptomatic (Class IIb). |
| Marked first-degree AV block | **Symptomatic individuals:**<br>• Symptoms of low output and hypotension similar to pacemaker syndrome in patients with left ventricular dysfunction or congestive heart failure. The symptoms should be improved by temporary AV pacing (Class IIa).<br>**Patients with neuromuscular disease:[a]**<br>• Patients may be symptomatic or asymptomatic (Class IIb). |

From the ACC/AHA/HRS 2008 Guidelines for Device-Based Therapy of Cardiac Rhythm Abnormalities. All the above recommendations for permanent pacemaker insertion are Class I indications unless specified.
[a]Neuromuscular diseases include myotonic muscular dystrophy, Erb dystrophy (limb-girdle), peroneal muscular atrophy, and Kearns-Sayre syndrome. AV, atrioventricular.

■ Figure 8.52 summarizes diagrammatically the different types of AV block.

## Indications for Permanent Pacing in AV Block

■ Unless specified, the following are Class I indications for implantation of permanent pacemakers in adult patients with acquired AV block according to the ACC/AHA/HRS guidelines (see Table 8.1).

## ECG Findings of Complete AV Block

1. In complete AV block, there is complete failure of the atrial impulses to capture the ventricles.
2. Only P waves will be present. Unless an escape rhythm comes to the rescue, ventricular asystole will occur.

## Summary of the Different Types of AV Block

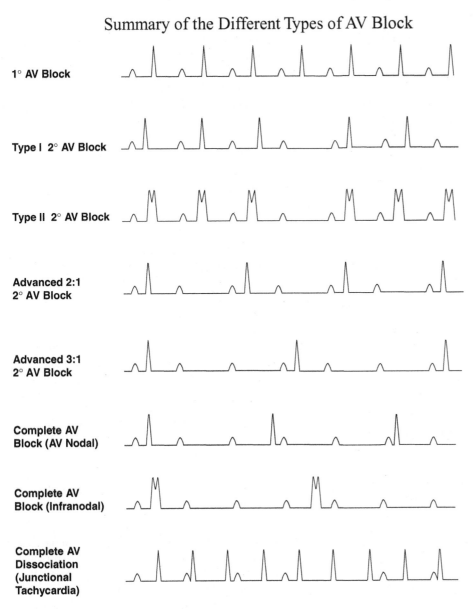

1° AV Block

Type I  2° AV Block

Type II  2° AV Block

Advanced 2:1
2° AV Block

Advanced 3:1
2° AV Block

Complete AV
Block (AV Nodal)

Complete AV
Block (Infranodal)

Complete AV
Dissociation
(Junctional
Tachycardia)

**Figure 8.52:    Atrioventricular (AV) Block.** The figure summarizes the different types of AV block.

3. The escape rhythm (the QRS complexes) can be narrow or wide.
4. The P waves and QRS complexes are completely dissociated.
5. The ventricular rate should be slower than the atrial rate and should be <50 bpm, usually in the mid- to low 40s.

## Mechanism

■ The intraventricular conduction system contains special cells with automatic properties that are capable of becoming pacemakers. These cells are called *latent pacemakers* because their rate of discharge is slower than the sinus node and do not become manifest because they are depolarized by the propagated sinus impulse. When the sinus impulse is blocked or when there is significant slowing of the sinus node, these latent pacemakers can become the dominant pacemaker of the heart. Cells in the middle portion of the AV node called the N region do not have automatic properties

and cannot become pacemakers. Cells at the upper portion of the AV node at its junction with the atria (AN region), lower portion of the AV node at its junction with the bundle of His (NH region) and His-Purkinje system have pacemaking properties. Cells with automatic properties that are located higher in the conduction system (closer to the AV node) have higher rates than cells that are located more distally. Thus, the intrinsic rate of the AV junction is 40 to 60 bpm and cells that are located more distally in the His-Purkinje system have slower rates of 20 to 40 bpm.

■ Complete AV block can occur anywhere in the AV conduction system. It can occur at the level of the AV node, bundle of His, both bundle branches, or the right bundle branch in combination with block involving both fascicular branches of the left bundle branch. If complete AV block is present, the sinus impulse will not be able to reach the ventricles because the AV conduction system is the only pathway by which the sinus impulse can reach the ventricles. This will result in syncope or sudden death unless an ectopic impulse comes to the rescue and initiates a ventricular rhythm. The escape rhythm has to originate below the level of the AV block. Thus, if the AV block is at the AV node, a junctional escape rhythm with narrow QRS complex usually comes to the rescue, and if the AV block is at the level of the His-Purkinje system, a ventricular escape rhythm with wide QRS complex is usually the escape mechanism. The presence of complete AV block is not certain unless the ventricles and AV conduction system are given enough time to recover from the previous impulse. For this to occur, the ventricular rate should be slower than the atrial rate and should be <50 bpm, usually in the mid- to low 40s.

## Clinical Implications

- Complete AV block can occur suddenly and can cause syncope or sudden death. The location of the AV block has prognostic significance and should be localized in all patients with AV block. The origin of the escape rhythm as well as the clinical setting in which the AV block occur are useful in localizing the AV block.

  - If the escape rhythm is AV junctional, the block is at the level of the AV node. In infranodal block, the escape rhythm is always ventricular.

  - The presence of bundle branch block before the onset of complete AV block suggests that there is distal conduction disease and favors an infranodal block.

  - If the patient is taking pharmacologic agents that block the AV node, such as digitalis, calcium channel blockers, or beta blockers, the block is AV nodal.

  - When complete AV block occurs in the setting of an acute inferior MI and the QRS complexes are narrow, the AV block is AV nodal.

  - When complete AV block occurs in the setting of acute anterior MI, the AV block is infranodal. When the AV block is infranodal, bundle branch block is usually present.

- There are multiple causes of complete AV block. Complete AV block may be congenital, occurring at birth, or advanced age resulting from calcification of the aortic ring and mitral annulus (also called Lev disease) and fibrosis or sclerodegenerative changes involving the conduction system (also called Lenègre disease). It could also be due to acute MI, inflammation of the conduction system as in Lyme disease, diphtheria, or Chagas disease, or from infiltrative diseases such as sarcoid or amyloid, hypothyroidism, and neuromuscular diseases. It could also be due to drugs that block the AV node or distal conducting system or during intracardiac surgery or ablation procedures.

- Physical examination of a patient with complete AV block will show cannon A waves in the jugular neck veins, variable intensity of the first heart sound, and variable pulse volume. This is similar to the physical findings of ventricular tachycardia (see Chapter 22, Wide Complex Tachycardia). These physical findings are due to the presence of complete AV dissociation.

- **Cannon A waves in the neck:** When there is complete AV dissociation, there is no relationship between atrial and ventricular contraction; thus, atrial contraction often occurs during systole when the tricuspid and mitral valves are closed, resulting in prominent jugular neck vein pulsations called cannon A waves. These cannon A waves occur intermittently, only when atrial and ventricular contractions are simultaneous.

- **Varying intensity of the first heart sound:** The intensity of the first heart sound depends on the position of the mitral and tricuspid valves at the onset of systole. When the valves are wide open, the first heart sound is markedly accentuated because of the wide distance the leaflets have to travel to their closure points. On the other hand, when the valves are near their coaptation points, the first heart sound will be very soft and hardly audible because the leaflets are almost in a semiclosed position at the onset of systole. During atrial contraction corresponding to the P wave in the ECG, the mitral and tricuspid leaflets are pushed wide open toward the ventricles away from their closure points. If this is immediately followed by ventricular contraction (as when the PR interval is short), closure of the mitral and tricuspid leaflets will be loud and often booming. On the other hand, if atrial contraction is not immediately followed by ventricular contraction (as when the PR interval is unduly prolonged), the closure of the leaflets will be soft or inaudible because the leaflets are allowed to drift back to a semiclosed position at the onset of ventricular contraction. Because the PR interval is variable when there is complete AV dissociation, the intensity of the first heart sound will also be variable.

- **Varying pulse volume:** When the P waves and the QRS complexes are completely dissociated, some ventricular beats will be preceded by atrial contraction, whereas other beats are not. When a P wave precedes a QRS complex, ventricular filling is augmented, resulting in a larger stroke volume, whereas QRS complexes without preceding P waves will have a lower stroke volume.

- **Jugular venous pulsations:** The jugular venous pulsations may be useful in the diagnosis of cardiac arrhythmias. In 1899, Wenckebach described the second-degree AV block that bears his name without using an ECG by examining jugular pulse tracings. The jugular pulse consists of three positive waves (a, c, and v waves) and two negative waves (x and y descents). To identify these waves and descents at bedside, the patient should be positioned properly and lighting should be adequate. The internal jugular veins lie deep behind the sternocleidomastoid muscle; thus, the venous column is not normally visible unless there is increased venous pressure because of right heart failure. The internal jugular pulsations, however, can be identified because they are transmitted superficially to the skin. Simultaneous auscultation of the heart or palpation of the radial pulse or opposite carotid artery is useful in timing the pulsations.

■ **Jugular versus carotid pulsations:** If there is difficulty in differentiating jugular venous from carotid arterial pulsations, the patient should be positioned more vertically upright because the venous pulse may disappear, whereas the arterial pulse does not disappear with any position. The venous pulse has two waves, with an inward motion corresponding to the x and y descents, whereas the arterial pulse has a single wave with an outward motion. If there is still doubt whether the pulse is venous or arterial, the base of the neck above the clavicle should be compressed. If the pulsation is venous, the pulse will disappear. Deep inspiration may enhance the venous pulsations, whereas the carotid pulse is not altered by pressure or by inspiration.

  □ **The "a" wave:** The "a" wave corresponds to the P wave in the ECG and is due to the rise in jugular venous pressure during atrial contraction. There is slight mechanical delay in the transmission of the atrial pulse to the neck; thus, the peak of the "a" wave usually coincides with the onset of the first heart sound. The "a" wave is prominent when there is increased resistance to the flow of blood to the right ventricle, as when there is tricuspid stenosis, right ventricular hypertrophy, pulmonic stenosis, or pulmonary hypertension. It is also prominent when there is left ventricular hypertrophy because the septum is shared by both ventricles. The "a" wave is absent if there is atrial fibrillation or the rhythm is AV junctional.

  □ **The x descent:** The x descent is the most conspicuous jugular motion occurring immediately after the "a" wave and is due to atrial relaxation and downward motion of the tricuspid annulus during systole. Because timing is systolic, it is easy to identify using the heart sounds or radial pulse. The x descent is prominent when the "a" wave is prominent. It is also prominent in constrictive pericarditis and in cardiac tamponade. The x descent is absent when there is no "a" wave, such as when there is AV junctional rhythm or atrial fibrillation.

  □ **The "c" wave:** The x descent in the jugular pulse is often interrupted by the "c" wave, which is due to transmitted pulsation from the carotid artery. Additionally, during right ventricular contraction, there is bulging of the tricuspid leaflets into the right atrium. The x descent continues as the x' descent after the c wave. The "c" wave is prominent when there is tricuspid regurgitation, often combining with the "v" wave to form a prominent "cv" wave. In some normal individuals, the "c" wave may not be demonstrable.

  □ **The "v" wave:** The "v" wave is due to the rise in right atrial pressure as blood accumulates in the atrium when the tricuspid valve is closed during systole. The peak of the "v" wave occurs with the onset of the second heart sound. The "v" wave becomes a large "cv" wave when there is tricuspid regurgitation. It is also prominent when there is increased right atrial pressure resulting from cardiomyopathy or increased volume due to atrial septal defect.

  □ **The y descent:** The y descent follows the downslope of the "v" wave and is due to the fall in right atrial pressure when the tricuspid valve opens during diastole. The y descent occurs after the second heart sound or after the radial pulse and is prominent in restrictive cardiomyopathy, constrictive pericarditis, right ventricular infarction, and tricuspid regurgitation. The y descent becomes diminished when there is tricuspid stenosis.

■ The jugular neck vein pulsations may be helpful in the diagnosis of certain arrhythmias:

  □ **First-degree AV block:** When the PR interval is prolonged, the "a" to "c" interval is wide.

  □ **Type I second-degree AV block or AV Wenckebach:** In AV Wenckebach, the interval between the "a" wave and "c" wave gradually widens until the "a" wave is not followed by a "v" wave. Additionally, as the PR interval becomes longer, the intensity of the first heart sound becomes softer until a dropped beat occurs.

  □ **Type II block:** When there is type II block, the interval between the "a" and "c" waves do not vary. The intensity of the first heart sound will not vary because the PR interval is fixed.

  □ **Other arrhythmias:** Cannon A waves are intermittently present when there is complete AV dissociation resulting from complete AV block or ventricular tachycardia. Cannon A waves are constantly present when the PR interval is markedly prolonged (see First-Degree AV Block in this chapter) when there is AV junctional rhythm, supraventricular tachycardia from AV nodal reentry, or AV reentry (see Chapter 16, Supraventricular Tachycardia.) or when there is ventricular tachycardia with retrograde conduction to the atria.

## Treatment

■ If complete AV block occurs at the level of the AV node and the patient is asymptomatic with narrow QRS complexes and a heart rate of at least 50 bpm, no treatment is necessary, other than further monitoring and observation. Any agent that can cause AV block should be discontinued.

■ Patients with AV block may become symptomatic because of bradycardia, which includes hypotension, altered mental status, ischemic chest pain, or signs of heart failure and low cardiac output. Treatment of the bradycardia includes airway and blood pressure support and identification of immediately reversible causes of AV block, including respiratory causes and blood gas and electrolyte abnormalities, hypovolemia, hypothermia, hypoglycemia, and acute coronary vasospasm.

■ The following intravenous agents may be useful in increasing the ventricular rate or improving AV conduction. These agents can enhance myocardial oxygen consumption and therefore should be used cautiously in the setting of acute MI because this may result in further extension of the myocardial infarct.

- **Atropine:** The drug of choice for the treatment of bradycardia is atropine. If there are no immediately reversible causes of AV block, this agent remains the drug of choice for symptomatic bradycardia and receives a Class IIa recommendation according to the AHA guidelines for cardiopulmonary resuscitation and emergency cardiovascular care.

  - Atropine 0.5 mg should be given intravenously every 3 to 5 minutes until a desired heart rate is achieved. Complete vagal blockade is expected when a total dose of 0.04 mg/kg or 3.0 mg is given intravenously over 2 hours.

  - Atropine should not be given in doses smaller than 0.5 mg because small doses stimulate the vagal nuclei and may enhance parasympathetic activity, resulting in paradoxical slowing and worsening of the AV block.

  - The drug can be given intratracheally during resuscitation, although subcutaneous or intramuscular administration should be avoided because these routes of administration can also result in paradoxical slowing.

  - Atropine is not effective in patients with AV block at the infranodal level. If the AV block is infranodal or the bradycardia does not respond to atropine, transcutaneous pacing should be instituted immediately in patients who are symptomatic.

- **Alternative medications:** There are other medications that can be tried for the treatment of bradycardia if atropine is not effective. These drugs are given only as alternative agents and receive a Class IIb recommendation according to the AHA guidelines.

  - **Epinephrine:** This can be given as an alternate to atropine if atropine is not effective or the AV block is infranodal and transcutaneous pacing is not available or has failed. This will serve as a temporizing measure before a transvenous pacemaker can be inserted. For the treatment of bradycardia and or hypotension, the infusion is prepared by adding 1 mg to 500 mL saline or $D_5W$ and started at an initial infusion of 1 µg/minute. The recommended dose is 1 to 10 µg/minute titrated according to the desired heart rate.

  - **Dopamine:** Dopamine may be given instead of atropine or epinephrine. It can be given as monotherapy or in combination with epinephrine. The dose is 2 to 10 µg/kg/minute titrated according to the desired heart rate.

  - **Glucagon:** If atropine is not effective, glucagon has been shown to improve symptomatic bradycardia induced by drugs such as beta blockers and calcium channel blockers. The dose is 3 mg given intravenously followed by infusion of 3 mg/hour if needed.

  - **Digibind:** If complete AV block is due to digitalis excess, digitalis should be discontinued and Digibind given as an antidote.

- **Transcutaneous pacing:** This intervention receives a Class I recommendation in patients who do not respond to atropine. Transcutaneous pacing is easier to perform than transvenous pacing and can be provided by most hospital personnel because the procedure is noninvasive.

- **Transvenous pacing:** Transvenous pacing should be performed if transcutaneous pacing is ineffective or unsuccessful or if the patient cannot tolerate transcutaneous pacing. This procedure is invasive and takes longer to accomplish, but provides more stable pacing.

- **Permanent pacing:** The following are indications for insertion of permanent pacemaker in complete AV block according to the ACC/AHA/HRS guidelines. In patients in whom the AV block is not reversible, a permanent pacemaker is indicated.

- **Symptomatic patients:** Patients with complete AV block at any anatomic level with symptoms related to the bradycardia, insertion of a permanent pacemaker is a Class I recommendation.

- **Asymptomatic patients:** Asymptomatic patients with complete AV block, permanent pacing is a Class I indication in the following conditions.

  - Patients with arrhythmias and other medical conditions that require drugs that can cause symptomatic bradycardia.

  - Documented asystole ≥3.0 seconds or any escape rate <40 bpm in patients with sinus rhythm who are awake and asymptomatic.

  - After catheter ablation of the AV junction.

  - Postcardiac surgery AV block that is not expected to resolve.

  - Neuromuscular diseases including myotonic muscular dystrophy, Kearns-Sayre syndrome, Erb dystrophy, and peroneal muscular atrophy with or without symptoms.

  - The recommendation is Class IIa in asymptomatic patients with complete AV block at any level with average awake ventricular rates of ≥40 bpm if cardiomegaly or left ventricular dysfunction is present.

- A permanent pacemaker should not be inserted if the AV block is expected to resolve or is unlikely to recur, such as those resulting from drug toxicity, Lyme disease, or during hypoxia related to sleep apnea in the absence of symptoms. These are Class III recommendations.

## Prognosis

- In patients with congenital complete AV block, the block is almost always at the level of the AV node. The escape rhythm is AV junctional and most patients remain stable and minimally symptomatic without therapy. These patients will eventually have permanent pacemakers implanted.

- When complete AV block is due to an acute inferior infarct, the block is AV nodal and is usually the result of enhanced parasympathetic activity when it occurs within 24 to 48 hours after the acute infarct. It is usually reversible and responds to atropine. If the onset of the AV block is after the second or third day, it is usually the result of continuing ischemia or structural damage to the AV node. Although the prognosis is good because the level of the block is AV nodal, inferior infarction with complete AV block generally indicates a larger infarct than one without AV block and therefore has a higher mortality.

- When complete AV block occurs in the setting of an acute anterior MI, the block is almost always infranodal and is very often preceded by bundle branch block. The mortality remains high even if a pacemaker is inserted because anterior infarct associated with AV block is usually extensive.

- The prognosis will also depend on the level of the AV block.
  - **AV nodal block:** AV nodal block has a better prognosis than an infranodal block because AV nodal block is usually reversible and a permanent pacemaker is often not needed. The AV junction can come to the rescue and has the highest firing rate among all potential pacemakers below the AV node. AV junctional rhythm has an intrinsic rate of 40 to 60 bpm and can be enhanced with atropine. It has narrow QRS complexes because the impulse originates above the bifurcation of the bundle of His. An AV junctional impulse is more effective than a ventricular impulse because it is able to activate both ventricles simultaneously. Finally, AV junctional rhythm is more stable than a ventricular escape rhythm. A pacemaker may be indicated if the AV block remains persistent and the patient becomes symptomatic. A permanent pacemaker is not needed and is a Class III indication if the AV block is transient and is not expected to recur.
  - **Infranodal:** When the block is infranodal, a ventricular escape rhythm usually comes to the rescue. The rhythm has inherently slower rate of 20 to 40 bpm. Unlike AV junctional rhythm, it cannot be enhanced with atropine. Additionally, the QRS complexes are wide because both ventricles are not activated synchronously. Thus, the ventricles do not contract simultaneously, the beat is ineffective, and a lower cardiac output than a junctional escape complex is generated. A ventricular rhythm, compared with AV junctional rhythm, is not a stable rhythm. Finally, an infranodal block is usually progressive and permanent

and is frequently associated with structural abnormalities not only of the conduction system, but also of the ventricles. Before the era of pacemaker therapy, complete AV block involving the distal conduction system was invariably fatal. Insertion of a permanent pacemaker is currently the only effective therapy available.

- The overall prognosis depends on the underlying cause of the AV block. If the AV block is isolated and no structural cardiac disease is present, the prognosis is similar to patients without AV block after a permanent pacemaker is implanted.

## Complete AV Dissociation

- **Complete AV dissociation:** Complete AV dissociation and complete AV block are not necessarily the same. Complete AV dissociation is a much broader term than complete AV block and includes any arrhythmia in which the atria and ventricles are completely independent from each other. Complete AV dissociation includes complete AV block as well as other arrhythmias not resulting from AV block such as ventricular tachycardia (Fig. 8.53), junctional tachycardia (Fig. 8.54), accelerated junctional rhythm (Fig. 8.55), and accelerated ventricular rhythm (Fig. 8.56). In junctional and ventricular tachycardia, the ventricular rate is faster than the atrial rate. Thus, the atrial impulse cannot conduct to the ventricles because the ventricles do not have ample time to recover before the arrival of the atrial impulse. In these examples, the dissociation between atria and ventricles is not the result of AV block.

- **Complete AV block:** In complete AV block, the ventricular rate is slower than the atrial rate. The ventricular rate is not only slower, but should be slow enough to allow sufficient time for the ventricles to recover so that it can be captured by the atrial impulse. Thus, the rate of the ventricles should be <50 bpm, usually in the low 40s before AV block is considered complete.

- **Accelerated rhythms:** In accelerated junctional or idioventricular rhythm, the atria and ventricles may be completely dissociated. The rate of the ventricles may not be slow enough and may not be able to recover on

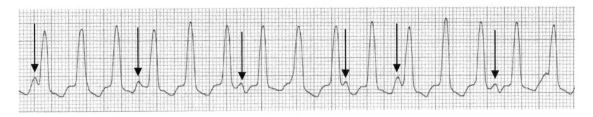

**Figure 8.53:    Complete Atrioventricular (AV) Dissociation from Ventricular Tachycardia.** The rhythm is ventricular tachycardia with complete AV dissociation. Note that the ventricular rate is faster than the atrial rate (*arrows*), which should be the other way around in complete AV block.

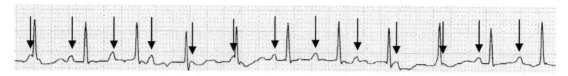

**Figure 8.54: Complete Atrioventricular (AV) Dissociation from Junctional Tachycardia.** The rhythm is junctional tachycardia with a rate of 101 beats per minute. Both P waves and QRS complexes are regular but are completely dissociated. Although the P waves have no relation to the QRS complexes, complete AV block is not present because the ventricular rate is not slow enough to be captured by the atrial impulse. The arrows identify the P waves, which have no relation to the QRS complexes.

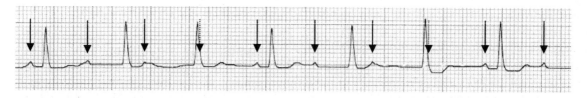

**Figure 8.55: Complete Atrioventricular (AV) Dissociation from Accelerated Junctional Rhythm.** Lead II rhythm strip showing complete AV dissociation with an atrial rate of 100 beats per minute and a ventricular rate at 80 beats per minute. The dissociation between the atria and ventricles may not be due to AV block. In complete AV block, the ventricular rate should be in the 40s to allow enough time for the conduction system and the ventricles to recover completely before the arrival of the next impulse. The P waves are marked by the arrows.

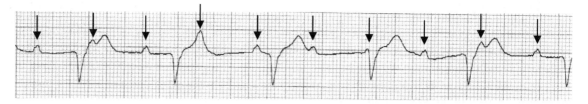

**Figure 8.56: Complete Atrioventricular (AV) Dissociation from Accelerated Idioventricular Rhythm.** There is complete AV dissociation with an atrial rate of almost 100 beats per minute and ventricular rate of 56 beats per minute. The QRS complexes are wide because of accelerated idioventricular rhythm. Although the dissociation between the P waves and QRS complex may be due to complete AV block, this cannot be certain because the ventricular rate is not slow enough. Thus, the rhythm is more appropriately complete AV dissociation rather than complete AV block. The arrows identify the sinus P waves.

**Figure 8.57: Complete Atrioventricular (AV) Dissociation.** Complete AV block is an example of complete AV dissociation. The other arrhythmias in which complete AV dissociation may occur are shown.

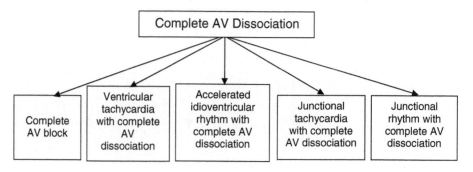

time before the arrival of the atrial impulse. This may result in complete AV dissociation, not necessarily AV block. Figure 8.57 shows the different arrhythmias that can result in AV dissociation.

## ECG Findings in Complete AV Dissociation

1. P waves and QRS complexes are completely dissociated and have no relation to each other.
2. In complete AV dissociation, the underlying rhythm may be ventricular tachycardia, junctional tachycardia, accelerated junctional rhythm, accelerated ventricular rhythm, or complete AV block.

## Mechanism

- Complete AV dissociation occurs when two completely independent pacemakers, one controlling the atria and the other controlling the ventricles, are present.
  - When there is ventricular tachycardia, junctional tachycardia or accelerated junctional, or ventricular rhythms, the sinus impulse may not be able to propagate to the ventricles because the ventricular rate is faster than the atrial rate. Absence of ventricular capture when the ventricular rate is faster than the atrial rate is not necessarily because of complete AV block, but may be from the ventricles being completely refractory every time atrial impulses arrive at the ventricles. This is a form of electrical interference resulting in AV dissociation. In these examples, complete AV block is not present.
  - In complete AV block, there is complete absence of AV conduction. The atrial impulse is unable to conduct through the ventricles because of an abnormality in the conduction system. The atrial impulse is given the opportunity to conduct to the ventricles, but is unable to do so when complete AV block is present.

## Clinical Implications

- Complete AV dissociation is a broader term that includes any rhythm where the atria and ventricles are completely independent from each other and includes complete AV block as well as other arrhythmias not resulting from complete AV block such as ventricular tachycardia, junctional tachycardia, AV junctional, or ventricular rhythm.
- Complete AV block is just one of the many examples of complete AV dissociation. For complete AV block to occur, the ventricular rate should be slower than the atrial rate and should be <50 bpm, usually in the low to mid-40s. This will allow enough time for the ventricles to recover before the next atrial impulse arrives. If the atrial impulse cannot capture the ventricles even when the ventricular

rate is slow, then complete AV block is the cause of the AV dissociation.

## Treatment and Prognosis

- Because there are other causes of complete AV dissociation other than complete AV block, treatment and prognosis will depend on the specific arrhythmia causing the AV dissociation.

## Suggested Readings

2005 American Heart Association guidelines for cardiopulmonary resuscitation and emergency cardiovascular care. Part 7.3: management of symptomatic bradycardia and tachycardia. *Circulation.* 2005;112:67–77.

2005 American Heart Association guidelines for cardiopulmonary resuscitation and emergency cardiovascular care. Part 7.4: monitoring and medications. *Circulation.* 2005;112:78–83.

Barold SS, Hayes DL. Second-degree atrioventricular block: a reappraisal. *Mayo Clin Proc.* 2001;76:44–57.

Chatterjee K. Physical examination. In: Topol EJ, ed. *Textbook of Cardiovascular Medicine.* 2nd ed. Philadelphia: Lippincott Williams & Wilkins; 2002:280–284.

Gregoratos G, Abrams J, Epstein AE, et al. ACC/AHA/NASPE 2002 guideline update for implantation of cardiac pacemakers and antiarrhythmia devices: summary article: a report of the American College of Cardiology/American Heart Association Task Force on Practice Guidelines (ACC/AHA/NASPE Committee to update the 1998 pacemaker guidelines). *Circulation.* 2002;106:2145–2161.

Epstein AE, DiMarco JP, Ellenbogen KA, et. al. ACC/AHA/HRS 2008 guidelines for device-based therapy of cardiac rhythm abnormalities: a report of the American College of Cardiology/American Heart Association Task Force on Practice Guidelines (Writing Committee to Revise the ACC/AHA/NASPE 2002 Guideline Update for Implantation of Cardiac Pacemakers and Antiarrhythmia Devices). *Circulation* 2008;117:e350-e408.

Mangrum JM, DiMarco JP. The evaluation and management of bradycardia. *N Engl J Med.* 2000;342:703–709.

Marriot HJL. Intra-atrial, sino-atrial and atrio-ventricular block. In: *Practical Electrocardiography.* 5th ed. Baltimore: Williams & Wilkins; 1972:194–211.

Marriott HJL, Menendez MM. A-V dissociation revisited. *Prog Cardiovas Dis.* 1966;8:522–538.

Narula OS, Scherlag BJ, Samet P, et al. Atrioventricular block. *Am J Med.* 1971;50:146–165.

Zipes DP, DiMarco JP, Gillette PC, et al. Guidelines for clinical intracardiac electrophysiological and catheter ablation procedures: a report of the American College of Cardiology/American Heart Association Task Force on Practice Guidelines (Committee on Clinical Intracardiac Electrophysiologic and Catheter Ablation Procedures), developed in collaboration with the North American Society of Pacing and Electrophysiology. *J Am Coll Cardiol.* 1995;26:555–573.

# Intraventricular Conduction Defect: Fascicular Block

## Fascicular Block

- **Intraventricular conduction system:** The intraventricular conduction system includes the bundle of His, the right and left bundle branches, the fascicular branches of the left bundle branch, and the distal Purkinje fibers (Fig. 9.1).
  - **Bundle of His:** The bundle of His is a continuation of the atrioventricular node. It is a short structure that immediately divides into two branches: the right and left bundle branches.
  - **Right bundle:** The right bundle branch follows the right side of the ventricular septum and terminates into a network of Purkinje fibers within the endocardium of the right ventricle.
  - **Left bundle:** The left bundle branch immediately fans into several branches, including a mid-septal branch and two main fascicles: the left anterior and left posterior fascicles.
    - **Left anterior fascicle:** The left anterior fascicle courses to the base of the anterior papillary muscle before terminating into a network of Purkinje fibers.

- **Left posterior fascicle:** The left posterior fascicle terminates into a network of Purkinje fibers after reaching the base of the posteromedial papillary muscle.
- Although the atria and ventricles are contiguous structures, the only pathway by which the sinus impulse can reach the ventricles is through the atrioventricular node. After exiting the atrioventricular node, conduction of the impulse through the intraventricular conduction system results in a fast and orderly sequence of ventricular activation. However, the sinus impulse can be pathologically delayed or interrupted anywhere within the intraventricular conduction system (Fig. 9.2).
  - **Bundle branch block:** If the sinus impulse is interrupted within the bundle branches, the abnormality is called bundle branch block.
    - **Right bundle branch block:** If the impulse is interrupted within the right bundle branch, the conduction abnormality is called right bundle branch block.
    - **Left bundle branch block:** If the sinus impulse is interrupted within the left bundle branch, the conduction abnormality is called left bundle branch block.

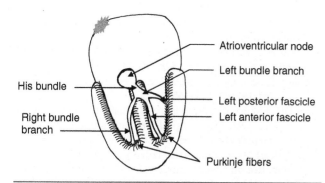

**Figure 9.1: The Intraventricular Conduction System.** The intraventricular conduction system consists of the bundle of His, right and left bundle branches, the fascicular branches of the left bundle branch, and the Purkinje fibers.

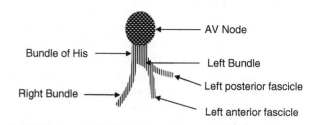

**Figure 9.2: Diagrammatic Representation of the Atrioventricular Node and Intraventricular Conduction System.** The sinus impulse can propagate to the ventricles only through the atrioventricular node and intraventricular conduction system, resulting in orderly sequence of ventricular activation. The sinus impulse can be blocked anywhere along this conduction pathway, resulting in different types of intraventricular conduction defect.

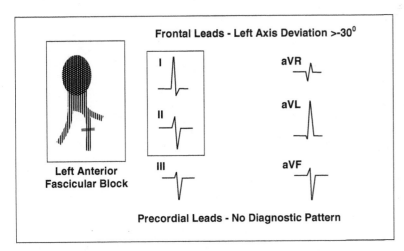

Frontal Leads - Left Axis Deviation >-30°

**Left Anterior Fascicular Block**

Precordial Leads - No Diagnostic Pattern

**Figure 9.3:  Left Anterior Fascicular Block.**
The hallmark of LAFB is the presence of left axis deviation >-30° with rS complexes in leads II, III, and aVF and tall R waves in leads I and aVL. Briefly, LAFB should always be suspected when there is negative or rS complex in lead II with a tall R wave in lead I (*the essential leads are framed*).

- ▪ **Fascicular block:** If the sinus impulse is interrupted within the fascicles, the conduction abnormality is called fascicular block.
  - □ **Left anterior fascicular block:** If the sinus impulse is interrupted within the left anterior fascicle, the conduction abnormality is called left anterior fascicular block (LAFB).
  - □ **Left posterior fascicular block:** If the sinus impulse is interrupted within the left posterior fascicle, the conduction abnormality is called left posterior fascicular block (LPFB).

## Left Anterior Fascicular Block

- ▪ **Left anterior fascicular block:** LAFB occurs when the sinus impulse is delayed or interrupted within the left anterior fascicle. LAFB is the most common intraventricular conduction abnormality because the left anterior fascicle is a long and thin structure that is more delicate and more vulnerable to injury than the rest of the conduction system.
- ▪ **Electrocardiogram findings:** LAFB alters the electrocardiogram (ECG) by abnormally shifting the axis of the QRS complex to the left of –30°. The most important leads in detecting the abnormal left axis deviation are leads II and aVL.
  - ▪ **Lead II:** This is the most important lead in suspecting that LAFB is present. In lead II, the QRS complex is negative with an rS configuration (r wave is smaller than the S wave). Leads III and aVF will also show an rS pattern.
  - ▪ **Lead aVL:** A tall R wave in lead I (Rs complex) and a qR pattern in aVL will confirm that the axis has shifted to the left.
- ▪ In LAFB, the right ventricle continues to be supplied by the right bundle branch, and the left ventricle continues to be supplied by the left posterior fascicle. Therefore,

activation of both ventricles remains synchronous and the duration of the QRS complex is not increased. It normally remains at 0.08 to 0.10 seconds.

- ▪ The ECG findings of LAFB are shown in Figures 9.3 and 9.4.
- ▪ **Common mistakes in left anterior fascicular block:**
  - ▪ **LAFB mistaken for anterior infarct:** LAFB may cause small q waves in $V_2$ and in $V_3$, which can be mistaken for anteroseptal infarct (Fig. 9.5). These micro–q waves may become more exaggerated if $V_1$ and $V_2$ are inadvertently positioned at a higher location on the patient's chest (at the 2nd rather than the 4th intercostal space).
  - ▪ **LAFB mistaken for inferior infarct:** LAFB may be confused with inferior myocardial infarction (MI) because both can shift the QRS axis to the left of –30°. However, inferior MI will show initial q waves in leads II, III, and aVF (Fig. 9.6), whereas the QRS complex in LAFB start with a small r wave in II, III, and aVF (Fig. 9.5).
- ▪ **LAFB and inferior MI:** LAFB and inferior MI may be difficult to recognize when they occur together unless the leads are recorded simultaneously (Fig. 9.7A).
  - ▪ **LAFB:** For LAFB to be present, (1) the axis of the QRS complex should exceed –30°, (2) both aVR and aVL should end with R waves, and (3) the peak of the R wave in aVL should occur earlier than the peak of the R wave in aVR (Fig. 9.7B).
  - ▪ **LAFB + inferior MI:** When LAFB is associated with inferior MI, a q wave in lead II should be present (Fig. 9.8A) in addition to criteria 1, 2, and 3 for LAFB listed previously (Fig. 9.8B).

### ECG of LAFB

1. Frontal or limb leads:
   - ▪ Left axis deviation >-30° (rS complexes in II, III, and aVF and qR in I and aVL).
   - ▪ Normal QRS duration.

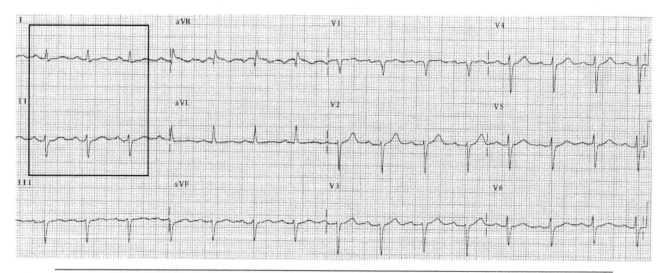

**Figure 9.4: Left Anterior Fascicular Block.** Twelve-lead electrocardiogram showing left anterior fascicular block (LAFB). The axis of the QRS complex is −60°. LAFB should always be suspected when a tall R wave is present in lead I and deep S wave is present in lead II (the leads are framed). The QRS complexes remain normal in duration. The precordial leads are not helpful in establishing the diagnosis, although poor R wave progression is usually present. The changes in the precordial leads are due to extreme deviation of the electrical axis superiorly. These changes may disappear if the leads are positioned two intercostal spaces higher than the standard location.

2. The horizontal or precordial leads are not needed for the diagnosis of LAFB.

## Mechanism

- The left anterior fascicle activates the anterior and superior portions of the left ventricle. When there is LAFB, the area supplied by the left anterior fascicle is the last to be activated. This causes the axis of the QRS complex to shift superiorly and to the left. The hallmark of LAFB is a shift in the QRS axis to the left of −30°. Although an axis of ≥−45° is the traditional criteria used in the diagnosis of LAFB, a QRS axis >−30° is accepted as LAFB.

- The QRS complex is not widened when there is LAFB because the left ventricle has two overlapping sets of Purkinje fibers: one from the left anterior fascicle and the other from the left posterior fascicle. When there is LAFB, the left ventricle is activated by the left posterior fascicle and the right ventricle by the right bundle branch, thus both ventricles remain synchronously activated. If there is any increased duration of

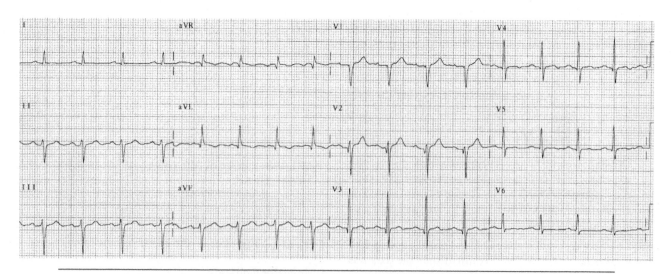

**Figure 9.5: Left Anterior Fascicular Block.** Left anterior fascicular block can cause small q waves in $V_2$ and $V_3$, which can be mistaken for anterior myocardial infarction. These micro–q waves become more pronounced if leads $V_1$ to $V_3$ are placed higher than the standard location and the patient is in a sitting position when the electrocardiogram is recorded.

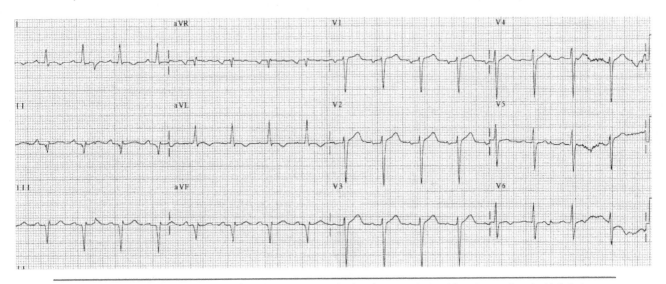

**Figure 9.6: Inferior Myocardial Infarction.** Left anterior fascicular block should not be confused with inferior myocardial infarction (MI). In inferior MI, leads II, III, and aVF start with a q wave as shown here, rather than with a small r.

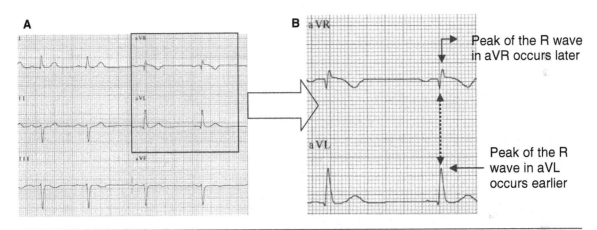

**Figure 9.7: Left Anterior Fascicular Block.** When leads aVR and aVL are simultaneously recorded **(A)**, left anterior fascicular block is present when there is left axis deviation >−30° and aVR and aVL both terminate with an R wave. **(B)** Magnified to show that the peak of the R wave in aVL occurs earlier than the peak of the R wave in aVR.

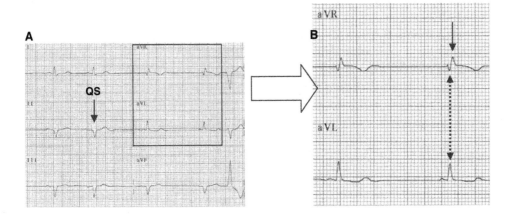

**Figure 9.8: Left Anterior Fascicular Block with Inferior MI.** **(A)** Leads aVR and aVL are recorded simultaneously and are magnified in **(B)**. Note that the terminal R wave in aVR (*arrow*) occurs later than the terminal R wave in aVL, consistent with left anterior fascicular block. In addition, q waves (QS) are present in lead II **(A)**, consistent with inferior myocardial infarction.

115

**Figure 9.9: Left Posterior Fascicular Block.** The most important feature of left posterior fascicular block (LPFB) is the presence of right axis deviation >90°. The diagnosis should be considered only after chronic obstructive pulmonary disease and other causes of right ventricular hypertrophy are excluded. The presence of LPFB is suspected when deep S wave is present in lead I (rS complex) and tall R wave (Rs complex) is present in lead II (*the leads are framed*).

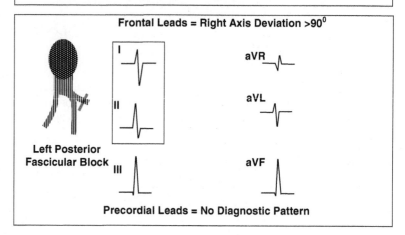

**Left posterior Fascicular Block**

- **Frontal leads:**
  - **Axis:** Right axis deviation >90°. Other causes are excluded.
    - Lead I: rS complex
    - Lead aVF: Tall R in aVF and lead III with qR pattern
  - The duration of the QRS complex remains normal
- **Precordial leads:** No diagnostic changes

**Frontal Leads = Right Axis Deviation >90°**

**Left Posterior Fascicular Block**

**Precordial Leads = No Diagnostic Pattern**

the QRS complex, it will be minimal and should not exceed 0.01 to 0.02 seconds above baseline. Thus, the total duration of the QRS complex will remain within 0.10 seconds unless there is MI or left ventricular hypertrophy.

- In LAFB, the left ventricle is initially activated by the left posterior fascicle. Thus, the initial QRS vector is directed inferiorly and to the right, often causing q waves in $V_2$ and $V_3$. This becomes exaggerated if the electrodes are positioned higher on the chest or if the heart is oriented vertically.

## Clinical Significance

- The left anterior fascicle is a long and thin structure that terminates into a network of Purkinje fibers at the base of the ante-

rior papillary muscle. It courses subendocardially in the direction of the outflow tract of the left ventricle, and thus is subject to higher intraventricular pressure than the rest of the conduction system. Because of its structure and location, LAFB is the most common intraventricular conduction abnormality.

- LAFB is a common cause of left axis deviation and should be considered immediately when left axis deviation exceeds −30°. LAFB may be difficult to recognize when combined with inferior MI because both can cause left axis deviation.
  - **LAFB:** In LAFB, the QRS axis is >−30° and leads II, III, and aVF start with small r waves. The terminal QRS vector loop in the frontal plane is directed superiorly and leftward in a counterclockwise direction. Thus, the peak of the R in aVL occurs earlier than the peak of the R in aVR.

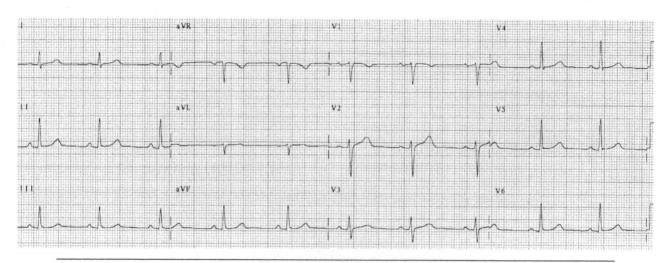

**Figure 9.10: Normal Electrocardiogram.** The QRS complexes are not widened, with normal axis of approximately 75°.

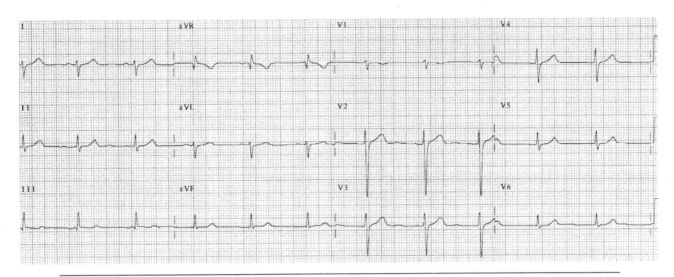

**Figure 9.11:    Left Posterior Fascicular Block.** Twelve-lead electrocardiogram showing left posterior fascicular block (LPFB). The QRS complexes are not widened and the axis is shifted to +120°. Before LPFB is diagnosed, other causes of right axis deviation should first be excluded.

- **Inferior MI:** In inferior MI, leads II, III, and aVF start with q waves.
- **LAFB and inferior MI:** There is LAFB if the QRS axis is >−30°, terminal R waves are present in aVR and aVL and the peak of the R wave in aVL occurs earlier than the peak of the R wave in aVR. If any q wave is present in lead II, inferior MI is also present.
- LAFB is commonly the result of hypertension, ischemic heart disease, cardiomyopathy, aortic valve disease, and sclerosis or fibrosis of the conduction system. Left ventricular hypertrophy is commonly associated with LAFB. Conversely, LAFB can augment the tall R waves in aVL, which can mimic left ventricular hypertrophy. In children, left axis deviation of ≥−30° is abnormal and is usually due to primum atrial septal defect.

## Treatment and Prognosis

- LAFB does not require any treatment. Therapy is directed to the underlying cause of the LAFB.
- The prognosis of LAFB depends on the underlying cause. If this is the only conduction abnormality and no associated cardiac disease is present, LAFB is generally benign.

## Left Posterior Fascicular Block

- **Left posterior fascicular block:** LPFB occurs when conduction across the left posterior fascicle is delayed or interrupted. It is the least common among all intraventricular conduction abnormalities.
- **ECG Findings:** The hallmark of LPFB is a shift in the electrical axis of the QRS complex to the right of 90°

(Fig. 9.9). Because LPFB is uncommon, other more common causes of right axis deviation should first be excluded before LPFB is diagnosed. The QRS complexes are not widened because the left ventricle continues to be activated by the left anterior fascicle. A normal ECG is shown in Fig. 9.10. For comparison, the ECG of LPFB is shown in Fig. 9.11.

- **Common mistakes in LPFB:**
  - **Right ventricular hypertrophy mistaken for LPFB:** LPFB is relatively uncommon and is considered a diagnosis of exclusion. Other causes of right axis deviation, such as right ventricular hypertrophy or pulmonary disease, should first be excluded before the diagnosis of LPFB is considered (Figs. 9.12 and 9.13). This contrasts with LAFB, where the diagnosis is considered immediately when the axis is >−30°.
  - **Lateral MI mistaken for LPFB:** High lateral MI can cause right axis deviation >90° and can be mistaken for LPFB. In LPFB, rS complexes are present in I and aVL (Fig. 9.11). In lateral MI, QS complexes are present in these leads (Fig. 9.14).

## ECG of LPFB

1. Frontal or limb leads:
   - Right axis deviation >90° with negative or rS complex in I and aVL and qR in III and aVF.
   - The QRS complexes are not widened.
   - Other causes of right axis deviation have been excluded.
2. Horizontal or precordial leads:
   - The precordial leads are not necessary in the diagnosis of LPFB.

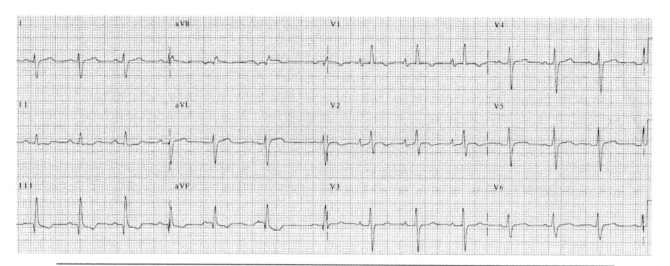

**Figure 9.12:** **Right Ventricular Hypertrophy.** The frontal leads show all features of left posterior fascicular block (LPFB). However, tall R waves are present in $V_1$, suggesting right ventricular hypertrophy and not LPFB.

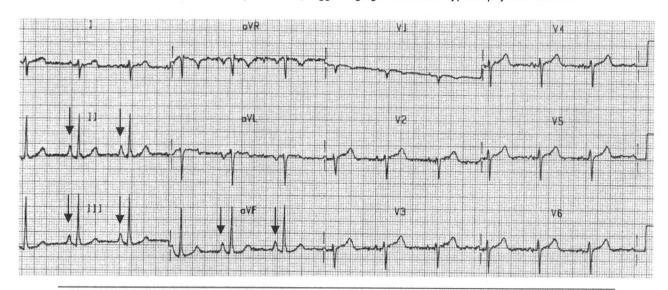

**Figure 9.13:** **Right Ventricular Hypertrophy.** There is right atrial enlargement with peaked P waves in leads II, III, and aVF (*arrows*). There is clockwise rotation of the QRS complexes in the precordial leads. This electrocardiogram is consistent with right ventricular hypertrophy and not left posterior fascicular block.

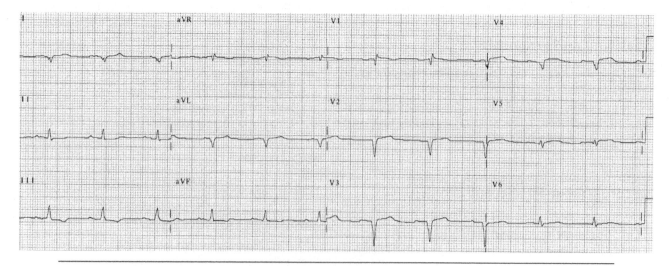

**Figure 9.14:** **Lateral Myocardial Infarction.** Lateral myocardial infarction (MI) with QS complexes in I and aVL can be mistaken for left posterior fascicular block (LPFB) as shown here. In LPFB, leads I and aVL have rS complexes, whereas in lateral MI, these leads start with q waves. Q waves are also present in $V_1$ to $V_4$ because of anterior MI.

## Mechanism

- The left posterior fascicle activates the posteroinferior left ventricular free wall, which is to the right and inferior to that activated by the left anterior fascicle. This portion of the left ventricle is the last to be activated when there is LPFB, thus causing the axis of the QRS complex to shift inferiorly and to the right. While a QRS axis $\geq 100°$ is traditionally used to identify LPFB, a QRS axis $>90°$ is generally accepted as LPFB.

- The QRS complex is not widened when there is LPFB because the left ventricle continues to be activated by the left anterior fascicle and the right ventricle by the right bundle branch, resulting in synchronous activation of both ventricles.

## Clinical Significance

- LPFB is a diagnosis of exclusion since LPFB is relatively uncommon. This contrasts with LAFB, in which the diagnosis is considered outright when there is left axis deviation $>-30°$. Before the diagnosis of LPFB is considered, other, more common, causes of right axis deviation such as pulmonary disease and other causes of right ventricular hypertrophy should first be excluded.

- In contrast to the left anterior fascicle, the left posterior fascicle has a dual blood supply, originating from the septal perforating branches of the left anterior descending coronary artery anteriorly and from the septal perforating branches of the posterior descending artery posteriorly. It is short, thick, and broad and courses along the inflow tract of the left ventricle before terminating into a network of Purkinje fibers at the base of the posteromedial papillary muscle. It is therefore protected and subjected to less intraventricular pressure compared with the left anterior fascicle. Because of its structure, location, and blood supply, LPFB is the least common among all intraventricular conduction abnormalities.

- The most important lead in recognizing LPFB is lead I. This will show a negative or rS complex, with the S wave deeper than the size of the r wave. This is accompanied by tall R waves in leads aVF and III.

- Right axis deviation due to high lateral MI can be mistaken for LPFB. Correspondingly, LPFB can obscure the ECG changes of inferior MI.

- The causes of LPFB are the same as that of LAFB and include coronary disease, hypertension, cardiomyopathy, acute myocarditis, valvular disease (especially aortic stenosis), and degenerative diseases of the conduction system.

## Treatment

- Treatment is directed toward the underlying cause of the LPFB.

## Prognosis

- Because the left posterior fascicle is the least vulnerable and the last to be involved when there is intraventricular conduction defect, LPFB seldom occurs independently and is frequently seen in combination with right bundle branch block or with LAFB. LPFB, therefore, indicates a more significant and more advanced form of conduction abnormality than LAFB. LPFB in combination with LAFB can result in left bundle branch block. The prognosis depends on the cause of the conduction abnormality.

## Suggested Readings

Dunn MI, Lipman BS. Abnormalities of ventricular conduction: fascicular block, infarction block, and parietal block. In: *Lippman-Massie Clinical Electrocardiography.* 8th ed. Chicago: Yearbook Medical Publishers, Inc.; 1989:148–159.

Elizari MV, Acunzo RS, Ferreiro M. Hemiblocks revisited. *Circulation.* 2007;115:1154–1163.

Marriott HJL. The hemiblocks and trifascicular block. In: *Practical Electrocardiography.* 5th ed. Baltimore: The Williams and Wilkins Company; 1972:86–94.

Sgarbossa EB, Wagner GS. Electrocardiography: In: Topol EJ, ed. *Textbook of Cardiovascular Medicine.* 2nd ed. Philadelphia: Lippincott Williams & Wilkins; 2002:1330–1354.

Warner RA, Hill NE, Mookherjee S, et al. Electrocardiographic criteria for the diagnosis of combined inferior MI and left anterior hemiblock. *Am J Cardiol.* 1983;51:718–722.

Warner RA, Hill NE, Mookherjee S, et al. Improved electrocardiographic criteria for the diagnosis of left anterior hemiblock. *Am J Cardiol.* 1983;51:723–726.

Willems JL, Robles de Medina EO, Bernard R, et al. Criteria for intraventricular conduction disturbances and pre-excitation. *J Am Coll Cardiol.* 1985;5:1261–1275.

# Intraventricular Conduction Defect: Bundle Branch Block

## Right Bundle Branch Block

- **Right bundle branch block:** Conduction of the sinus impulse can be interrupted at the level of the right bundle branch resulting in right bundle branch block (RBBB) (Fig. 10.1).
- **ECG findings:** Unlike fascicular blocks in which the electrocardiogram (ECG) findings are best seen in the frontal leads, the ECG changes of RBBB are best recognized in the precordial leads $V_1$ and $V_6$. The hallmark of RBBB is the presence of wide QRS complexes measuring ≥0.12 seconds with large terminal R' waves in $V_1$ and wide terminal S waves in $V_6$ as well as in leads I and aVL. The septal Q waves are preserved.

- Bundle branch block is a more extensive conduction abnormality than the fascicular blocks. In RBBB, the QRS complex is widened by ≥0.12 seconds because activation of the entire right ventricle is delayed.
- The axis of the QRS complex is not significantly changed and remains normal when there is RBBB (Fig. 10.2, Fig. 10.3). The axis may shift to the left if left anterior fascicular block (LAFB) is present or to the right if left posterior fascicular block (LPFB), pulmonary hypertension, or right ventricular hypertrophy is present.
- In the setting of RBBB, only the first 0.06 to 0.08 seconds of the QRS complex should be used in calculating the axis of the QRS complex because the terminal portion of the QRS complex represents delayed activation of the right ventricle (Fig. 10.3).

**Figure 10.1: Right Bundle Branch Block.** In right bundle branch block, the QRS complexes are wide measuring ≥0.12 seconds. Large terminal R' waves are present in $V_1$ with rR' or rsR' configuration. $V_6$ shows wide S wave with a qRS or RS configuration. The onset of the intrinsicoid deflection also called R peak time is prolonged in $V_1$ but normal in $V_6$.

---

**Right Bundle Branch Block**

- Wide QRS complexes measuring ≥0.12 second.
  - **$V_1$:**
    - Large terminal R' waves with rR' or rsR' configuration.
    - Onset of intrinsicoid deflection (R peak time) >0.05 sec.
  - **$V_6$ and leads on left side of ventricular septum (I and aVL):**
    - Wide terminal S waves are present.
    - Septal q waves are preserved.

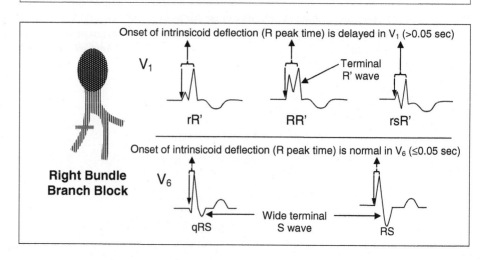

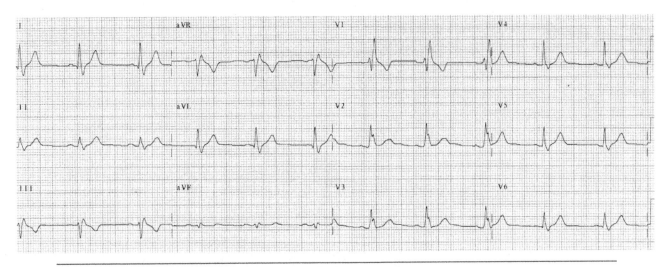

**Figure 10.2:    Complete Right Bundle Branch Block.** The QRS complexes are wide measuring ≥0.12 seconds. rsR′ configuration is present in V₁ and qRs configuration is present in V₆. Wide S waves are present in leads I and V₆. The axis of the QRS complex in the frontal plane is normal.

## RBBB + LAFB

- **Right bundle branch block + left anterior fascicular block:** RBBB can occur in combination with a fascicular block. Thus, RBBB + LAFB are present if the sinus impulse is simultaneously interrupted at the right bundle branch and left anterior fascicular branch. RBBB in combination with LAFB is an example of a bifascicular block because two conduction pathways are interrupted. Activation of the ventricles can occur only through the remaining left posterior fascicle.

- **ECG findings:** The typical features of RBBB are seen in the precordial leads and that of LAFB in the frontal leads (Fig. 10.4).
  - **RBBB:** The QRS complexes are wide measuring ≥0.12 seconds because of the presence of RBBB. The characteristic rR′ or rsR′ pattern is present in V₁, and wide S waves are present in V₆.
  - **LAFB:** In the frontal plane, the axis of the QRS complex is >−30° with rS in lead II and tall R wave in aVL.
- **RBBB + LPFB:** RBBB + LPFB can occur when conduction across the right bundle and left posterior fascicle is

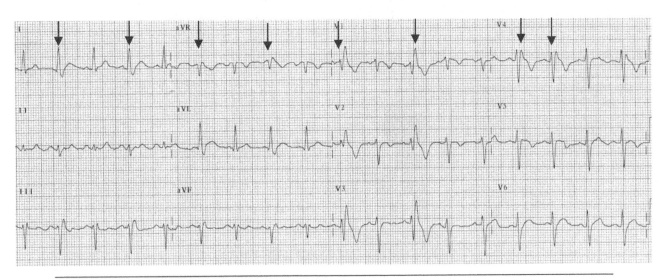

**Figure 10.3:    Right Bundle Branch Block Alternating with Normal Conduction.** Note that when right bundle branch block occurs (*arrows*), the axis of the QRS complex using only the first 0.06 to 0.08 seconds is not significantly changed when compared with the normally conducted QRS complexes.

**Figure 10.4:   Diagrammatic Representation of Right Bundle Branch Block + Left Anterior Fascicular Block.** The QRS complexes are wide. The precordial leads show classical RBBB with rR′, RR′, or rsR′ in $V_1$ and qRS in $V_6$. The limb leads show left axis deviation >−30° with deep rS complex in lead II and tall R in aVL.

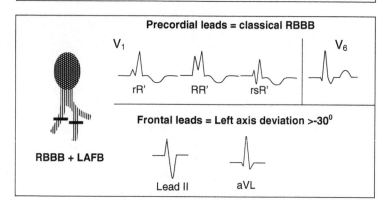

**RBBB + LAFB**

- The QRS complexes measure ≥0.12 second due to RBBB
  o **Precordial leads:** RBBB in $V_1$ and in $V_6$
  o **Frontal leads:** LAFB with left axis deviation >-30⁰

simultaneously interrupted. RBBB + LPFB is also an example of bifascicular block (Fig. 10.5, Fig. 10.6, Fig. 10.7, Fig. 10.8).

■ **ECG findings:** The presence of RBBB and LPFB is recognized separately.

　■ **RBBB:** The typical features of RBBB are best recognized in the precordial leads as widening of the QRS complex (≥0.12 seconds) with a characteristic large terminal R′ (rR′ or rsR′) in $V_1$ and wide S in $V_6$.

■ **LPFB:** LPFB is best recognized in the frontal plane as a shift in the QRS axis >90°. Deep S waves are present in lead I, with tall R waves in leads III and aVF. For LPFB to be considered, other causes of right axis deviation should first be excluded.

**Figure 10.5:   Diagrammatic Representation of Right Bundle Branch Block + Left Posterior Fascicular Block.** The classical pattern of right bundle branch block is recognized in the precordial leads with rR′ or rsR′ in $V_1$ and qRS in $V_6$. The limb leads show right axis deviation >90° with rS in lead I and tall R wave in lead aVF from left posterior fascicular block.

**RBBB + LPFB**

- Wide QRS complexes measuring ≥0.12 seconds due to RBBB
  o **Precordial leads:** RBBB in $V_1$ and in $V_6$
  o **Frontal leads:** LPFB with right axis deviation >90⁰

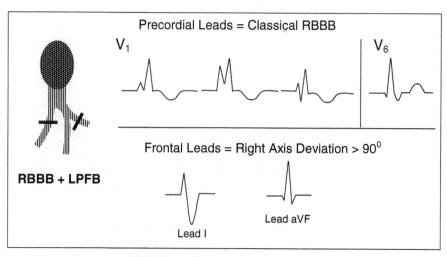

RBBB and Fascicular Block

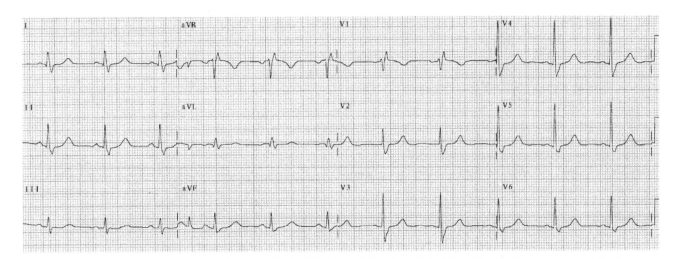

**Figure 10.6: Uncomplicated Right Bundle Branch Block.** The QRS complexes are wide measuring ≥0.12 seconds with rsr' configuration in $V_1$ and qRs configuration in $V_6$. Wide S waves are noted in leads I and $V_6$. The axis of the QRS complex in the frontal plane is normal.

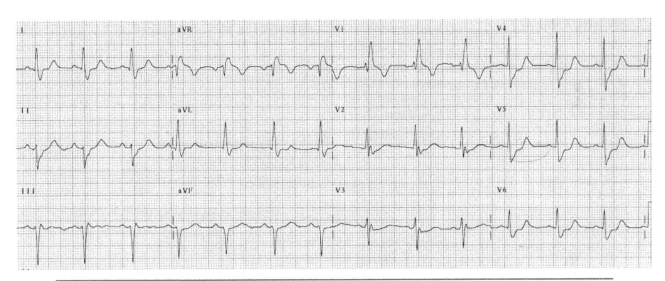

**Figure 10.7: Right Bundle Branch Block + Left Anterior Fascicular Block.** Right bundle branch block is recognized by the presence of wide QRS complexes measuring ≥0.12 seconds with rR' or rsR' in $V_1$ and wide S waves in $V_6$. Left anterior fascicular block is diagnosed by the presence of left axis deviation of –60° in the frontal leads.

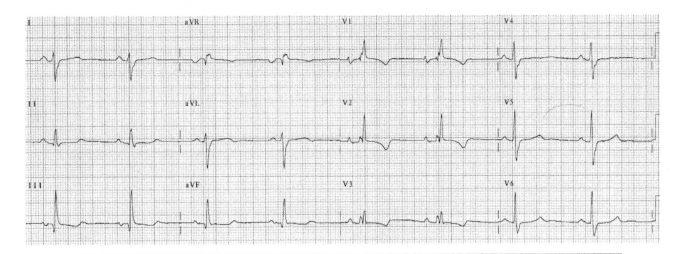

**Figure 10.8: Right Bundle Branch Block + Left Posterior Fascicular Block.** There is right bundle branch block with rR' pattern in $V_1$ and RS in $V_6$. Left posterior fascicular block is diagnosed by the presence of right axis deviation of 120° in the frontal plane.

**Figure 10.9:   ST and T Wave Changes in Right Bundle Branch Block.** **(A)** When uncomplicated right bundle branch block is present, the terminal portion of the QRS complex and the ST segment and T waves are discordant. Note that the small arrows (pointing to the terminal QRS complex) are opposite in direction to the large arrows, which is pointing to the direction of the T wave. **(B)** When the ST and T waves are concordant (arrows are pointing in the same direction), the ST and T wave changes are primary and indicate the presence of a myocardial abnormality.

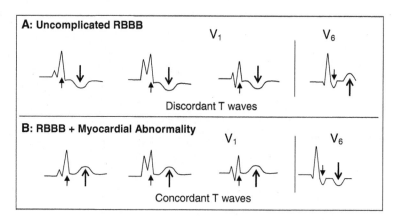

## RBBB: Concordant and Discordant T Waves

- **Secondary repolarization changes:** In uncomplicated RBBB, the ST segment and T wave are normally *discordant* and opposite in direction to the terminal portion of the QRS complex (Fig. 10.9A). These ST-T changes are *secondary* to the abnormal activation of the ventricles. They are not included as criteria in the diagnosis of RBBB.

  - **V$_1$:** Because the terminal portion of the QRS complex is an R′ wave in V$_1$ (which is upright), the ST segment is isoelectric or depressed and the T wave is normally inverted (Fig. 10.9A).

  - **V$_6$:** Because the terminal portion of the QRS complex is an S wave in V$_6$, the ST segment is isoelectric or elevated and the T wave is normally upright.

- **Primary repolarization changes:** When the ST and T waves are *concordant* (in the same direction as the terminal portion of the QRS complex; Fig. 10.9B), in the setting of RBBB, these changes are *primary* and due to the presence of an intrinsic myocardial disorder such as cardiomyopathy or myocardial ischemia rather than secondary to the abnormal activation of the ventricles.

## Incomplete RBBB

- **Incomplete RBBB:** Incomplete RBBB has all the features of complete RBBB except that the duration of the QRS complex is <0.12 seconds. In incomplete RBBB, there is delay rather than complete interruption of the impulse to the right ventricle.

  - **ECG Findings:** The ECG findings of incomplete RBBB are identical to those of complete RBBB except

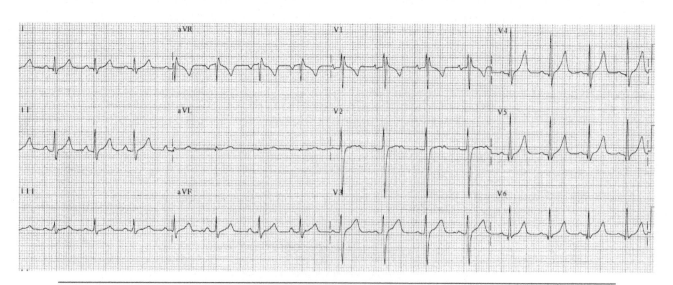

**Figure 10.10:   Incomplete Right Bundle Branch Block.** The QRS complexes are only minimally widened, measuring <0.12 seconds, with rSr′ in V$_1$ and a minimally wide S wave in leads I and V$_6$. This electrocardiogram is otherwise similar to that of complete right bundle branch block, as shown in Figure 10.6.

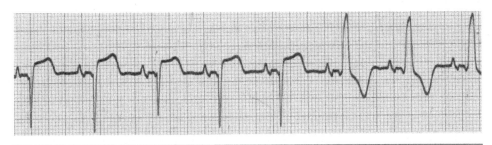

**Figure 10.11: Intermittent Right Bundle Branch Block.** Lead V₁ rhythm strip showing intermittent right bundle branch block (RBBB). Note the change in the width and configuration of the QRS complex in V₁ with the onset of RBBB.

that the QRS complexes measure <0.12 seconds (Fig. 10.10). The axis of the QRS complex is normal unless there is LAFB or LPFB.

- ☐ **V₁:** Right precordial lead V₁ shows an rsr′ or rR′ pattern very similar to that of complete RBBB.
- ☐ **V₆:** Left precordial lead V₆ will show a slightly widened S wave.

- **Intermittent RBBB:** RBBB often occurs intermittently before it becomes fixed (Fig. 10.11). Intermittent RBBB is usually rate related meaning that it usually occurs when the heart rate exceeds a certain level.

## Common Errors in RBBB

- **Ectopic ventricular impulses:** Ectopic impulses originating from the ventricles have wide QRS complexes. These ectopic impulses are wide because they do not follow the normal conduction system and spread to the ventricles by muscle cell to muscle cell conduction. The wide complexes may be mistaken for bundle branch block.
  - **Ventricular tachycardia:** A common example is ventricular tachycardia with RBBB configuration. Although the QRS complexes are wide with tall R waves in V₁, it is erroneous to conclude that there is RBBB during ventricular tachycardia. The ventricular tachycardia may originate from the left ventricle and spread to the right ventricle, causing the QRS complexes to have a RBBB pattern. Despite this appearance, RBBB is not present.
  - **Accelerated idioventricular rhythm (AIVR):** When ventricular impulses resulting from accelerated idioventricular rhythm occur, the wide QRS complexes may have a RBBB pattern and may be mistaken for RBBB (Fig. 10.12).
- In true RBBB, the impulse should be sinus or supraventricular. When the impulse originates from the ventricles or below the bifurcation of the bundle of His, the impulse is ventricular. A ventricular impulse

may demonstrate an RBBB configuration, even though RBBB is not present.

## ECG Findings in RBBB

1. Wide QRS complexes measuring ≥0.12 seconds.
   - Right-sided precordial leads V₁.
     - ☐ Large terminal R′ waves with rSR′ or rR′ often in an M-shaped configuration.
     - ☐ Onset of intrinsicoid deflection or R peak time is prolonged and is >0.05 seconds.
   - Left-sided precordial leads V₆.
     - ☐ Wide S wave with qRS, RS, or rS pattern.
     - ☐ Septal Q waves are preserved.
     - ☐ Onset of intrinsicoid deflection or R peak time is normal and is ≤0.05 seconds.
   - Frontal or limb leads:
     - ☐ Wide S waves in leads I and aVL.
     - ☐ The axis of the QRS complex is normal.
2. ST segment and T wave are opposite in direction (normally discordant) to the terminal QRS complex. These ST and T wave changes are not included as criteria for the diagnosis of RBBB.
   - Right-sided precordial leads V₁ or V₂:
     - ☐ ST segment isoelectric or depressed.
     - ☐ T wave inverted.
   - Left sided precordial leads V₅ or V₆:
     - ☐ ST segment isoelectric or elevated.
     - ☐ T wave is upright.

## Mechanism of RBBB

- **Wide QRS complex:** The intraventricular conduction system activates both ventricles synchronously, resulting in a narrow QRS complex. When RBBB occurs, conduction of the impulse through the right bundle branch is delayed or interrupted, whereas conduction to the left bundle branch and left ventricle is preserved. Activation of the right ventricle is

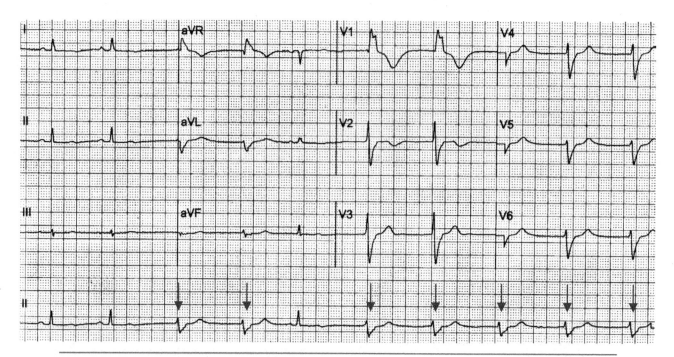

**Figure 10.12: Accelerated Idioventricular Rhythm.** The rhythm is normal sinus as shown by the first two complexes on the left. The wide QRS complexes that follow (*arrows*) look like intermittent right bundle branch block with tall R waves in $V_1$. The wide QRS complexes are ventricular escape complexes because of accelerated idioventricular rhythm. Note that the wide QRS complexes are not preceded by P waves and occur only when there is slowing of the sinus node.

abnormal because the impulse must originate from the left ventricle by muscle cell to muscle cell conduction. Because the ventricles are activated sequentially instead of synchronously, the QRS complexes are wide measuring ≥0.12 seconds. The wide QRS complex can be divided into two halves: the initial half representing left ventricular activation and the terminal half representing right ventricular activation.

- **Vector 1:** In RBBB, vector 1 or septal activation is not altered, thus the initial portion of the QRS complex remains preserved. A small r wave is normally recorded in lead $V_1$, and a normal septal q wave is recorded in $V_6$ as well as in leads located on the left side of the ventricular septum (leads I and aVL).

- **Vector 2:** Activation of the left ventricular free wall or vector 2 is also preserved and normally occurs from endocardium to epicardium in a right to left direction. This result in deep S waves in $V_1$ and tall R waves in $V_6$. Activation of the right side of the septum, however, is no longer possible because the right bundle branch is blocked. Thus, septal activation continues unopposed in a left to right direction, which is opposite the direction of activation of the left ventricular free wall. Because the septum and left ventricular free wall are activated in opposite directions, the depth of the S wave in $V_1$ and the height of the R wave in $V_6$ are smaller than normal.

- **Vector 3:** Whenever there is an intraventricular conduction abnormality, the area with the conduction abnormality is always the last to be activated. Activation of the

right ventricle, therefore, is the last to occur in RBBB (vector 3). Because the right bundle branch supplies the right ventricle, and the right ventricle is located anterior and to the right of the left ventricle, the terminal impulse will be directed to the right and anteriorly. This results in a large terminal R' in $V_1$ and wide terminal S in $V_6$ (and also in leads I and aVL). This is the most distinctive abnormality of RBBB. This terminal impulse is slow because it is conducted by direct myocardial spread and is unopposed because activation of the right ventricle is still ongoing, whereas activation of the rest of the ventricle is already completed.

- **Delayed onset of the intrinsicoid deflection or R peak time:** The ventricular activation time is the time from onset of the ventricular impulse to the arrival of the impulse at the recording precordial electrode. It is measured from the onset of the QRS complex to the height of the R or R' wave. The turning point or abrupt downward deflection of the R or R' wave toward baseline is called the intrinsicoid deflection (see Chapter 6, Depolarization and Repolarization). For practical purposes, the R peak time has been recommended by the Cardiology Task Force of the World Health Organization/International Society and Federation to represent the onset of the intrinsicoid deflection. The normal onset of the intrinsicoid deflection in $V_1$ is ≤0.03 seconds. When there is RBBB, the onset of the intrinsicoid deflection in $V_1$ is prolonged and measures >0.05 seconds because conduction of the impulse across the right ventricle is delayed. The onset of the intrinsicoid deflection in leads $V_5$ or $V_6$ is preserved (normal ≤0.05 seconds) because the left bundle branch is intact.

■ **Abnormal ST-T changes:** The ST and T abnormalities in RBBB are secondary to abnormal activation of the ventricles and are normally discordant to the terminal portion of the QRS complex. The ST-T changes are not considered criteria for the diagnosis of RBBB.

■ **QRS Axis:** In uncomplicated RBBB, the axis of the QRS complex is within normal limits. However, when RBBB occurs in association with pulmonary hypertension or conditions that can cause right ventricular hypertrophy, the axis of the QRS complex may shift to the right. The axis of the QRS complex can also become abnormal when there is fascicular block or previous myocardial infarct.

## Clinical Significance

■ Incomplete RBBB with a terminal r′ wave in $V_1$ or $V_2$ does not always imply that a conduction block is present in the right bundle branch. This ECG pattern could also be due to delayed conduction of the impulse to the right ventricle, causing the right ventricle to be partly activated by the left bundle branch. It could also be due to delayed activation of the base of the right or left ventricle due to a focal area of hypertrophy. For example, in infants and children, the terminal r′ in $V_1$ may be due to hypertrophy of the outflow tract of the right ventricle, a condition that may persist through adulthood. It has also been shown than an rSr′ pattern in $V_1$ or $V_2$ may occur if the precordial leads $V_1$ and $V_2$ are inadvertently positioned higher than the correct location at the 4th intercostal space, a common error among house officers or technicians who are not properly trained to record ECGs.

■ Because the right bundle branch is partially subendocardial in location, it is vulnerable to sudden and severe increases in right ventricular pressure. RBBB can therefore occur in the setting of pulmonary hypertension or acute pulmonary embolism. The right bundle branch is also vulnerable to local injury during right heart catheterization. Thus, extreme caution should be exercised when inserting a pulmonary artery catheter in a patient who has preexistent left bundle branch block (LBBB).

■ RBBB may initially occur intermittently before it becomes fixed. When RBBB is intermittent, it is usually rate related. In rate-related bundle branch block, bundle branch block occurs only when the heart rate increases above a certain threshold. Normal conduction is restored when the heart rate slows down to baseline. The presence of rate-related bundle branch block is often suspected when the wide QRS complexes normalize after a long compensatory pause of a premature ectopic impulse.

■ **Clinical significance:** RBBB can occur as an isolated finding in the general population, including young individuals without evidence of cardiac disease. Among 110,000 subjects screened for cardiovascular disease during a 25-year period, isolated RBBB (no evidence of heart disease or hypertension) occurred in 198 cases (0.18%) and was associated with an excellent prognosis. In another study consisting of 1,142 elderly men followed in the Baltimore Longitudinal Study on Aging, 39 or 3.4% had complete RBBB. Twenty-four of these patients had no evidence of heart disease. Long-term follow-up of patients who are apparently healthy and completely asymptomatic had not shown any adverse effects on mortality and morbidity.

■ RBBB and LAFB is a common combination because the right bundle and left anterior fascicle are adjacent to each other, straddling both sides of the ventricular septum. Both are supplied by the left anterior descending coronary artery. Thus, a concurrent RBBB and LAFB is a common complication of acute anteroseptal myocardial infarction (MI). When RBBB with fascicular block is due to acute anterior MI, the myocardial damage is usually extensive, resulting in a higher incidence of atrioventricular (AV) block, pump failure, and ventricular arrhythmias. However, if the RBBB is due to degenerative disease of the conduction system with preservation of myocardial function, progression to complete AV block is slow, and long-term prognosis is good.

■ **RBBB and MI:** The presence of RBBB generally does not conceal the ECG changes associated with Q wave MI. This contrasts with LBBB, where ECG changes of acute MI are usually masked by the conduction abnormality. Thus, Q waves will continue to be useful in signifying acute or remote MI in patients with RBBB.

■ **RBBB and stress testing:** According to the American College of Cardiology/American Heart Association guidelines for chronic stable angina, the presence of RBBB on a baseline ECG during exercise stress testing will not interfere with the detection of myocardial ischemia. The ST segment depression in leads $V_1$ to $V_3$ may not be related to myocardial ischemia; however, ST depression in leads $V_5$, $V_6$, II, and aVF is as reliable in indicating myocardial ischemia as in ECGs without RBBB. Thus, patients with RBBB on baseline ECG may undergo ECG exercise stress testing similar to patients without the conduction abnormality. This contrasts with patients with LBBB in whom ST depression does not necessarily imply the presence of myocardial ischemia (see Left Bundle Branch Block section in this chapter). Unlike patients with RBBB, patients with LBBB should undergo imaging in conjunction with ECG stress testing.

■ **RBBB and congestive heart failure:** In patients with severe left ventricular dysfunction with ongoing symptoms of congestive heart failure intractable to standard medical therapy, the presence of wide QRS complexes—including patients with RBBB—may be candidates for resynchronization therapy (see Left Bundle Branch Block section in this chapter).

■ **Causes of RBBB:** RBBB can be due to several causes, including acute MI, cardiomyopathy, pulmonary hypertension, pulmonary embolism, cor pulmonale, acute myocarditis, valvular heart disease (especially aortic stenosis), sclerodegenerative changes involving the conduction system, infiltrative diseases such as sarcoidosis and amyloidosis, Chagas disease, and congenital heart disease such as tetralogy of Fallot and Ebstein's anomaly. It may occur as a complication of cardiac surgery or interventional procedures such as cardiac catheterization, percutaneous coronary intervention, radiofrequency ablation, or alcohol ablation of the ventricular septum in patients with idiopathic hypertrophic subaortic stenosis. It may also be a normal finding in young individuals.

■ **Auscultatory findings:** Auscultatory findings associated with RBBB include delayed closure of the pulmonic valve resulting in wide splitting of the second heart sound. There may also be delay in the closure of the tricuspid valve resulting in wide splitting of the first heart sound.

## Treatment and Prognosis

■ The overall prognosis of patients with RBBB depends on the associated cardiac abnormality.

   ■ Asymptomatic RBBB does not require any therapy and may be a normal finding in younger asymptomatic individuals or in older patients without evidence of cardiac disease. When RBBB is an isolated abnormality, progression to complete AV block is uncommon, occurring <1% per year. Even patients with isolated RBBB who subsequently go on to develop complete AV block can expect to have a normal life span after placement of a permanent pacemaker.

   ■ RBBB with or without fascicular block complicating acute anterior MI is associated with a mortality of >20%. Most of these patients have extensive myocardial damage and will succumb to ventricular arrhythmias and pump failure rather than complete AV block. Thus, insertion of a permanent pacemaker in these patients may prevent AV block, but may not alter the overall prognosis. Practice guidelines recommend that patients who survive an acute

MI with a final ejection fraction ≤35% should have an automatic defibrillator implanted regardless of the presence or absence of arrhythmias or conduction abnormality. The underlying cardiac disease, therefore, is most important in defining the prognosis of patients with RBBB.

## Left Bundle Branch Block

■ **LBBB:** Conduction of the sinus impulse can be interrupted at the main left bundle or more distally at the level of both fascicles resulting in LBBB (Fig. 10.13).

■ **ECG findings:** When the left bundle branch is blocked, activation of the left ventricle is delayed resulting in wide QRS complexes that measure ≥0.12 seconds. The ECG findings of LBBB are best recognized in precordial leads $V_1$ and $V_6$. In lead $V_1$, a QS or rS complex is recorded. In $V_6$, the septal q wave is no longer present. A tall monophasic R wave often with initial slurring or M-shaped configuration is present, and onset of intrinsicoid deflection or R peak time is prolonged (>0.05 seconds).

■ **Incomplete LBBB:** Incomplete LBBB is similar to complete LBBB except that the duration of the QRS complex is <0.12 seconds. In incomplete LBBB, there is a delay (rather than a complete interruption) in the conduction of the impulse to the left bundle branch.

**Figure 10.13:   Left Bundle Branch Block.** $V_1$ and $V_6$ are the most important leads in recognizing left bundle branch block. The QRS complexes in $V_1$ will show deep QS or rS complexes and $V_6$ will show rR', monophasic R, or RR' often M-shaped configuration. The R peak time or onset of the intrinsicoid deflection in $V_6$ is shown by the arrows and is delayed (>0.05 seconds). No septal Q waves are present.

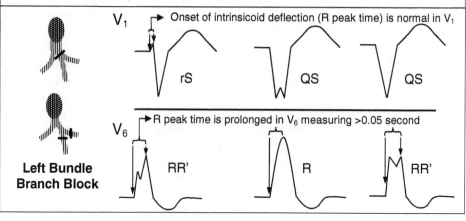

**Left Bundle Branch Block**

- Wide QRS complexes measuring ≥0.12 second
   o **$V_1$:**
      ▪ QS or rS complexes
   o **$V_6$ and leads on left side of ventricular septum (I and aVL):**
      ▪ Septal q waves are absent
      ▪ Monophasic R, RR', slurred R or M-shaped R
      ▪ Onset of intrinsicoid deflection or R peak time is prolonged (>0.05 sec)

$V_1$   Onset of intrinsicoid deflection (R peak time) is normal in $V_1$

rS          QS          QS

$V_6$   R peak time is prolonged in $V_6$ measuring >0.05 second

**Left Bundle Branch Block**          RR'          R          RR'

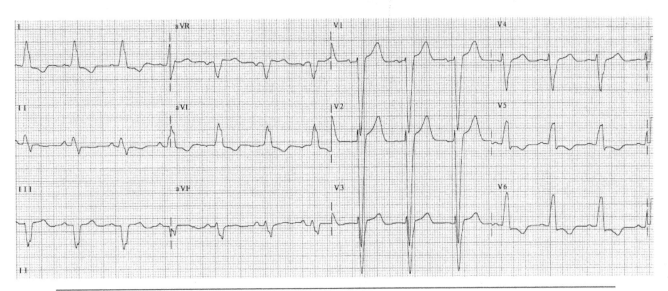

**Figure 10.14:  Left Bundle Branch Block.** In left bundle branch block, the QRS complexes are wide with a QS or rS complex in $V_1$ and tall monophasic R wave in $V_6$ without septal q waves. The ST segment and T waves are normally discordant.

■ **ECG Findings:** In incomplete LBBB, the QRS complexes are slightly widened, measuring <0.12 seconds. All the features of LBBB are present; septal q waves in $V_5$ or $V_6$ are absent, and either a QS complex or a small r wave (rS complex) is present in $V_1$ (Fig. 10.14, Fig. 10.15).

■ The left ventricle is supplied by two main fascicles: the left anterior and left posterior fascicles. LBBB is therefore considered a bifascicular block. Although a midseptal fascicle also exists, its significance is uncertain and there are presently no diagnostic criteria for lesions involving the mid-septal branch.

■ In LBBB, the abnormal activation of the left ventricle can result in ECG abnormalities that may be mistaken for left ventricular hypertrophy. The presence of abnormal q waves and ST-T abnormalities can mimic MI. Conversely, LBBB can mask the ECG changes of acute MI.

■ The abnormal activation of the left ventricle can cause wall motion abnormalities, even in patients without myocardial disease. It may also result in mitral regurgitation because of asynchrony in the contraction of the anterior and posterior papillary muscles. These abnormalities are enhanced when myocardial disease is superimposed on

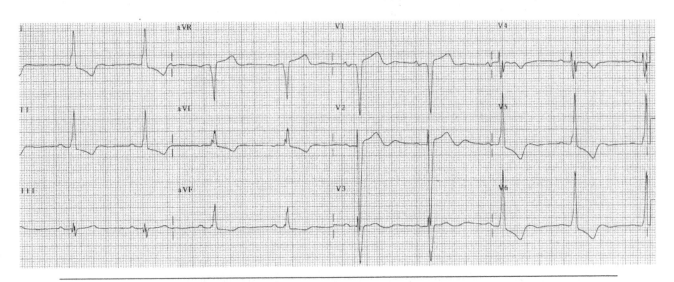

**Figure 10.15:  Incomplete Left Bundle Branch Block.** In incomplete left bundle branch block (LBBB), the QRS complexes have all the features of LBBB. QS or rS configuration is present in $V_1$, tall monophasic R waves are present in $V_6$, and no septal q waves in $V_6$. The duration of the QRS complex, however, is <0.12 seconds.

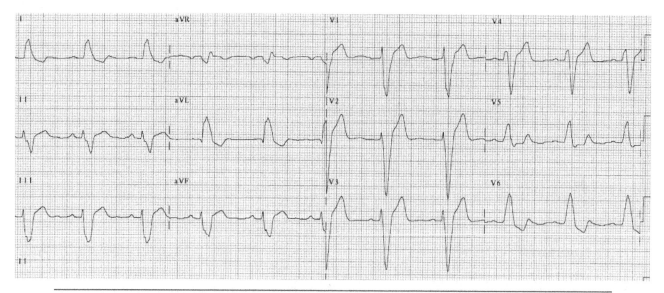

**Figure 10.16:   Left Bundle Branch Block with Unusually Wide QRS Complexes.** The QRS complexes measure almost 0.20 seconds and the axis is shifted to the left. The unusual width of the QRS complexes is often a marker of severe myocardial disease, especially when there is right or left axis deviation.

the conduction defect. In general, patients with LBBB with very wide QRS complexes (Fig. 10.16) have more severe contraction abnormalities and lower ejection fractions compared with patients with LBBB with narrower complexes.

■ The axis of the QRS complex in LBBB is variable. When LBBB is associated with left axis deviation, the conduction abnormality is more widespread and may involve the distal fascicles and Purkinje system. When right axis deviation is present, it may be associated with diffuse myocardial disease and biventricular enlargement.

■ **Secondary ST and T wave changes:** Similar to RBBB, the ST-T changes are not included as criteria in the ECG diagnosis of LBBB. The ST-T changes associated with uncomplicated LBBB are *secondary* to abnormal activation of the left ventricle. The direction of the ST segment and T wave is normally *discordant* or opposite that of the QRS complex (Fig. 10.17A).

  ■ **$V_1$:** In $V_1$, the ST segment is normally elevated and the T wave upright because the terminal portion of the QRS complex is an S wave, which is negative or downward.

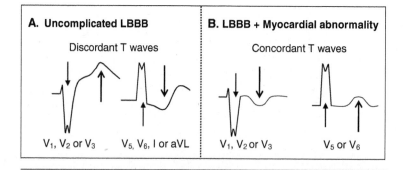

**Figure 10.17:   ST Segment and T Waves in Left Bundle Branch Block. (A)** The ST segment and T wave are normally opposite in direction (discordant) from that of the QRS complex when there is uncomplicated left bundle branch block. Note that the small arrow (pointing to the QRS complex) is opposite in direction to the large arrow, which is pointing to the T wave. **(B)** When there is myocardial disease, such as myocardial ischemia or cardiomyopathy, the ST segments and T waves become concordant and follow the direction of the QRS complex. Note that the small and large arrows are pointing in the same direction.

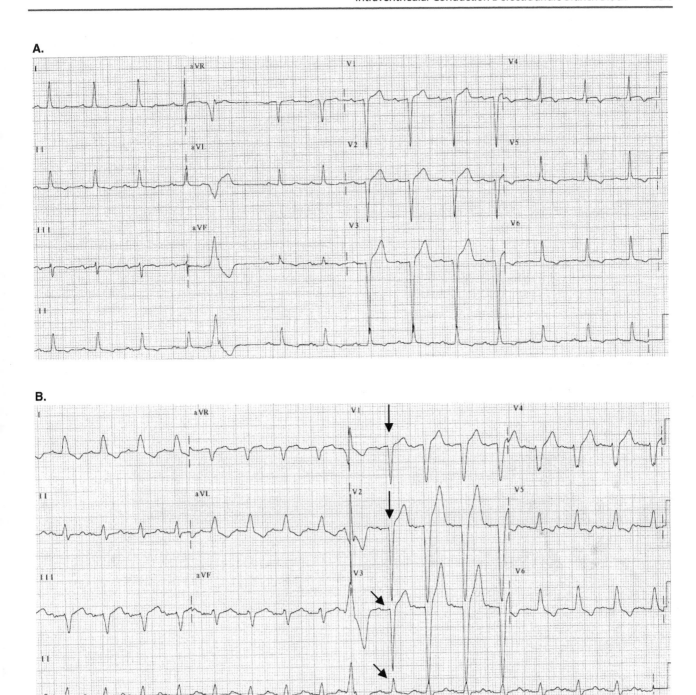

**Figure 10.18:  Rate-Related Left Bundle Branch Block (LBBB).** Electrocardiogram **(ECG) A** shows sinus rhythm, 83 beats per minute with narrow QRS complexes. **ECG B** is from the same patient showing sinus tachycardia of 102 beats per minute and LBBB. The LBBB is rate related developing only during tachycardia. Note that after the compensatory pause of the PVC in **ECG B**, there is narrowing of the QRS complex (*arrows*) similar to the QRS complex in **ECG A**. The long pause after the PVC allows the left bundle branch to recover and conducts the next impulse normally.

- **V$_6$:** In V$_5$ or V$_6$, the ST segment is isoelectric or depressed and the T wave inverted because the terminal portion of the QRS complex is upright.
- **Primary ST and T wave changes:** When the ST segment and T wave changes are *concordant* in the setting of LBBB, they are *primary* and due to the presence of an intrinsic myocardial disorder such cardiomyopathy

or myocardial ischemia rather than secondary to the abnormal activation of the ventricles (Fig. 10.17B).
- LBBB may be rate related (Figs. 10.18, 10.19, and 10.20). In rate-related LBBB, the bundle branch block becomes manifest only when there is tachycardia or bradycardia. This contrasts with fixed bundle branch block, which is present regardless of the heart rate.

■ Table 10.1 is a diagrammatic representation of the different intraventricular conduction abnormalities using only the minimum leads necessary for diagnosis.

## ECG Findings in LBBB

1. Wide QRS complexes measuring ≥0.12 seconds
   ■ Right-sided precordial lead $V_1$
     □ Deep QS or rS complex often with slurring of the downstroke or upstroke of the S wave
     □ Onset of intrinsicoid deflection is normal measuring ≤0.03 seconds
   ■ Left sided precordial lead $V_6$
     □ Monophasic R or slurred upstroke of the R wave with rR′, RR′, or M-shaped configuration
     □ R peak time or onset of intrinsicoid deflection is prolonged measuring >0.05 seconds
2. ST segments and T waves are opposite in direction (normally discordant) to the QRS complexes
   ■ Right-sided precordial lead $V_1$
     □ ST segment elevated
     □ T wave upright
   ■ Left-sided precordial lead $V_6$
     □ ST segment depressed
     □ T wave inverted

## Mechanism

■ **Wide QRS complex:** When there is LBBB, conduction of the electrical impulse to the right bundle branch occurs normally and conduction of the impulse through the left bundle branch is delayed or interrupted. This results in wide QRS complexes measuring ≥0.12 seconds because of asynchronous activation of the ventricles.

■ **Delayed onset of the intrinsicoid deflection or R peak time in $V_5$ or $V_6$:** The intrinsicoid deflection refers to the abrupt downward deflection of the R wave on arrival of the impulse at the recording electrode. When there is LBBB, activation of the right ventricle is preserved because conduction through the right bundle branch is intact. Thus the onset of the intrinsicoid deflection in $V_1$ is normal, measuring ≤0.03 seconds. Activation of the left ventricle is delayed because there is a block in the left bundle branch. Thus the onset of the intrinsicoid deflection in $V_5$ and $V_6$ is delayed, measuring >0.05 seconds.

**TABLE 10.1**

**Summary of the ECG Findings of the Different Intraventricular Conduction Abnormalities**

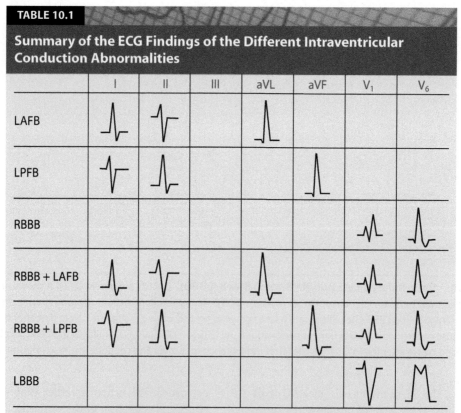

| | I | II | III | aVL | aVF | $V_1$ | $V_6$ |
|---|---|---|---|---|---|---|---|
| LAFB | | | | | | | |
| LPFB | | | | | | | |
| RBBB | | | | | | | |
| RBBB + LAFB | | | | | | | |
| RBBB + LPFB | | | | | | | |
| LBBB | | | | | | | |

The table summarizes the different ECG features of the different intraventricular conduction abnormalities using only the minimum leads for diagnosis. ECG, electrocardiogram; LAFB, left anterior fascicular block; LPFB, left posterior fascicular block; LBBB, left bundle branch block; RBBB, right bundle branch block.

## A. Baseline ECG

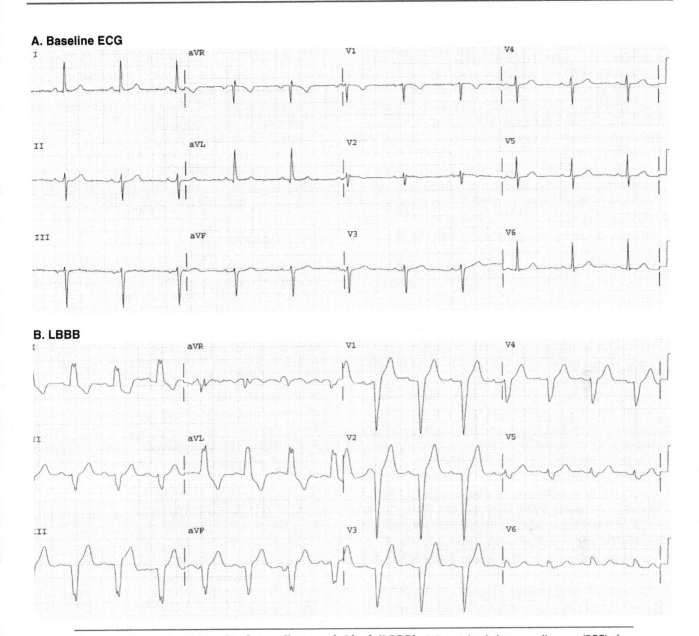

## B. LBBB

**Figure 10.19:   Rate-Related Left Bundle Branch Block (LBBB).  (A)** A 12-lead electrocardiogram (ECG) obtained a few hours before **(B)**. The QRS complexes are narrow with left axis deviation because of left anterior fascicular block. **(B)** ECG from the same patient a few hours later showing LBBB. QS complexes with tall voltages are present in $V_1$ to $V_3$, which can be mistaken for anteroseptal myocardial infarction or left ventricular hypertrophy. Marked ST depression is noted in I and aVL and marked ST elevation is noted in $V_1$ to $V_3$, which can be mistaken for acute coronary syndrome.

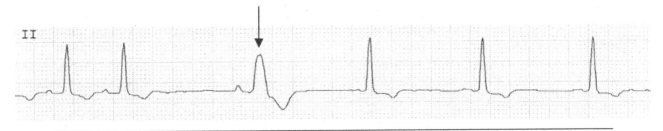

**Figure 10.20:   Bradycardia-Dependent Bundle Branch Block.**  Rhythm strip showing widening of the QRS complex (*arrow*) after a pause from bradycardia-dependent bundle branch block.

- **Absence of septal q wave in V₅ or V₆:** Normally, the ventricular septum is activated by the left bundle branch in a left to right direction (vector 1) resulting in a small septal q wave in $V_5$ or $V_6$ and a small r wave in $V_1$. When there is LBBB, the ventricular septum is no longer activated in a left-to-right direction. Rather, it is activated by the right bundle branch in a right-to-left direction, which is the reverse of normal. The normal septal q wave in $V_5$ or $V_6$ is no longer recorded and should not be present when there is LBBB. $V_1$ and $V_2$ may record a small r wave, representing activation of the right ventricular wall and apex. The small r wave in $V_1$ does not represent septal activation.

- **Slurring of the upstroke of the R wave with rR′ or RR′ (M-shaped) configuration of the QRS complex in V₆:** After the right ventricle is activated, the impulse moves from right ventricle to left ventricle across the interventricular septum by myocardial cell to myocardial cell conduction. This results in tall R waves in $V_6$ and deep S waves in $V_1$ and $V_2$. The initial R wave in $V_6$ represents activation of the ventricular septum, and the larger terminal R′ deflection represents activation of the left ventricular free wall. The dip or notch between the initial R and terminal R′ is due to activation of a smaller mass of myocardium between the septum and left ventricular free wall. Deep S waves often with slurred downstroke are recorded in $V_1$ and $V_2$.

- **Absence of terminal r′ in V₁ and absence of terminal s waves in V₆:** Whenever there is an intraventricular conduction abnormality, the area supplied by the blocked bundle branch is delayed and will be the last to be activated. Because the left bundle branch supplies the left ventricle and the left ventricle is located to the left and posterior to the right ventricle, the terminal impulse will be directed to the left and posteriorly. Right-sided precordial leads such as $V_1$ or $V_2$ should not record a terminal r′ wave, and left sided precordial leads $V_5$ or $V_6$ should not record a terminal S or s wave.

- **Rate-related bundle branch block:** Bundle branch block, left or right, may be rate related before it becomes fixed. When LBBB is rate related, LBBB occurs only when the heart rate becomes increased or decreased. When LBBB is fixed or permanent, LBBB persists regardless of the heart rate.

  - **Bradycardia-dependent bundle branch block:** In bradycardia-dependent bundle branch block, RBBB or LBBB occurs only when there is bradycardia or slowing of the heart rate. Bradycardia-dependent bundle branch block is due to phase 4 diastolic depolarization, which is inherently present in cells with automatic properties, including cells within the intraventricular conduction system. When there is a long R-R interval, cells with automatic properties undergo spontaneous phase 4 diastolic depolarization resulting in a transmembrane potential that slowly becomes less and less negative. Thus, the sinus impulse may not be able to conduct across a bundle branch that is partially depolarized.

  - **Tachycardia-related bundle branch block:** The refractory period of one bundle branch is usually longer than the refractory period of the other bundle branch.

When the heart rate is relatively slow, both bundle branches are given enough time to repolarize. However, when the heart rate is faster, the impulses may arrive well before the bundle branch with a longer refractory period has a chance to recover. This may result in bundle branch block that is evident during tachycardia, that resolves when the heart rate slows down to baseline. The longer refractory period of one bundle branch is due to its longer action potential duration when compared with the other bundle branch. This type of rate-related bundle branch block is called phase 3 aberration.

## Clinical Significance

- Unlike the right bundle branch, which is long and thin, the left bundle branch immediately divides into two main fascicles: the left anterior and left posterior fascicles. A midseptal branch also exists, although there are no criteria diagnostic of a midseptal lesion. LBBB therefore is an example of bifascicular block. LBBB can occur in the main left bundle (predivisional) or at the level of the fascicles (postdivisional). It can also occur at the level of the bundle of His.

- **Clinical significance:** LBBB can occur as an isolated finding in normal, asymptomatic individuals without evidence of cardiac disease but is rare.

  - In a study of 122,043 asymptomatic and healthy airmen, only 17 individuals were noted to have LBBB compared with 231 with RBBB. In this study, none of 44,231 men younger than age 25 had LBBB.

  - In another study of 110,000 individuals, isolated LBBB occurred in 112 cases (0.1%) without apparent or suspected heart disease, compared with 198 cases of isolated RBBB (0.28%). The overall mortality in patients with isolated LBBB was not increased when compared with patients with RBBB during a mean follow-up of 9.5 years. However, patients with isolated LBBB but not RBBB had increased risk of developing overt cardiovascular disease, which may, in the long run, translate into a higher morbidity and mortality.

    - In the Framingham study, 55 of 5,209 individuals (1%) developed new-onset LBBB during a follow-up period of 18 years. The mean age of onset was 62 years. LBBB was associated with hypertension (defined as blood pressure of ≥160/95 mm Hg), ischemic heart disease, or primary myocardial disease among 47 of the 55 patients. Only 9 of 55 patients (16%) were free of cardiovascular disease during a mean follow-up period of 6 years after the onset of LBBB.

    - A 40-year follow-up study of 17,361 subjects in Hiroshima and Nagasaki, Japan, who underwent biennial health examinations showed 110 subjects with LBBB. The average age at diagnosis was 69.6 ± 10 years in men and 68.3 ± 10.9 years in women, with progressive increase in the incidence of LBBB with age. There was a higher incidence of hypertension, ischemic heart disease, left ventricular hypertrophy with ST-T abnormalities, and increased cardiothoracic ratio among patients who developed LBBB when compared with controls. Age at death was similar for patients with LBBB and controls, although mortality from congestive heart failure and myocardial infarction was significantly higher in patients with LBBB.

☐ Finally, among 723 asymptomatic patients with normal left ventricular ejection fraction incidentally diagnosed to have bundle branch block (58.1% LBBB and 41.9% RBBB) in a community-based patient population, retrospective analysis of computerized medical records after 24 years' follow-up showed that isolated bundle branch block is not a benign finding. Cardiac-related morbidity and mortality is similar to patients with known conventional risk factors without bundle branch block.

■ **Etiology:** LBBB is an acquired conduction disorder and is usually a marker of an underlying cardiac abnormality in contrast to RBBB, which may be congenital and may remain as an isolated finding. The majority of patients with LBBB, but not RBBB, have cardiac disease. If cardiac disease is not apparent, it is very likely that overt cardiac abnormality will subsequently develop. The common causes of LBBB include hypertension, coronary artery disease, valvular diseases (especially aortic stenosis), cardiomyopathy, acute myocarditis, and degenerative disease of the conduction system. LBBB is generally a marker of left ventricular disease and is the most common conduction abnormality in patients with primary cardiomyopathy.

■ **Hemodynamic abnormalities:** LBBB can diminish cardiac performance even in the absence of associated myocardial disease. In LBBB, the ventricles are activated sequentially rather than synchronously. Thus, left and right ventricular contraction is not simultaneous. Furthermore, because conduction of the impulse within the left ventricle is by direct myocardial spread, contraction of the left ventricle is not synchronized and can result in wall motion abnormalities. Mitral regurgitation can occur when the two papillary muscles are not simultaneously activated. The significance of these contraction abnormalities may not be apparent in patients with reasonably good left ventricular systolic function. However, in patients who have myocardial disease and severe left ventricular dysfunction, the presence of LBBB can make systolic dysfunction even more pronounced.

■ **LBBB makes diagnosis of certain disorders difficult:** When LBBB is present, the ECG becomes unreliable as a diagnostic tool for identifying a variety of clinical entities.

■ **Left ventricular hypertrophy:** Left ventricular hypertrophy will be difficult to diagnose when there is LBBB because of the tall voltage and secondary ST-T changes associated with LBBB. Nevertheless, approximately 85% of patients with LBBB will have left ventricular hypertrophy.

■ **Acute MI:** Acute MI is difficult to diagnose when LBBB is present because q waves and ST-T abnormalities associated with acute MI can be obscured by the LBBB. Conversely, when LBBB is present, Q waves or QS complexes may occur in the anterior precordial leads and may mimic a myocardial infarct. The ST-T changes of LBBB can also be mistaken for current of injury (see acute MI and LBBB Chapter 23, Acute Coronary Syndrome: ST Elevation Myocardial Infarction). The following findings suggest the presence of MI when there is LBBB.

☐ Acute MI should be suspected when there is concordant ST segment depression or concordant ST segment elevation $\geq 1$ mm in a patient with symptoms of myocardial ischemia. Concordant ST segment depression is present when the QRS complex is negative and the ST segment is depressed. Concordant ST segment elevation is present when the QRS complex is positive and the ST segment is elevated.

☐ Acute MI should also be suspected when there is discordant ST segment elevation $\geq 5$ mm accompanied by symptoms of ischemia. This implies that ST segment elevation of at least 5 mm is present in leads with deep S waves such as $V_1$, $V_2$, or $V_3$.

☐ Notching of the upstroke of the S wave in $V_3$ or $V_4$, also called Cabrera sign, or the upstroke of the R wave in $V_5$ or $V_6$, also called Chapman sign, are highly specific but not very sensitive for MI.

☐ Q waves in leads $V_5$ or $V_6$ or leads located at the left side of the ventricular septum (I or aVL) indicate an MI, which may be recent or remote.

■ **During stress testing:** LBBB can cause a false-positive or a false-negative stress test.

☐ **ECG stress testing:** During stress testing, LBBB may mask the ECG changes of myocardial ischemia resulting in a false-negative stress test. Conversely, LBBB can result in a false-positive stress test because it can cause secondary ST-T changes in the ECG, which may be misinterpreted as being due to ischemia. Thus, the American College of Cardiology/American Heart Association guideline on chronic stable angina does not recommend stress testing in patients with LBBB using ECG alone as a marker for myocardial ischemia. This is a Class III indication, meaning that there is evidence that the procedure is not useful. Stress testing of patients with complete LBBB on baseline ECG should always include an imaging modality, preferably a nuclear perfusion scan.

☐ **Stress testing with imaging:** Nuclear scan uses perfusion mismatch, whereas echo uses wall motion abnormality as the end point for detecting myocardial ischemia. Because left ventricular wall motion abnormalities inherently occur when there is LBBB, a nuclear perfusion scan is preferred over echocardiography as the imaging modality during stress testing. Pharmacologic stress testing is preferred over exercise when LBBB is present because exercise can further augment the wall motion abnormalities of LBBB even in the absence of ischemia. Dipyridamole or adenosine (but not dobutamine) are preferred because both agents do not alter contractility.

☐ **Auscultatory findings:** The presence of LBBB will delay closure of the mitral and aortic valves. This will cause the first heart sound to become single and the second heart sound to be paradoxically split. When paradoxical splitting of the second heart sound is present, the second heart sound becomes single or narrowly split with inspiration and widely split with expiration. This pattern is the opposite of normal. A short murmur of mitral regurgitation may be audible during early systole because of asynchrony in contraction of the papillary muscles. The presence of mild mitral regurgitation from LBBB, however, is better shown with color Doppler imaging during echocardiography.

## Treatment

■ LBBB is usually associated with cardiac disease more commonly coronary disease, hypertension, valvular disease, or cardiomyopathy. Overall treatment depends on the underlying cardiac condition. In completely asymptomatic patients without known cardiac disease, no treatment is required.

■ LBBB is a bifascicular block that may progress to trifascicular block or complete AV block. In patients with trifascicular block, insertion of a permanent pacemaker is warranted (see Chapter 11, Intraventricular Conduction Defect: Trifascicular Block; see also the American College of Cardiology/American Heart Association/Heart Rhythm Society guidelines on permanent pacemaker implantation in patients with bifascicular and trifascicular block).

■ Patients with systolic left ventricular dysfunction who continue to have symptoms of heart failure despite receiving optimal medical therapy may benefit from cardiac resynchronization therapy if they have LBBB. Cardiac resynchronization involves insertion of a biventricular pacemaker that can stimulate both right and left ventricles simultaneously. Pacing both ventricles simultaneously significantly decreases the delay in the spread of electrical impulse in patients with wide QRS complexes and has been shown to improve cardiac output and diminish mitral regurgitation. The patient should be in normal sinus rhythm so that timing of atrial and ventricular contraction can be synchronized. Although most patients who have received biventricular pacemakers have LBBB, the width of the QRS complex rather than the type of bundle branch block is the main indication for biventricular pacing. Patients who are candidates for cardiac resynchronization therapy should have all of the following features:

■ Patients with wide QRS complexes ($\geq 0.12$ seconds)

■ Normal sinus rhythm

■ Systolic dysfunction (ejection fraction $\leq 35\%$) because of ischemic or nonischemic cardiomyopathy

■ New York Heart Association functional class III or IV heart failure

■ Patients continue to have heart failure in spite of optimal medical therapy

## Prognosis

■ Similar to RBBB, the overall prognosis depends on the etiology of the LBBB.

▪ In the Framingham study, patients who did well were those with normal axis of the QRS complex (to the right of $0°$), those without any left atrial abnormality or left atrial conduction delay and those who did not have changes in the ECG before the development of LBBB.

▪ Among older patients with LBBB, majority had antecedent cardiomegaly, hypertension, or coronary disease. If they did not have any of these findings, the majority went on to develop one of these cardiovascular abnormalities. The presence of these cardiovascular diseases will translate into a higher mortality.

▪ Finally, long-term follow-up studies show that patients with LBBB have a higher incidence of cardiovascular disease with higher mortality from congestive heart failure and acute MI, although all-cause mortality may not be significantly different among patients with LBBB compared with those who do not.

## Suggested Readings

Bax JJ, Ansalone G, Breithardt OA, et al. Echocardiographic evaluation of cardiac resynchronization therapy: ready for routine clinical use? A critical appraisal. *J Am Coll Cardiol.* 2004;44: 1–9.

Dunn MI, Lipman BS. Abnormalities of ventricular conduction: right bundle-branch block. In: *Lippman-Massie Clinical Electrocardiography.* 8th ed. Chicago: Yearbook Medical Publishers, Inc.; 1989:117–132.

Dunn MI, Lipman BS. Abnormalities of ventricular conduction: left bundle-branch block. In: *Lippman-Massie Clinical Electrocardiography.* 8th ed. Chicago: Yearbook Medical Publishers, Inc.; 1989:133–147.

Epstein AE, DiMarco JP, Ellenbogen KA, et al. ACC/AHA/HRS 2008 guidelines for device-based therapy of cardiac rhythm abnormalities: a report of the American College of Cardiology/American Heart Association Task Force on Practice Guidelines (Writing Committee to Revise the ACC/AHA/ NASPE 2002 Guideline Update for Implantation of Cardiac Pacemakers and Antiarrhythmia Devices). *Circulation.* 2008;117: e350–e408.

Fahy GJ, Pinski SL, Miller DP, et al. Natural history of isolated bundle branch block. *Am J Cardiol.* 1996;77:1185–1190.

Fleg JL, Das DW, Lakatta EG. Right bundle branch block: long term prognosis in apparently healthy men. *J Am Cardiol.* 1983;1:887–892.

Francia P, Balla C, Paneni F, et al. Left bundle-branch block—pathophysiology, prognosis, and clinical management. *Clin Cardiol.* 2007;30:110–115.

Gibbons RJ, Abrams J, Chatterjee K, et al. ACC/AHA 2002 guideline update for the management of patients with chronic stable angina: a report of the American College of Cardiology/American Heart Association Task Force on

Practice Guidelines (Committee to Update the 1999 Guidelines for the Management of Patients with Chronic Stable Angina. www.acc.org/clinical/guidelines/stable/stable.pdf.

Goldberger AL, Arnsdorf MF. Electrocardiographic diagnosis of myocardial infarction in the presence of bundle branch block or a paced rhythm. 2008 UpToDate. www. uptodate.com.

Hiss RG, Lamb LE. Electrocardiographic findings in 122,043 individuals. *Circulation*. 1962;25:947–961.

Imanishi R, Seto S, Ichimaru S, et al. Prognostic significance of incident left bundle branch block observed over a 40-year period. *Am J Cardiol*. 2006;98:644–648.

Marriott HJL. The hemiblocks and trifascicular block. In: *Practical Electrocardiography*. 5th ed. Baltimore: The Williams and Wilkins Company, 1972:86–94.

Miller WL, Ballman KV, Hodge DO, et al. Risk factor implications of incidentally discovered uncomplicated bundle branch block. *Mayo Clinic Proc*. 2005;80:1585–1590.

Schneider JF, Thomas Jr HE, McNamara PM, et al. Clinical-electrocardiographic correlates of newly acquired left bundle branch block: the Framingham study. *Am J Cardiol*. 1985; 55:1332–1338.

Sgarbossa EB, Pinski SL, Barbagelata A, et al. Electrocardiographic diagnosis of evolving acute myocardial infarction in the presence of left bundle branch block. *N Engl J Med*. 1996;334:481–487.

Sgarbossa EB, Wagner GS. Electrocardiography: In: Topol EJ, ed. *Textbook of Cardiovascular Medicine*. 2nd ed. Philadelphia: Lippincott Williams & Wilkins; 2002:1330–1354.

Strickberger SA, Conti J, Daoud EG, et al. Patient selection for cardiac resynchronization therapy. *Circulation*. 2005;111: 2146–2150.

Trevino AJ, Beller BM. Conduction disturbance of the left bundle branch system and their relationship to complete heart block I. A review of experimental, electrophysiologic and electrocardiographic aspects. *Am J Med*. 1971;51:362–373.

Trevino AJ, Beller BM. Conduction disturbance of the left bundle branch system and their relationship to complete heart block II.A review of differential diagnosis, pathology and clinical significance. *Am J Med*. 1971;51:374–382.

Willems JL, Robles de Medina EO, Bernard R, et al. Criteria for intraventricular conduction disturbances and pre-excitation. *J Am Coll Cardiol*. 1985;5:1261–1275.

# Intraventricular Conduction Defect: Trifascicular Block

## Trifascicular Block

- **Types of intraventricular conduction defect:** Instead of two main branches, the bundle of His can be simplified as dividing into three discrete pathways; namely, the right bundle branch, the left anterior, and the left posterior fascicles. Thus, the following abnormalities can occur:
  - **Unifascicular block** (block involves one fascicle):
    - ☐ Left anterior fascicular block (LAFB)
    - ☐ Left posterior fascicular block (LPFB)
    - ☐ Right bundle branch block (RBBB)
  - **Bifascicular block** (block involves two fascicles):
    - ☐ Left bundle branch block (LBBB)
    - ☐ RBBB + LAFB
    - ☐ RBBB + LPFB
  - ***Definite* trifascicular block** (block involves all three fascicles). The following are examples of definite trifascicular block.
    - ☐ Alternating bundle branch block
    - ☐ RBBB + alternating fascicular block
    - ☐ RBBB + Mobitz type II second-degree atrioventricular (AV) block
    - ☐ LBBB + Mobitz type II second-degree AV block
  - ***Possible* trifascicular block:** The following are examples of possible trifascicular block.
    - ☐ Complete AV block with ventricular escape rhythm
    - ☐ Any bifascicular block + first-degree or second-degree AV block
      - ☐ RBBB + LAFB + first-degree or second-degree AV block
      - ☐ RBBB + LPFB + first-degree or second-degree AV block
      - ☐ LBBB + first-degree or second-degree AV block
  - **Nonspecific intraventricular block:** This type of electrocardiogram (ECG) abnormality does not conform to any of the above intraventricular blocks.

- Trifascicular block indicates that some form of conduction abnormality is present in all three fascicles. The conduction abnormality may be due to simple delay (first-degree block), intermittent block (second-degree block), or complete interruption (third-degree block) of the sinus impulse to all three fascicles. Trifascicular block does not imply that the block is always complete in all three fascicles.

## Bilateral Bundle Branch Block

- **Alternating bundle branch block:** Whether it is a RBBB alternating with LBBB, or a RBBB recorded at one time and a LBBB recorded at some other time, such a block would constitute a trifascicular block because there is evidence that both bundle branches, and therefore all three fascicles of the conduction system, are involved. Example of RBBB and LBBB occurring in the same patient is shown in Figure 11.1. Another example of LBBB and RBBB occurring in the same patient is shown in Figure 11.2A, B. When LBBB and RBBB occur in the same patient, bilateral bundle branch block is present. This is an example of trifascicular block.

- **RBBB + alternating fascicular block:** When RBBB is fixed and is accompanied by LAFB that alternates with LPFB, a trifascicular block is present because all three fascicles are involved (Fig. 11.3). This is a rare presentation of trifascicular block.

- **RBBB or LBBB + Mobitz type II second-degree AV block:** Mobitz type II second-degree AV block is an infranodal block (see Chapter 8, Atrioventricular Block). When there is RBBB or LBBB with a type II second-degree AV block, the AV block is at the level of the His-Purkinje system. Thus, a RBBB or LBBB with a type II second-degree AV block suggests the presence of a trifascicular block (Fig. 11.4).

- **Complete AV block with ventricular escape rhythm:** The ultimate manifestation of trifascicular block is complete block involving all three fascicles or

**A.**

**B.**

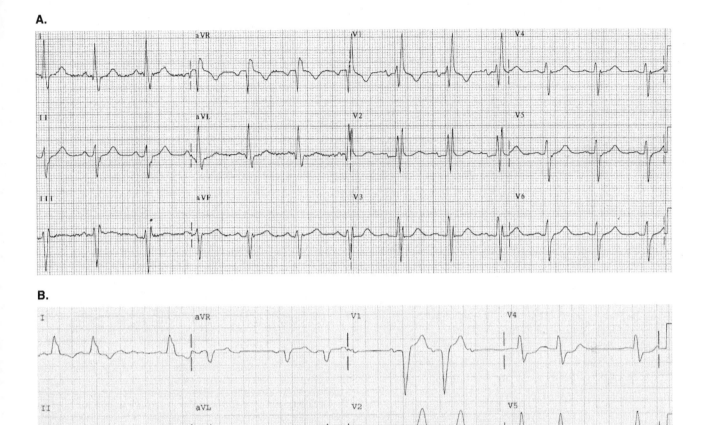

**Figure 11.1:    Bilateral Bundle Branch Block.** Electrocardiogram (ECG) **A** and ECG **B** are from the same patient taken 6 months apart. **(A)** Right bundle branch block (RBBB) with left anterior fascicular block. **(B)** Left bundle branch block (LBBB) with type II second-degree AV block. The presence of RBBB and LBBB in the same patient suggests bilateral bundle branch block. **(B)** also shows Mobitz type II second-degree AV block. Mobitz type II second-degree AV block in addition to LBBB is also indicative of trifascicular block.

both bundle branches. When this occurs, only a ventricular escape impulse can maintain the cardiac rhythm (Fig. 11.5A). Complete AV block with ventricular escape rhythm is most often a trifascicular block. However, should the complete block occur at the level of the AV node, it would not constitute a trifascicular block.

■ **Complete AV block with ventricular escape rhythm:** Another example of complete AV block with ventricular escape rhythm is shown in Figure 11.6. The initial ECG showed LBBB with first-degree AV block. When a bifascicular or trifascicular block deteriorates into complete AV block with ventricular escape rhythm, the AV block is almost always trifascicular.

**A.**

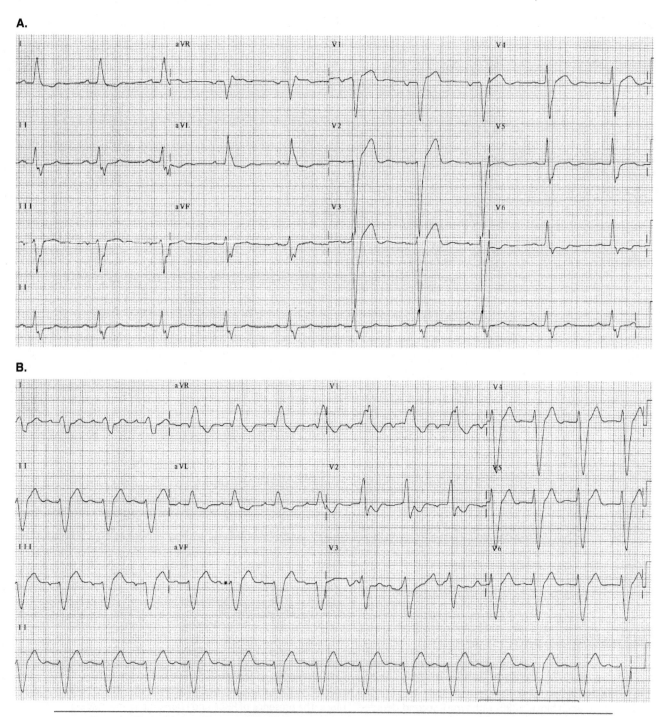

**B.**

**Figure 11.2:    Bilateral Bundle Branch Block.  (A, B)** From the same patient. The initial electrocardiogram (ECG) **(A)** shows left bundle branch block (LBBB) with deep S waves in V$_1$. Subsequent ECG taken a year later **(B)** shows right bundle branch block (RBBB) + left anterior fascicular block. The presence of LBBB and RBBB in the same patient is consistent with bilateral bundle branch block. Note also that there is first-degree atrioventricular block in both ECGs, which in the presence of bifascicular block, is also indicative of trifascicular block.

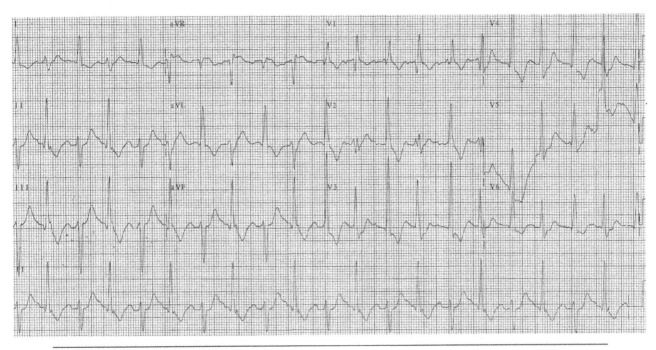

**Figure 11.3:   Fixed Right Bundle Branch Block (RBBB) + Left Anterior Fascicular Block Alternating with Left Posterior Fascicular Block.** The precordial leads show RBBB. The frontal leads show left anterior fascicular block alternating with left posterior fascicular block. This conduction abnormality is an example of trifascicular block.

- **Any bifascicular block + first-degree or second-degree AV block:** RBBB + LAFB + second-degree AV block (Fig. 11.7), RBBB + LPFB + second-degree AV block (Fig. 11.8), and LBBB + second-degree AV block are all possible examples of trifascicular block. Bifascicular block with second-degree AV block is not always the result of trifascicular block because the AV block can occur at the AV node instead of the remaining fascicle.

- When there is a bifascicular block such as RBBB + LAFB, the only pathway by which the atrial impulse can reach the ventricles is through the remaining posterior fascicle. Note that the atrial impulse may be delayed or interrupted at the level of the AV node or at the distal conducting system resulting in first-degree or second-degree AV block. Should the first-degree or second-degree AV block involve the remaining fascicle, a trifascicular block would be present. Should the first-degree or second-degree AV block occur at the AV node, it would not qualify as a trifascicular block. This latter condition must therefore be excluded before diagnosing a trifascicular block. RBBB + LAFB + type I second-degree AV block is shown in Figure 11.9. This is usually an AV nodal block, but it is also possible that the block is trifascicular, involving the remaining fascicle.

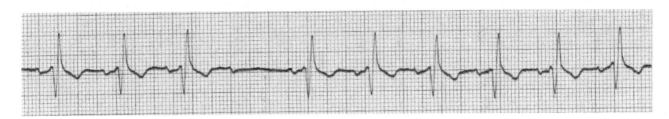

**Figure 11.4:   Mobitz Type II Second-Degree Atrioventricular (AV) Block.** Mobitz type II second-degree AV block is a disease of the distal conduction system. The rhythm strip above was recorded in lead $V_1$. It shows right bundle branch block (RBBB) and second-degree AV block with a fixed PR interval from Mobitz type II AV block. The presence of RBBB and Mobitz type II AV block is consistent with trifascicular block.

**A.**

**B.**

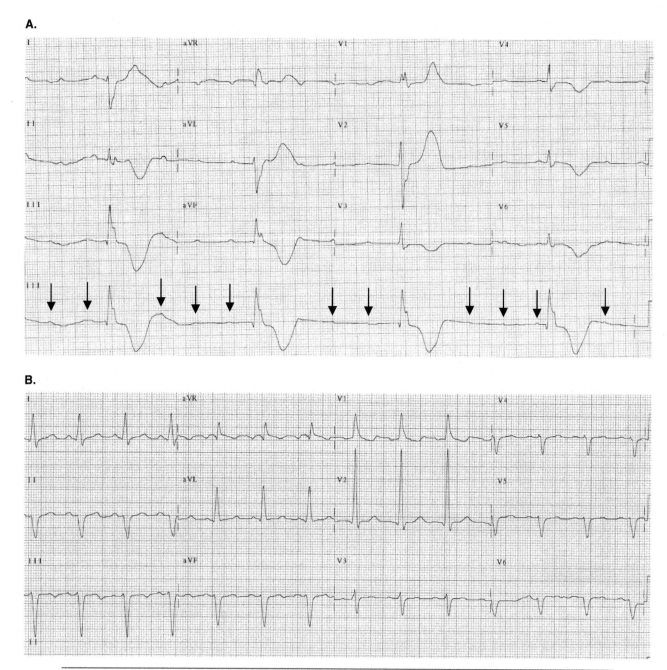

**Figure 11.5:   Complete Atrioventricular (AV) Block with Ventricular Escape Rhythm.** Electrocardiogram (ECG) **A** shows complete AV block with ventricular escape rhythm. ECG **B** was obtained from the same patient several hours earlier showing right bundle branch block + left anterior fascicular block. The presence of ventricular escape rhythm and a previous ECG showing bifascicular block suggests that the complete AV block is infranodal.

**A.**

**B.**

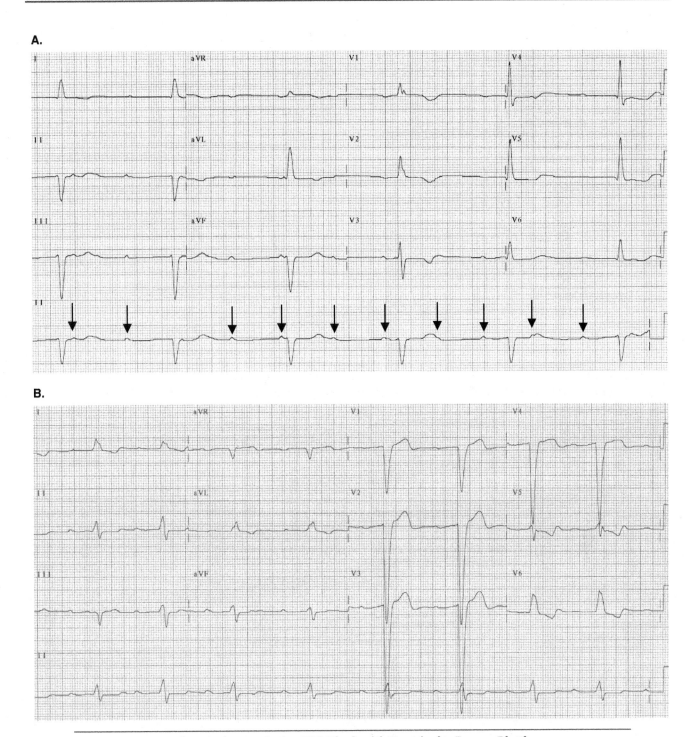

**Figure 11.6:   Complete Atrioventricular (AV) Block with Ventricular Escape Rhythm.**
Electrocardiogram (ECG) **(A)** shows complete AV block with ventricular escape rhythm. The P waves are nonconducted (*arrows*). ECG **(B)** taken 2 months earlier shows left bundle branch block with first-degree AV block, which is consistent with trifascicular block.

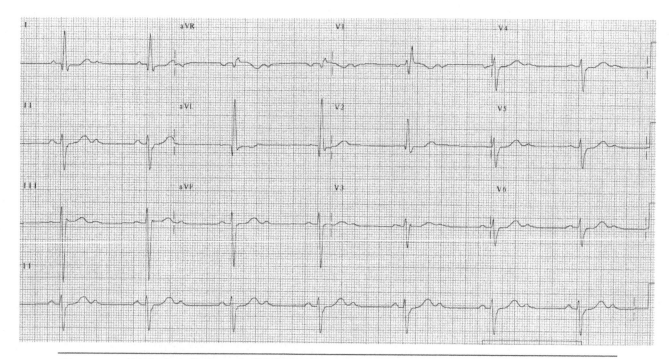

**Figure 11.7:  Right Bundle Branch Block (RBBB) + Left Anterior Fascicular Block (LAFB) + Second-Degree Atrioventricular (AV) Block.**  This 2:1 second-degree AV block combined with RBBB and LAFB is almost always a trifascicular block.

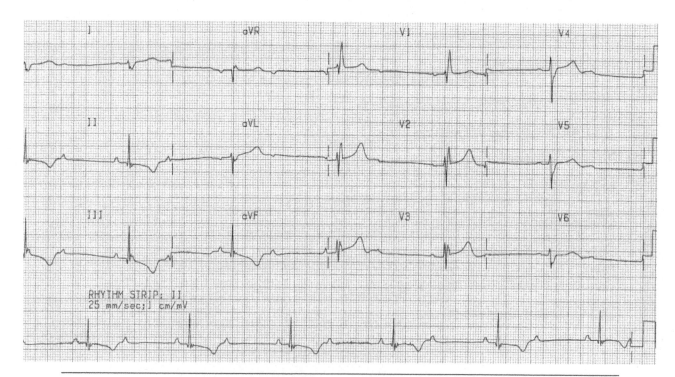

**Figure 11.8:  Right Bundle Branch Block (RBBB) + Left Posterior Fascicular Block (LPFB) + Second-Degree Atrioventricular (AV) Block.**  A 2:1 second-degree AV block in association with RBBB and LPFB is almost always a trifascicular block.

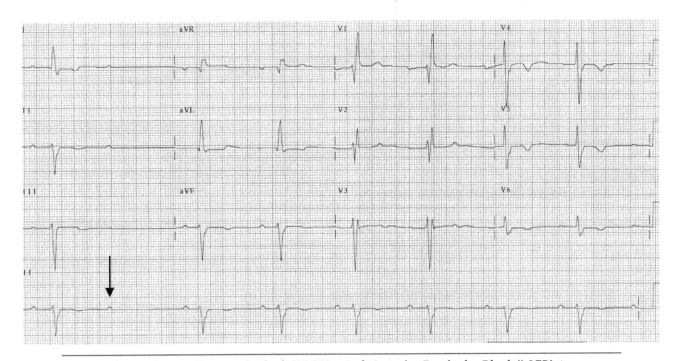

**Figure 11.9:   Right Bundle Branch Block (RBBB) + Left Anterior Fascicular Block (LAFB) + First-Degree and Second-Degree Atrioventricular (AV) Block = Trifascicular Block.** The 12-lead electrocardiogram (ECG) shows RBBB + LAFB. There is also first-degree and type I second-degree AV block (*arrow*). This combination of ECG abnormalities may be due to trifascicular block.

- Complete AV block resulting from trifascicular block is invariably fatal unless a permanent pacemaker is implanted. The presence of trifascicular disease therefore should be recognized so that a permanent pacemaker can be implanted before the conduction abnormality progresses to complete AV block. Bifascicular or trifascicular block with subsequent development of intermittent or persistent complete AV block is a Class I indication for permanent pacemaker implantation regardless of the presence or absence of symptoms according to American College of Cardiology/American Heart Association/Heart Rhythm Society guidelines.

## ECG Findings in Trifascicular Block

1. The following are definite examples of trifascicular block:
   - Alternating bundle branch block
   - RBBB + alternating fascicular block
   - RBBB + Mobitz type II second-degree AV block
   - LBBB + Mobitz type II second-degree AV block
2. The following are possible examples of trifascicular block:
   - Bifascicular block + first-degree AV block
     - RBBB + LAFB + first-degree AV block
     - RBBB + LPFB + first-degree AV block
     - LBBB + first-degree AV block

- Bifascicular block + second-degree AV block
  - RBBB + LAFB + second-degree AV block
  - RBBB + LPFB + second-degree AV block
  - LBBB + second-degree AV block
- Complete AV block with ventricular escape rhythm

## Mechanism

- **Definite trifascicular block:**
  - **Alternating bundle branch block:** Before complete AV block develops, trifascicular block may manifest as a more subtle abnormality, such as RBBB alternating with LBBB. When this occurs, a delay in the impulse (first-degree block) in one bundle branch alternates with delay in the other bundle branch, resulting in alternating bundle branch block. The presence of RBBB alternating with LBBB suggests disease of both bundle branches and is consistent with bilateral bundle branch block or trifascicular block.
  - **RBBB + alternating fascicular block:** RBBB is constantly present in the precordial leads with the axis in the frontal plane alternating between left axis deviation $>-30°$ and right axis deviation $>90°$. This is due to a delay in one fascicle alternating with a delay in the other fascicle. This is consistent with trifascicular block.
  - **Type II second-degree AV block:** If LBBB or RBBB (with or without fascicular block) is associated with type II second-degree AV block, it is very likely that there is bilateral

bundle branch block because type II second-degree AV block involves only the distal conduction system.

- **Possible trifascicular block:**
  - **Bifascicular block + first-degree or second-degree AV block:** First-degree AV block as well as type 1 second-degree AV block can occur anywhere within the conduction system including the AV node or more distally within the bundle branches or fascicles. When AV block occurs in the setting of bifascicular block, the AV block may involve the third or remaining fascicle, in which case a trifascicular block would be present. It is also possible that the AV block may not be in the third fascicle, but at the level of the AV node, in which case it would not be a trifascicular block. The block is trifascicular only if the first-degree or second-degree AV block involves the remaining fascicle.
  - **Complete AV block with ventricular escape rhythm:** Trifascicular block is present when there is simultaneous block involving both bundle branches or all three fascicles of the conduction system. The ECG will show complete AV block. The escape rhythm can originate only from the ventricles. If bifascicular or trifascicular block is present in previous ECGs, complete AV block with a ventricular escape rhythm is almost always the result of a block in the His-Purkinje system.

## Clinical Implications

- Patients with trifascicular block are at risk for developing complete AV block. The AV block can occur suddenly and can result in syncope (Stokes-Adams syndrome) or sudden death. The presence of trifascicular block should be recognized before complete AV block develops.
- When complete AV block occurs, the level of the AV block should always be localized. AV block at the level of the AV node is often reversible and has a better prognosis than AV block occurring more distally at the level of the His-Purkinje system. The patient's history, previous ECG, presence and location of the acute myocardial infarction (MI), and the origin of the escape rhythm are helpful in localizing the level of the AV block.
  - **History:** The block is most likely AV nodal if the patient gives a history of taking medications that can block the AV node such as beta blockers, calcium channel blockers (verapamil and diltiazem), and digitalis.
  - **Previous ECG:** The presence of distal conduction system disease such as bundle branch block, bifascicular block, or trifascicular block suggest that the AV block is in the distal conduction system.
  - **Acute MI:** When acute MI is associated with AV block, the AV block is at the level of the AV node if the MI is inferior. It is infranodal and at the level of the His-Purkinje system if the MI is anterior.
  - **Escape rhythm:** When the AV block is infranodal, the escape rhythm is always ventricular. When the AV block is at the level of the AV node, the escape rhythm is usually AV junctional.

- The presence of bundle branch block (especially LBBB) may be a marker of severe myocardial disease and left ventricular systolic dysfunction. When a patient with bifascicular or trifascicular block presents with syncope, progression to complete AV block is likely. However, one should not overlook the possibility that ventricular tachycardia rather than complete AV block may be the cause of the syncope. Insertion of a permanent pacemaker to prevent bradyarrhythmia may not alter the prognosis of patients with severe myocardial disease if the cause of the syncope is a ventricular arrhythmia.

- The causes of trifascicular block include idiopathic cardiomyopathy, ischemic heart disease, hypertension, valvular heart diseases (especially calcific aortic stenosis), fibrosis or calcification of the conduction system, infiltrative cardiac diseases such as sarcoidosis, hypothyroidism, myocarditis, and other inflammatory heart diseases such as Dengue fever, diphtheria, leishmania, and Lyme disease.

## Treatment

The following are the indications for implantation of permanent pacemakers in patients with chronic bifascicular and trifascicular block according to the American College of Cardiology/American Heart Association/Heart Rhythm Society guidelines.

**Class I:** Condition in which there is evidence or agreement that a given procedure or treatment is useful and effective.

Symptomatic and Asymptomatic Patients:

1. Advanced second-degree or intermittent third-degree AV block
2. Type II second-degree AV block
3. Alternating bundle branch block

**Class IIa:** The weight of evidence is in favor of usefulness or efficacy of a procedure or treatment.

Symptomatic Patients:

1. Syncope not demonstrated to be due to AV block when other likely causes have been excluded, specifically ventricular tachycardia.

Asymptomatic Patients:

1. Incidental finding at electrophysiological study of markedly prolonged HV interval ($\geq$100 milliseconds).
2. Incidental finding at electrophysiological study of pacing induced infra-His block that is not physiological.

**Class IIb:** Usefulness or efficacy of the procedure or treatment is less well established.

Symptomatic or Asymptomatic Patients:

1. Neuromuscular diseases with bifascicular block or any fascicular block with or without symptoms. These include myotonic muscular dystrophy, Erb dystrophy, and peroneal muscular atrophy.

**Class III:** The procedure is not useful or effective and in some cases may be harmful.

Asymptomatic Patients:

Permanent pacemaker implantation is not indicated for:

1. Fascicular block without AV block or symptoms.

2. Fascicular block with first-degree AV block without symptoms.

- Complete AV block involving the distal conducting system is often sudden and unexpected. Thus, the ECG manifestations of trifascicular block should be recognized before complete AV block becomes manifest. When there is evidence of trifascicular block, a permanent pacemaker should be inserted, even in asymptomatic patients, because there is no effective medical therapy for complete AV block at the level of the distal conduction system.

- Therapy should target the underlying cause of the conduction abnormality, such as ischemic cardiomyopathy, hypothyroidism, sarcoidosis, myocarditis, or other inflammatory diseases. Whenever there is a need for permanent pacing in patients with bifascicular or trifascicular disease, left ventricular systolic function should be evaluated with an imaging procedure such as echocardiography. In this era of advanced technology, the need for permanent pacing for bradycardia should also take into consideration the need for biventricular pacing and automatic defibrillation in patients with severe left ventricular systolic dysfunction.

## Prognosis

- Prognosis depends on the cause of the trifascicular block. If the conduction abnormality is an isolated abnormality resulting from sclerosis or degenerative disease of the conduction system, prognosis after insertion of a permanent pacemaker is the same as for patients without the conduction abnormality. Most patients with trifascicular disease may have associated myocardial disease. The prognosis of these patients depends on the etiology of the conduction abnormality.

## Suggested Readings

Dunn MI, Lipman BS. Abnormalities of ventricular conduction: fascicular block, infarction block, and parietal block. In: *Lippman-Massie Clinical Electrocardiography*. 8th ed. Chicago: Yearbook Medical Publishers, Inc; 1989:148–159.

Epstein AE, DiMarco JP, Ellenbogen KA, et al. ACC/AHA/HRS 2008 guidelines for device-based therapy of cardiac rhythm abnormalities: a Report of the American College of Cardiology/ American Heart Association Task Force on Practice Guidelines (Writing Committee to Revise the ACC/AHA/NASPE 2002 Guideline Update for Implantation of Cardiac Pacemakers and Antiarrhythmia Devices). *J Am Coll Cardiol*. 2008;51:2085-2105.

Marriott HJL. The hemiblocks and trifascicular block. In: *Practical Electrocardiography*. 5th ed. Baltimore: The Williams and Wilkins Company; 1972:86–94.

Sgarbossa EB, Wagner GS. Electrocardiography: In: Topol EJ, ed. *Textbook of Cardiovascular Medicine*. 2nd ed. Philadelphia: Lippincott Williams & Wilkins; 2002:1330–1354.

Willems JL, Robles de Medina EO, Bernard R, et al. Criteria for intraventricular conduction disturbances and pre-excitation. *J Am Coll Cardiol*. 1985:1261–1275.

# Sinus Node Dysfunction

## Sick Sinus Syndrome

- The sinus node is the pacemaker of the heart. It contains cells with automatic properties that are capable of generating electrical impulses. When the sinus node discharges, it does not leave any imprint in the electrocardiogram (ECG). The sinus impulse is recognized only when it has propagated to the atria causing a small deflection called a P wave. The impulse from the sinus node is called normal sinus rhythm.

- **Sinus node dysfunction:** Sinus node dysfunction occurs when the sinus node fails to function as the pacemaker of the heart. Slowing of the heart because of sinus node dysfunction should not be confused with slowing of the heart because of atrioventricular (AV) block.

  - **Sinus dysfunction:** When the sinus node completely fails as the pacemaker of the heart, a long period of asystole will occur. The ECG will record a long flat line without P waves (Fig. 12.1A). The long pause is frequently terminated by escape complexes from the atria or ventricles.

  - **AV block:** When there is complete AV block, sinus P waves are present, but are not conducted to the ventricles. The presence of sinus P waves indicates that

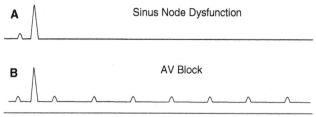

**Figure 12.1: Sinus Node Dysfunction versus Atrioventricular (AV) Block. (A)** When bradycardia or asystole is due to sinus node dysfunction, no P waves will be recorded in the electrocardiogram. **(B)** When bradycardia or ventricular asystole is due to AV block, sinus P waves are present but are not followed by QRS complexes because the atrial impulses are blocked on their way to the ventricles.

the sinus node is functioning normally and is generating impulses that conduct to the atria, but is blocked on its way to the ventricles (Fig. 12.1B).

- **Sinus node dysfunction:** Sinus node dysfunction can be due to intrinsic or extrinsic causes.

  - **Intrinsic causes of sinus node dysfunction:** Intrinsic disease of the sinus node is associated with structural changes in the sinus node itself or the surrounding atria resulting in progressive deterioration in sinus node function. This may be due to ischemia, inflammation, infection, infiltrative, metastatic or rheumatic diseases, surgical injury, collagen disease, sclerosis, fibrosis, or idiopathic degenerative diseases that often involve the whole conduction system. Sinus node dysfunction can be manifested by a number of arrhythmias, although the underlying rhythm disorder is always a bradycardia. About half of all permanent pacemakers in the United States are implanted because of sinus node dysfunction. Before sinus node dysfunction is attributed to sick sinus syndrome, which is progressive and usually irreversible, extrinsic causes, which are reversible, should be excluded.

  - **Extrinsic and reversible sinus node dysfunction:** The sinus node can be suppressed by neurocardiogenic reflexes; enhanced vagal tone; hypothermia; hypoxia and hypercapnia (especially during sleep apnea); increased intracranial pressure; hypothyroidism; hyperkalemia; and drugs that can suppress the sinus node such as lithium, amitriptyline, clonidine, methyldopa, beta blockers, nondihydropyridine calcium channel blockers, amiodarone, sotalol, and digitalis. Sinus suppression from extrinsic causes is usually reversible and should be differentiated from intrinsic disease of the sinus node.

- **Arrhythmias associated with sick sinus syndrome:** Sick sinus syndrome should be suspected when any of the following arrhythmias occur. Except for the tachycardia-bradycardia syndrome, these arrhythmias may be difficult to differentiate from extrinsic and reversible causes of sinus node dysfunction.

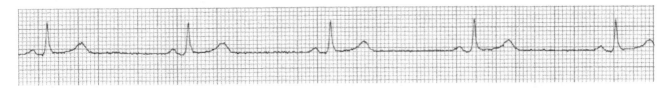

**Figure 12.2: Sinus Bradycardia.** The rhythm is sinus bradycardia with a rate of 42 beats per minute. Although sinus bradycardia is commonly seen in normal healthy and well-conditioned individuals, the slow sinus rate may also be a sign of sick sinus syndrome.

- Inappropriate sinus bradycardia
- Sinus arrest, sinus pause, and sinoatrial (SA) exit block
- Tachycardia-bradycardia syndrome
- Chronic atrial fibrillation
- Escape rhythms arising from the atria, AV junction, or ventricles

- **Inappropriate sinus bradycardia:** When there is structural disease of the sinus node, one of the manifestations is abnormal slowing of the sinus rate, resulting in sinus bradycardia. Sinus bradycardia is defined as a sinus rate of <60 beats per minute (bpm). It is a normal finding during rest or sleep. Sinus bradycardia is seldom a cause of concern until it becomes unusually slow at <50 bpm. Sinus bradycardia of 40 to 50 bpm is often seen in normal healthy, well-conditioned athletes (Fig. 12.2). Thus, marked sinus bradycardia occurring in healthy individuals may be difficult to differentiate from inappropriate sinus bradycardia occurring in patients with sick sinus syndrome. The sinus bradycardia is inappropriate when it is unusually slow, is persistent, and does not increase sufficiently with exercise. For example, sinus bradycardia of <50 bpm may be appropriate for a patient who is asleep, but not for an individual who is physically active.

- **Chronotropic incompetence:** A patient with sick sinus syndrome may or may not be bradycardic at rest, although there may be failure of the heart rate to increase sufficiently with exercise or with physical activity because of chronotropic incompetence. Chronotropic incompetence is diagnosed during exercise testing when the patient is unable to reach a heart rate equivalent to at least 80% of the maximum heart rate predicted for the patient's age. Although chronotropic incompetence may be a manifestation of sick sinus syndrome, there are so many other causes of failure to reach a certain target heart rate during exercise—most commonly, the use of pharmacologic agents that can suppress the sinus node (beta blockers and calcium channel blockers) as well as autonomic influences. Patients with chronotropic incompetence resulting from sick sinus syndrome with symptoms of low cardiac output is a Class I indication for permanent pacing according to the American College of Cardiology (ACC), American Heart Association (AHA), and Heart Rhythm Society (HRS) guidelines on implantation of permanent pacemakers.

## Sinoatrial Exit Block

- **Sinoatrial exit block and sinus arrest:** Another manifestation of sinus node dysfunction is failure of the sinus impulse to conduct to the atria (SA exit block) or failure of the sinus node to generate an impulse (sinus arrest).

  - **Sinoatrial exit block:** In SA exit block, the sinus node continues to discharge at regular intervals, but some impulses are blocked and are unable to reach the surrounding atria. This can result in complete absence of an entire P-QRS-T complex. If two or more consecutive sinus impulses are blocked, the long P-P intervals representing the pauses are exact multiples of the shorter P-P intervals representing the basic rhythm (Fig. 12.3). The long pauses should be terminated by another sinus impulse and not by an escape complex, so that the P-P intervals can be measured. Thus, in SA exit block, a mathematical relation exists between the shorter P-P intervals and the long pauses.

  - **Sinus arrest:** In sinus arrest, the sinus node is unable to generate impulses regularly. Because the abnormality is one of impulse formation rather

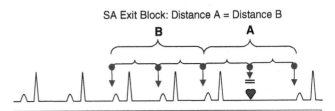

SA Exit Block: Distance A = Distance B

**Figure 12.3: Sinoatrial Exit Block.** In sinoatrial exit block, the P-P interval straddling a pause **(A)** is equal to two basic P-P intervals **(B)**. The red heart represents an entire P-QRS-T that is missing.

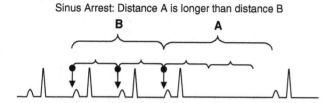

Sinus Arrest: Distance A is longer than distance B

**Figure 12.4:** **Sinus Arrest.** The long pause **(A)** contains a P-P interval that is not equal to two basic P-P intervals **(B)**. The pause represents sinus arrest.

than impulse conduction, the pauses represented by the long P-P intervals, are not exact multiples of the shorter P-P intervals representing the basic sinus rhythm (Fig. 12.4).

- **Sinus pause:** Sinus pause and sinus arrest are similar and either one can be used interchangeably to describe the other. Additionally, sinus arrest may be difficult to differentiate from SA exit block when the P-P intervals are irregular, such as when there is sinus arrhythmia or when an escape complex terminates a pause (Fig. 12.5). When these occur, the pause is simply a sinus pause because it cannot be identified as sinus arrest or exit block (Figs. 12.6 and 12.7).

- **Sinoatrial exit block:** Similar to AV block, SA exit block can be divided into first-degree, second-degree, and third-degree block. First- and third-degree SA exit block are not recognizable in the surface ECG because the sinus node does not leave any imprint when it discharges. Only second-degree SA exit block can be identified.

- **Second-degree SA exit block:** Second-degree SA exit block is further subdivided into type I, also called SA Wenckebach, and type II, SA exit block. The difference between type I and type II exit block is shown in Figure 12.8B, C.

## Sinoatrial Wenckebach

- **SA Wenckebach:** Second-degree type I SA block or SA Wenckebach should always be suspected when there is group beating. In this group beating, some QRS com-

plexes are clustered together because they are separated by pauses representing sinus impulses not conducted to the atria. Group beating is commonly seen in type I block because this type of block has a tendency to be repetitive. In SA Wenckebach, there is gradual delay in conduction between the sinus node and the atrium. Because sinus node to atrial interval cannot be measured, only the gradual shortening of the P-P or R-R intervals before the pause may be the only indication that SA Wenckebach is present (Fig. 12.9).

- Thus, group beating with shortening of the P-P interval before the pause should always raise the possibility of SA Wenckebach as shown in Figures 12.8B, 12.9, and 12.10. In Figure 12.9, there is group beatings labeled #1 to #3. The shortening of the R-R (or P-P) intervals before the pause is better appreciated by the distances between the arrows at the bottom of the tracing, which represent the R-R intervals.

## Tachycardia-Bradycardia Syndrome

- **Tachycardia-bradycardia syndrome:** When the sinus node fails to function as the pacemaker of the heart, ectopic rhythms come to the rescue, which enhances the vulnerability of the patient to develop atrial arrhythmias, including atrial tachycardia, atrial flutter, or atrial fibrillation. These arrhythmias are usually sustained and most often become the dominant rhythm. During tachycardia or during atrial flutter or fibrillation, the presence of sinus node dysfunction is not obvious until the atrial arrhythmia terminates spontaneously. If there is sick sinus syndrome, the sinus node is unable to take over the pacemaking function of the heart and the long pause that follows is a frequent cause of syncope in tachycardia-bradycardia syndrome (Figs. 12.11 and 12.12).

## Chronic Atrial Fibrillation

- **Chronic atrial fibrillation:** Atrial fibrillation is not an uncommon sequela of sick sinus syndrome. Before the

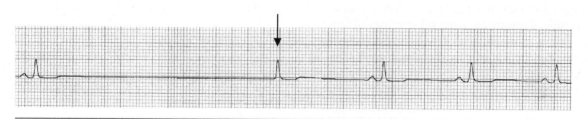

**Figure 12.5:** **Sinus Pause.** A long pause of more than 3 seconds is terminated by a junctional escape complex (*arrow*). A long pause is usually due to sinus arrest. It is also called sinus pause.

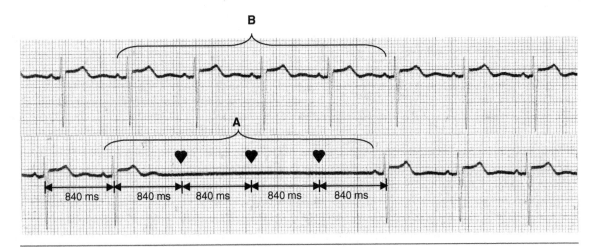

**Figure 12.6:    Sinoatrial Exit Block.** The rhythm strips are continuous. A long period of asystole labeled distance **A** is equal to distance **B. A** contains three P-QRS-T complexes that are missing, which are marked by the red hearts. The long pause is due to sinoatrial exit block. ms, milliseconds.

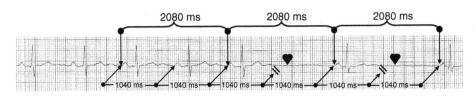

**Figure 12.7:    Sinoatrial Exit Block.** In sinoatrial exit block, the P-P intervals are fixed. Note that the longer P-P intervals measure 2,080 milliseconds and are equal to two shorter P-P intervals, which measure 1,040 milliseconds. This is due to SA exit block. Each red heart represents an entire P-QRS-T complex that is missing. ms, milliseconds.

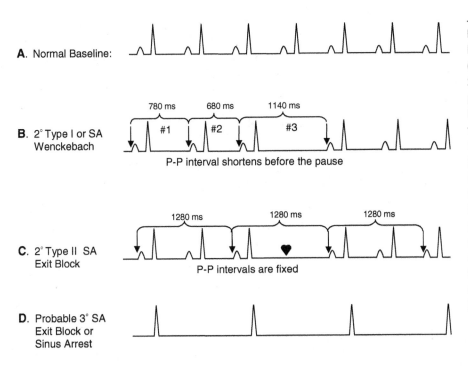

**A**. Normal Baseline:

**B**. 2° Type I or SA Wenckebach

P-P interval shortens before the pause

**C**. 2° Type II SA Exit Block

P-P intervals are fixed

**D**. Probable 3° SA Exit Block or Sinus Arrest

**Figure 12.8:    Sinoatrial (SA) Exit Block. (A)** Normal sinus rhythm. **(B)** Type I second degree SA Wenckebach. Shortening of the P-P intervals before a pause is the hallmark of SA Wenckebach. P-P interval #2 is shorter than P-P interval #1. The pause is represented by P-P interval #3. **(C)** Type II second-degree SA exit block. An entire P-QRS-T complex represented by the red heart is missing. This long P-P interval is equivalent to two P-P intervals straddling a sinus complex. **(D)** This rhythm is consistent with third-degree SA exit block, although this cannot be distinguished from sinus arrest. The sinus impulse cannot conduct to the atria hence sinus P waves are not present.

#1               #2             #3

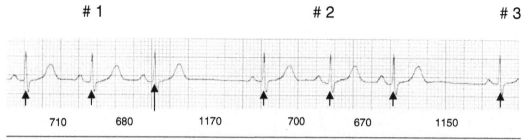

710     680     1170     700     670     1150

**Figure 12.9: Sinoatrial (SA) Wenckebach.** The rhythm strips were recorded in lead II. SA Wenckebach should always be suspected when there is group beating labeled #1 to #3. These QRS complexes are grouped together because they are separated by pauses, which represent the sinus impulses that are not conducted to the atrium. Note also that there is gradual shortening of the R-R (or P-P) intervals before the pause as shown by the distances between the arrows. This is the hallmark of SA Wenckebach. The numbers between the arrows (between the QRS complexes) are in milliseconds.

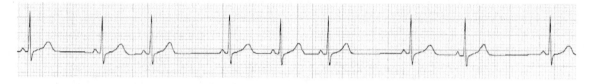

**Figure 12.10: Group Beating in Sinoatrial (SA) Wenckebach.** Lead II rhythm strip showing group beating similar to the electrocardiogram in Figure 12.9. There is also shortening of the R-R (or P-P) intervals before the long pauses consistent with SA Wenckebach.

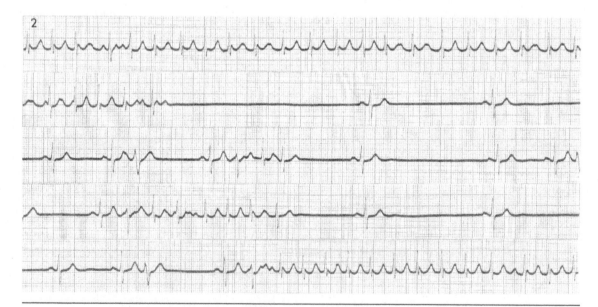

**Figure 12.11: Tachycardia-Bradycardia Syndrome.** The rhythm strips are continuous. Note that the atrial tachycardia is paroxysmal with sudden onset and termination. When the tachycardia terminates abruptly, long pauses follow, which are terminated by marked sinus bradycardia.

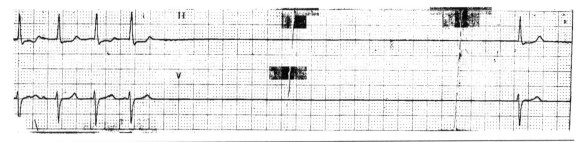

**Figure 12.12: Prolonged Asystole as a Result of Tachycardia-Bradycardia Syndrome.** The two rhythm strips are simultaneous showing a supraventricular tachycardia followed by a long pause of more than 5 seconds before a junctional escape complex comes to the rescue.

era of cardiac pacemakers, atrial fibrillation may have been the only spontaneous cure for patients with significant bradycardia resulting from sinus node dysfunction. Unfortunately, atrial fibrillation may be intermittent and impermanent. When it terminates spontaneously, the sinus node is unable to provide any rhythm and a long asystole can occur (Figs. 12.13 and 12.14).

■ Patients with chronic atrial fibrillation frequently undergo electrical cardioversion to convert the atrial fibrillation to normal sinus rhythm. After the atrial fibrillation is terminated by an electrical shock, the sinus node is unable to provide a sinus impulse, thus a long period of asystole may occur if the atrial fibrillation is due to sick sinus syndrome. Sick sinus syndrome should be suspected in patients with chronic atrial fibrillation when the ventricular rate is slow but are not on AV nodal blocking agents because sick sinus syndrome is often due to degenerative disease that involves not only the sinus node, but also the whole AV conduction system.

## Escape Rhythms

■ **Escape rhythms:** When the rate of the sinus node becomes unusually slow, escape rhythms may originate from the atria, AV junction, or ventricles. These cells have intrinsically slower rates than the sinus node and usually do not become manifest because they are depolarized by the propagated sinus impulse. When there is sinus node dysfunction or when there is AV block (see Chapter 8, Atrioventricular Block), these latent pacemakers may become the dominant pacemaker of the heart.

 ▪ **Atrial escape rhythm:** The atrial impulse originates from cells in the atria usually at the area of the coronary sinus and is followed by a narrow QRS complex (Fig. 12.15).

 ▪ **AV junctional rhythm:** The AV junction includes the AV node down to the bifurcation of the bundle of His. The escape impulse usually originates below

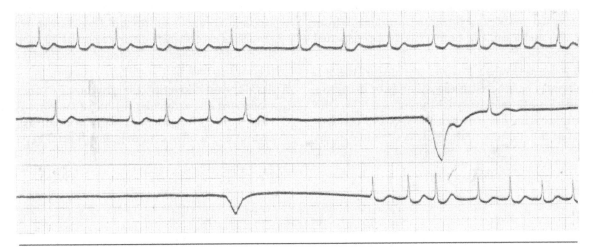

**Figure 12.13: Sick Sinus Syndrome Manifesting as Atrial Fibrillation.** Lead II rhythm strip showing atrial fibrillation. Long pauses can occur when there is sick sinus syndrome because the sinus node is unable to provide a sinus impulse when the atrial fibrillation terminates spontaneously. These long pauses can cause syncope or sudden death.

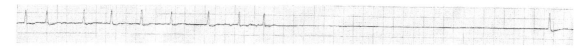

**Figure 12.14:   Sick Sinus Syndrome and Atrial Fibrillation.** Rhythm strip showing atrial fibrillation followed by a long period of asystole of >5 seconds spontaneously terminated by a junctional escape complex.

the AV node at its junction with the bundle of His and has a rate of 40 to 60 bpm 12.16).

- **Ventricular escape rhythm:** Instead of the atria or AV junction, the ventricles may be the origin of the escape complex. A ventricular escape complex is wide, measuring ≥0.12 seconds because it originates below the bifurcation of the bundle of His (Fig. 12.17).

## Junctional Escape Rhythms

- **AV junctional escape complex:** AV junctional escape rhythms are the most common escape rhythms when there is bradycardia resulting from sinus node dysfunction or AV block (Fig. 12.18). The ectopic impulse may or may not be associated with retrograde P waves. When retrograde P waves are present, they may occur before or after the QRS complex and are inverted in leads II, III, and aVF (Fig. 12.19).

  - **P waves before the QRS complex:** Retrograde P waves will occur in front of the QRS complex if conduction of the impulse to the atria is faster than conduction of the impulse to the ventricles. This type of junctional escape rhythm may be difficult to differentiate from an atrial escape complex. If the impulse is junctional, the PR interval is usually short, measuring <0.12 seconds, and the retrograde P waves are usually narrow because the impulse originates from the AV node, causing both atria to be activated simultaneously.

  - **No P waves:** When P waves are absent, the impulse may be blocked at the AV node or the retrograde P wave may be synchronous with the QRS complex. This occurs when the speed of conduction of the impulse to the atria is the same as the

speed of conduction of the impulse to the ventricles (Fig. 12.18).

  - **P waves after the QRS complex:** The retrograde P waves may occur after the QRS complex if conduction of the impulse to the ventricles is faster than conduction of the impulse to the atria.

- The 12-lead ECG of a patient with AV junctional escape rhythm resulting from sinus node dysfunction (Fig. 12.20) and another patient with ventricular escape rhythm also from sinus node dysfunction (Fig. 12.21) are shown.

- **Wandering atrial pacemaker:** Escape complexes may originate from two or more locations in the atria and compete with the sinus node as the pacemaker of the heart (Fig. 12.22). Ectopic impulses from the AV junction may also compete as pacemaker as shown in Figure 12.23. In wandering atrial pacemaker, the ectopic atrial impulses have the same rate as the sinus node (Figs. 12.22 and 12.23) and may even be late or slower (Fig. 12.24). Thus, the rhythm passively shifts from sinus node to ectopic atrial. They should not be confused with multifocal or chaotic atrial rhythm where the atrial complexes are premature and anticipate the next sinus impulse.

- **Accelerated rhythms:** Very often, these escape rhythms become accelerated and develop a rate that is faster than their intrinsic rates. Thus, when the rate of the AV junction is >40 to 60 bpm, the rhythm is called accelerated junctional rhythm (Fig. 12.25); when the ventricles exceed their intrinsic rate of 20 to 40 bpm, the rhythm is called accelerated idioventricular rhythm (Figs. 12.26 and 12.27).

- **Accelerated idioventricular rhythm:** Two examples of accelerated idioventricular rhythm are shown in Figures 12.26 and 12.27. Accelerated idioventricular rhythm is a rhythm that is often confusing and difficult to recognize

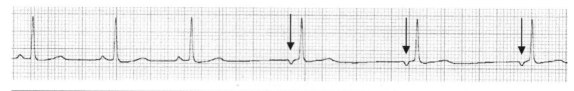

**Figure 12.15:   Atrial Escape Rhythm.** Atrial escape complexes (*arrows*) can become the dominant pacemaker when there is slowing of the sinus impulse.

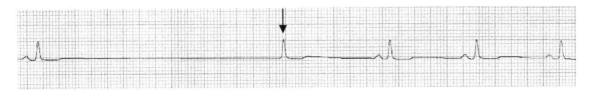

**Figure 12.16:** **Atrioventricular (AV) Junctional Escape Complex.** Arrow points to an AV junctional escape complex. The escape complex terminates a long pause.

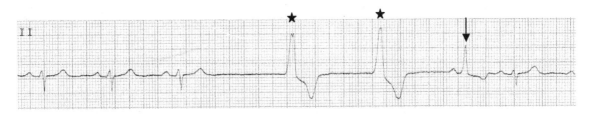

**Figure 12.17:** **Ventricular Escape Rhythm.** Rhythm strip showing ventricular escape complexes (*stars*) terminating a sinus pause. The third complex (*arrow*) is a ventricular fusion complex.

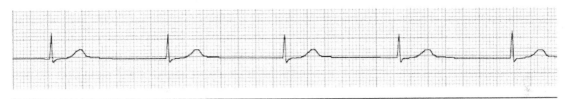

**Figure 12.18:** **Junctional Escape Rhythm.** Lead II rhythm strip showing junctional rhythm with a rate of 46 bpm with narrow QRS complexes and no P waves because of sinus node dysfunction.

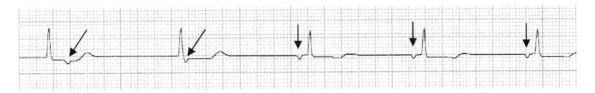

**Figure 12.19:** **Junctional Escape Rhythm.** Lead II rhythm strip showing junctional escape rhythm. The retrograde P waves are narrow and occur after (*first arrow*), within (*second arrow*), and before the QRS complexes (*third, fourth, and fifth arrows*). The retrograde P wave in the second complex deforms the terminal portion of the QRS complex and can be mistaken for an S wave.

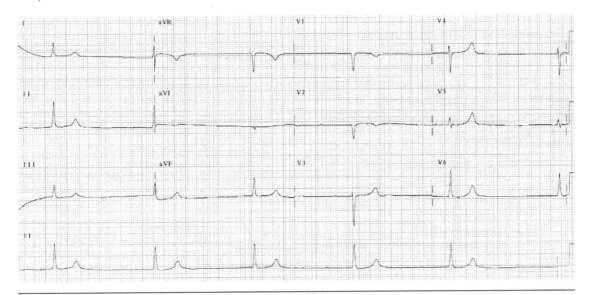

**Figure 12.20:** **Atrioventricular (AV) Junctional Rhythm.** Twelve-lead electrocardiogram showing total absence of sinus node activity. The rhythm is AV junctional with narrow QRS complexes.

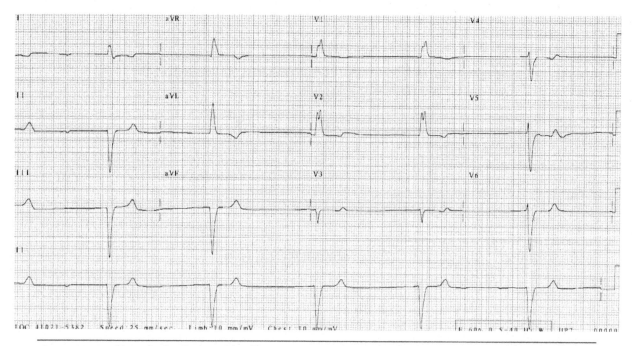

**Figure 12.21:   Ventricular Escape Rhythm.**   Twelve-lead electrocardiogram showing ventricular escape rhythm. The QRS complexes are wide with a regular rate of 34 bpm. There is no evidence of sinus node activity (no P waves) in the whole tracing.

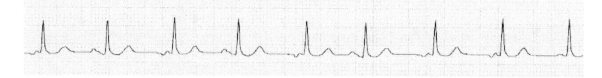

**Figure 12.22:   Wandering Atrial Pacemaker.**   The P waves have different morphologies and originate from different locations from the atria. The rate is approximately 80 beats per minute.

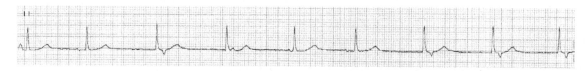

**Figure 12.23: Wandering Pacemaker.**   The morphology of the P waves is variable because the escape impulses originate from different locations in the atria and atrioventricular junction.

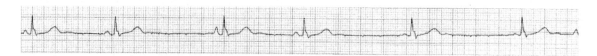

**Figure 12.24:   Wandering Atrial Pacemaker.**   Lead II rhythm strip showing P waves with varying morphologies. The complexes originate from different foci in the atria and are late.

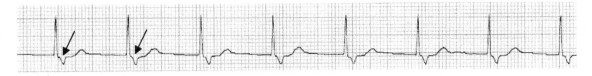

**Figure 12.25:   Accelerated Junctional Rhythm.**  Lead II rhythm strip showing accelerated AV junctional rhythm, 73 bpm with retrograde P waves after the QRS complexes (*arrows*).

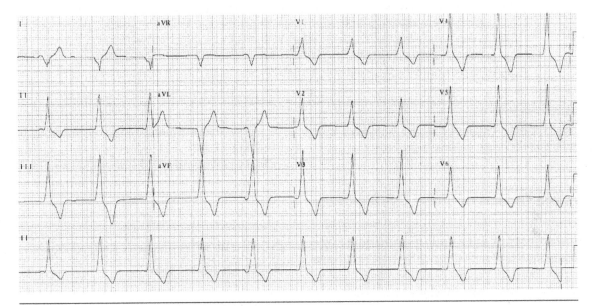

**Figure 12.26:   Accelerated Idioventricular Rhythm (AIVR).**  The ventricular rate is 70 bpm. The QRS complexes are wide measuring ≥0.12 seconds, consistent with AIVR. The QRS complexes have right bundle branch block configuration and no P waves are present.

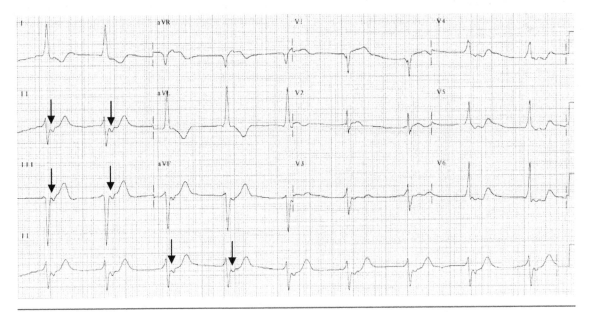

**Figure 12.27:   Accelerated Idioventricular Rhythm (AIVR) with Ventriculoatrial Conduction.**  The ventricular rate is 54 bpm with wide QRS complexes consistent with AIVR. The configuration of the QRS complexes is different when compared with that shown in Figure 12.26. In addition, there is ventriculoatrial conduction with retrograde P waves after the QRS complexes (*arrows*).

4 seconds

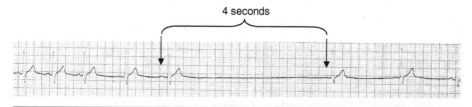

**Figure 12.28:  Hypersensitive Carotid Sinus.** Sinus dysfunction is often due to vagal influences, including the presence of hypersensitive carotid sinus. When the carotid sinus is stimulated as shown, the pauses that follow generally do not last more than 3 seconds because they are normally terminated by escape complexes. Pauses of >3 seconds that occur spontaneously or during carotid sinus stimulation are abnormal, as in this example, indicating the presence of hypersensitive carotid sinus without adequate escape complexes.

because the configuration of the QRS complexes varies depending on the origin of the ectopic impulse.

## Reversible Causes of Sinus Dysfunction

■ **Extrinsic causes of sinus node dysfunction:** Examples of sinus node dysfunction not from sick sinus syndrome are shown in Figs. 12.28 and 12.29.

   ■ **Hypersensitive carotid sinus:** Extrinsic or reversible causes of sinus node dysfunction include autonomic reflexes as well as the presence of hypersensitive carotid sinus. During carotid sinus stimulation, a long period of asystole can occur. In normal individuals, the pause should not exceed 3 seconds. A pause of 3 seconds or more is abnormal and sug-

gests that a hypersensitive carotid sinus is present (Fig. 12.28).

■ **Hyperkalemia:** Hyperkalemia can also suppress sinus node function resulting in junctional escape rhythm as shown in Figure 12.29.

## Common Mistakes in Sinus Node Dysfunction

■ **Blocked premature atrial complex (PAC):** One of the most common errors in the diagnosis of sinus node dysfunction is the presence of blocked PACs. When a PAC is blocked, a pause follows because the atrial impulse is not conducted to the ventricles and is not followed by a QRS complex (see Chapter 13, Premature Supraventricular

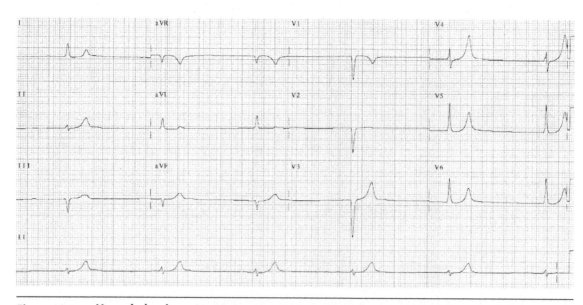

**Figure 12.29:  Hyperkalemia.** In hyperkalemia, P waves may disappear because of sinus suppression or marked slowing in the conduction of the sinus impulse in the atria. Impairment in sinus node function associated with hyperkalemia is reversible.

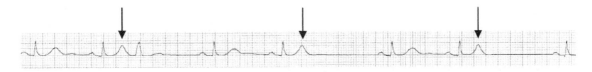

**Figure 12.30:   Blocked Premature Atrial Complexes (PACs).** The long R-R intervals are not due to sinus pauses but are due to blocked PACs. The first PAC (*first arrow*) is conducted with aberration. The last two PACs (*middle and last arrows*) are blocked. The PACs can be identified by the presence of P waves riding on top of the T wave of the previous complex (compare the T wave with arrows and those without). Thus, the T wave with a PAC looks taller when compared to the other T waves without PACs.

Complexes). The ectopic P wave is visible because it usually deforms the ST segment or T wave before the pause. Before sinus node dysfunction is considered as the cause of a sudden pause, a blocked PAC should always be excluded first because this is the most common cause of sudden lengthening of the R-R interval as shown in several examples (Figs. 12.30–12.33).

■ **Blocked PACs in bigeminy mistaken for sinus bradycardia:** Blocked PACs occurring in bigeminy can be mistaken for sinus bradycardia as shown in Figure 12.34A, B. Figure 12.34A starts with normal sinus rhythm at 74 bpm. The third complex is a PAC conducted aberrantly followed by normal sinus rhythm and a succession of blocked PACs in bigeminy (arrows). The 12-lead ECG in Figure 12.34B is from the same patient showing a slow rhythm with a rate of 44 bpm. The rhythm is slow not because of sinus bradycardia but because of blocked PACs in bigeminy. The atrial rate, including the blocked PACs, is actually double and is 88 beats per minute.

■ **Sinus arrhythmia:** Another common error that can be confused with sinus node dysfunction is sinus arrhythmia. In sinus arrhythmia, the sinus rate is irregular. Although sinus arrhythmia is a normal finding, the long P-P (or R-R) intervals can be easily mistaken for sinus pauses (Fig. 12.35). Sinus arrhythmia is more frequent and much more pronounced in infants and in young children.

■ In sinus arrhythmia, the difference between the longest and shortest P-P interval should be >10% or >0.12 seconds.

■ All P waves originate from the sinus node. Thus, the P waves are generally uniform in configuration and the P-R interval is usually the same throughout

(Fig. 12.35). In Figure 12.36, the rhythm is not sinus arrhythmia because the P waves have different morphologies; thus, not all P waves are of sinus node origin. This is due to wandering atrial pacemaker and not sinus arrhythmia.

■ The shortening and lengthening of the P-P intervals are usually cyclic because sinus arrhythmia is commonly respiratory related, causing the intervals to shorten during inspiration and widen during expiration. This changing P-P interval is due to vagal effects. During inspiration, vagal influence is diminished causing the rate to increase. During expiration, the rate decreases as vagal influence is enhanced. Sinus arrhythmia may not be respiratory related when there is enhanced vagal tone, as would occur in patients who are taking digitalis.

## Permanent Pacemakers and Sinus Node Dysfunction

■ **Permanent pacemakers and sinus node dysfunction:** The following are the indications for implantation of permanent pacemakers in patients with sinus node dysfunction according to the ACC/AHA/NASPE guidelines (Fig. 12.38).

### ECG Findings

The ECG findings of sinus node dysfunction are summarized diagrammatically in figure 12.37 and include the following:
1. Inappropriate sinus bradycardia
2. Sinoatrial block, sinus arrest, and sinus pauses

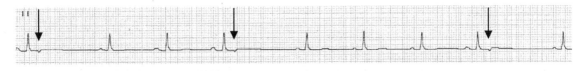

**Figure 12.31:   Blocked Premature Atrial Complexes (PACs).** Note that whenever there is a long pause, the ST segment of the previous complex is deformed by a dimple marked by the arrows. The dimples represent nonconducted PACs. Note that there are no dimples in complexes without pauses.

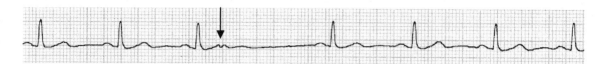

**Figure 12.32:    Blocked Premature Atrial Complexes (PACs).**  The arrow points to a nonconducted PAC, the most common cause of sudden lengthening of the P-P and R-R intervals.

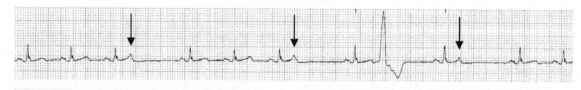

**Figure 12.33:    Blocked Premature Atrial Complexes (PACs) Resembling Sinus Pauses.**  The arrows point to nonconducted PACs superimposed on the T wave of the previous complex. The tall QRS complex is a premature ventricular impulse.

**Figure 12.34:    Blocked Premature Atrial Complexes (PACs) in Bigeminy Resembling Sinus Bradycardia. (A)** The rhythm is normal sinus at 74 beats per minute (first two sinus complexes on the left). The first arrow shows a PAC that is conducted with aberration. The subsequent PACs are blocked PACs occurring in bigeminy (*arrows*). **(B)** Twelve-lead electrocardiogram obtained from the same patient showing blocked PACs (*arrows*) in bigeminy. The slow heart rate can be mistaken for sinus bradycardia.

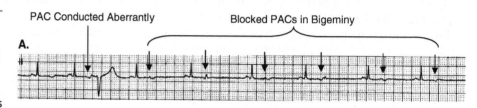

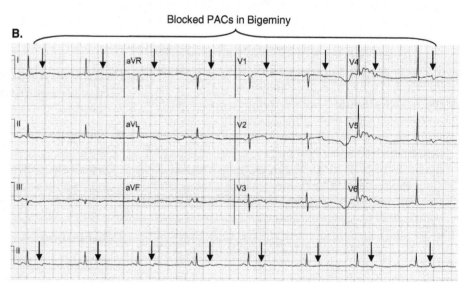

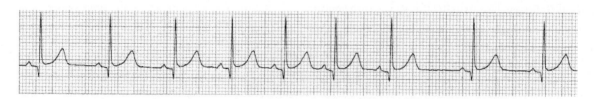

**Figure 12.35:    Sinus Arrhythmia.**  The variation in P-P interval is due to sinus arrhythmia. In sinus arrhythmia, the longest P-P interval should measure >0.12 seconds when compared with the shortest P-P interval. The longer intervals may be mistaken for sinus arrest or sinus pause.

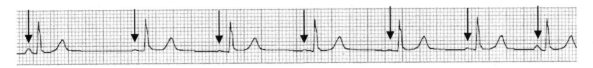

**Figure 12.36:    This is not Sinus Arrhythmia.** The rhythm strip shows irregular R-R intervals; however, the P waves (*arrows*) are not the same throughout because some are ectopic in origin. The rhythm is wandering atrial pacemaker. In sinus arrhythmia, all P waves should originate from the sinus node and should have the same configuration throughout.

3. Tachycardia-bradycardia syndrome
4. Chronic atrial fibrillation
5. Escape rhythms from the atria, AV junction, or ventricles

## Mechanism

■ The sinus node is the pacemaker of the heart and is the origin of the sinus impulse. Because the electrical impulse from the sinus node is not of sufficient magnitude, it does not cause any deflection in the surface ECG. The sinus impulse is

recognized only when it has spread to the atria and is inscribed as a P wave in the ECG. The anatomy and electrophysiology of the sinus node and normal sinus rhythm has already been discussed elsewhere (see Chapter 1, Basic Anatomy and Electrophysiology).

■ When the sinus node fails to function as the pacemaker of the heart, supraventricular or ventricular escape impulses usually come to the rescue. If there are no escape impulses, the ultimate expression of total sinus failure is complete absence of P waves in the ECG, which is represented by a long

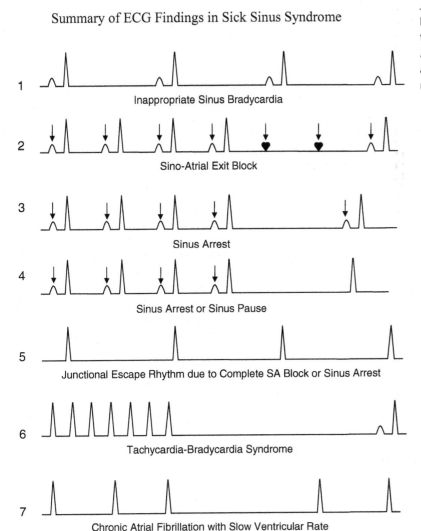

Summary of ECG Findings in Sick Sinus Syndrome

1  Inappropriate Sinus Bradycardia

2  Sino-Atrial Exit Block

3  Sinus Arrest

4  Sinus Arrest or Sinus Pause

5  Junctional Escape Rhythm due to Complete SA Block or Sinus Arrest

6  Tachycardia-Bradycardia Syndrome

7  Chronic Atrial Fibrillation with Slow Ventricular Rate

**Figure 12.37:    Diagrammatic Representation of the Different Arrhythmias Associated with Sick Sinus Syndrome.** The arrows point to sinus P waves and the red hearts represent sinus impulses that are blocked.

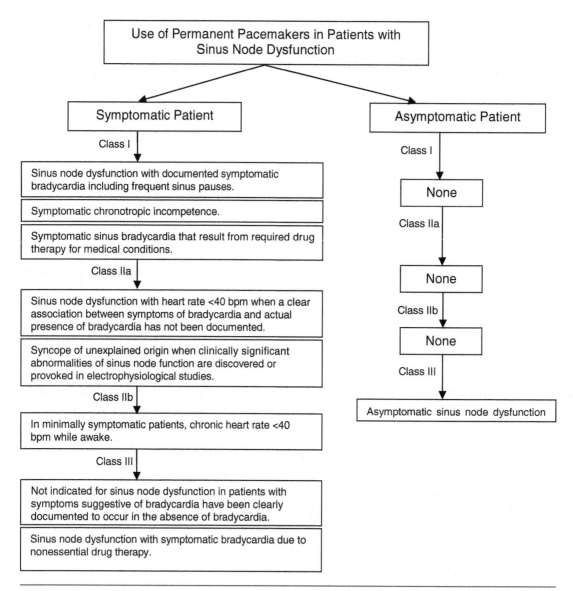

**Figure 12.38: Implantation of Permanent Pacemakers in Patients with Sinus Node Dysfunction According to the American College of Cardiology/American Heart Association/Heart Rhythm Society Guidelines.** Class I: Condition in which there is evidence or agreement that a given procedure is useful and effective. Class IIa: The weight of evidence is in favor of usefulness or efficacy of the procedure or treatment. Class IIb: Efficacy of the procedure or treatment is less well established. Class III: The procedure or treatment is not useful or effective and in some cases may be harmful. Note that in patients with sinus node dysfunction, implantation of a permanent pacemaker is generally reserved for patients who are symptomatic.

flat line without any electrical activity. Unless an escape rhythm originating from the atria, AV junction, or ventricles comes to the rescue, syncope or sudden death can occur.

■ Escape rhythms usually originate anywhere in the specialized AV conduction system except the middle portion of the AV node. These pacemakers are called latent pacemakers because they have a slower rate than the sinus impulse. They do not become manifest because they are normally discharged by the propagated sinus impulse. However, when the sinus node fails to function appropriately, these latent pacemakers may take over and become the dominant pacemaker of the heart.

■ The intrinsic rate of these latent or subsidiary pacemakers is slower than the intrinsic rate of the sinus node. For example, impulses originating from the AV junction have a rate of 40 to 60 bpm and impulses originating from the distal His-Purkinje system and ventricles have a rate of 20 to 40 bpm. The intrinsic rate of these ectopic impulses can become accelerated by sympathetic and parasympathetic influences. Thus, an AV junctional rhythm with a rate of >60 bpm is called *accelerated junctional rhythm* and a ventricular rhythm with a rate >40 is called *accelerated idioventricular rhythm*.

## Clinical Implications

- Sick sinus syndrome refers to the presence of sinus node dysfunction associated with structural abnormalities in the sinus node. It should not include extrinsic causes of sinus dysfunction, such as those resulting from pharmacologic agents that can suppress the SA node, hyperkalemia, neurocardiogenic reflexes including vagally mediated syncope, hypersensitive carotid sinus, increased intracranial pressure, sleep apnea, or hypothyroidism and other physiologic or functional changes that affect the sinus node, which are transient or reversible. Thus, the presence of sinus node dysfunction should always trigger a workup for reversible causes before the diagnosis of sick sinus syndrome is suspected.

- **Inappropriate sinus bradycardia:** The manifestations of sick sinus syndrome may be very subtle and intermittent and may be difficult to differentiate from reversible sinus dysfunction. Between normal sinus function and total sinus node failure are varying gradations of sinus node dysfunction. One of the earliest manifestations is inappropriate sinus bradycardia. This arrhythmia is often difficult to differentiate from sinus bradycardia occurring in normal individuals, especially those who are athletic or well conditioned. When there is inappropriate sinus bradycardia, the rate of the sinus node is unusually slow and does not increase sufficiently with exercise.

- **Chronotropic incompetence:** Chronotropic incompetence is failure of the sinus node to increase in rate during exercise. Most patients with chronotropic incompetence will not be able to attain 80% of their maximum predicted heart rate during exercise testing. The maximum (100%) predicted heart rate is calculated by subtracting the patients' age from 220. Thus, if the patient is 70 years of age, the maximum heart rate that is expected during maximal exercise is approximately 150 bpm (220 − 70 = 150 bpm). If the patient is unable to attain 80% of the predicted maximum heart rate, which is 120 bpm (150 × 0.80 = 120), the patient has chronotropic incompetence.

- Other arrhythmias resulting in sinus node dysfunction include the following.
  - **SA exit block:** In SA exit block, the sinus node is able to generate impulses, but some impulses are blocked as they exit out to the surrounding atria. The main abnormality in SA exit block is one of impulse conduction. If one impulse is blocked, a whole P-QRS-T complex will be missing. The P-P interval can be measured if the pause is terminated by another sinus impulse but not by an escape rhythm. If the P-P interval of the long pauses is mathematically related to the shorter P-P intervals, the diagnosis is SA exit block.
  - **Sinus arrest:** In sinus arrest, the sinus node is unable to generate impulses intermittently; thus, the main abnormality is one of impulse formation. Sudden long pauses also occur, but these pauses are not mathematically related to the shorter P-P intervals; thus, the long P-P interval is not exact multiples of the shorter P-P intervals.

- **Sinus pause:** Sinus pauses can be used interchangeably with sinus arrest because long pauses are most commonly the result of sinus arrest. In normal individuals, sinus pauses are commonly present but are short and do not exceed 3 seconds. When sinus pauses are longer than 3 seconds, sinus dysfunction should be suspected even if no symptoms are present.

- **Tachycardia-bradycardia syndrome and chronic atrial fibrillation:** When the sinus node fails, sinus rhythm is often replaced by atrial fibrillation or atrial tachycardia. The atrial arrhythmia can further suppress sinus function because the atrial impulses do not only activate the atria, but can also penetrate and repeatedly depolarize the sinus node during atrial fibrillation or atrial tachycardia. When the atrial arrhythmia terminates spontaneously, the tachycardia is often followed by a long pause because sinus node function is suppressed. Unless the pause is terminated by an escape rhythm, the patient will become completely asystolic, resulting in syncope or sudden death. This can also occur when a patient with sinus dysfunction presents with chronic atrial fibrillation and is electrically cardioverted. After termination of the atrial fibrillation, a long asystolic period terminated by escape impulses usually occurs.

- **Escape rhythms originating from the atria, AV junction, or ventricles:** These escape rhythms may become manifest when the sinus node defaults as the pacemaker of the heart or when there is complete AV block. These escape rhythms may be enhanced by sympathetic or parasympathetic influences and may become accelerated. Although accelerated junctional and ventricular rhythms may occur in normal healthy individuals as well as in patients with structural heart disease, these accelerated rhythms may be a sign of sinus node dysfunction.

- The presence of sinus dysfunction is usually diagnosed by cardiac monitoring. The type of monitoring depends on the frequency of symptoms.
  - **Holter monitor:** Ambulatory Holter recording for 24 to 48 hours may be sufficient for most patients with frequent symptoms that occur almost on a daily basis. In other patients with intermittent symptoms, longer monitoring may be necessary.
  - **Event recorder:** The use of an event recorder that lasts 30 to 60 days may be necessary if symptoms are infrequent.
  - **Implantable loop recorder:** The use of an implantable monitoring device inserted subcutaneously may be necessary if the patient continues to be symptomatic and other monitoring techniques have not been useful. This is capable of monitoring the patient for 12 to 14 months. The loop recorder can also correlate whether the symptoms are related to other causes or other arrhythmias.

- Other tests to identify the presence of sinus node dysfunction may include the following.
  - **Exercise testing:** Exercise stress testing may confirm the diagnosis of chronotropic incompetence, but is usually

not useful in the diagnosis of other arrhythmias resulting from sinus node dysfunction.

- **Electrophysiologic testing:** This is an invasive test in which electrodes are introduced transvenously into the heart. Sinus node function is evaluated by measuring sinus node recovery time. This is performed by rapid atrial pacing resulting in overdrive suppression of the sinus node. When atrial pacing is abruptly discontinued, sinoatrial recovery time is measured from the last paced beat to the next spontaneously occurring sinus impulse, which is prolonged when there is sick sinus syndrome. The sensitivity of electrophysiologic testing in the diagnosis of bradyarrhythmias is generally low and is not routinely recommended. This is more commonly used to exclude ventricular arrhythmias in patients with coronary disease, especially when there is history of syncope.

- Sick sinus syndrome may be due to ischemia, inflammation, infection including Lyme disease, rheumatic heart disease, pericarditis, collagen disease, muscular dystrophy, infiltrative diseases such as amyloid, sarcoid, hemochromatosis, hypothyroidism, and vascular diseases due to ischemia or myocardial infarction. It also includes sclerosis and other degenerative changes that involve not only the sinus node but the whole AV conduction system.

- Sick sinus syndrome may manifest abruptly with frank syncope or sudden death. It can also occur more insidiously and may remain asymptomatic for several years before it becomes fully manifests. Thus, it may be difficult to differentiate sick sinus syndrome from reversible causes of sinus node dysfunction.

- Among the more common conditions that can be mistaken for sinus node dysfunction are blocked PACs and sinus arrhythmia.

  - **Blocked PACs:** When a premature atrial complex or PAC occurs too prematurely, before the AV node or the rest of the conduction system has fully recovered from the previous impulse, the PAC can be blocked at the AV node resulting in premature ectopic P wave that is not followed by a QRS complex. This is usually identified by the presence of nonconducted P wave superimposed on the T wave of the previous complex. Nonconducted PACs and not sinus pauses are the most common causes of sudden lengthening of the P-P or R-R intervals. Nonconducted PACs should be recognized because they are benign and do not have the same prognosis as patients with sinus node dysfunction. The pause caused by the nonconducted PAC is not an indication for pacemaker therapy.

  - **Sinus arrhythmia:** Sinus arrhythmia is present when the difference between the shortest and longest P-P interval is >10% or 0.12 seconds (120 milliseconds). Sinus arrhythmia is a normal finding; however, the irregularity in the heart rate can be mistaken for sinus pauses, especially when there is marked variability in the R-R (or P-P) intervals. The pause resulting from sinus arrhythmia is not an indication for pacemaker therapy.

    - **Respiratory sinus arrhythmia:** Sinus arrhythmia is usually cyclic because it is respiratory related, resulting in increase in sinus rate with inspiration and decrease in rate with expiration. This has been ascribed to reduction of vagal inhibition during inspiration, resulting in shortening of the P-P and R-R intervals. The marked variability in the sinus rate is more pronounced in infants and young children.

    - **Nonrespiratory:** Sinus arrhythmia may be nonrespiratory related as would occur with digitalis therapy.

    - **Absence of sinus arrhythmia:** Absence of heart rate variability is more common in the elderly and in patients with diabetic neuropathy, which increases the risk of cardiovascular events. Thus, absence of sinus rate variability is often used as a marker for increased risk of sudden cardiovascular death similar to patients with low ejection fraction or nonsustained ventricular arrhythmias after acute myocardial infarction or in patients with cardiomyopathy and poor left ventricular systolic function.

- **Hypersensitive carotid sinus syndrome:** Hypersensitive carotid sinus syndrome should always be excluded in a patient with history of syncope who is suspected to have sinus node dysfunction as the cause of the syncope. The symptoms are often precipitated by head turning. The diagnosis of hypersensitive carotid sinus can be confirmed by carotid sinus pressure while a rhythm strip is being recorded (see technique of performing carotid sinus pressure in Chapter 16, Supraventricular Tachycardia due to Reentry). A pause that exceeds 3 seconds during carotid stimulation is considered abnormal.

## Treatment

- The presence of sinus dysfunction does not always indicate sick sinus syndrome. Extrinsic causes of sinus dysfunction are often reversible and should always be excluded. If sinus dysfunction is due to extrinsic causes such as hypothyroidism or sleep apnea, treatment of the hypothyroid state or the sleep apnea may not only prevent or delay progression of sinus node dysfunction, but may be able to reverse the process. Medications that can cause slowing of sinus rhythm such as beta blockers, non-dihydropyridine calcium channel blockers, rauwolfia alkaloids, digitalis, and antiarrhythmic and antipsychotic agents should be eliminated. Thus, treatment should be directed to the underlying condition, which is often successful in reversing the arrhythmia.

- In patients with sinus bradycardia, sinus pauses, or supraventricular and ventricular rhythms with rates ≥50 bpm who remain asymptomatic, no therapy is indicated other than to identify and correct the cause of the bradycardia. Although sinus pauses of 3 or more seconds is considered pathologic, it does not necessarily imply that a permanent pacemaker should be implanted if the patient is completely asymptomatic.

- When prolonged asystole occurs during cardiac monitoring and the patient is still conscious, forceful coughing should be instituted immediately. Forceful coughing is commonly used to terminate bradyarrhythmias in patients undergoing coronary angiography but is seldom tried in other clinical settings. Because it needs the cooperation of a conscious patient, it should be tried as early as possible. Cough may be able to maintain the level of consciousness for 90 seconds and can serve as a self-administered cardiopulmonary resuscitation.

- When there is symptomatic bradyarrhythmia because of sinus dysfunction, atropine is the initial drug of choice. Atropine is given intravenously with an initial dose of 0.5 mg. The dose can be repeated every 3 to 5 minutes until a total dose of 0.04 mg/kg or approximately 3 mg is given within 2 to 3 hours. This dose will result in full vagal blockade. If the bradycardia remains persistent in spite of atropine, transcutaneous pacing should be instituted. If a transcutaneous pacemaker is not effective, is not tolerable, or is not available, sympathetic agents such as epinephrine, dopamine, isoproterenol, or dobutamine may be given until a temporary transvenous pacemaker can be inserted. The treatment of symptomatic bradycardia is discussed in more detail in Chapter 8, Atrioventricular Block.

- The use of permanent pacemakers is the only effective treatment available but is usually reserved for symptomatic patients with sick sinus syndrome. The symptoms should be related to the sinus node dysfunction before a permanent pacemaker is inserted. In patients with the tachycardia-bradycardia syndrome, insertion of a permanent pacemaker is the only therapy that is appropriate, because there is generally no effective therapy for bradycardia. Furthermore, pharmacologic treatment to control tachycardia or to control the ventricular rate in atrial fibrillation will result in further depression of the sinus node, in turn resulting in more pronounced bradycardia when the patient converts to normal sinus rhythm. The indications for insertion of permanent pacemakers in patients with sinus node dysfunction according to the ACC/AHA/HRS guidelines on permanent pacemakers are summarized in Figure 12.38.

- Sick sinus syndrome from idiopathic degenerative disease is usually progressive and may involve not only the sinus node, but also the whole conduction system. Thus, atrial pacing combined with ventricular pacing should be considered in these patients. When AV conduction is intact, a single-channel AAI pacemaker may be sufficient. Dual-chamber programmable pacemaker with automatic mode switching from AAI to DDD may be more appropriate in anticipation of AV block or atrial fibrillation that often develops in patients with sick sinus syndrome (see Chapter 26, The ECG of Cardiac Pacemakers).

- The use of dual-chamber pacemakers compared with single-chamber VVI devices may diminish the incidence of atrial fibrillation in patients with sick sinus syndrome. Mode switching pacemaker, capable of automatically switching from DDD to VVI, may be advantageous in patients with intermittent atrial fibrillation.

- Anticoagulation should be given to patients with chronic atrial fibrillation to prevent thromboembolism. This is one of the common causes of death in patients with sick sinus syndrome manifesting with chronic atrial fibrillation (see Chapter 19, Atrial Fibrillation).

- In patients with sinus node dysfunction who are completely asymptomatic, there are no clear-cut indications for insertion of a permanent pacemaker according to the ACC/AHA/HRS guidelines.

- Although there is no effective chronic oral therapy for bradycardia associated with sick sinus syndrome, some patients with sinus pauses >2.5 seconds who are symptomatic but refuse permanent pacemaker insertion, slow-release theophylline, 200 to 400 mg daily given in two divided doses, may be tried. This is based on the observation that sick sinus syndrome is associated with increased sensitivity to adenosine. Thus, theophylline, which is the antidote to adenosine, may be able to reverse the bradycardia resulting from sinus pauses. Hydralazine in small doses of 15 to 100 mg daily in divided doses has also been tried with varying results.

## Prognosis

- When sinus dysfunction is due to isolated degenerative disease of the conduction system, the prognosis in these patients with sick sinus syndrome who receive permanent pacemakers is good and is similar to patients in the same age group without sick sinus syndrome.

- The prognosis of other patients depends on the underlying disease causing the sick sinus syndrome.

## Suggested Readings

2005 American Heart Association guidelines for cardiopulmonary resuscitation and emergency cardiovascular care: Part 7.3, Management of symptomatic bradycardia and tachycardia. *Circulation.* 2005;112:67–77.

Belic N, Talano JV. Current concepts in sick sinus syndrome II. ECG manifestation and diagnostic and therapeutic approaches. *Arch Intern Med.* 1985;145:722–726.

Blaufuss AH, Brown DC, Jackson B, et al. Does coughing produce cardiac output during cardiac arrest? [abstract] *Circulation.* 1978;55–56 (Suppl III):III-68.

Buxton AE, Calkins H, Callans DJ, et al. ACC/AHA/HRS 2006 key data elements and definitions for electrophysiology studies and procedures: a report of the American College of Cardiology/American Heart Association Task Force on Clinical Data Standards (ACC/AHA/HRS Writing Committee to Develop Data Standards on Electrophysiology. *J Am Coll Cardiol.* 2006;48:2360–2396.

Criley JM, Blaufuss AH, Kissel GL. Cough-induced cardiac compression. *JAMA.* 1976;236:1246–1250.

Ferrer MI. *The Sick Sinus Syndrome.* Mount Kisco, NY: Futura Publishing Company; 1974:7–122.

Epstein AE, DiMarco JP, Ellenbogen KA, et al. ACC/AHA/HRS 2008 guidelines for device-based therapy of cardiac rhythm abnormalities: a Report of the American College of Cardiology/American Heart Association Task Force on Practice Guidelines (Writing Committee to Revise the ACC/AHA/NASPE 2002 Guideline Update for Implantation of Cardiac Pacemakers and Antiarrhythmia Devices). *Circulation.* 2008;117:e350–e408.

Lamas GA, Lee KL, Sweeney MO, et al. Ventricular pacing or dual-chamber pacing for sinus-node dysfunction. *N Engl J Med.* 2002;346:1854–1862.

Mangrum JM, DiMarco JP. The evaluation and management of bradycardia. *N Engl J Med.* 2000;342:703–709.

Olgin JE, Zipes DP. Specific arrhythmias: diagnosis and treatment. In: Libby P, Bonow RO, Mann DL, et al. eds. *Braunwald's Heart Disease, A Textbook of Cardiovascular Medicine.* 7th ed. Philadelphia: Elsevier Saunders; 2005:803–810.

Saito D, Matsubara K, Yamanari H, et al. Effects of oral theophylline on sick sinus syndrome. *J Am Coll Cardiol.* 1993;21:1199–1204.

Strickberger SA, Benson W, Biaggioni I, et al. AHA/ACCF scientific statement on the evaluation of syncope. *J Am Coll Cardiol.* 2006;47:473–484.

Vijayaraman P, Ellenbogen KA. Bradyarrhythmias and pacemakers. In: Fuster V, Alexander RW, O'Rourke RA, eds. *Hurst's The Heart.* 11th ed. New York: McGraw-Hill Medical Publishing Division; 2004:893–907.

Weiss AT, Rod JL, Lewis BS. Hydralazine in the management of symptomatic sinus bradycardia. *Eur J Cardiol.* 1981;12:261.

Wolbrette DL, Naccarelli GV. Bradycardias: sinus nodal dysfunction and atrioventricular conduction disturbances. In: Topol EJ, ed. *Textbook of Cardiovascular Medicine.* 2nd ed. Philadelphia: Lippincott Williams and Wilkins; 2002:1385–1402.

# Premature Supraventricular Complexes

## Premature Atrial Complex

- **Ectopic impulse:** Any impulse that does not originate from the sinus node is an ectopic impulse. The ectopic impulse may be supraventricular or ventricular in origin.
  - **Supraventricular impulse:** The impulse is supraventricular if it originates from the atria or atrioventricular (AV) junction or anywhere above the bifurcation of the bundle of His (Fig. 13.1). Supraventricular impulses have narrow QRS complexes because they follow the normal AV conduction system and activate both ventricles synchronously.
  - **Ventricular impulse:** The impulse is ventricular if it originates in the ventricles or anywhere below the bifurcation of the bundle of His. The ventricular impulse has wide QRS complex because the impulse does not follow the normal AV conduction system. It activates the ventricles sequentially by spreading from one ventricle to the other by muscle cell to muscle cell conduction. Ventricular complexes will be further discussed in Chapter 21, Ventricular Arrhythmias.
  - Supraventricular complexes may be premature or they may be late.
    - **Premature supraventricular complex:** The supraventricular complex is premature if it occurs earlier than the next expected normal sinus impulse (Fig. 13.2A). The premature supraventricular impulse may originate from the atria or AV junction.
      - □ **Premature atrial complex:** An early impulse originating from the atria is called a premature atrial complex (PAC).
      - □ **Premature junctional complex:** An early impulse originating from the AV junction is called a premature junctional complex (PJC).
    - **Late or escape supraventricular complex:** The supraventricular impulse is late if it occurs later than the next expected normal sinus impulse (Fig. 13.2B). Similar to premature complexes, late complexes may originate from the atria or AV junction. Late impulses are also called escape complexes. Late or escape complexes were previously discussed in Chapter 12, Sinus Node Dysfunction.
  - **Premature atrial complex:** A PAC is easy to recognize because the impulse is premature and is followed by a pause.
    - **Typical presentation:** The typical presentation of a PAC is shown in Figure 13.2A. Because the PAC originates from the atria, the atria are always activated earlier than the ventricles; thus, the P wave always precedes the QRS complex. The P wave is not only premature, but also looks different in size and shape compared with a normal sinus P wave. The

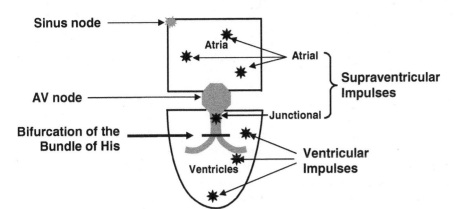

Sinus node
Atria
Atrial
AV node
Junctional
Bifurcation of the Bundle of His
Ventricles
Ventricular Impulses
Supraventricular Impulses

**Figure 13.1: Ectopic Impulses.** Ectopic impulses may be supraventricular or ventricular in origin. Supraventricular impulses originate anywhere above the bifurcation of the bundle of His and could be atrial or atrioventricular junctional. Ventricular impulses originate from the ventricles or anywhere below the bifurcation of the bundle of His. The stars represent the origin of the ectopic impulses.

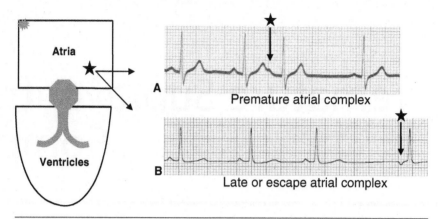

**Figure 13.2: Premature and Late Atrial Complexes.** The diagram on the left shows an impulse originating from the atria (*star*). This ectopic impulse may be premature or late. A premature atrial impulse is shown in rhythm strip **A**. The atrial impulse occurs earlier than the next normal sinus impulse. The premature P wave is recognized as a notch superimposed on the down slope of the T wave of the previous complex (*arrow*). This premature impulse is followed by a narrow QRS complex. The lower rhythm strip **B** shows a late atrial complex (*arrow*). The atrial complex occurs later than the next expected sinus impulse with a P wave configuration that is different from the sinus P waves. This late impulse is also called an escape atrial complex.

QRS complex is typically narrow similar to a normally conducted sinus impulse (Fig. 13.2A).

- **Other presentations:**
  - □ **Blocked or nonconducted PAC:** The PAC may be completely blocked, meaning that the atrial impulse may not be conducted to the ventricles.
  - □ **PAC conducted with prolonged PR interval:** The PAC may be conducted to the ventricles with a prolonged PR interval.
  - □ **PAC conducted with aberration:** The PAC may be conducted to the ventricles with a wide QRS complex and mistaken for PVC.
- **Blocked PAC:** A premature atrial impulse may not be conducted to the ventricles because of a refractory AV node or His-Purkinje system. This usually occurs when the PAC is too premature and the AV node or His-Purkinje system has not fully recovered from the previous impulse. This is seen as a premature P wave without a QRS complex (Fig. 13.3). The P wave may be difficult to recognize if it is hidden in the T wave of the previous complex or the P wave is flat or isoelectric and is not visible in the lead used for recording.

- **PAC with prolonged PR interval:** Instead of the premature P wave being completely blocked without a QRS complex, the atrial impulse may be delayed at the AV node resulting in a prolonged PR interval measuring >0.20 seconds (Fig. 13.4).
- **PAC conducted with aberration:** The premature atrial impulse may be conducted normally across the AV node and bundle of His, but may find one of the

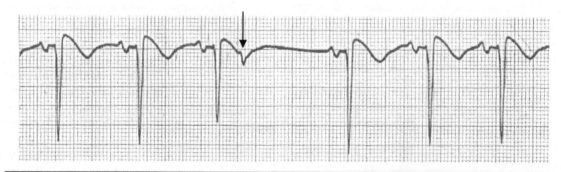

**Figure 13.3: Blocked PAC.** The arrow points to a premature P wave without a QRS complex. This is an example of a blocked or nonconducted PAC. The premature P wave can not conduct across the AV node because the AV node is still refractory from the previous impulse. The premature P wave may not be apparent because it is hidden by the T wave of the previous complex, thus the pause following the PAC may be mistaken for sinus arrest or sinoatrial block.

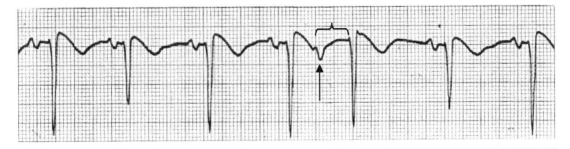

**Figure 13.4:    Premature Atrial Complex (PAC) Conducted with a Prolonged PR Interval.** The PAC marked by the arrow, is conducted with a prolonged PR interval (*bracket*). The P wave is premature and has a different configuration when compared to the normal sinus P waves. In spite of the prolonged PR interval, the impulse is conducted normally to the ventricles resulting in a narrow QRS complex.

bundle branches still refractory from the previous impulse. Thus, the PAC will be conducted across one bundle branch (but not the other branch that is still refractory), resulting in a wide QRS complex. PACs that are conducted with wide QRS complexes are aberrantly conducted PACs. Aberrantly conducted PACs usually have a right bundle branch block configuration because the right bundle branch has a longer refractory period than the left bundle branch in most individuals. Aberrantly conducted PACs are frequently mistaken for PVCs because they have wide QRS complexes (Fig. 13.5).

- PACs may also occur in bigeminy or in trigeminy (Figs. 13.6–13.9) or they may occur in pairs or couplets or in short bursts of atrial tachycardia.
- **Atrial tachycardia:** The rhythm is atrial tachycardia if three or more PACs occur consecutively with a rate >100 beats per minute (bpm) (Fig. 13.10).
  - **Multifocal atrial tachycardia:** The tachycardia is multifocal if the P waves have different morphologies (Fig. 13.11).

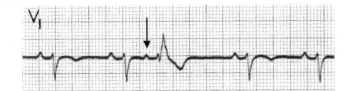

**Figure 13.5:    Premature Atrial Complex (PAC) Conducted with Aberration.** The third QRS complex is premature and is wide and may be mistaken for a premature ventricular contraction (PVC). Note, however, that there is an ectopic P wave preceding the wide QRS complex (*arrow*), suggesting that the wide QRS complex is a PAC, not a PVC. This type of PAC with wide QRS complex is aberrantly conducted. Aberrantly conducted PACs usually have right bundle branch block configuration and the QRS complexes are triphasic with rsR′ configuration in $V_1$ as shown.

- **Multifocal atrial rhythm:** Multifocal atrial rhythm is present if three or more consecutive PACS are present with a rate ≤100 bpm (Fig. 13.12).
- A single PAC can precipitate a run of atrial tachycardia, atrial flutter, or atrial fibrillation when there is appropriate substrate for reentry (Fig. 13.13).
- **Compensatory pause:** The pause after a PAC is usually not fully compensatory in contrast to the pause after a PVC, which is usually fully compensatory. A pause is fully compensatory if the distance between two sinus complexes straddling a PAC is the same as the distance between two sinus complexes straddling a normal sinus impulse.
  - **PAC:** The PAC does not have a fully compensatory pause because the PAC activates not only the atria, but also resets the sinus node by discharging it earlier than normal. Thus, the duration of two sinus cycles straddling a PAC is shorter than the duration of two similar sinus cycles straddling another sinus impulse (Fig. 13.14).
  - **PVC:** The pause after a PVC is usually fully compensatory because the PVC does not reset the sinus node (Fig. 13.15). Thus, the sinus node continues to discharge on time. However, if the PVC is retrogradely conducted to the atria, it might reset the sinus node and the pause may not be fully compensatory.

## Common Mistakes Associated with PACs

- PACs are commonly mistaken for other arrhythmias.
  - **Blocked PACs may be mistaken for sinus arrest or sinoatrial block:** The pauses caused by blocked PACs may be mistaken for sinus node dysfunction and may result in an erroneous decision to insert a temporary pacemaker (Fig. 13.16A, B).

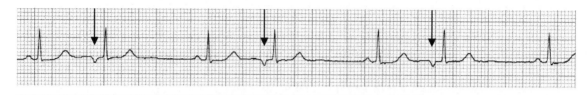

**Figure 13.6:    Premature Atrial Complex (PAC) Occurring in Bigeminy.** Every other complex is a PAC (*arrows*).

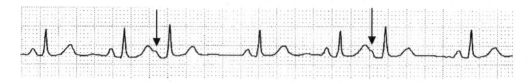

**Figure 13.7:    Premature Atrial Complex (PAC) in Trigeminy.** Every third complex is a PAC. The ectopic P waves are seen as small bumps deforming the T waves of the previous complexes (*arrows*). The PACs are conducted normally and the QRS complexes are narrow.

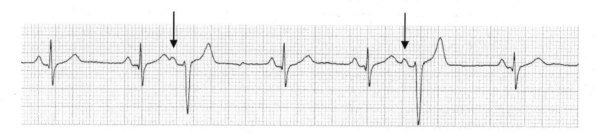

**Figure 13.8:    Aberrantly Conducted Premature Atrial Complex (PAC) in Trigeminy.** Every third complex is a PAC. The ectopic P waves are marked by the arrows and are followed by wide QRS complexes that are different from the sinus complexes. These PACs are aberrantly conducted.

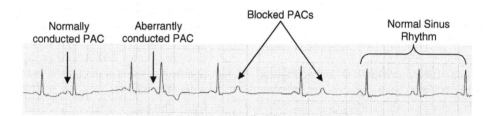

**Figure 13.9:    Normally Conducted, Aberrantly Conducted, and Blocked Premature Atrial Complex (PAC).** The arrows point to the PACs. The first PAC is normally conducted. The PR interval is short and the QRS complex is narrow. The second PAC is conducted with aberration. An ectopic P wave is followed by a wide QRS complex. The third and fourth PACs are blocked and are followed by pauses. The blocked PACs can be identified by the presence of deformed T waves of the previous complexes. Note that the T waves of the QRS complexes during normal sinus rhythm are flat (*right side of the tracing*), whereas the T waves with blocked PACs are peaked and are followed by pauses.

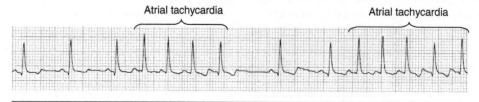

**Figure 13.10:    Atrial Tachycardia.** Three or more consecutive premature atrial complexes in a row is considered atrial tachycardia if the rate exceeds 100 beats per minute.

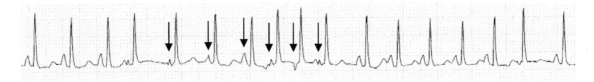

**Figure 13.11:    Multifocal Atrial Tachycardia.** When three or more consecutive multifocal premature atrial complexes are present (*arrows*) with a rate >100 beats per minute, the rhythm is called multifocal atrial tachycardia.

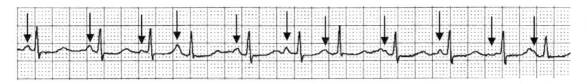

**Figure 13.12:    Multifocal Atrial Rhythm or Chaotic Atrial Rhythm.** The rhythm shows P waves with varying sizes and shapes (*arrows*) similar to the arrhythmia shown in Figure 13.11. The rate, however, is ≤100 beats per minute and does not qualify as tachycardia. The arrhythmia is called multifocal atrial rhythm, chaotic atrial rhythm, or simply sinus rhythm with multifocal premature atrial complexes.

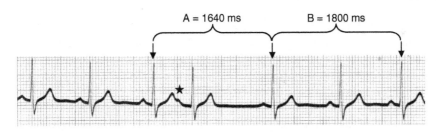

**Figure 13.13:    Premature Atrial Complexes (PACs) Causing Atrial Fibrillation.** A single PAC (*arrow*) can precipitate atrial tachycardia, atrial flutter, or atrial fibrillation when there is appropriate substrate for reentry.

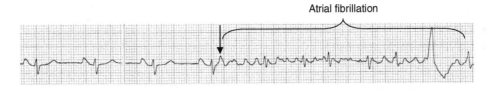

**Figure 13.14:    The Pause after a Premature Atrial Complex (PAC) is not Fully Compensatory.** The rhythm strip shows a PAC followed by a pause that is not fully compensatory. The fourth P wave, marked by the star, is a PAC. Distance **A**, which includes two sinus impulses straddling the PAC is shorter than distance **B**, which includes two sinus impulses straddling another sinus complex. ms, milliseconds.

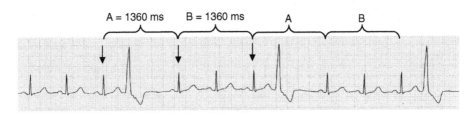

**Figure 13.15:    The Pause after a Premature Ventricular Contraction (PVC) is Usually Fully Compensatory.** The rhythm strip shows frequent PVCs. The pause after each PVC is fully compensatory. Note that the distance between two sinus impulses straddling a PVC (distance **A**) is the same as the distance between two sinus impulses straddling another sinus impulse (distance **B**). ms, milliseconds.

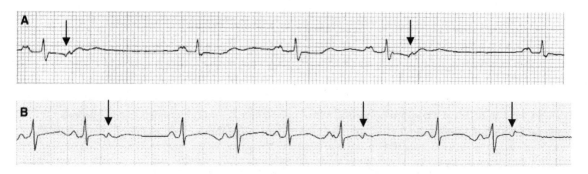

**Figure 13.16:    Blocked Premature Atrial Complexes (PACs) Resembling Sinus Pauses.** Rhythm strips **A** and **B** are examples of blocked PACs (*arrows*). The premature P waves (*arrows*) are barely visible because they are superimposed on the T wave of the previous complex. What is striking when PACs are blocked is the appearance of sudden pauses. The pauses can be mistaken for sinus arrest or sinus pause.

■ **Blocked PACs may also be mistaken for second-degree AV block:** The blocked PACs look like sinus P waves that are not conducted and may be mistaken for second-degree AV block. This may also result in an erroneous decision to insert a pacemaker (Fig. 13.17).

**Aberrantly conducted PACs may be mistaken for PVCs:** Aberrantly conducted PACs have wide QRS complexes that can be mistaken for PVCs (Fig. 13.18).

■ **Blocked PACs in bigeminy mistaken for sinus bradycardia:** In Fig. 13.19A, the rhythm starts as normal sinus with a rate of 74 bpm. The third complex is a PAC conducted aberrantly. This is followed by normal sinus rhythm with a normally conducted QRS complex and a succession of blocked PACs in bigeminy (arrows), which can be mistaken for sinus bradycardia. The 12-lead electrocardiogram (ECG) in Fig. 13.19B is from the same patient showing a slow rhythm with a rate of 44 bpm. The rhythm is slow not because of sinus bradycardia, but because of blocked PACs in bigeminy. The atrial rate, including the blocked PACs, is actually double and is 88 bpm.

## ECG Findings of Premature Atrial Complexes

### P wave and PR interval

1. The P wave is premature and is inscribed before the QRS complex. The P wave may be difficult to recognize if it is hid-

den in the T wave of the previous complex or is isoelectric in the lead used for monitoring.

2. The P wave is ectopic and therefore has a different contour when compared with the sinus impulse.

3. The PR interval may be normal (≥0.12 seconds) or it may be prolonged (>0.20 seconds).

4. The P wave may be blocked and not followed by a QRS complex; thus, only a pause may be present.

### QRS complex

1. The QRS complex is narrow, similar to a normally conducted sinus impulse.

2. The QRS complex may be wide when the impulse is conducted to the ventricles aberrantly or there is preexistent bundle branch block.

3. A QRS complex may not be present if the PAC is blocked.

### Compensatory pause

■ The pause after the PAC is usually not fully compensatory.

### Mechanism

■ **P wave:** The PAC may originate anywhere in the atria including veins draining into the atria such as the coronary sinus, pulmonary veins, and vena cava. The impulse originates from cells that are capable of firing spontaneously. The

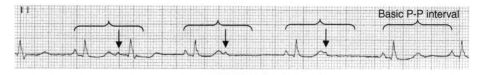

**Figure 13.17:    Blocked Premature Atrial Complexes (PACs) Resembling Atrioventricular (AV) Block.** The PACs are marked by the arrows. The first PAC is conducted to the ventricles. The second and third PACs are blocked. The nonconducted PACs may be mistaken for sinus P waves and the rhythm mistaken for second-degree AV block.

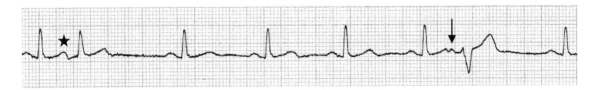

**Figure 13.18:  Premature Atrial Complex (PAC) Conducted with Aberration.**  The first PAC (*star*) is conducted to the ventricles normally. The QRS complex is narrow, similar to a normally conducted sinus impulse. Another PAC is marked with an arrow. This PAC is conducted with aberration. The QRS complex after the P wave is wide and can be mistaken for premature ventricular contraction.

ectopic P wave has a different contour compared with the normal sinus impulse and always precedes the QRS complex.

- **QRS complex:** The impulse follows the normal AV conduction system, resulting in a narrow QRS complex similar to a normally conducted sinus impulse. The premature atrial impulse may be delayed or blocked on its way to the ventricles, depending on the prematurity of the PAC and state of refractoriness of the AV node and conducting system.

  - **Blocked PAC:** If the AV node or distal conduction system is still refractory (has not fully recovered) from the previous impulse, the PAC will activate only the atria, but will not be able to conduct to the ventricles resulting in a premature P wave without a QRS complex.

  - **Aberrantly conducted:** The PAC is followed by a wide QRS complex and can be mistaken for PVC. When the

PAC is too premature, it may be able to conduct through the AV node, but finds either the right or left bundle branch still refractory from the previous impulse. If the right bundle branch is still refractory, the premature atrial impulse will reach the ventricles only through the left bundle branch instead of both bundle branches, resulting in a wide QRS complex.

- **Compensatory pause:** The PAC activates not only the atria but also resets the sinus node by discharging it prematurely. Thus, the pause after a PAC is not fully compensatory. Occasionally, however, the sinus node may be suppressed by the PAC preventing it from recovering immediately. This may result in a pause that is fully compensatory, similar to a PVC, or the pause may even be longer than a full compensatory pause.

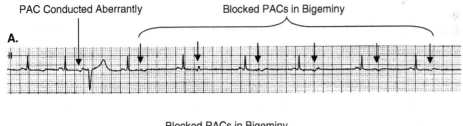

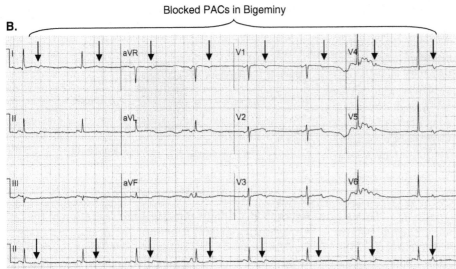

**Figure 13.19:  Blocked Premature Atrial Complexes (PACs) in Bigeminy Resembling Sinus Bradycardia. (A)** The rhythm is normal sinus at 74 bpm (first two sinus complexes on the left). The first arrow shows a PAC that is conducted with aberration. The subsequent PACs are blocked PACs occurring in bigeminy (*arrows*). **(B)** Twelve-lead electrocardiogram obtained from the same patient showing blocked PACs (*arrows*) in bigeminy. The slow heart rate can be mistaken for sinus bradycardia.

## Clinical Significance

- PACs frequently occur in normal individuals as well as those with structural heart disease. These extra heartbeats may cause symptoms of palpitations. Most PACs, however, do not cause symptoms and most individuals are not aware that they have premature atrial impulses. They may be detected during routine ECG, which may be taken for reasons other than palpitations.

- PACs, especially when frequent, may be caused by excessive coffee or tea, smoking, diet pills, thyroid hormones, digitalis, antiarrhythmic agents, isoproterenol, theophylline, and albuterol. They can also occur in the presence of electrolyte abnormalities, congestive heart failure, coronary disease, valvular heart disease (especially mitral valve prolapse), cardiomyopathy and other noncardiac conditions such as pulmonary diseases, infections, thyroid disorders, and other metabolic abnormalities.

- PACs may be mistaken for PVCs when they are aberrantly conducted or sinus pauses when they are nonconducted. Blocked PACs is the most common cause of sudden lengthening of the P-P or R-R interval and should always be suspected before sinus node dysfunction is considered.

- Although single or repetitive PACs are benign, they may trigger sustained arrhythmias (atrial tachycardia, atrial flutter, or atrial fibrillation) when there is appropriate substrate for reentry. Similar to the ventricles, the atria have a vulnerable period in which a premature atrial impulse can precipitate atrial fibrillation. This often occurs when the PAC is very premature with coupling interval that is <50% of the basic P-P interval (P to PAC interval is <50% of the basic rhythm). Thus, overall treatment of atrial tachycardia, flutter, or fibrillation may include suppression or elimination of ectopic atrial impulses.

## Treatment

- Ectopic atrial impulses generally do not cause symptoms. If the patient is symptomatic and the palpitations have been identified as resulting from PACs, treatment usually involves correction of any underlying abnormality, electrolyte disorder, or any precipitating cause that can be identified such as exposure to nicotine, caffeine, or any pharmacologic agent that can cause the arrhythmia. Treatment also includes reassurance that the arrhythmia is benign. Pharmacologic therapy is not necessary. When reassurance is not enough, especially if the patient is symptomatic, beta blockers may be tried and if contraindicated because of reactive airway disease, nondihydropyridine calcium channel blockers (diltiazem or verapamil) may be used as alternative.

## Prognosis

- Single or repetitive atrial complexes are benign in patients without cardiac disease. In patients with known cardiac disease, the prognosis depends on the nature of the cardiac abnormality and not the presence of atrial ectopy.

## Premature Junctional Complex

- **Atrioventricular junction:** The AV junction includes the AV node down to the bifurcation of the bundle of His. It is the center of the heart because it is located midway between the atria and ventricles.

- **Atrioventricular node:** The AV node can be divided into three distinct areas with different electrophysiologic properties. These include the upper, middle, and lower AV node (Fig. 13.20).

  - **Upper AV node:** The upper portion or head of the AV node is directly contiguous to the atria. This portion is called AN, or atrionodal region. It receives impulses from the atria and relays it to the rest of the conduction system. This area of the AV node contains cells that are capable of firing spontaneously.

  - **Middle AV node:** The middle portion of the AV node is also called the N (nodal) region. This is the body or AV node proper. This portion of the AV node contains cells that conduct slowly and is responsible for the delay in the spread of the atrial impulse to the ventricles. This portion of the AV node does not contain cells that are capable of firing spontaneously and therefore can not initiate an ectopic impulse.

  - **Lower AV node:** The tail or lower portion of the AV node is directly contiguous with the bundle of His and is called NH or nodo-His region. This portion of the AV node contains cells with pacemaking properties and is usually the site of origin of the junctional impulse.

- The AV junction is the only pathway by which the sinus impulse is conducted to the ventricles. The AV junction is also the origin of the junctional impulse.

- Any impulse originating from the AV node or bundle of His is a junctional impulse.

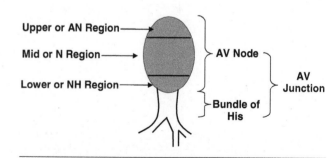

**Figure 13.20:    Diagrammatic Representation of the Atrioventricular (AV) Junction.** The AV junction includes the AV node down to the bifurcation of the bundle of His. The AV node consists of the upper (AN region), mid- or AV node proper (N region), and lower AV node (nodo-His) region.

**A**

PJC —

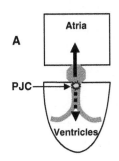
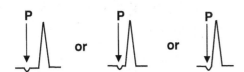

Retrograde P wave is in front of the QRS complex (the atria are activated before the ventricles). The PR interval is usually short measuring <0.12 second and can be mistaken for a Q wave although it can be longer if the impulse is delayed on its way to the atria.

**B**

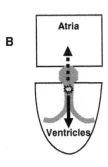
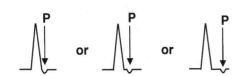

Retrograde P wave follows the QRS complex (the ventricles are activated before the atria). The retrograde P wave can be mistaken for an S wave or it may be further away from the QRS complex.

**C**

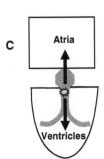

No P wave. The atria and ventricles are activated simultaneously and the retrograde P wave is buried within the QRS complex.

**Figure 13.21: Premature Junctional Complex (PJC).** The different patterns of PJC are shown. **(A)** Retrograde P wave is inscribed before the QRS complex. **(B)** Retrograde P wave is inscribed after the QRS complex. **(C)** Retrograde P wave is synchronous with the QRS complex or the impulse is blocked on its way to the atria, but is normally conducted to the ventricles.

- **Atrial activation:** An impulse originating from the AV junction will activate the atria retrogradely from below upward because the AV junction is located below the atria. This causes the P wave to be inverted in leads II, III, and aVF. Both left and right atria are activated synchronously, causing the P wave to be narrow.
- **Ventricular activation:** Because the AV junction is located above the ventricles, an impulse originating from the AV junction will activate the ventricles anterogradely through the normal AV conduction system, resulting in narrow QRS complexes similar to a normally conducted sinus impulse.
- **ECG findings:** A PJC can manifest in several different patterns, depending on the speed of conduction of the junctional impulse to the atria and to the ventricles. Thus, the retrograde P wave may occur before or after the QRS complex or it may occur synchronously with the QRS complex.
  - **Retrograde P wave before the QRS complex:** Retrograde P wave occurring in front of the QRS

complex suggests that the speed of conduction of the junctional impulse to the atria is faster than the speed of conduction of the impulse to the ventricles (Fig. 13.21A).
- **Retrograde P wave after the QRS complex:** Retrograde P wave occurring after the QRS complex suggests that the speed of conduction of the junctional impulse to the ventricles is faster than the speed of conduction of the impulse to the atria (Fig. 13.21B).
- **Retrograde P wave synchronous with the QRS complex:** When there is simultaneous activation of the atria and ventricles, the retrograde P wave will be superimposed on the QRS complex and will not be visible. Only a QRS complex will be recorded (Fig. 13.21C). The retrograde P wave may also be absent if the junctional impulse is blocked at the AV node on its way to the atria but is conducted normally to the ventricles.
- Figure 13.21 shows the different patterns of premature junctional impulse when recorded in lead II.

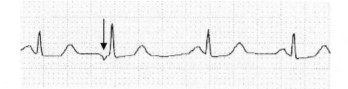

**Figure 13.22: Premature Junctional Complex (PJC) with a P Wave Before the QRS Complex.** Lead II rhythm strip showing a PJC. When an ectopic P wave precedes the QRS complex, a PJC may be difficult to differentiate from a premature atrial complex (PAC). In PJC, the P wave is always retrograde and inverted in leads II, III, and aVF, which is not always the case if the ectopic impulse is a PAC. The PR interval is usually short measuring <0.12 seconds, although it could be longer if the retrograde impulse is delayed at the atrioventricular (AV) node. The retrograde P wave is narrow because the AV node is located inferiorly, midway between the atria, thus both atria are activated retrogradely simultaneously. An atrial impulse is wider, especially if it originates from the lateral border of either atrium because the impulse has to activate the atria sequentially instead of simultaneously.

■ Examples of single premature junctional complexes are shown (Figs. 13.22–13.24). When P waves are present, the P waves are always retrograde and are inverted in leads II, III, and aVF and can occur before or after the QRS complex.

## Accelerated Junctional Rhythm

■ **Accelerated junctional rhythm:** The AV junction has an intrinsic rate of approximately 40 to 60 bpm. If the rate is 61 to 100 bpm, accelerated junctional rhythm is the preferred terminology (Figs. 13.25–13.28). This rhythm is also traditionally accepted as junctional tachycardia even if the rate is ≤100 bpm because junctional rhythm with a rate that is >60 bpm is well above the intrinsic rate of the AV junction. This is further discussed in Chapter 17, Supraventricular Tachycardia due to Altered Automaticity.

■ A summary of the different supraventricular complexes is shown diagrammatically in Figure 13.29.

### Summary of ECG Findings

#### P wave

1. When P waves are present, they are always retrograde and are inverted in leads II, III, and aVF.
2. The retrograde P wave may occur before the QRS complex.
3. The retrograde P wave may occur after the QRS complex.
4. The P wave may be entirely absent; thus, only a premature QRS complex is present.

#### QRS complex

1. The QRS complex is narrow, similar to a normally conducted sinus impulse.
2. The QRS complex is wide if there is pre-existent bundle branch block or the impulse is aberrantly conducted.

#### No P wave or QRS complex

■ A unique and unusual presentation of PJC is absence of P wave or QRS complex and is thus concealed.

### Mechanism

■ The AV junction includes the AV node and bundle of His. The AV node consists of three areas with different electrophysiologic properties: the AN (atrionodal), N (nodal), and NH (nodo-His) regions corresponding to the top, middle, and caudal portions, respectively. A premature junctional impulse may originate anywhere in the AV junction except the middle portion of the AV node because this portion of the AV node does not contain cells with pacemaking properties. Junctional impulses usually originate from the NH region.

■ Because the AV junction lies midway between the atria and ventricles, the atria are activated retrogradely from below upward in the direction of −60° to −150°. Thus the P waves are inverted in leads II, III, and aVF and are upright in leads aVR and aVL. The ventricles are activated anterogradely through the bundle of His and normal intraventricular conduction system. The QRS complexes are narrow, similar to a normally conducted sinus impulse, but may be wide if there is preexistent bundle branch block or if the impulse is conducted aberrantly.

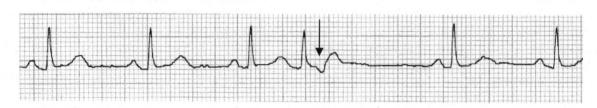

**Figure 13.23: Premature Junctional Complex (PJC) with a P Wave After the QRS Complex.** Lead II rhythm strip showing a PJC (fourth complex). The premature impulse starts with a QRS complex followed by a retrograde P wave (*arrow*).

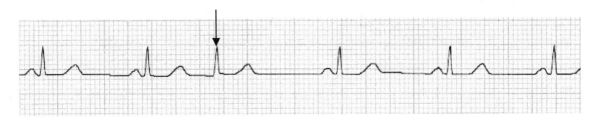

**Figure 13.24:  Premature Junctional Complex (PJC) Without a P Wave.** Lead II rhythm strip showing PJC without a retrograde P wave. The P wave is buried within the QRS complex or the junctional impulse may have been blocked retrogradely on its way to the atria. It is also possible that an ectopic P wave is present but the axis of the P wave is isoelectric in this lead used for recording.

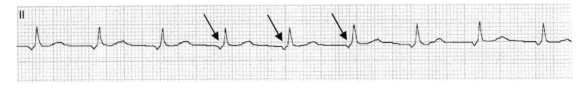

**Figure 13.25:  Accelerated Junctional Rhythm With P Waves Before the QRS Complexes.** Lead II rhythm strip showing accelerated junctional rhythm with retrograde P waves preceding the QRS complexes (*arrows*) with very short PR intervals. The retrograde P waves can be mistaken for Q waves. Although the rate is <100 bpm, the rhythm is traditionally accepted as junctional tachycardia because it exceeds its intrinsic rate of 40 to 60 bpm.

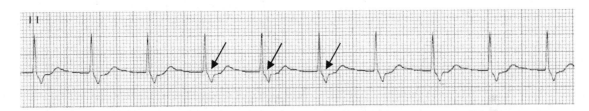

**Figure 13.26:  Accelerated Junctional Rhythm With P Waves After the QRS Complexes.** Lead II rhythm strip showing accelerated junctional rhythm with retrograde P waves immediately after the QRS complexes (*arrows*). The retrograde P wave can be mistaken for S waves. Note that the P waves are narrow.

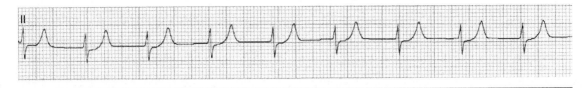

**Figure 13.27:  Accelerated Junctional Rhythm Without P Waves.**  Retrograde P waves are not present.

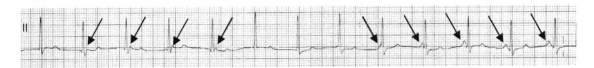

**Figure 13.28:  Junctional Rhythm with Complete Atrioventricular (AV) Dissociation.** The rhythm is accelerated junctional rhythm, also called junctional tachycardia (rate 80 beats per minute) with complete AV dissociation. Note that the QRS complexes are regular and are completely dissociated from the P waves (*arrows*). The P waves are regular and are normal sinus in origin (P waves are upright in lead II).

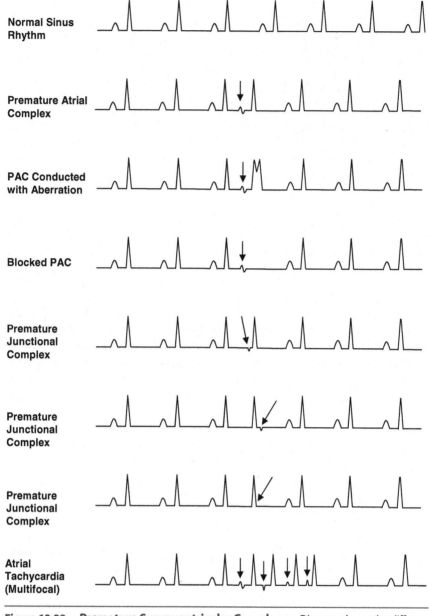

**Figure 13.29:** **Premature Supraventricular Complexes.** Diagram shows the different types of supraventricular impulses. Arrows point to the ectopic supraventricular complexes.

■ The retrograde P wave is usually narrow because both atria are activated simultaneously. The P wave may occur before, after, or within the QRS complex. The position of the P wave in relation the QRS complex depends on the speed of conduction of the junctional impulse retrogradely to the atria and anterogradely to the ventricles and not from the area of origin of the impulse within the AV junction. There are other possible ECG presentations of junctional rhythm. These include the following.

■ **Complete AV dissociation:** When there is junctional rhythm, the junctional impulse may control the ventricles, but not the atria. Thus, the P wave and the QRS complex may be completely dissociated. When this occurs, the

atria are independently controlled by normal sinus rhythm or by atrial fibrillation. The ventricles are independently controlled by the junctional impulse.

■ **Concealed junctional impulses—no P wave, no QRS complex:** It is possible that the junctional impulse is blocked retrogradely on its way to the atria and anterogradely on its way to the ventricles; thus, no P wave or QRS complex will be recorded. When this occurs, the PJC is concealed or is nonconducted. The presence of a nonconducted junctional impulse is not visible in the ECG, but its presence can be inferred because it will affect the next sinus impulse by rendering the AV node refractory. This may result in varying degrees of pseudo-AV block.

Thus, sudden and unexpected lengthening of the PR interval or intermittent second-degree AV block may be the only abnormality indicating the presence of concealed junctional ectopic impulses.

## Clinical Significance and Treatment

- PJCs are much less common than PACs. Similar to PACs, they can occur in normal individuals as well as those with structural heart disease. Unlike PAC, in which the P wave always precedes the QRS complex, single or repetitive PJCs have varying ECG presentations.

- When the retrograde P wave is in front of the QRS complex, a PJC may look like a PAC. The following findings suggest that the ectopic impulse is AV junctional rather than atrial.

  - AV junctional impulses always conduct to the atria retrogradely, thus the P waves are always inverted in leads II, III, and aVF. On the other hand, PACs may originate anywhere in the atria and may or may not be inverted in these leads.

  - Junctional P waves are usually narrow because the AV node lies in the lower mid-atria; thus, both atria are activated simultaneously.

  - The PR interval is usually short measuring <0.12 seconds. The PR interval however may be longer if the junctional impulse is delayed on its way to the atria.

- Accelerated junctional rhythm is the preferred terminology if the rate exceeds 60 bpm. This rhythm is also accepted as nonparoxysmal junctional tachycardia because it is above the intrinsic rate of the AV junction, which is 40 to 60 bpm. Although the tachycardia may be seen in perfectly normal hearts, it is more commonly associated with inferior myocardial infarction, rheumatic carditis, cardiac surgery, and digitalis toxicity—especially when there is associated hypokalemia. Digitalis toxicity should be strongly considered when there is atrial fibrillation with regularization of the R-R interval in a patient who is taking digitalis. The arrhythmia may also be an escape mechanism when there is primary sinus node dysfunction or when there is hyperkalemia. Thus, the significance and treatment of nonparoxysmal junctional tachycardia depends on the underlying condition, which may be cardiac or noncardiac (see Nonparoxysmal Junctional Tachycardia in Chapter 17, Supraventricular Tachycardia due to Altered Automaticity).

- Retrograde P waves occurring within or after the QRS complex may cause cannon A waves in the neck because of simultaneous contraction of both atria and ventricles. Patients therefore may complain of recurrent neck vein pulsations rather than palpitations.

- The clinical significance and treatment of single or repetitive but nonsustained PJCs is the same as for PACs.

## Prognosis

- The prognosis of single and repetitive but nonsustained PJCs is benign because these ectopic complexes are present in structurally normal hearts.

- Junctional ectopic rhythms, including accelerated junctional rhythm, may be a sign of sinus node dysfunction or presence of underlying heart disease or digitalis toxicity. The treatment and prognosis of this rhythm depends on the underlying cardiac condition.

## Suggested Readings

Marriott HJL. Atrial arrhythmias. In: *Practical Electrocardiography*. 5th ed. Baltimore: The William & Wilkins Co; 1972: 128–152.

Wilkinson Jr DV. Supraventricular (atrial and junctional) premature complexes. In: Horowitz LN, ed. *Current Management of Arrhythmias*. Philadelphia: BC Decker Inc; 1991;47–50.

# Sinus Tachycardia

## Electrocardiogram Findings

- **Sinus tachycardia:** Sinus tachycardia refers to impulses that originate from the sinus node with a rate that exceeds 100 beats per minute (bpm). The 12-lead electrocardiogram (ECG) is helpful in identifying the presence of sinus tachycardia as well as excluding other causes of tachycardia such as supraventricular tachycardia (SVT), atrial flutter, and atrial fibrillation.

- **ECG findings:** The classic ECG finding of sinus tachycardia is the presence of sinus P wave in front of every QRS complex with a PR interval of ≥0.12 seconds. The morphology of the P wave in the 12-lead ECG differentiates a sinus P wave from a P wave that is not of sinus origin.

  - **Frontal plane:** Because the sinus node is located at the upper right border of the right atrium close to the entrance of the superior vena cava, the sinus impulse spreads from right atrium to left atrium and from top to bottom in the direction of 0° to 90°, resulting in upright P waves in leads I, II, and aVF (Fig. 14.1). The axis of the sinus P wave is approximately 45° to 60°; thus, the P wave is expected to be upright in lead II. The hallmark of normal sinus rhythm therefore is a positive P wave in lead II. If the P wave is not upright in lead II, the P wave is probably ectopic (not of sinus node origin).

  - **Horizontal plane:** In the horizontal plane, the sinus node is located at the posterior and right border of the right atrium. Thus, the impulse travels anteriorly and leftward causing the P waves to be upright in $V_3$ to $V_6$ (Fig. 14.2). This was previously discussed in Chapter 7, Chamber Enlargement and Hypertrophy.

## Pathologic Sinus Tachycardia

- **Sinus tachycardia:** Sinus tachycardia accelerates and decelerates gradually and is a classic example of a tachycardia that is nonparoxysmal. Sinus tachycardia usually has an identifiable cause, which could be physiologic, such as exercise, emotion, fear, or anxiety. The underlying condition may be pathologic, such as acute pulmonary embolism, acute pulmonary edema, thyrotoxicosis, infection, anemia, hypotension, shock, or hemorrhage. It may be due to the effect of pharmacologic agents such as atropine, hydralazine, epinephrine, norepinephrine and other catecholamines.

- **Pathologic sinus tachycardia:** Although sinus tachycardia is appropriate and physiologic, it should be differentiated from other types of sinus tachycardia that are not associated with any identifiable cause. These other types of tachycardia are primary compared with normal sinus tachycardia, which is secondary to an underlying condition or abnormality. Sinus tachycardia without an identifiable cause is abnormal and can occur in the following conditions.

  - **Inappropriate sinus tachycardia:** This type of sinus tachycardia is not associated with any underlying condition and no definite causes can be identified.

**Figure 14.1: Sinus Tachycardia.** Because the sinus node is located at the upper border of the right atrium, activation of the atria is from right to left and from top to bottom (*arrows*) resulting in upright P waves in leads I, II, and aVF. RA, right atrium; LA, left atrium.

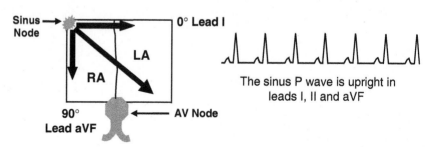

The sinus P wave is upright in leads I, II and aVF

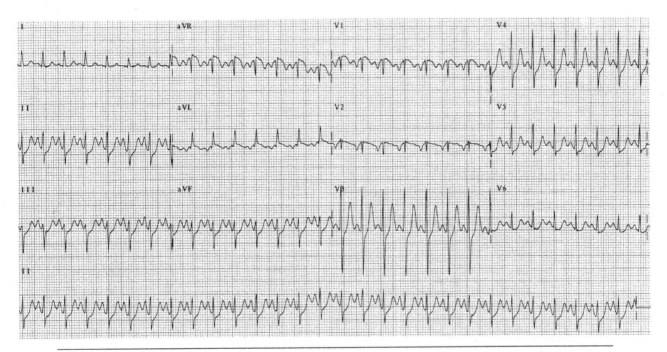

**Figure 14.2: Sinus Tachycardia.** Twelve-lead electrocardiogram showing sinus tachycardia. Sinus tachycardia is identified by the presence of upright P waves in leads I, II, and aVF and also in $V_3$ to $V_6$. The axis of the P wave is closest to lead II, which is the most important lead in identifying the presence of sinus rhythm.

Very often, the rate of the tachycardia is inappropriately high at rest or during physical activity. Increase in sinus rate during exercise is very often out of proportion to the expected level of response. The sinus tachycardia is due to enhanced automaticity of the cells within the sinus node.

- **Postural orthostatic tachycardia syndrome (POTS):** This is similar to inappropriate sinus tachycardia except that the tachycardia is initiated by the upright posture and is relieved by recumbency. In POTS, there should be no significant orthostatic hypotension or autonomic dysfunction because sinus tachycardia becomes appropriate when these entities are present.
- **Sinoatrial reentry:** This tachycardia is a type of SVT resulting from re-entry where the sinus node is part of the reentrant pathway. When this occurs, the P waves resemble that of sinus tachycardia. It is paroxysmal in contrast to the other types of sinus tachycardia that are nonparoxysmal. This tachycardia will be discussed in more detail under SVT from sinoatrial reentry.

## Sinus Tachycardia

- The 12-lead ECG alone cannot differentiate physiologic sinus tachycardia from sinus tachycardia that is pathologic and inappropriate because the ECG findings of

these two clinical entities are identical. The diagnosis of pathologic sinus tachycardia therefore is based on additional clinical information demonstrating that the sinus tachycardia is not associated with any underlying condition. Continuous monitoring is often helpful in demonstrating that the tachycardia is inappropriate. It is also helpful in showing that the sinus tachycardia can be paroxysmal and can be precipitated or terminated by premature atrial complexes, suggesting that the tachycardia is due to sinoatrial reentry.

- The following ECG shows sinus tachycardia (Fig. 14.2). The P waves are upright in leads I, II, and aVF and in $V_3$ to $V_6$. Each P wave is in front of the QRS complex with a PR interval of ≥0.12 seconds.

### Summary of ECG Findings

1. Sinus P waves are present with a rate >100 bpm.
2. The sinus P waves precede each QRS complex with a PR interval ≥0.12 seconds.
3. The morphology of the P wave should be upright in leads I, II, and aVF and in $V_3$ to $V_6$.

### Mechanism

- The sinus impulse arises from the sinus node, which contains automatic cells with pacemaking properties. Pacemaking cells exhibit slow spontaneous diastolic depolarization during phase 4 of the action potential (see Chapter 1, Basic Anatomy and Electrophysiology). The sinus node has the fastest rate of spontaneous depolarization occurring more than one per second. As a result, the rhythm originating from the sinus node is the most dominant and is the pacemaker of the heart.

- The rate of the sinus node is usually modified by a number of stimuli, most notably sympathetic and parasympathetic events, but it could also be influenced by other conditions such as stretch, temperature, and hypoxia. It responds appropriately to physiologic as well as pathologic stimuli. When the sinus tachycardia is inappropriate, it may be due to enhance firing rate of the automatic cells in the sinus node or autonomic regulation of the sinus node may be abnormal with increased response to sympathetic stimuli or decreased response to parasympathetic influences.

- Pacemaker cells are not localized to a specific area, but are widely distributed throughout the sinus node. Cells with faster rates occupy the more cranial portion, whereas cells with slower rates occupy the more caudal portion of the sinus node. During sinus tachycardia, the impulses do not originate from a single stationary focus, but migrate from a caudal area to a more cranial location as the rate of the tachycardia increases. This shift in the origin of the sinus impulse to a more cranial location may change the morphology of the P wave, resulting in a P wave axis that is slightly more vertical (toward 90°) during faster heart rates and slightly more horizontal (toward 0°) during slower sinus rates. This change in the origin of the impulse during sinus tachycardia has clinical and therapeutic implications. Patients with inappropriate sinus tachycardia, where the primary abnormality is due to inappropriate increase in automaticity in the sinus node cells and are refractory to medical therapy, may respond to selective ablation of certain portions of the sinus node.

## Clinical Implications

- Sinus tachycardia is a physiologic mechanism occurring appropriately in response to known stimuli. This includes hypotension, fever, anemia, thyrotoxicosis, and pain, among other things.

- Sinus tachycardia is appropriate when it is due to a secondary cause. Sinus tachycardia however may be difficult to differentiate from SVT, especially if the P waves are obscured by the T waves of the preceding complex. The clinical significance and therapy of sinus tachycardia are different from that of SVT, and every attempt should be made to differentiate one from the other.

- Although sinus tachycardia is usually physiologic and appropriate in response to a variety of clinical conditions, sinus tachycardia may result in unnecessary increase in heart rate without a definite secondary cause. When this occurs, the sinus tachycardia is abnormal and could be due to inappropriate sinus tachycardia, postural orthostatic tachycardia syndrome, or sinoatrial reentrant tachycardia.

  - **Inappropriate sinus tachycardia:** Sinus tachycardia is inappropriate when there is no known cause for the sinus tachycardia. Inappropriate sinus tachycardia occurs usually in young females in their 30s. Most are health care workers. Inappropriate sinus tachycardia is important to differentiate from appropriate sinus tachycardia because the abnormality may reside in the sinus node itself due to inappropriate enhancement in automaticity of the sinus node cells rather than due to secondary causes.

  - **POTS:** This type of sinus tachycardia is similar to inappropriate sinus tachycardia except that the tachycardia is triggered by the upright posture and is relieved by recumbency. The tilt table test may result in increase in heart rate ≥30 bpm from baseline or increase in heart rate ≥120 bpm without significant drop in blood pressure. The drop in blood pressure should not be ≥30 mm Hg systolic or ≥20 mm Hg mean blood pressure within 3 minutes of standing or tilt. The cause of POTS is multifactorial and approximately half of patients have antecedent viral infection. It may be due to the presence of a limited autonomic neuropathy associated with postganglionic sympathetic denervation of the legs, resulting in abnormality in vasomotor tone and blood pooling. It may also be due to a primary abnormality of the sinus node cells similar to inappropriate sinus tachycardia. Other secondary causes such as venous pooling in the splanchnic bed, hypovolemia, or failure to vasoconstrict have also been implicated. Because the abnormality in POTS may be in the sinus node itself (primary), but could also be due to abnormalities outside the sinus node (secondary causes), response to therapy may be difficult to predict. Thus, therapy to suppress sinus node automaticity with the use of pharmacologic agents or radiofrequency modification of the sinus node may be appropriate if the abnormality is in the sinus node itself, but may not be effective if the abnormality is due to secondary causes.

  - **Sinoatrial reentrant tachycardia:** This is further discussed in Chapter 17, Supraventricular Tachycardia due to Reentry. The tachycardia can be precipitated or terminated by a premature ectopic atrial impulse. Unlike the other types of sinus tachycardia, sinoatrial reentrant tachycardia is usually associated with structural cardiac disease.

## Treatment

- **Sinus tachycardia:** Appropriate sinus tachycardia does not need any pharmacologic therapy to suppress the arrhythmia. The underlying cause of the tachycardia should be recognized and corrected.

  - Occasionally, sinus tachycardia may occur in a setting that is not advantageous to the patient. For example, sinus tachycardia may be related to pericarditis, acute myocardial infarction, congestive heart failure, or thyrotoxicosis. In these patients, it may be appropriate to slow down the heart rate with beta blockers and identify other causes of sinus tachycardia that can be corrected. Beta blockers are standard drugs for congestive heart failure resulting from systolic dysfunction as well as for patients with acute myocardial infarction, whether or not sinus tachycardia is present. It is also commonly used to control sinus tachycardia associated with thyrotoxicosis.

- **Inappropriate sinus tachycardia:** If secondary causes have been excluded and the sinus tachycardia is deemed inappropriate, therapy includes beta blockers and nondihydropyridine calcium channel blockers such as diltiazem and verapamil. Beta blockers may be used as first-line therapy unless these agents are contraindicated. In patients who are resistant to pharmacologic therapy or patients who are unable to take oral therapy, sinus node modification using radiofrequency ablation has been used successfully. This carries a risk of causing sinus node dysfunction and permanent pacing and should be considered only as a last resort.

- **POTS:** Because the cause of POTS may be a primary sinus node abnormality but could also be due to secondary causes, response to therapy is unpredictable.

  - **Nonpharmacologic therapy:** Volume expansion may be required with proper regular oral hydration combined with high-sodium intake of up to 10 to 15 g daily, use of compressive stockings, sleeping with the head of the bed tilted up, and resistance training such as weight lifting.

  - **Pharmacologic therapy:** Pharmacologic therapy has been shown to provide short-term, partial relief of symptoms in approximately half of patients, regardless of the agent used.

    - ☐ **Beta blockers:** If nonpharmacologic therapy is not effective, low-dose beta blockers such as propranolol 20 to 30 mg three to four times daily may be tried because the abnormality may be in the sinus node cells or the result of hypersensitivity to endogenous beta agonists.

    - ☐ **Calcium channel blockers:** If beta blockers are not effective or are contraindicated because of bronchospastic pulmonary disease, calcium channel blockers such as diltiazem or verapamil may be given. These drugs are contraindicated when there is left ventricular systolic dysfunction.

    - ☐ **Mineralocorticoids:** Mineralocorticoids, such as fludrocortisone 0.1 to 0.3 mg orally once daily, may be useful when there is hypovolemia, which is often seen in POTS. This should be considered only after nonpharmacologic therapy has been tried. These agents are usually combined with hydration and high sodium intake.

    - ☐ **Adrenoceptor agonists:** Adrenoceptor agonist such as midodrine 2.5 to 10 mg three times daily orally has been shown to improve symptoms during tilt table testing, although its efficacy during long-term therapy is not known.

    - ☐ **Serotonin reuptake inhibitors:** Response to selective serotonin reuptake inhibitors is similar to that of other pharmacologic agents.

  - **Catheter ablation:** Although catheter ablation or catheter modification has been performed in some patients with POTS, response to this type of therapy may be difficult to predict because the abnormality may be primarily in the sinus node but could also be due to secondary causes.

## Prognosis

- **Appropriate sinus tachycardia:** Sinus tachycardia is physiologic and is an expected normal response to a variety of clinical situations. The overall prognosis of a patient with sinus tachycardia depends on the underlying cause of the sinus tachycardia and not the sinus tachycardia itself.

- **Pathologic sinus tachycardia:** Therapy for pathologic sinus tachycardia is given primarily to improve the quality of life rather than to prolong survival. In supraventricular tachycardia from sinoatrial reentry, the tachycardia may be associated with structural cardiac disease. The prognosis will depend on the nature of the underlying cause. Pathologic sinus tachycardia has not been shown to cause tachycardia mediated cardiomyopathy.

- **POTS:** Up to 80% of patients with POTS improve with most returning to normal functional capacity. Those with antecedent viral infection seem to have a better outcome.

## Suggested Readings

Blomstrom-Lundqvist C, Scheinman MM, Aliot EM, et al. ACC/AHA/ESC guidelines for the management of patients with supraventricular arrhythmias—executive summary: a report of the American College of Cardiology/American Heart Association Task Force on Practice Guidelines, and the European Society of Cardiology Committee for Practice Guidelines (Writing Committee to Develop Guidelines for the Management of Patients With Supraventricular Arrhythmias). *J Am Coll Cardiol.* 2003;42:1493–531.

Freeman R, Kaufman H. Postural tachycardia syndrome. 2007 UptoDate. www.utdol.com.

Sandroni P, Opfer-Gehrking TL, McPhee BR, et al. Postural tachycardia syndrome: clinical features and follow-up study. *Mayo Clin Proc.* 1999;74:1106–1110.

Singer W, Shen WK, Opfer-Gehrking TL, et al. Evidence of an intrinsic sinus node abnormality in patients with postural tachycardia syndrome. *Mayo Clin Proc.* 2002;77:246–252.

Thieben MJ, Sandroni P, Sletten DM, et al. Postural orthostatic tachycardia syndrome: the Mayo Clinic experience. *Mayo Clin Proc.* 2007;82:308–313.

Yussuf S, Camm J. Deciphering the sinus tachycardias. *Clin Cardiol.* 2005;28:267–276.

# Supraventricular Tachycardia

## Introduction

- Tachycardia refers to a heart rate >100 beats per minute (bpm). The tachycardia may be supraventricular or ventricular depending on the origin of the arrhythmia.
  - **Supraventricular tachycardia (SVT):** If the tachycardia originates above the bifurcation of the bundle of His, usually in the atria or atrioventricular (AV) junction, the tachycardia is supraventricular (Fig. 15.1A). Supraventricular impulses follow the normal AV conduction system, activate the ventricles synchronously and will have narrow QRS complexes measuring <120 milliseconds. The QRS may be wide if there is preexistent bundle branch block, ventricular aberration, or the impulse is conducted through a bypass tract.

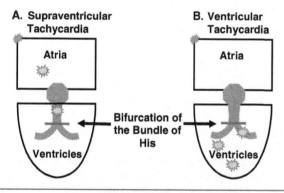

**A. Supraventricular Tachycardia**
Atria
Ventricles

**B. Ventricular Tachycardia**
Atria
Ventricles

Bifurcation of the Bundle of His

**Figure 15.1: Supraventricular and Ventricular Tachycardia (VT).** **(A)** In supraventricular tachycardia, the impulses originate above the bifurcation of the bundle of His, follow the normal AV conduction system, and activate both ventricles synchronously resulting in narrow QRS complexes. **(B)** In VT, the impulses originate below the bifurcation of the bundle of His. Activation of the ventricles is not synchronous because the impulse has to spread outside the normal conduction system resulting in wide QRS complexes. The stars represent the origin of the impulse. The horizontal line represents the bifurcation of the bundle of His.

- **Ventricular tachycardia (VT):** If the tachycardia originates below the bifurcation of the bundle of His, the tachycardia is ventricular (Fig. 15.1B). The impulse will spread to the ventricles outside the normal AV conduction system. Activation of the ventricles will not be synchronous resulting in wide QRS complexes measuring ≥120 milliseconds.
- There are other types of tachycardias with narrow QRS complexes other than SVT. These include sinus tachycardia, atrial flutter, and atrial fibrillation. These tachycardias should be distinguished from each other because the treatment of these various arrhythmias is different.
  - **Sinus tachycardia:** Sinus tachycardia implies that the rhythm originates from the sinus node with a rate that exceeds 100 bpm. Sinus tachycardia is a normal finding, which is usually an appropriate response to a physiologic or pathologic condition. This was previously discussed in Chapter 14, Sinus Tachycardia.
  - **Atrial flutter:** The diagnosis of atrial flutter is based on the presence of a very regular atrial rate of 300 ± 50 bpm. This will be discussed separately in Chapter 18.
  - **Atrial fibrillation:** The diagnosis of atrial fibrillation is based on an atrial rate of 400 ± 50 bpm with characteristic baseline fibrillatory pattern and irregularly irregular R-R intervals. This will also be discussed separately.
- Table 15.1 classifies the different types of narrow complex tachycardias.
- **SVT:** SVT is a narrow complex tachycardia originating outside the sinus node but above the bifurcation of the bundle of His, with a rate that exceeds 100 bpm. Several types of SVT are present and are classified according to three general mechanisms: reentry, enhanced automaticity, and triggered activity.
  - **Reentry:** SVT due to reentry is an abnormality in the propagation of the electrical impulse resulting from the presence of two separate pathways with different electrophysiologic properties (Fig. 15.2A).

| TABLE 15.1 | | | | |
|---|---|---|---|---|
| **Narrow Complex Tachycardia** | | | | |
| Sinus Tachycardia | SVT | | Atrial Flutter | Atrial Fibrillation |
| **Sinus Rate >100** | Reentrant<br>• AVNRT<br>• AVRT<br>• Intraatrial<br>• Sinoatrial | Automatic<br>• Atrial<br>  ◦ Focal or unifocal<br>  ◦ Multifocal<br>• Junctional<br>  ◦ Paroxysmal<br>  ◦ Nonparoxysmal | **Atrial Rate 300 ± 50** | **Atrial Rate 400 ± 50** |
| | **Atrial Rate 200 ± 50** | | | |

Table shows the different tachycardias that can result in narrow QRS complexes. Generally, the atrial rate of atrial fibrillation is 400 ± 50 bpm, for atrial flutter 300 ± 50 bpm, for SVT approximately 200 ± 50 and for sinus tachycardia >100 bpm. AVNRT, atrioventricular nodal reentrant tachycardia; AVRT, atrioventricular reciprocating tachycardia; SVT, supraventricular tachycardia.

■ **Enhanced automaticity:** This is an abnormality in initiation rather than conduction of the electrical impulse. Some cells in the atria or AV junction may exhibit phase 4 diastolic depolarization and may spontaneously discharge faster than that of the sinus node if the discharge rate is enhanced (Fig. 15.2B).

■ **Triggered activity:** This is also an abnormality in initiation of the electrical impulse resulting from occurrence of afterdepolarizations. Afterdepolarizations are secondary depolarizations that are triggered by the initial impulse (Fig. 15.2C). The afterdepolarization does not always reach threshold potential, but when it does, it may be followed by repetitive firing of the membrane voltage. Triggered activity is usually seen in association with digitalis toxicity, calcium excess, or increased catecholamines.

■ SVT from reentry usually occurs in normal individuals without evidence of structural cardiac disease. SVT from enhanced automaticity may occur in normal individuals, although they are more frequently associated with structural cardiac diseases, abnormalities in electrolytes and blood gasses, or use of pharmacologic agents. SVT from triggered activity usually occurs with digitalis excess or after cardiac surgery. The differences between SVT from reentry, from enhanced automaticity, and from triggered activity are summarized in Table 15.2.

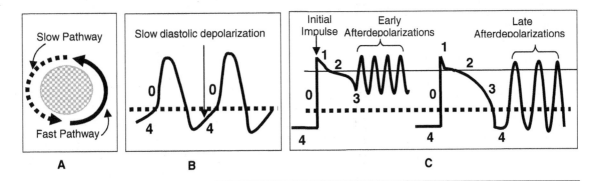

A          B          C

**Figure 15.2:    Mechanisms of Supraventricular tachycardia (SVT). (A)** Reentry is the most common mechanism of all SVT. In reentry, two separate pathways with different electrophysiologic properties are present. **(B)** Diagram of action potential of a cell with automatic properties. These cells exhibit slow phase 4 diastolic depolarization, which may dominate as the pacemaker if the discharge rate is enhanced. **(C)** Diagram of action potential of a cell with triggered activity. Oscillations occur early during phase 2 or phase 3, or late during phase 4 of the action potential. The dotted horizontal lines in **(B)** and **(C)** represent threshold potential. Numbers 0 to 4 represent the different phases of the action potential. Adapted and modified from Wellens and Conover.

**TABLE 15.2**

## Differences between SVT because of Reentry, Enhanced Automaticity, and Triggered Activity

| | Reentry | Enhanced Automaticity | Triggered Activity |
|---|---|---|---|
| Mechanism | This is an abnormality in impulse conduction. A reentrant circuit is present. | This is an abnormality in impulse initiation. Cells with automatic properties become the dominant pacemaker. | Early or late after-depolarizations are present. |
| Initiation | Initiated by premature impulses or by rapid pacing. | Initiated by increased firing rate of automatic cells in the atria or AV junction. | Initiation is not well defined. |
| Termination \ | Terminated by vagal maneuvers, AV nodal blockers, ectopic impulses, overdrive pacing, or electrical cardioversion. | Not usually terminated by vagal maneuvers, AV nodal blockers, ectopic impulses, overdrive pacing or electrical cardioversion. | May be terminated by premature impulses, overdrive pacing, or electrical cardioversion. |
| Underlying Condition | Frequently seen in structurally normal hearts. | Frequently seen in patients with metabolic or pulmonary disorders or patients on adrenergic drugs, caffeine, theophylline, or other agents. | Frequently seen in patients with digitalis toxicity or postcardiac surgery. |
| Examples of SVT | • AV nodal reentry<br>• AV reentry<br>• Sinoatrial reentry<br>• Intraatrial reentry | • AT<br>  ○ Focal AT<br>  ○ Multifocal AT<br>• Junctional tachycardia<br>  ○ Focal or paroxysmal<br>  ○ Nonparoxysmal | • Atrial tachycardia with 2:1 AV block<br>• Nonparoxysmal junctional tachycardia |

SVT, supraventricular tachycardia; AT, atrial tachycardia; AV, atrioventricular.

## Suggested Readings

Conover MB. Arrhythmogenesis. In: *Understanding Electrocardiography*. 5th ed. St. Louis: Mosby; 1988:31–41.

Wellens HJJ, Conover M. Drug induced arrhythmic emergencies. In: *The ECG in Emergency Decision Making*. 2nd ed. St. Louis: Saunders Elsevier; 2006:178.

Wit AL, Rosen MR. Cellular electrophysiology of cardiac arrhythmias. Part I. Arrhythmias caused by abnormal impulse generation. *Mod Concepts Cardiovasc Dis.* 1981; 50:1–6.

Wit AL, Rosen MR. Cellular electrophysiology of cardiac arrhythmias. Part II. Arrhythmias caused by abnormal impulse conduction. *Mod Concepts Cardiovasc Dis.* 1981; 50:7–12.

# Supraventricular Tachycardia due to Reentry

## Types of Reentrant Supraventricular Tachycardia

- **Supraventricular tachycardia (SVT) from reentry:** This accounts for approximately 80% to 90% of all sustained SVT in the general population. Reentrant SVT results from abnormal propagation of the electrical impulse because of the presence of two separate pathways with different electrophysiologic properties.
- There are four types of SVT from reentry. They are diagrammatically shown in Figure 16.1A–D.
  - **Atrioventricular nodal reentrant tachycardia (AVNRT):** The reentrant circuit consists of a slow and fast pathway that circles around the AV node (Fig. 16.1A).
  - **Atrioventricular reciprocating (or reentrant) tachycardia (AVRT):** The tachycardia is associated with a bypass tract connecting the atrium directly to the ventricle (Fig. 16.1B).
  - **Sinoatrial reentrant tachycardia (SART):** The tachycardia involves the sinus node and contiguous atrium (Fig. 16.1C).
  - **Intra-atrial reentrant tachycardia (IART):** The tachycardia is confined to a small circuit within the atrium (Fig. 16.1D).

## Atrioventricular Nodal Reentrant Tachycardia

- **AVNRT:** AVNRT is the most common SVT occurring in the general population. It usually affects young and healthy individuals without evidence of structural heart disease and is twice more common in women than in men.

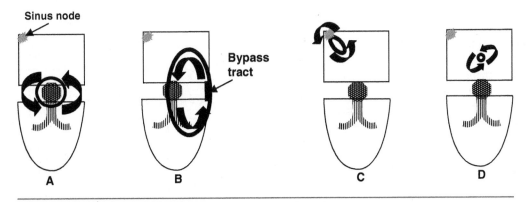

**Figure 16.1:   Supraventricular Tachycardia (SVT) from Reentry.  (A)** AV nodal reentrant tachycardia. The two pathways circle the AV node. This is the most common, occurring in more than 60% of all reentrant narrow complex tachycardia. **(B)** AV reciprocating tachycardia. This type of SVT is associated with a bypass tract connecting the atrium and ventricle. This is the next common occurring in approximately 30% of all reentrant SVT. **(C)** Sinoatrial reentrant tachycardia. The reentrant circuit involves the sinus node and adjacent atrium. This type of SVT is rare. **(D)** Intraatrial reentrant tachycardia. A microreentrant circuit is present within the atria. This type of SVT is also rare. The red circles represent the reentrant circuit. The arrows point to the direction of the reentrant circuit. AV, atrioventricular.

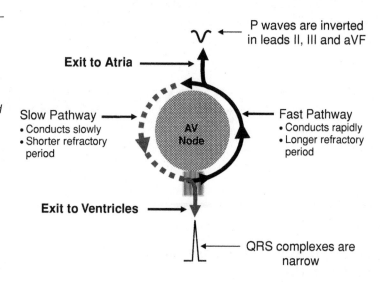

**Figure 16.2:   Diagrammatic Representation of the Electrical Circuit in Atrioventricular Nodal Reentrant Tachycardia (AVNRT).** Two separate pathways are present around the AV node, the slow pathway (*dotted line*), which conducts the impulse slowly and has a shorter refractory period and the fast pathway (*solid line*), which conducts rapidly and has a longer refractory period. The impulse circles the AV node repeatedly using these two separate pathways causing a reentrant tachycardia called AVNRT.

■ AVNRT is a type of reentrant SVT with two separate pathways. These two pathways have different electrophysiologic properties and are both located within or around the AV node.

■ **Slow pathway:** The slow pathway has a shorter refractory period.

■ **Fast pathway:** The fast pathway has a longer refractory period.

■ The slow pathway conducts the impulse anterogradely from atrium to ventricles. The QRS complex is narrow because the impulse follows the normal AV conduction system. The fast pathway conducts the impulse retrogradely to the atria. Because the atria are activated from below upward in a caudocranial direction, the P waves are inverted in leads II, III, and aVF (Fig. 16.2).

## AVNRT

■ **Mechanism of AVNRT:** AVNRT is triggered by a premature impulse originating from the atria or ventricles.

■ The premature atrial impulse should be perfectly timed to occur when the slow pathway has fully recovered from the previous impulse and the fast pathway is still refractory because of its longer refractory period. The premature atrial impulse enters the slow pathway, but is blocked at the fast pathway (Fig. 16.3, #1 and #2).

■ When the impulse reaches the end of the slow pathway, it can exit through the bundle of His to activate the ventricles (#3) and at the same time

**Figure 16.3:   Mechanism of AV Nodal Reentrant Tachycardia.** A premature atrial complex (PAC) is conducted anterogradely through the slow pathway but is blocked at the fast pathway. The impulse activates the ventricles and at the same time is conducted retrogradely through the fast pathway to activate the atria resulting in reentry (see text). AVNRT, atrioventricular nodal reentrant tachycardia.

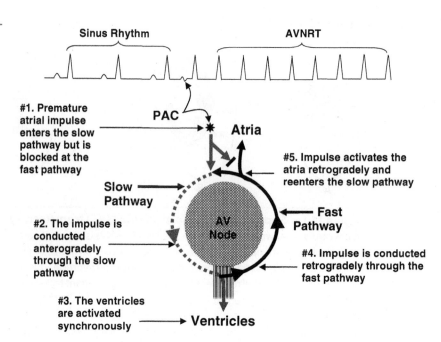

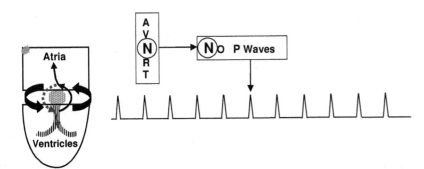

Figure 16.4: **Diagrammatic Representation of Atrioventricular Nodal Reentrant Tachycardia (AVNRT).** AVNRT is classically recognized as a narrow complex tachycardia with regular R-R intervals and no P waves. A complete 12-lead electrocardiogram of AVNRT is shown in Figure 16.5.

circles back through the fast pathway, which by now is fully recovered, to activate the atria retrogradely (#4 and #5).

■ The impulse can reenter the slow pathway and travels the same circuit repetitively causing a reentrant tachycardia called AVNRT.

■ **Electrocardiogram (ECG) findings:** The most common ECG presentation of AVNRT is the presence of a narrow complex tachycardia with regular R-R intervals and no visible P waves (Figs. 16.4 and 16.5). The P waves are retrograde and are inverted in leads II, III, and aVF, but are not visible in the ECG because the atria and ventricles are activated simultaneously; hence, the P waves are buried within the QRS complexes. This is the most common presentation occurring in 66% of all cases of AVNRT.

■ **Other ECG patterns of AVNRT:** In AVNRT, activation of the atria and ventricles may not be perfectly synchronous. If the retrograde P wave occurs immediately after the QRS complex, it may be mistaken for S wave in leads II, III, and aVF or r′ in V₁. If the retrograde P wave occurs immediately before the QRS complex, it may be mistaken for q wave in lead II, III, or aVF (Fig. 16.6). These pseudo-Q, pseudo-S, and pseudo-r′ waves should resolve on conversion of the tachycardia to normal sinus rhythm (Fig. 16.7).

■ Examples of pseudo-S waves in leads II or pseudo-r′ in V₁ are shown (See Figs 16.8 to 16.10). This pattern is diagnostic of AVNRT and is seen in approximately 30% of all cases. The pseudo-S waves in lead II and pseudo-r′ in V₁ are retrograde P waves, but are commonly mistaken as part of the QRS complex. These P waves should resolve when the AVNRT converts to normal sinus rhythm, as shown in Figures 16.7 and 16.8.

■ AVNRT can also manifest in the ECG by the presence of retrograde P waves much further away from the QRS

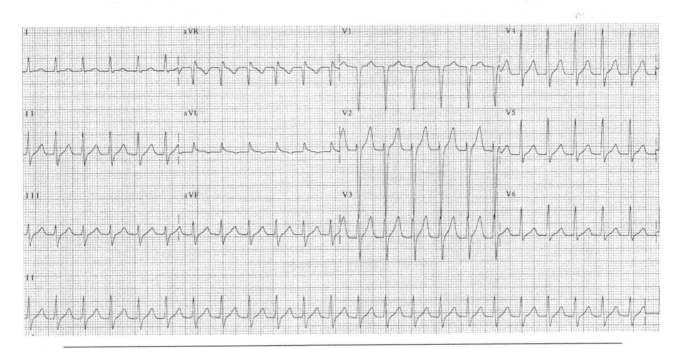

Figure 16.5: **Twelve-Lead Electrocardiogram of Atrioventricular Nodal Reentrant Tachycardia (AVNRT).** "No P waves." Twelve-lead electrocardiogram showing AVNRT. The retrograde P waves are superimposed within the QRS complexes and are not visible in any of the 12 leads. This is the most common presentation of AVNRT.

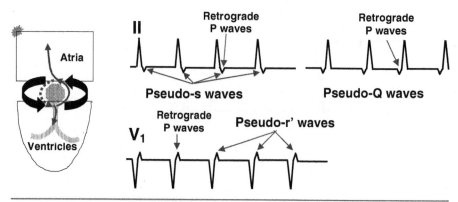

**Figure 16.6:   Pseudo-S and Pseudo-R' waves in Atrioventricular Nodal Reentrant Tachycardia (AVNRT).** In AVNRT, the retrograde P waves may emerge at the beginning or terminal portion of the QRS complexes and can be mistaken for pseudo-Q or pseudo-S waves in leads II, III, and aVF or as pseudo r' waves in V₁. These pseudo-q and pseudo-s waves in lead II and pseudo-r' in V₁ should resolve upon conversion of the tachycardia to normal sinus rhythm (see Fig. 16.7).

complexes. The retrograde P waves may distort the ST segment rather than the terminal portion of the QRS complex as shown in Figures 16.11 and 16.12. Generally, when the P waves are no longer connected to the QRS complexes, the SVT is more commonly the result of AVRT rather than AVNRT.

■ **Atypical AVNRT:** Finally, AVNRT can also manifest with retrograde P waves preceding each QRS complex (Figs. 16.13 and 16.14). This type of AVNRT is called atypical or uncommon and occurs infrequently. The tachycardia is initiated by an ectopic ventricular (rather than atrial) impulse. The impulse is retrogradely conducted to the atria through the slow pathway and anterogradely conducted to the ventricles through the fast pathway. This type of SVT may be difficult to differentiate from other narrow complex tachycardias, especially focal atrial tachycardia.

■ AVNRT therefore has many possible ECG presentations and should be considered in any narrow complex tachycardia with regular R-R intervals whether or not retrograde P waves can be identified.

■ **Summary of ECG findings:** Figure 16.15 is a summary of the different ECG patterns of AVNRT as recorded in lead II.

   ▪ **Typical AVNRT:** Figures 16.15A–D are examples of typical AVNRT. The impulse is conducted anterogradely to the ventricles through the slow pathway and retrogradely to the atria through the fast pathway (slow/fast circuit).

   ▪ **Atypical AVNRT:** Figure 16.15E is an example of atypical AVNRT. The impulse is conducted anterogradely to the ventricles through the fast pathway and retrogradely to the atria through the slow pathway (fast/slow circuit).

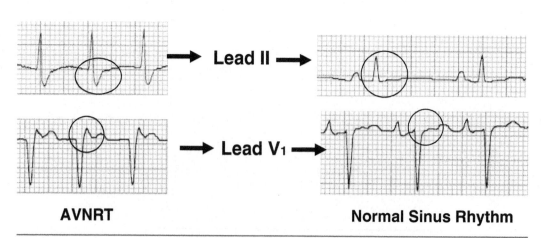

**Figure 16.7:   Atrioventricular Nodal Reentrant Tachycardia (AVNRT) Before and After Conversion to Sinus Rhythm.** Note the presence of pseudo-S waves in lead II and pseudo r' waves in V₁ (*left panel, circled*) during AVNRT, which resolve on conversion to normal sinus rhythm.

**A.** During tachycardia

Pseudo-r' waves

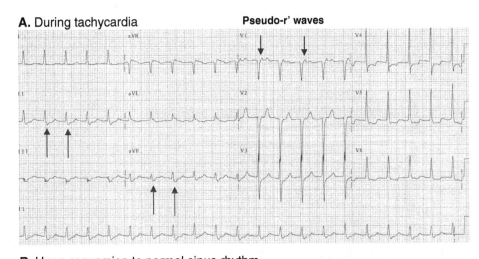

**B.** Upon conversion to normal sinus rhythm

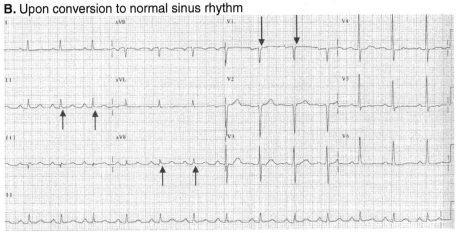

**Figure 16.8:    Atrioventricular Nodal Reentrant Tachycardia (AVNRT) with Pseudo-S and Pseudo-R' waves.** Complete 12-lead electrocardiogram during AVNRT is shown **(A)**. Note the pseudo-S waves in leads II and aVF and pseudo-r' in $V_1$ (*arrows*), which are no longer present on conversion of the AVNRT to normal sinus rhythm **(B)**.

**A.** During Tachycardia

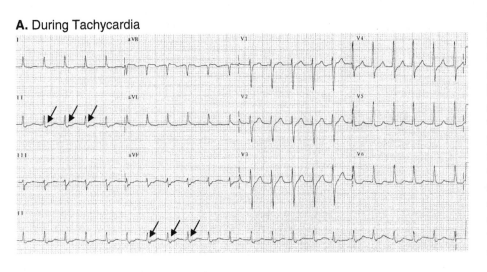

**B.**

Pseudo-S waves          Pseudo-S waves have disappeared upon conversion to sinus rhythm

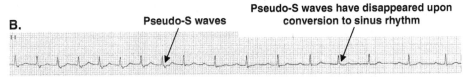

**Figure 16.9:    Spontaneous Conversion of Atrioventricular Nodal Reentrant Tachycardia (AVNRT) to Normal Sinus Rhythm.   (A)** A 12-lead ECG during AVNRT showing pseudo-S waves in lead II (*arrows*). **(B)** Lead II rhythm strip recorded from the same patient during tachycardia (*left half of rhythm strip*) and after spontaneous conversion to normal sinus rhythm (*right half of rhythm strip*). Note that the pseudo-S waves during AVNRT have disappeared (*arrow*).

**Lead II**

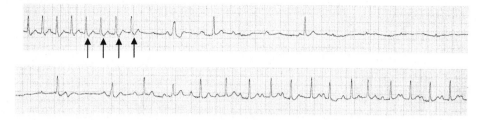

**Figure 16.10: Conversion of Atrioventricular Nodal Reentrant Tachycardia (AVNRT) to Normal Sinus Rhythm with Adenosine.** Adenosine is the drug of choice in converting AVNRT to normal sinus rhythm. The initial portion of the rhythm strip shows a narrow complex tachycardia with pseudo-S waves (*arrows*) in lead II consistent with AVNRT. Note the disappearance of the pseudo-S waves on conversion to sinus rhythm. Note also that the tachycardia terminated with a pseudo-S wave (*last arrow*), implying that the reentrant circuit was blocked at the slow pathway.

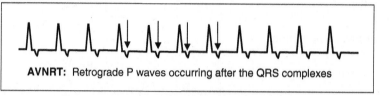

**AVNRT:** Retrograde P waves occurring after the QRS complexes

**Figure 16.11: Other Patterns of Atrioventricular Nodal Reentrant Tachycardia (AVNRT).** Retrograde P waves (*arrows*) occur immediately after the QRS complexes and distort the ST segment or T waves of the previous complex. Although this pattern is consistent with AVNRT, this is more commonly the result of atrioventricular reentrant tachycardia.

**A.**

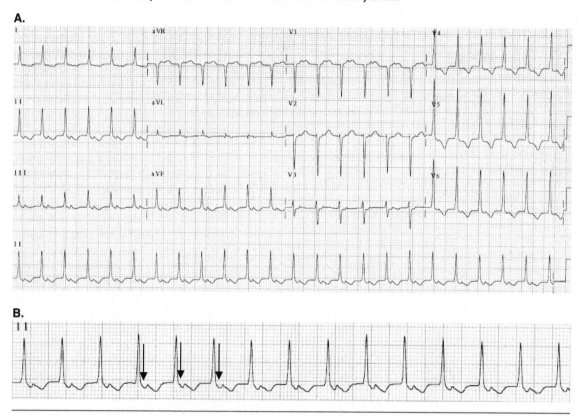

**B.**

**Figure 16.12: Twelve-lead Electrocardiogram Showing Other Presentations of Atrioventricular Nodal Reentrant Tachycardia (AVNRT).** Twelve-lead electrocardiogram **(A)** and lead II rhythm strip from the same patient **(B)** showing retrograde P waves that are further away from the QRS complexes (*arrows*). Although this pattern is more typically seen in atrioventricular reentrant tachycardia, electrophysiologic study in this patient confirmed the presence of AVNRT with successful ablation of the slow pathway.

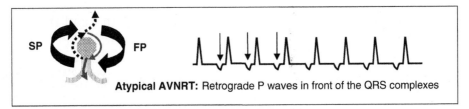

**Atypical AVNRT:** Retrograde P waves in front of the QRS complexes

**Figure 16.13:    Diagrammatic Representation of Atypical Atrioventricular Nodal Reentrant Tachycardia (AVNRT).** Retrograde P waves (*arrows*) occur before the next QRS complex with R-P interval longer than PR interval. The impulse is conducted retrogradely through the slow pathway (SP) and anterogradely through the fast pathway (FP).

## ECG Findings of AVNRT

1. AVNRT is typically a narrow complex tachycardia with regular R-R intervals and no P waves.

2. When P waves are present, they are always retrograde because the atria are activated from below upward. The P waves therefore are inverted in leads II, III, and aVF.

3. Retrograde P waves may be present but may not be recognized when they are embedded within the QRS complexes. When the retrograde P waves distort the terminal portion of the QRS complexes, they can be mistaken for S waves in II, III, and aVF or r′ in $V_1$. In rare instances, the retrograde P waves may distort the initial portion of the QRS complex and mistaken for q waves in lead II, III, and aVF.

4. The retrograde P waves may be inscribed immediately after the QRS complexes deforming the ST segment or T wave of the previous complex.

5. The retrograde P waves may be inscribed before the QRS complex. This type of AVNRT is called atypical or uncommon. Other atypical forms may be associated with retrograde P waves midway or almost midway between the QRS complexes.

6. The presence of second-degree AV block during tachycardia is possible but is rare and makes the diagnosis of AVNRT highly unlikely.

7. The ventricular rate in AVNRT varies from 110 to 250 beats per minute (bpm). The rate, however, is not helpful in distinguishing AVNRT from other types of SVT.

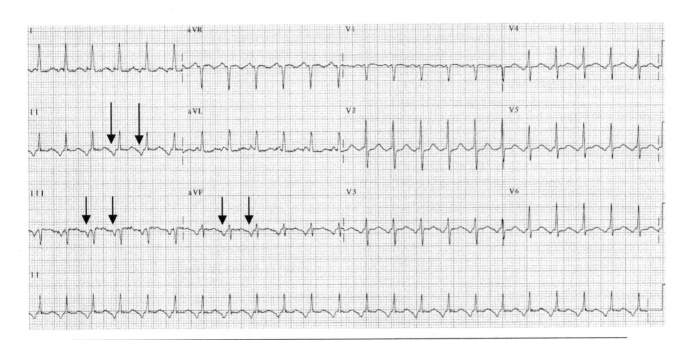

**Figure 16.14:    Twelve-lead Electrocardiogram of Atypical Atrioventricular Nodal Reentrant Tachycardia (AVNRT).** Inverted P waves are seen before the QRS complexes in leads II, III and aVF (*arrows*). Although this pattern is more commonly seen in other types of supraventricular tachycardia such as focal atrial or junctional tachycardia, this type of electrocardiogram can also occur in patients with atypical AVNRT.

**Figure 16.15: Summary of the Different Patterns of Atrioventricular Nodal Reentrant Tachycardia (AVNRT). (A–E)** The different possible electrocardiogram patterns of AVNRT in lead II. Arrows identify the retrograde P waves.

## ECG of AVNRT in Lead II

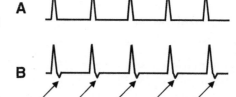

A — No P waves. This is the most common presentation of AVNRT occurring in 66% of all cases. The P waves are centered within the QRS complexes.

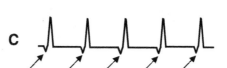

B — Pseudo S waves: 30%

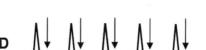
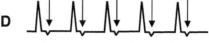

C — Pseudo q waves: 4%.

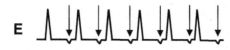

D — Retrograde P waves after the QRS complex. This is rare and is almost always due to AVRT.

E — Atypical AVNRT: This is rare and is more commonly due to focal atrial tachycardia.

8. AVNRT should always be considered as a possible diagnosis in any narrow complex tachycardia with regular R-R intervals, regardless of the presence or absence of retrograde P waves because this is the most common type of SVT.

## Mechanism

■ AVNRT is an example of microreentry associated with a circuit within or around the AV node. The reentrant circuit consists of two separate pathways with different electrical properties. The slow pathway has a short refractory period and the fast pathway has a longer refractory period. The tachycardia is precipitated by an ectopic impulse originating from the atria or ventricles. The impulse has to occur when one pathway is still refractory and the other has completely recovered. The tachycardia has a narrow QRS complex because the impulse follows the normal conduction system and activates the ventricles normally. The rate of the tachycardia is very regular because the impulse follows a fixed circuit.

■ Second-degree AV block is unusual but is possible during AVNRT. It can potentially occur at the level of the His bundle or more distally, which is extremely rare when the tachycardia has narrow QRS complexes.

■ There are two types of AVNRT: typical and atypical.

■ **Typical presentation:** This is the most common presentation of AVNRT occurring in more than 90% of all cases. The slow pathway conducts the impulse to the ventricles and the fast pathway conducts the impulse to the atria. This type of AVNRT is often called the slow/fast circuit.

☐ **No P Waves:** This is the most typical and most common presentation, occurring in approximately 66% of all AVNRT. The atrial impulse is conducted anterogradely to the ventricles through the slow pathway and retrogradely to the atria through the fast pathway. Activation of both atria and ventricles are simultaneous; thus, the P waves and QRS complexes are inscribed synchronously and no P waves are evident in the ECG.

☐ **Retrograde P waves:** When P waves are present, they are inverted in leads II, III, and aVF because the atria are activated from below upward. The P waves may deform the terminal portion of the QRS complexes and mistaken for S waves in II, III, and aVF or r′ in V₁. This occurs in approximately 30% of all AVNRT. The retrograde P waves may deform the initial portion of the QRS complex and mistaken for q waves in II, III, and aVF. This occurs in 4% of all AVNRT. The retrograde P waves may also deform the ST segment or the initial portion of the T wave, although this type of AVNRT is rare.

■ **Atypical presentation:** The fast pathway conducts the impulse to the ventricles and the slow pathway conducts the impulse to the atria. This fast/slow circuit is rare.

☐ The atypical form is characterized by retrograde P waves in front of the QRS complexes. This is often precipitated by an ectopic ventricular impulse retrogradely conducted to the atria through the slow pathway and anterogradely conducted to the ventricles through the fast pathway.

☐ Other atypical forms may be associated with retrograde P waves midway or almost midway between the QRS complexes.

## Clinical Significance

■ SVT from reentry is the most common sustained narrow complex tachycardia in the general population accounting for approximately 80% to 90% of all SVT. Among the SVT due to reentry, AVNRT is the most common occurring in more than 60% of all reentrant SVT. AVNRT is frequently seen in normal healthy individuals without structural cardiac disease and is more common in females.

■ AVNRT can occur suddenly and terminate abruptly and is therefore paroxysmal. This contrasts with sinus tachycardia where the tachycardia is nonparoxysmal with gradual onset and gradual termination. SVT from reentry are usually episodic occurring for a few minutes to a few hours and are recurrent. Unlike SVT from enhanced automaticity, they are rarely incessant, meaning that the tachycardia rarely persists for >12 hours a day.

■ AVNRT is generally tolerable except in patients with stenotic valves, ischemic heart disease, left ventricular (LV) dysfunction, or cardiomyopathy. In these patients, hypotension or symptoms of low cardiac output, myocardial ischemia, heart failure, or actual syncope may occur during tachycardia. It can also cause symptoms even among healthy patients when the tachycardia is unusually rapid; thus, syncope can occur when the tachycardia starts abruptly with a very fast rate or terminates with a very long pause because of overdrive suppression of the sinus node. The latter occurs when the tachycardia is associated with sinus node dysfunction. It is rarely associated with mortality or morbidity in otherwise healthy individuals.

■ Although physical examination is usually not helpful in the diagnosis of SVT, prominent neck vein pulsations are often present and may be the patient's chief complaint during tachycardia. These neck vein pulsations are due to cannon A waves, which occur when atrial contraction is simultaneous with ventricular contraction due to retrograde P waves occurring within or immediately after the QRS complex. The tachycardia causes atrial stretch, which may be followed by a period of diuresis due to release of atrial natriuretic peptide.

## Acute Treatment

■ Unless the patient is severely hypotensive or in cardiogenic shock, immediate electrical cardioversion is rarely necessary in patients with AVNRT because the tachycardia is well tolerated. Vagal maneuvers and pharmacologic therapy are usually very effective in terminating the tachycardia.

■ **Vagal maneuvers:** Vagal stimulation should be attempted as the initial therapeutic maneuver before any pharmacologic agent is given. The ECG should be recorded when vagal stimulation is performed because vagal stimulation is not only effective in terminating the tachycardia, but is also helpful as a diagnostic maneuver if the tachycardia turns out to be due to other arrhythmias.

■ **Carotid sinus pressure:** The most commonly used and most effective vagal maneuver in terminating SVT is carotid sinus pressure. Carotid sinus pressure is always performed under cardiac monitoring in the recumbent position. With the neck hyperextended, the common carotid artery is identified by its pulsations and followed distally as close to the mandible as possible, usually at the angle of the jaw where the artery bifurcates into external and internal carotid arteries. It is at this bifurcation where the carotid sinus is located. Carotid sinus pressure is performed by applying gentle but constant pressure to the pulsating artery using both middle and index fingers. Pressure should be applied initially only for a few seconds until slowing of the heart rate can be identified in the cardiac monitor. The maneuver can be repeated several more times by pressing the artery at longer intervals if needed, especially if the previous maneuvers are unsuccessful in eliciting any response. There is no need to rub or massage the artery or press the pulsating artery for longer than 5 seconds at a time. Constant gentle pressure on the artery is all that is necessary. Only one artery should be pressed at any time. If there is no response, the same maneuver should be tried on the other carotid artery. This maneuver can also be repeated if the SVT persists after a pharmacologic agent has been given, but is not effective in terminating the tachycardia. Occasionally, a tachycardia that is previously unresponsive to carotid sinus pressure may become more responsive after an intravenous medication such as calcium channel blocker or digoxin has been given. If carotid stenosis is suspected by the presence of a carotid bruit, carotid sinus pressure should not be attempted.

■ **Pharyngeal stimulation:** A tongue blade is positioned at the back of the tongue as if performing a routine oropharyngeal examination. The tongue blade is gently brushed to the pharynx to make the patient gag.

■ **Valsalva maneuver:** This can be performed by several methods. The simplest is to instruct the patient to tense the abdominal muscles by exhaling forcefully against a closed glottis. The examiner can also make a fist, which is gently placed on the patient's abdomen. The patient, who is recumbent, is instructed to resist by tensing the abdominal muscles as the examiner's fist is gently pressed on the abdomen. The procedure can also be performed by blowing forcefully through a spirometer, balloon, or brown bag. This can also be done by straining, as if the patient is lifting a heavy object. The patient, who is recumbent, is asked to cross both legs on top of one another and instructed to lift them together while resistance is being applied to prevent the legs from being lifted. The Valsalva maneuver should not be performed if the patient is severely hypertensive, in congestive failure, or if an acute coronary event is suspected or patient is hemodynamically unstable.

■ **Forceful coughing.**

■ **Diving reflex:** When the face comes in contact with cold water, bradycardia usually occurs and is known as the diving reflex. This can be done at bedside by immersing the face in iced water.

- **Ocular pressure:** This vagal maneuver is not recommended since retinal detachment may occur as a potential complication of the procedure especially if done forcefully.

- **Pharmacologic therapy:** ABCD are the drugs of choice for the treatment of AVNRT. (A, adenosine; B, beta blockers; C, calcium channel blockers; D, digoxin). These drugs are not necessarily given in alphabetical order.

- **Adenosine:** If vagal maneuvers are not successful in terminating the tachycardia, adenosine is the drug of choice for terminating AVNRT.

  - Adenosine should not be given if the patient has bronchospastic pulmonary disease because adenosine can precipitate asthma.

  - The initial dose of adenosine is 6 mg given as an intravenous bolus. The injection should be given rapidly within 1 to 2 seconds preferably to a proximal vein followed by a saline flush. If a peripheral vein is used, the arm where the injection was given should be immediately raised. If the arrhythmia has not converted to normal sinus rhythm, another bolus using a bigger dose of 12 mg is given IV. A third and final dose of 12 mg may be repeated if the tachycardia has not responded to the two previous doses. Approximately 60% of patients with AVNRT will convert with the first dose within 1 minute and up to 92% after a 12-mg dose.

  - Adenosine is very effective in terminating AVNRT, but is also helpful in the diagnosis of other arrhythmias especially atrial flutter with 2:1 block. A 12-lead ECG or a rhythm strip should be recorded when adenosine is injected. When adenosine converts AVNRT to normal sinus rhythm, the tachycardia ends with a retrograde P wave, implying that the tachycardia was blocked at the slow pathway, which is usually the most vulnerable part of the reentrant circuit. The response of AVRT to adenosine is similar, ending with a retrograde P wave because both tachycardias are AV node–dependent. Focal atrial tachycardia is not AV node–dependent, although it may respond to adenosine. When focal atrial tachycardia terminates, the tachycardia ends with a QRS complex rather than a P wave. Atrial flutter with 2:1 block will not respond to adenosine, but will slow the ventricular rate significantly allowing the diagnosis of atrial flutter to become obvious by the presence of a regular sawtooth, wavy undulating baseline between the QRS complexes.

  - Adenosine is potentiated by dipyridamole, since dipyridamole prevents the metabolic breakdown of adenosine. It is also potentiated by carbamazepine, which may result in prolonged asystole on conversion of the tachycardia to normal sinus rhythm. If the patient is taking dipyridamole or carbamazepine, the initial dose should be cut in half to 3 mg.

  - Theophylline is the antidote for adenosine. If the patient is on theophylline, higher doses of adenosine may be given to treat the SVT if there is no history of bronchospastic pulmonary disease. If the patient has reactive airway disease, adenosine can cause bronchospasm.

- If the SVT has not responded after three doses of adenosine or if adenosine is contraindicated, another pharmacologic agent should be tried. The choice of the next pharmacologic agent will depend on the presence or absence of LV dysfunction or clinical congestive heart failure.

- **Preserved LV function**

  - **Calcium channel clockers:** In patients with preserved LV function, the next drug of choice after failure to terminate AVNRT with adenosine is verapamil or diltiazem. If the patient is not hypotensive, 2.5 to 5 mg of verapamil is given IV slowly over 2 minutes under careful ECG and blood pressure monitoring. If there is no response and the patient remains stable, additional doses of 5 to 10 mg may be given every 15 to 30 minutes until a total dose of 20 mg is given. Alternate dosing with verapamil is to give 5 mg boluses every 15 minutes not to exceed 30 mg. Verapamil is effective in up to 90% of patients. Verapamil is a hypotensive and negatively inotropic agent and should not be given when there is congestive heart failure or LV dysfunction. Diltiazem is another calcium channel blocker that can be given at an initial dose of 0.25 mg per kg (equivalent to approximately 15 to 20 mg in a 70-kg patient) over 2 minutes. If the tachycardia has not terminated with the first bolus, a higher dose of 0.35 mg/kg or 25 mg is given after 15 minutes. This is followed by a maintenance IV dose of 5 to 15 mg/hour if needed. Diltiazem is shorter acting and less hypotensive than verapamil and may be better tolerated in some patients. In patients who become hypotensive with verapamil or diltiazem, calcium gluconate or calcium chloride 5% 10 mL may be given intravenously to reverse the hypotension. For more detailed dosing of verapamil or diltiazem, see Appendix.

  - **Beta Blockers:** Beta blockers (metoprolol, atenolol, propranolol, or esmolol) may be tried if the patient has not responded to the above therapy. Beta blockers should not be given when there is congestive heart failure or evidence of LV systolic dysfunction, hypotension, or bronchospastic pulmonary disease.

    - Metoprolol is given intravenously slowly at a dose of 5 mg and repeated two more times every 5 minutes if necessary for a total dose of 15 mg in 15 minutes.

    - Atenolol is given IV slowly 5 mg over 5 minutes and repeated once after 10 minutes if needed if the first dose was well tolerated.

    - Propranolol is given at a dose of 0.1 mg/kg. The drug is given IV slowly not to exceed 1 mg per minute until the arrhythmia is terminated. A second dose may be repeated after 2 minutes if needed.

    - Esmolol is given at an initial dose of 0.5 mg/kg infused over a minute. This is followed by a maintenance infusion of 0.05 mg/kg/min for the next 4 minutes (see Appendix for further dosing). If immediate control of SVT is necessary intraoperatively, a higher dose of 1 mg/kg may be given over 30 seconds followed by 150 mcg/kg/min maintenance infusion.

☐ **Digoxin:** Digoxin has a slow onset of action and is not as effective as the previously discussed agents. The initial dose of digoxin in a patient who is not on oral digoxin is 0.5 mg given slowly IV for 5 minutes or longer. Subsequent doses of 0.25 mg IV should be given after 4 hours and repeated if needed for a total dose of no more than 1.5 mg over a 24-hour period.

☐ **Other Agents:**

☐ Other antiarrhythmic agents that should be considered include type IA (procainamide), type IC (propafenone), or type III agents (amiodarone, ibutilide). The use of these agents requires expert consultation. These agents should be considered only if the SVT is resistant to the above pharmacologic agents. For more detailed dosing of these agents, see Appendix.

☐ An old remedy, now seldom used, that should be considered when there is hypotension is acute elevation of systolic blood pressure with arterial vasopressors such as phenylephrine. Intravenous vasopressors may cause bradycardia and AV block by reflex vagal stimulation of baroreceptors in the carotid sinus. This may be considered when the patient is hypotensive but not when there is heart failure. The initial dose of phenylephrine is 100 mcg given as an IV bolus over 20 to 30 seconds and repeated in increments of 100 to 200 mcg. A total dose of 100 to 500 mcg is usually given, usual dose 200 mcg. The maximal dose depends on the blood pressure response, which should not exceed an arbitrary level of 180 mm Hg systolic.

☐ **Electrical cardioversion:** In stable patients, synchronized electrical cardioversion is not encouraged. It should be attempted only as a last resort.

■ **Presence of heart failure or LV systolic dysfunction (ejection fraction ≤40%).**

☐ **Digoxin:** Although digoxin may not be the most effective agent, it is the preferred agent when there is LV dysfunction, decompensated congestive heart failure, or hypotension. If the patient is not on oral digoxin, 0.5 mg is given intravenously as described previously.

☐ **Other agents:** Nondihydropyridine calcium channel blockers (diltiazem or verapamil) should not be given when there is decompensated heart failure or LV dysfunction. Verapamil is contraindicated because it is negatively inotropic and has a longer half-life than diltiazem. Diltiazem may be more tolerable because of its shorter half-life and may be tried unless there is decompensated heart failure. The drug is given IV slowly at an initial dose of 15 to 20 mg (0.25 mg/kg).

Intravenous beta blockers (metoprolol, atenolol, propranolol, esmolol) should not be given in the presence of LV dysfunction, heart failure, or bronchospastic pulmonary disease. Although beta blockers are indicated as long-term therapy for chronic congestive heart failure from systolic LV dysfunction, they are given orally in small doses and titrated slowly over several days. They should not be given in intravenous doses such as those used for the emergency treatment of SVT with preserved systolic LV function.

☐ **Antiarrhythmic agents:** Amiodarone, a Class III agent, may be the only intravenous antiarrhythmic drug that may be tried when there is LV dysfunction. This agent, however, should be considered only if the SVT has not responded to the other agents.

☐ **Electrical cardioversion:** Synchronized electrical cardioversion is rarely necessary and should be attempted only as a last resort.

■ **Long-term therapy:** Long-term oral therapy is generally given to prevent further recurrence of the arrhythmia, minimize symptoms, and improve quality of life rather than to prolong survival.

▨ For patients with minimal or no symptoms during tachycardia, especially if the arrhythmia occurs only infrequently, no oral medications are needed.

▨ For patients who develop symptoms of hemodynamic instability during AVNRT or those with recurrent and prolonged arrhythmias, chronic oral medical therapy may be tried. In patients without LV dysfunction, oral medications include calcium channel blockers (verapamil or diltiazem), beta blockers (atenolol, metoprolol, or propranolol), or digoxin. Although digoxin is less effective than the other agents, it may be the only oral agent that is appropriate for long-term maintenance therapy in patients with LV dysfunction. Beta blockers, such as carvedilol and metoprolol succinate, are standard agents for the treatment of systolic LV dysfunction and should be titrated slowly orally until an adequate maintenance dose is given that is also effective for controlling or preventing the tachycardia.

▨ Catheter ablation of the reentrant circuit with a chance of permanent cure should be considered in patients who do not respond to medical therapy or those not willing to take oral medications. The success rate of catheter ablation is approximately 96% with a recurrence rate of 3% to 7% after successful ablation. Because the reentrant circuit is close to the AV node, there is a 1% or more chance of developing second- or third-degree AV block, which may require implantation of a permanent pacemaker.

## Prognosis

■ Because most AVNRT occurs in young patients with structurally normal hearts, the tachycardia is usually tolerable and overall prognosis is excellent with a chance of permanent cure among patients who are willing to undergo electrical ablation.

**Figure 16.16:** **Orthodromic and Antidromic Atrioventricular Reentrant Tachycardia (AVRT).** In orthodromic AVRT **(A)**, the QRS complexes are narrow since the ventricles are activated through the normal AV conduction system. In antidromic AVRT **(B)**, the QRS complexes are wide because the ventricles are activated through the bypass tract.

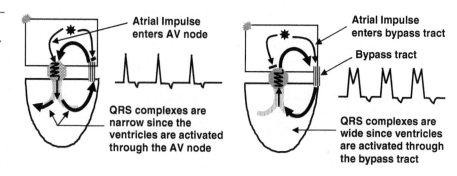

A. Orthodromic AVRT          B. Antidromic AVRT

## Atrioventricular Reciprocating Tachycardia

- **AVRT:** AVRT is the second most common SVT occurring in approximately 30% of all reentrant SVT. This type of SVT is associated with a bypass tract that connects the atrium directly to the ventricle.

- Normally, an atrial impulse can conduct to the ventricles only through the AV node. When a bypass tract is present, a second pathway is created for reentry to occur. Thus, an atrial impulse can enter the ventricles through the AV node and return to the atria through the bypass tract (Fig. 16.16A) or enter the ventricle through the bypass tract and return to the atria through the AV node (Fig. 16.16B).

- AVRT may have narrow or wide QRS complexes:

  - **AVRT with narrow QRS complexes:** When the atrial impulse enters the ventricles through the AV node and returns to the atria through the bypass

tract, the QRS complex will be narrow. This type of tachycardia is called orthodromic AVRT (Fig. 16.16A).

  - **AVRT with wide QRS complexes:** When the atrial impulse enters the ventricles through the bypass tract and returns to the atria through the AV node, the QRS complex will be wide. This type of tachycardia is called antidromic AVRT (Fig. 16.16B). Antidromic AVRT is an example of SVT with wide QRS complexes and will be further discussed in Chapter 20, Wolff-Parkinson-White Syndrome.

- **Mechanism:** AVRT with narrow QRS complexes is triggered by a premature impulse originating from the atria or ventricles. The diagram below illustrates how the tachycardia is initiated by a premature atrial complex (PAC) (Fig. 16.17).

  - The PAC should be perfectly timed to occur when the AV node (the slow pathway) has fully recovered, while the bypass tract (the fast pathway) is still refractory from the previous impulse. Because the AV node has a shorter refractory period, the premature

**Figure 16.17:** **Mechanism of Narrow Complex Atrioventricular Reentrant Tachycardia (AVRT).** The diagram shows how a narrow complex AVRT is initiated by a premature atrial complex (PAC). The PAC finds the bypass tract still refractory because of its longer refractory period but is conducted through the AV node, which has a shorter refractory period, resulting in AVRT with narrow QRS complexes (see text).

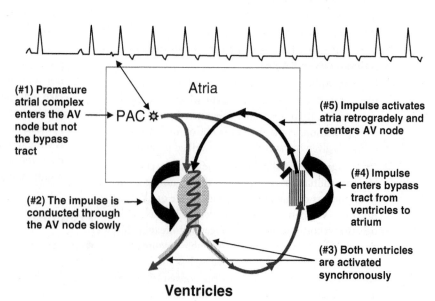

(#1) Premature atrial complex enters the AV node but not the bypass tract

Atria

PAC ☼

(#5) Impulse activates atria retrogradely and reenters AV node

(#4) Impulse enters bypass tract from ventricles to atrium

(#2) The impulse is conducted through the AV node slowly

(#3) Both ventricles are activated synchronously

**Ventricles**

atrial impulse will enter the AV node but not the bypass tract (Fig. 16.17, #1).

- The impulse conducts slowly through the AV node (#2) and activates the ventricles normally resulting in a narrow QRS complex (#3). After the ventricles are activated, the impulse circles back through the bypass tract (#4) and activates the atria retrogradely (#5).
- After the atria are activated, the impulse can again enter the AV node and the circuit starts all over again.
- In AVRT, the reentrant circuit involves a large mass of tissue consisting of the atria, AV node, bundle of His, bundle branches and fascicles, ventricles, and bypass tract before returning to the atria. AVRT therefore is a form of macro-reentry.
- **ECG Findings:** Narrow complex AVRT has the following features:
  - The atria and ventricles are essential components of the circuit; thus, activation of the atria and ventricles cannot be simultaneous. The P wave, therefore, cannot be buried within the QRS complex. It should always be inscribed outside the QRS complexes.
  - Because the atria are activated from the bypass tract, the P waves are inscribed retrogradely. The P waves are usually inverted in II, III, and aVF although the configuration of the P wave may vary depending on the location of the bypass tract.
  - Typically, the retrograde P waves are inscribed immediately after the QRS complexes and deform the ST segments. Thus, the R-P interval is shorter than the PR interval (Fig. 16.18). This is the typical or most common presentation of AVRT.
  - AV block is not possible during AVRT because the atria and ventricles are essential components of the circuit; thus, every retrograde P wave is always followed by a QRS complex during tachycardia. When AV block occurs, the reentrant circuit (and therefore the tachycardia) will terminate.
- An example of AVRT is shown in Figure 16.19. Note that the P waves are retrograde and are inverted in leads II, III, and aVF and also in $V_4$ to $V_6$. The retrograde P

wave is inscribed immediately after the QRS complex, deforming the ST segment of the previous QRS complex with an R-P interval that is shorter than the PR interval.

- Other examples of narrow complex tachycardia with retrograde P waves immediately after the QRS complex are shown in Figs. 16.20 to 16.22. The retrograde P waves may be mistaken for inverted T waves.
- There are two types of narrow complex (orthodromic) AVRT: typical and atypical (see Figs. 16.22 to 16.25).
  - **Typical AVRT:** AVRT is typical when the retrograde P waves are inscribed immediately after the QRS complex and deform the ST segment or T wave of the preceding complex (Figs. 16.21 and 16.22). Conduction from ventricle to atrium across the bypass tract (R-P interval) is faster than conduction from atrium to ventricle across the AV node (PR interval); thus, the R-P interval is shorter than the PR interval. In typical AVRT, the AV node is the slow pathway and the bypass tract is the fast pathway (slow/fast activation). Virtually all cases of AVRT present in this manner.
  - **Atypical AVRT:** AVRT is atypical when the retrograde P waves occur in front of the QRS complexes (Fig. 16.23); thus, the R-P interval is longer than the PR interval. Atypical AVRT is associated with a slowly conducting bypass tract. Conduction from ventricle to atrium across the bypass tract (R-P interval) is slower than conduction from atrium to ventricle (PR interval) across the AV node (fast/slow activation). This type of AVRT is rare. The ECG of atypical AVRT is similar to that of atypical AVNRT.
- **Typical AVRT versus AVNRT:** When retrograde P waves are inscribed immediately after the QRS complexes during tachycardia, AVRT may be difficult to differentiate from AVNRT (Fig. 16.24). One clue in differentiating AVRT from AVNRT is the duration of the R-P interval (Figs. 16.21 and 16.22A). The R-P interval in AVRT should measure ≥80 milliseconds in the surface ECG because this is the minimum time required for the impulse to travel from ventricles to atria across the bypass tract. If the retrograde P wave is too close to the QRS complex and the R-P interval is <80 milliseconds, as

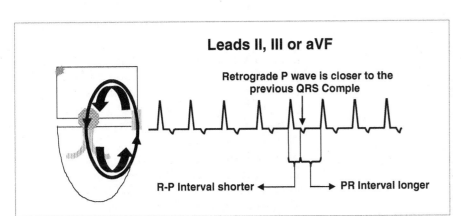

### Leads II, III or aVF

Retrograde P wave is closer to the previous QRS Comple

R-P Interval shorter ← → PR Interval longer

**Figure 16.18: Typical Atrioventricular Reentrant Tachycardia (AVRT).** In AVRT, the retrograde P wave is inscribed immediately after the QRS complex with the R-P interval shorter than the PR interval. This is the typical or most common presentation of AVRT.

**A.** During Tachycardia

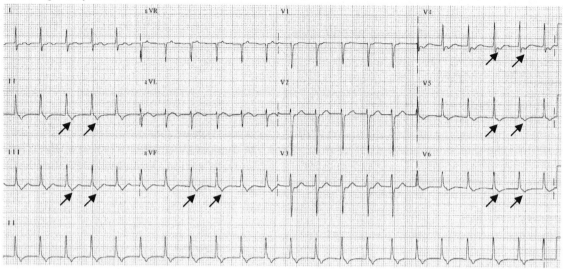

**B.** During Normal Sinus Rhythm

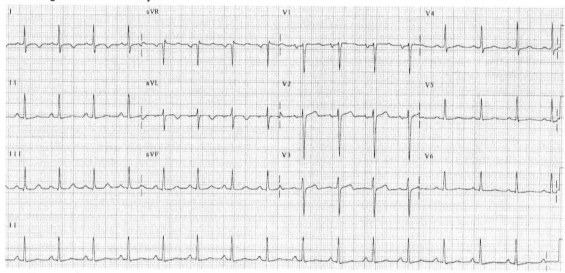

**Figure 16.19:    Twelve-lead Electrocardiogram in Atrioventricular Reentrant Tachycardia (AVRT).**
**(A)** A narrow complex tachycardia with retrograde P waves in II, III, aVF, and in V₄ to V₆ (*arrows*). The retrograde P waves are inscribed after the QRS complexes and deform the ST segments or T waves of the previous complex with an R-P interval shorter than PR interval. **(B)** The same patient after conversion to normal sinus rhythm. The retrograde P waves are no longer present.

shown in Figure 16.22A, AVRT is unlikely and AVNRT is the more likely diagnosis.

- Because the R-P interval in AVRT measure ≥80 milliseconds, the retrograde P waves are usually inscribed separately from the QRS complexes, whereas in AVNRT, the retrograde P waves are usually connected to the terminal portion of the QRS complexes.

- **Concealed bypass tract:** In 30% to 40% of patients with AVRT, the bypass tract is concealed, indicating that the bypass tract is capable of conducting only in a retrograde fashion from ventricle to atrium but not

from atrium to ventricle (see Chapter 20, Wolff-Parkinson-White Syndrome). Thus, the baseline ECG during normal sinus rhythm or upon conversion of the AVRT to normal sinus rhythm will not show any preexcitation (no delta wave or short PR interval). The presence of a bypass tract is suspected only when tachycardia from AVRT occur.

- **Manifest bypass tract:** Patients with AVRT with manifest bypass tracts have preexcitation (delta wave and short PR interval) in baseline ECG during normal sinus rhythm. These bypass tracts are capable of

**A.** During AVRT

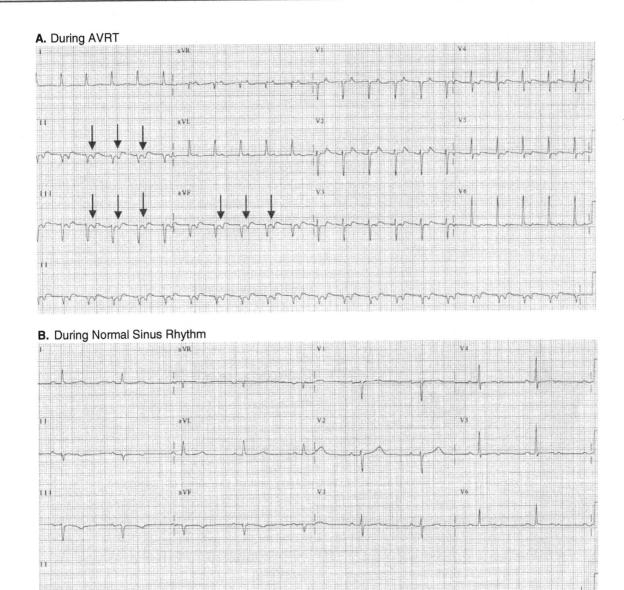

**B.** During Normal Sinus Rhythm

**Figure 16.20: Retrograde P Waves can be Mistaken for Inverted T Waves in Atrioventricular Reentrant Tachycardia (AVRT). (A)** A 12-lead electrocardiogram (ECG) during tachycardia. The retrograde P wave is inscribed immediately after the QRS complex with the R-P interval shorter than the PR interval. This is the most common presentation of AVRT. The retrograde P waves may be mistaken for inverted T waves in II, III, and aVF (*arrows*). **(B)** A 12-lead ECG of the same patient upon conversion to normal sinus rhythm. The retrograde P waves are no longer present.

Typical AVRT

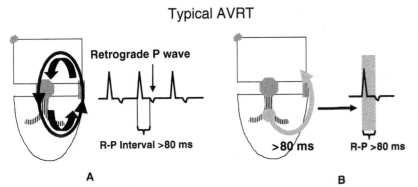

**A**                                          **B**

**Figure 16.21: The R-P Interval in Typical Atrioventricular Reentrant Tachycardia (AVRT).** In typical AVRT, the R-P interval (measured from the onset of QRS complex to the onset of the retrograde P wave) should measure ≥80 ms. This is the time required for the impulse to travel from ventricles to atria retrogradely through the bypass tract. The length of the arrow in **(B)** indicates the R-P interval, which is the time required for the impulse to travel from ventricle to atrium across the bypass tract and is ≥80 ms. ms, milliseconds.

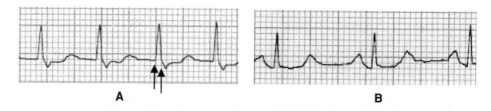

**Figure 16.22: Atrioventricular Nodal Reentrant Tachycardia (AVNRT). (A)** Retrograde P waves are inscribed immediately behind the QRS complexes during tachycardia. Note that the R-P interval is <80 ms (distance between the two arrows), hence the tachycardia is AVNRT and not atrioventricular reentrant tachycardia (AVRT). In AVRT, at least 80 ms is required for the impulse to travel from ventricle to atrium across the bypass tract in the surface electrocardiogram. **(B)** Same patient on conversion to normal sinus rhythm. ms, milliseconds.

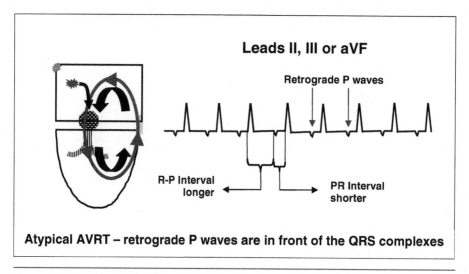

**Figure 16.23: Atypical Atrioventricular Reentrant Tachycardia (AVRT).** In atypical AVRT, the retrograde P waves are inscribed in front of the QRS complexes with the R-P interval longer than PR interval. Atypical AVRT is associated with a slowly conducting bypass tract resulting in a long R-P interval.

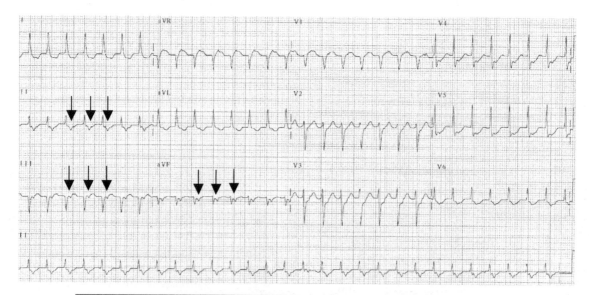

**Figure 16.24: Typical Atrioventricular Reentrant Tachycardia (AVRT).** Twelve-lead electrocardiogram showing typical AVRT. Retrograde P waves are present in leads II, III, and aVF (*arrows*) with R-P interval measuring 80 milliseconds. The R-P interval is shorter than the PR interval.

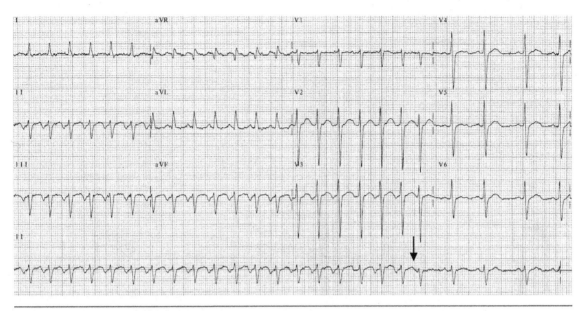

**Figure 16.25:    Atypical Atrioventricular Reentrant Tachycardia (AVRT).** In atypical AVRT, retrograde P waves are in front of the QRS complex (R-P interval longer than PR interval) because of the presence of a slowly conducting bypass tract. The supraventricular tachycardia is terminated by a perfectly timed premature atrial complex (*arrow*).

conducting from atrium to ventricle and also from ventricle to atrium. This will be discussed more extensively in Chapter 20, Wolff-Parkinson-White Syndrome.

- **Electrical alternans:** In electrical alternans, the amplitude of the QRS complexes alternates by more than 1 mm. Although electrical alternans is more commonly seen in AVRT (Fig. 16.26), electrical alternans can also occur with other types of SVT. Electrical alternans is more commonly a function of the heart rate rather than the type or mechanism of the SVT.

- **Localizing the bypass tract:** Most bypass tracts are located at the free wall of the left ventricle (50% to 60%) followed by the posteroseptal area (20% to 30%), free wall of the right ventricle (10% to 20%), and the anteroseptal area (5%). The atrial insertion of the bypass tract can be localized by the configuration of the P wave during AVRT. The bypass tract can also be localized during sinus rhythm if the baseline ECG shows ventricular preexcitation. This is further discussed in Chapter 20, Wolff-Parkinson-White Syndrome.

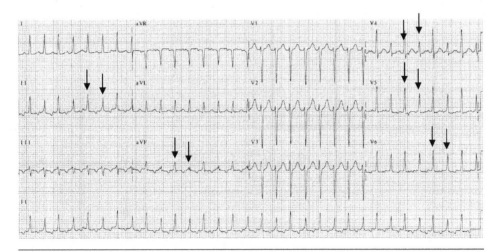

**Figure 16.26:    Electrical Alternans.** In electrical alternans, taller QRS complexes alternate with shorter QRS complexes by more than 1 mm. Arrows point to a tall QRS complex alternating with a smaller QRS complex. Electrical alternans is more commonly seen in atrioventricular reentrant tachycardia (AVRT) than with other types of supraventricular tachycardia (SVT) because the ventricular rate of AVRT is generally faster when compared with other types of SVT.

**Figure 16.27:    Localizing the Bypass Tract.**
If the P waves are inverted in lead I during tachycardia **(A)**, the bypass tract is left sided. If the P waves are upright in lead I during the tachycardia **(B)**, the bypass tract is right sided. Arrows represent the direction of atrial activation.

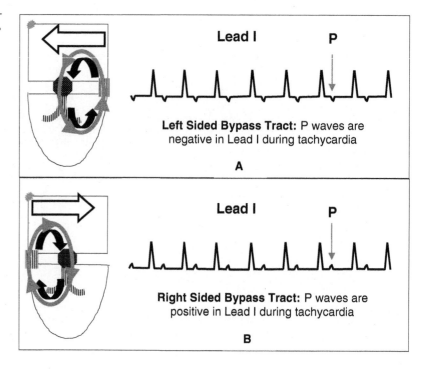

**Left Sided Bypass Tract:** P waves are negative in Lead I during tachycardia

**A**

**Right Sided Bypass Tract:** P waves are positive in Lead I during tachycardia

**B**

- **Left-sided bypass tract:** If the P waves are inverted in lead I during tachycardia, the direction of atrial activation is from left atrium to right atrium. This indicates that the bypass tract is left sided since the left atrium is activated earlier than the right atrium (Fig. 16.27A).
- **Right-sided bypass tract:** If the P waves are upright in lead I, the direction of atrial activation is

from right atrium to left atrium. Because the right atrium is activated earlier than the left atrium, the bypass tract is right sided (Figs. 16.27B and 16.28).

- **Localizing the bypass tract:** In a patient with known Wolff-Parkinson-White (WPW) syndrome, rate-related bundle branch block may occasionally develop during narrow complex AVRT. If the rate of the tachycardia

**Figure 16.28:    Atrioventricular Reentrant Tachycardia (AVRT).    (A)** A 12-lead electrocardiogram during AVRT. The P waves are inverted in II, III, and aVF and upright in I and aVL (*arrows*). Retrograde P waves are also present in V$_3$ to V$_5$. The presence of upright P waves in I and aVL during AVRT suggests that atrial activation is from right to left consistent with a right sided bypass tract. Note that on conversion to normal sinus rhythm **(B)**, no evidence of pre-excitation is present. This type of AVRT is associated with a concealed bypass tract.

**A.** During Tachycardia

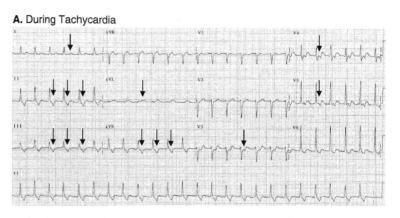

**B.** Normal Sinus Rhythm

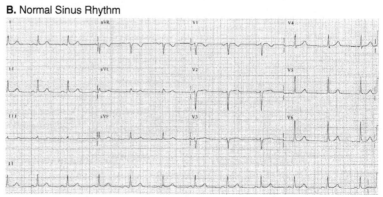

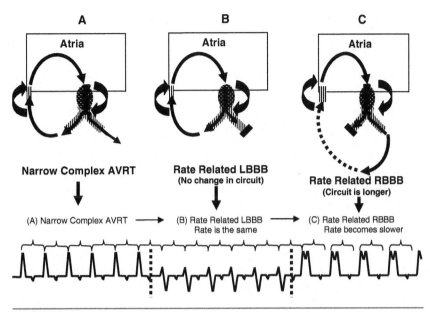

**Figure 16.29:   Localizing the Bypass Tract.** The diagrams explain how a rate-related bundle branch block will slow down the ventricular rate during AVRT if the bypass tract is on the same side as the bundle branch block. **(A)** Narrow complex AVRT with a right-sided bypass tract. **(B)** If a rate-related LBBB develops during tachycardia, the circuit is not altered by the bundle branch block and the rate of the tachycardia remains unchanged. **(C)** If a rate-related right bundle branch block occurs, the rate of the tachycardia will become slower if the bypass tract is right sided because the right ventricle and bypass tract have to be activated from the left bundle branch, resulting in a longer and slower circuit. AVRT, atrioventricular reentrant tachycardia; LBBB, left bundle branch block; RBBB, right bundle branch block.

becomes slower when the rate-related bundle branch block occurs, the bypass tract is on the same side as the bundle branch block. For example:

- **RBBB:** If a rate-related RBBB occurs during tachycardia and the ventricular rate becomes slower, the bypass tract is right sided (Fig. 16.29).
- **LBBB:** If a rate-related LBBB occurs and the ventricular rate becomes slower during the tachycardia, the bypass tract is left sided. Conversely, if the heart rate does not become slower, the bypass tract is at the opposite side.

## ECG Findings of Orthodromic AVRT

1. Orthodromic AVRT is a narrow complex tachycardia with regular R-R intervals.
2. The P waves and QRS complexes are inscribed separately because the atria and ventricles are part of the reentrant circuit.
3. The configuration of the retrograde P waves may be different, depending on the location of the bypass tract. The P waves are commonly inverted in leads II, III, and aVF because the atria are activated by the bypass tract from below upward.
4. In typical AVRT, the retrograde P wave may be inscribed at the ST segment or T wave of the previous complex, thus, the retrograde P wave is closer to the previous QRS complex

than the next QRS complex (R-P interval is shorter than the PR interval).
5. In atypical AVRT, the retrograde P waves are inscribed before the QRS complex and are closer to the next QRS complex than to the previous QRS complex (R-P interval longer than PR interval).
6. AV block is not possible during tachycardia. AVRT is excluded if AV block occurs.
7. Electrical alternans favors AVRT but does not exclude other types of SVT.

## Mechanism

- AVRT is a reentrant tachycardia associated with a bypass tract. The bypass tract connects the atrium directly to the ventricle and provides an alternate route by which the atrial impulse can conduct anterogradely to the ventricles and the ventricular impulse retrogradely to the atrium.
- The tachycardia is precipitated by an ectopic impulse originating from the atria or ventricles. The ectopic impulse should occur when one pathway (either the AV node or bypass tract) has fully recovered and the other pathway is still refractory.
- The tachycardia is very regular because the impulse follows a fixed pathway consisting of the AV node, bundle of His, a bundle branch, ventricle, bypass tract, and atrium. Second-degree

AV block is not possible since the AV node is an essential component of the reentrant circuit. If the impulse is blocked at the AV node, the reentrant circuit will terminate.

- The tachycardia may have wide or narrow complexes depending on how the ventricles are activated.

  - **Antidromic AVRT:** Antidromic AVRT is associated with wide QRS complexes. The QRS complex is wide because the atrial impulse activates the ventricles anterogradely through the bypass tract. Because the impulse is conducted outside the normal conduction system, the QRS complexes are wide measuring ≥0.12 seconds. Antidromic AVRT is a classic example of wide complex tachycardia due to SVT. This type of SVT can be mistaken for ventricular tachycardia. This is further discussed in Chapter 20, Wolff-Parkinson-White Syndrome.

  - **Orthodromic AVRT:** Orthodromic AVRT is associated with narrow QRS complexes. The QRS complex is narrow because the atrial impulse activates the ventricles anterogradely through the AV node. Because the ventricles are activated normally, the QRS complexes are narrow measuring <0.12 seconds. Orthodromic AVRT can be typical or atypical.

    - **Typical AVRT:** The P waves deform the ST segment or early portion of the T wave of the previous complex, thus the R-P interval is shorter than the PR interval. In typical AVRT, the AV node is the slow pathway and the bypass tract the fast pathway (slow/fast activation).

    - **Atypical AVRT:** The P waves precede the QRS complexes, thus, the R-P interval is longer than the PR interval. In atypical AVRT, the AV node is the fast pathway and the bypass tract the slow pathway (fast/slow activation). This type of AVRT is rare.

## Clinical Significance

- AVRT is the second most common SVT, occurring in approximately 30% of all reentrant SVT. It is another classic example of a tachycardia that is paroxysmal with abrupt onset and abrupt termination.

- The bypass tract may be capable of conducting only retrogradely (ventricle to atrium) but not anterogradely (atrium to ventricle). Such bypass tracts are called concealed bypass tracts. When the bypass tract is concealed, preexcitation (presence of short PR interval and delta wave) is not present in the 12-lead ECG during normal sinus rhythm. Patients with AVRT with preexcitation during normal sinus rhythm have manifest bypass tracts. These patients with preexcitation and symptoms of tachycardia have WPW syndrome.

- The location of the bypass tract can be diagnosed by the morphology of the P waves during SVT.

  - If the bypass tract is left sided, activation of the left atrium occurs earlier than the right atrium resulting in inverted P waves in lead I during the tachycardia.

  - If the bypass tract is right sided, the right atrium is activated before the left atrium, resulting in upright P waves in lead I during the tachycardia.

  - When a rate-related bundle branch block occurs and the rate of the tachycardia slows down, the bypass tract is on the same side as the bundle branch block. Thus, if rate-related RBBB occurs and the rate of the tachycardia is slower, the bypass tract is right sided. If LBBB occurs and the rate of the tachycardia is slower, the bypass tract is left sided.

- **Atypical AVRT:** Although AVRT is almost always precipitated by an ectopic impulse, there is a subset of atypical AVRT in which the tachycardia may occur spontaneously during an abrupt onset of sinus tachycardia—such as during exertion, excitement, or enhanced sympathetic activity. This type of SVT should be recognized because it is usually incessant (the tachycardia lasts more than 12 hours per day) and may result in tachycardia mediated cardiomyopathy. This type of tachycardia is also called permanent junctional reciprocating tachycardia or PJRT. The tachycardia is associated with a slowly conducting bypass tract; thus, the P waves are in front of the QRS complex with R-P interval longer than PR interval. The bypass tract is located at the posteroseptal area very close to the orifice of the coronary sinus and may be treated successfully with radiofrequency ablation. The tachycardia is usually poorly responsive to medical therapy.

- Because the retrograde P waves occur at the ST segment or T waves during tachycardia, contraction of the atria occurs during systole when the mitral and tricuspid valves are closed. This can cause cannon A waves, which are prominent jugular neck vein pulsations during tachycardia. The presence of cannon A waves in the neck during SVT suggests AVNRT or AVRT as the cause of the tachycardia.

## Acute Treatment

- The acute treatment of narrow complex AVRT is identical to that of AVNRT (see Treatment of AVNRT). Because AVRT is dependent on the AV node for perpetuation of the arrhythmia, treatment includes vagal maneuvers and pharmacologic agents that block the AV node. Similar to AVNRT, adenosine given intravenously is the drug of choice to terminate the tachycardia. The tachycardia ends with a retrograde P wave, meaning that the last part of the tachycardia to be recorded before the rhythm becomes sinus is a retrograde P wave. This implies that the tachycardia was blocked at the level of the AV node, regardless whether the AV node is a fast or slow pathway. Similar to adenosine, AV nodal blockers such as verapamil and diltiazem terminate the tachycardia at the level of the AV node causing a P wave to be inscribed last, before the rhythm converts to normal sinus.

- Although adenosine is the drug of choice among patients with paroxysmal SVT, adenosine can precipitate asthma and should not be given to patients with history of severe reactive airway disease. Some of these patients with asthma may

**A.** Diagrammatic Representation of SART

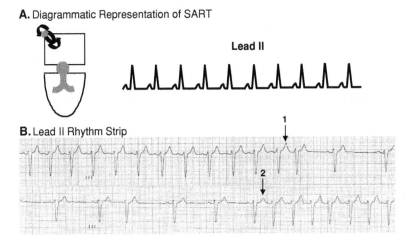

Lead II

**B.** Lead II Rhythm Strip

**Figure 16.30:   Sinoatrial Reentrant Tachycardia (SART). (A)** Diagrammatic representation of SART. Because the sinus node is part of the reentrant circuit, the P waves resemble sinus tachycardia and are upright in leads II, III, and aVF. **(B)** Continuous lead II rhythm strip of a patient thought to have SART. The SART can be terminated (*arrow 1*) or precipitated (*arrow 2*) by premature atrial complexes and is paroxysmal.

already be on theophylline, which is the antidote for adenosine. Adenosine is less effective for the treatment of SVT in patients who are already on theophylline.

- Adenosine can potentially cause atrial fibrillation in 1% to 10% of patients. This can result in potential lethal complication among patients with AVRT with manifest bypass tracts (preexcitation or WPW pattern is present in baseline ECG). Atrial fibrillation in these patients can result in very rapid ventricular responses, which can result in hemodynamic collapse. This complication should be anticipated when treating AVRT so that a defibrillator is available if needed.

## Prognosis

- The prognosis of patients with orthodromic AVRT with concealed bypass tracts (no evidence of preexcitation in baseline ECG) is good. Similar to AVNRT, the arrhythmia can be permanently cured with electrical ablation. Patients should be referred to a facility with extensive experience. Early referral should be done if the tachycardia is recurrent or the patient cannot tolerate medications.

- Patients with evidence of preexcitation during normal sinus rhythm may have a different prognosis (see Chapter 20, Wolff-Parkinson-White Syndrome). These patients may develop atrial fibrillation as a complication of the SVT and therefore can potentially develop arrhythmias that are more lethal. These patients with manifest bypass tracts and known WPW syndrome should be referred to an electrophysiologist for further evaluation.

## Other Types of SVT from Reentry

- There are two other types of SVT due to reentry: sinoatrial reentrant tachycardia (SART) and intra-atrial reentrant tachycardia (IART). These two types of reentrant SVT are relatively uncommon.

- **SART:** SART is a type of micro-reentrant tachycardia involving the sinus node and contiguous atrium. The tachycardia is difficult to differentiate from sinus tachycardia because the sinus node is part of the reentrant circuit. During tachycardia, the P waves are identical to sinus P waves (Figs. 16.30 and 16.31) and easily mistaken for sinus tachycardia.

- The tachycardia is usually precipitated and terminated by a premature atrial impulse and is therefore paroxysmal with an abrupt onset and abrupt termination (Fig. 16.30). This is in contrast to sinus tachycardia, which has a slow onset and gradual termination and is nonparoxysmal. SART can also be terminated by vagal maneuvers as well as agents that block the AV node because AV nodal blocking agents also inhibit the sinus node. This includes adenosine, beta blockers, calcium blockers, and digoxin.

- Figure 16.31A,B show the difficulty in making a diagnosis of SART. Except for the abrupt onset and termination, the tachycardia is identical and easily mistaken for sinus tachycardia.

## ECG Findings of SART

1. The ECG of SART is identical to that of sinus tachycardia. The P waves precede the QRS complexes and are upright in leads I, II, and aVF.

2. The tachycardia is paroxysmal with abrupt onset and termination.

3. It is usually precipitated and can be terminated by premature atrial complexes.

4. The atrial rate is usually not very rapid and is usually 120 to 150 bpm but can be <100 bpm.

## Mechanism

- SART is another example of microreentry. The reentrant SVT includes the sinus node and surrounding atrial tissue. Because the sinus node is part of the reentrant pathway, the

**Figure 16.31:    Twelve-lead Electrocardio-gram of Sinoatrial Reentrant Tachycardia (SART).  (A, B)** From the same patient. **(A)** A 12-ead electrocardiogram (ECG) during SART. **(B)** A 12-lead ECG immediately on conversion of the SART to normal sinus rhythm. Note that the P waves are virtually identical during tachycardia and during normal sinus rhythm. Most patients with SART are difficult to diagnose because the tachycardia is easily mistaken for sinus tachycardia.

**A.** During SART

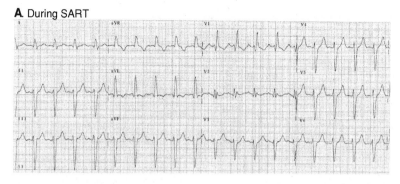

**B. During normal sinus rhythm**

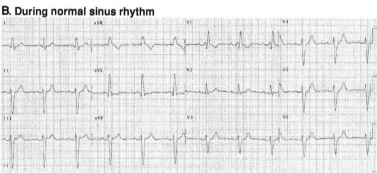

P waves during tachycardia resemble sinus P waves and may be difficult to differentiate from sinus tachycardia. Unlike sinus tachycardia, ectopic atrial impulses can terminate or precipitate SART. SART can also be precipitated or terminated by programmed electrical stimulation of the atrium similar to the other reentrant tachycardia and is paroxysmal with abrupt onset and abrupt termination. This is in contrast to sinus tachycardia, which is nonparoxysmal.

## Clinical Implications

- SART is uncommon, occurring in <5% of all reentrant SVT. SART is usually associated with structural cardiac disease.
- SART is difficult to differentiate from sinus tachycardia. Because SART involves the sinus node as part of the reentrant circuit, the morphology of the P waves resemble sinus tachycardia and are upright in leads I, II, and aVF.
- The tachycardia can cause symptoms of lightheadedness but usually not syncope because the atrial rate is usually <120 to 150 bpm, rarely exceeds 180 bpm and can be slower than 100 bpm. P waves precede each QRS complex; thus, atrial contribution to LV filling is preserved during tachycardia.

## Acute Treatment

- Appropriate therapy is usually not instituted early because the tachycardia is easily mistaken for sinus tachycardia, which is a physiologic response to a variety of clinical situations. Because the sinus node is part of the reentrant circuit, it can be terminated by vagal maneuvers such as carotid sinus stimulation. It can also be terminated by AV nodal blockers

including adenosine, beta blockers, calcium channel blockers, and digoxin because these agents also inhibit the sinus node.

- In symptomatic patients, long-term therapy is usually effective in preventing recurrences. This may include oral beta blockers, nondihydropyridine calcium channel blockers such as diltiazem and verapamil, and digoxin.
- Sinus node modification using radiofrequency ablation is often useful if the tachycardia is intractable to medications.

## Prognosis

- SART is usually well tolerated and therapy is given primarily to improve symptoms and prevent recurrence of the tachycardia. Because SART is associated with structural cardiac disease, prognosis will depend primarily on the underlying cardiac condition.

## IART

- **Intraatrial Reentrant Tachycardia:** IART is another SVT due to reentry. The electrical circuit is confined to a small area in the atrium and therefore is a form of micro-reentry (Fig. 16.32). The reentrant circuit may be larger if it circles around a scar tissue or around a healed surgical incision such as a previous atrial septal defect repair.
- The tachycardia starts from a focal area and spreads circumferentially to activate the whole atria. The morphology of the P wave will depend on the origin of the tachycardia; thus, the P wave may be upright, inverted,

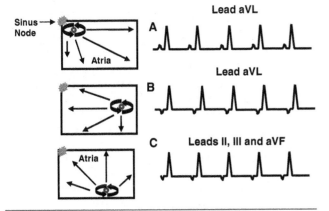

**Figure 16.32: Intraatrial Reentrant Tachycardia (IART).** In IART, a micro-reentrant circuit is present in the atrium, which spreads circumferentially to activate the whole atria. IART is therefore included as an example of focal atrial tachycardia. The morphology of the P wave will depend on the origin of the tachycardia. **(A)** The P waves are upright or biphasic in lead aVL because the reentrant circuit originates from the right atrium close to the sinus node. **(B)** The P waves are inverted in lead aVL because the impulse originates from the left atrium. **(C)** The P waves are inverted in lead II, III, and aVF because the tachycardia originates from the bottom of the atria (see also Figs. 13.6 and 13.7).

or biphasic in lead II. Because the tachycardia originates from the atria, the P waves are inscribed before the QRS complexes with a PR interval ≥0.12 seconds.

■ Atrial tachycardia from IART is difficult to distinguish from atrial tachycardia resulting from enhanced or triggered automaticity using the surface ECG. Because these tachycardias all look alike electrocardiographically, they are all included as examples of focal atrial tachycardia regardless of the mechanism and will be further discussed in Chapter 17, Supraventricular Tachycardia due to Altered Automaticity.

## ECG Findings of IART

1. The P waves are uniform in configuration and precede each QRS complex with a rate of 110 to 200 bpm.

2. The configuration of the P waves depends on the origin of the tachycardia and may be upright, biphasic or inverted in leads II, III, or aVF.

3. The atrial impulse is conducted to the ventricles through the normal AV conduction system; thus, the PR interval is usually ≥0.12 seconds. Because the tachycardia is not dependent on the AV node, AV block can occur.

## Mechanism

■ IART is another example of microreentry within the atria. The reentrant circuit may be confined to a small area in the atrium because of inflammation, scarring, or previous sur-

gery. The impulse spreads circumferentially until the whole atria are activated. The P waves are uniform in configuration since the impulse originates from a focal area in the atria. The P waves precede each QRS complex with PR interval shorter than R-P interval.

## Clinical Significance, Treatment, and Prognosis

■ Although IART is an example of reentrant tachycardia, the ECG findings cannot be differentiated from other types of atrial tachycardia because of enhanced or triggered automaticity. Thus IART is included as an example of focal atrial tachycardia. The clinical significance, treatment, and prognosis of focal atrial tachycardia will be further discussed in Chpater 17, Supraventricular Tachycardia due to Altered Automaticity, under Focal Atrial Tachycardia.

## Suggested Readings

2005 American Heart Association Guidelines for Cardiopulmonary Resuscitation and Emergency Cardiovascular Care: part 7.3: management of symptomatic bradycardia and tachycardia. *Circulation.* 2005;112:67–77.

Bar FW, Brugada P, Dassen WRM, et al. Differential diagnosis of tachycardia with narrow QRS complex (shorter than 0.12 second). *Am J Cardiol.* 1984;54:555–560.

Blomstrom-Lundqvist C, Scheinman MM, Aliot EM, et al. ACC/AHA/ESC guidelines for the management of patients with supraventricular arrhythmias—executive summary: a report of the American College of Cardiology/American Heart Association Task Force on Practice Guidelines, and the European Society of Cardiology Committee for Practice Guidelines (Writing Committee to Develop Guidelines for the Management of Patients With Supraventricular Arrhythmias). *J Am Coll Cardiol.* 2003;42:1493–531.

Botteron GW, Smith JM. Cardiac arrhythmias. In: Carey CF, Lee HH, Woeltje KF, eds. *Washington Manual of Medical Therapeutics.* 29th ed. Philadelphia: Lippincott; 1998:130–156.

Chauhan VS, Krahn AD, Klein GJ, et al. Supraventricular tachycardia. *Med Clin N Am.* 2001;85:193–223.

Dresing TJ, Schweikert RA, Packer DL. Atrioventricular nodal-dependent tachycardias. In: Topol EJ, ed. *Textbook of Cardiovascular Medicine.* 2nd ed. Philadelphia: Lippincott; 2002:1453–1478.

Engelstein ED, Lippman N, Stein KM, et al. Mechanism-specific effects of adenosine on atrial tachycardia. *Circulation.* 1994; 89:2645–2654.

Esberger D, Jones S, Morris F. ABC of clinical electrocardiography: junctional tachycardias. *BMJ.* 2002;324:662–665.

Ganz LI, Friedman PL. Supraventricular tachycardia. *N Engl J Med.* 1995;332:162–173.

Guidelines 2000 for Cardiopulmonary Resuscitation and Emergency Cardiovascular Care: 7D: the tachycardia algorithms. *Circulation.* 2000;102(suppl I):I-158–I-165.

Kay GN, Pressley JC, Packer DL, et al. Value of the 12-lead electrocardiogram in discriminating atrioventricular nodal reciprocating tachycardia from circus movement atrioventricular tachycardia utilizing a retrograde accessory pathway. *Am J Cardiol.* 1987;59:296–300.

Manolis AS, Mark Estes III NA. Supraventricular tachycardia mechanisms and therapy. *Arch Intern Med.* 1987;147:1706–1716.

Olgen JE, Zipes DE. Specific arrhythmias: diagnosis and treatment. In: Libby P, Bonow RO, Mann DL, et al. eds. *Braunwald's Heart Disease, A Textbook of Cardiovascular Medicine.* 7th ed. Philadelphia: Elsevier Saunders; 2005:803–863.

Saoudi N, Cosio F, Waldo A, et al. Classification of atrial flutter and regular atrial tachycardia according to electrophysiological mechanisms and anatomical bases. *Eur Heart J.* 2001;22:1162–1182.

Sinai Policies and Procedures on Intravenous Medications. LBH-Web at Sinai Hospital. Belvedere Avenue, Greenspring, Baltimore, MD: Sinai Policy and Procedures; January 15, 2003.

Wagner GS. Reentrant junctional tachyarrhythmias. In: *Marriott's Practical Electrocardiography.* 10th ed. Philadelphia: Lippincott; 2001:328–344.

Waldo AL, Biblo LA. Atrioventricular nodal-independent supraventricular tachycardias. In: Topol EJ, ed. *Textbook of Cardiovascular Medicine.* 2nd ed. Philadelphia: Lippincott; 2002:1453–1478.

Waxman MB, Wald RW, Sharma AD, et al. Vagal techniques for termination of paroxysmal supraventricular tachycardia. *Am J Cardiol.* 1980;46:655–664.

Wellens HJJ, Conover MB. Narrow QRS tachycardia. In: *The ECG in Emergency Decision Making.* 2nd ed. St. Louis: Saunders/Elsevier; 2006:92–126.

Xie B, Thakur RK, Shah CP, et al. Clinical differentiation of narrow QRS complex tachycardias. In: Thakur RK, Reisdorff EJ, eds. Emergency Medicine Clinics of North America. Emergency Management of Cardiac Arrhythmias. 1998:295–330.

Webb JG, Kerr CR. Paroxysmal supraventricular tachycardia and bundle branch block. *Arch Intern Med.* 1987;147:367–369.

# Supraventricular Tachycardia due to Altered Automaticity

## Introduction

- Other mechanisms by which supraventricular tachycardia (SVT) can occur include enhanced automaticity and triggered activity.

- **SVT from enhanced automaticity:** Unlike reentrant SVT, which is dependent on the presence of a reentrant circuit, SVT from enhanced automaticity is dependent on cells with automatic properties. Cells with pacemaking properties exhibit diastolic depolarization characterized by a slowly rising slope during phase 4 of the action potential. Once threshold potential is reached, the cells discharge automatically. This is in contrast to non-pacemaking cells, in which phase 4 is flat and therefore the resting potential never reaches threshold (Fig. 17.1A, B).

- Examples of cells with automatic properties are cells within the sinus node, atrioventricular (AV) junction, and throughout the AV conduction system except the midportion of the AV node. Although the cells of the AV conduction system have automatic properties and are capable of discharging spontaneously, their rate of discharge is slower than that of the sinus node. These cells therefore are depolarized

by the propagated sinus impulse and serve as backup or latent pacemakers.

- Ordinary working myocytes in the atria and ventricles do not exhibit phase 4 diastolic depolarization, but may develop this property when they become pathologic, as would occur during ischemia or injury.

- The following types of SVT are due to enhanced automaticity (see Figure 17.2):

  - **Pathologic sinus tachycardia:** This tachycardia is due to enhanced automaticity of the sinus node cells and may be clinically difficult to differentiate from physiologic sinus tachycardia (Fig. 17.2A).

  - **Atrial tachycardia:** The atria, including the atrial appendage, large veins draining into the atria (pulmonary veins, vena cava, and coronary sinus) or even the mitral or tricuspid annulus, may contain cells with properties of automaticity. The rate of discharge of these cells may be enhanced, resulting in atrial tachycardia. The tachycardia may be unifocal or focal (Fig. 17.2B) or it may be multifocal (Fig. 17.2C).

    - ☐ **Focal atrial tachycardia:** The tachycardia originates from a single focus in the atria or from a venous connection contiguous to the atria such as the pulmonary veins or vena cava.

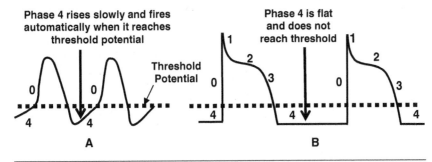

**Figure 17.1:   Pacemaking and Non-pacemaking Cell. (A)** Action potential of pacemaking cells. Pacemaking cells exhibit slow diastolic depolarization during phase 4 and discharge automatically when phase 4 reaches threshold potential. **(B)** Action potential of non-pacemaking cells. In non-pacemaking cells, phase 4 is flat and the action potential never reaches threshold. The numbers 0, 1, 2, 3, and 4 represent the different phases of the transmembrane action potential.

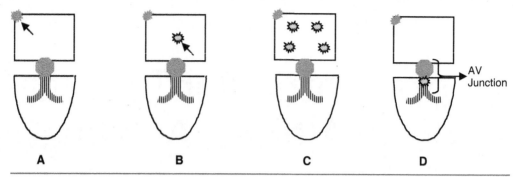

**Figure 17.2:    Automatic Supraventricular Tachycardia (SVT).** Automatic SVT can occur anywhere in the atria or atrioventricular junction. **(A)** Pathologic or inappropriate sinus tachycardia. **(B)** Focal atrial tachycardia arising from a single focus in the atria. **(C)** Multifocal atria tachycardia showing multiple foci in the atria. **(D)** Junctional tachycardia, which can be paroxysmal or nonparoxysmal.

- ☐ **Multifocal atrial tachycardia:** The tachycardia is multifocal if several ectopic foci are present in the atria.
- ■ **AV junctional tachycardia:** The tachycardia arises from the AV junction, which includes the AV node down to the bifurcation of the bundle of His (Fig. 17.2D). Junctional tachycardia can be paroxysmal or nonparoxysmal.
  - ☐ **Nonparoxysmal junctional tachycardia:** The tachycardia arises from a focus in the AV junction and has a relatively slow rate of 70 to 120 beats per minute (bpm).
  - ☐ **Paroxysmal junctional tachycardia:** The tachycardia is paroxysmal because it starts abruptly and terminates suddenly. The tachycardia has a faster rate varying from 120 to 180 bpm.

## Focal Atrial Tachycardia

- ■ **Focal atrial tachycardia:** Focal atrial tachycardia implies that the tachycardia arises from a single location in the atria. The atrial impulse spreads in a circumferential manner regardless of the mechanism of the tachycardia. Thus, the tachycardia may be due to enhanced automaticity (automatic atrial tachycardia), intra-atrial micro-reentry (intraatrial reentrant tachycardia), or triggered automaticity (atrial tachycardia with 2:1 AV block). The mechanisms underlying these tachycardias cannot be differentiated from one another with a 12-lead electrocardiogram (ECG). Because these tachycardias all look similar, any tachycardia originating from a single focus in the atria that spreads circumferentially is focal atrial tachycardia (Figure 17.3).
- ■ The ECG findings of focal atrial tachycardia include the following:

- ■ Presence of a regular narrow complex tachycardia >100 bpm.
- ■ Ectopic P waves, which are different from sinus P waves, precede the QRS complexes usually with a PR interval ≥0.12 seconds.
- ■ The P waves are uniform and the atrial rate varies to as high as 250 bpm. The baseline between the P waves is usually flat or isoelectric and not wavy or undulating as in atrial flutter.
- ■ Second-degree or higher grades of AV block may occur because the tachycardia is not dependent on the AV node.
- ■ The tachycardia terminates with a QRS complex in contrast to reentrant SVT (atrioventricular nodal reentrant tachycardia [AVNRT] and atrioventricular reentrant tachycardia [AVRT]), which usually terminates with a retrograde P wave (Fig. 17.4).
- ■ Although nonsustained focal atrial tachycardia is frequently seen during cardiac monitoring in the coronary or intensive care units, sustained focal atrial tachycardia is rare, occurring in <0.5% of symptomatic patients. The sustained form is slightly more common in children than in adults but is also a rare clinical entity. The tachycardia can be incessant (persists more than 12 hours per day), which can result in tachycardia-mediated cardiomyopathy.
- ■ Focal atrial discharges do not occur randomly. They frequently cluster in certain areas in the atria such as the mitral or tricuspid annulus, atrial appendages, ostium of the coronary sinus, and along the crista terminalis. Spontaneous focal discharges from the pulmonary veins are too small to be recorded in the surface ECG, but have been recorded by intracardiac techniques. These focal discharges can result in SVT and have also been implicated as an important cause of atrial fibrillation.

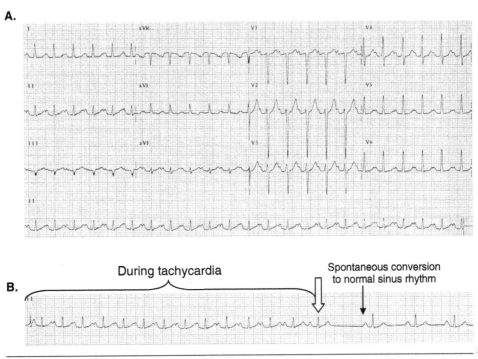

**Figure 17.3:    Focal Atrial Tachycardia. (A)** A 12-lead electrocardiogram showing focal atrial tachycardia with a rate of 136 beats per minute. The P waves are uniform in configuration and are upright in I, II, III, aVF, and $V_1$. The tachycardia can be mistaken for sinus tachycardia. **(B)** Lead II rhythm strip showing spontaneous conversion of the tachycardia to normal sinus rhythm. Note that the P wave morphology is different during tachycardia and during normal sinus rhythm. Note also that the tachycardia terminated with a QRS complex (*block arrow*) rather than a retrograde P wave, suggesting that the SVT is due to focal atrial tachycardia.

- **Localizing the origin of the tachycardia:** In focal atrial tachycardia, the origin of the tachycardia may be localized by the morphology of the P waves. The most useful lead is $V_1$ followed by lead aVL (see Fig. 17.5).

  - **Right atrial vs left atrial origin:**

    □ **Right atrial origin:** If the tachycardia is of right atrial origin, the P waves are inverted in $V_1$. If biphasic in $V_1$, the P waves are initially positive

(upright) and terminally negative (inverted). In lead aVL, the P waves are upright or biphasic (Fig. 17.5A).

    □ **Left atrial origin:** If the tachycardia is left atrial in origin, the P waves are upright in $V_1$. If $V_1$ is biphasic, the P waves are initially negative (inverted) and terminally positive (upright). In aVL, the P waves are negative or isoelectric (flat) (Fig. 17.5B).

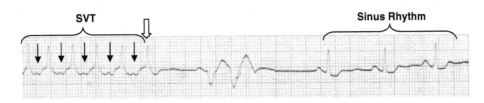

**Figure 17.4:    Focal Atrial Tachycardia.** The rhythm strip was recorded in lead II. The left side of the rhythm strip shows focal atrial tachycardia with P waves between QRS complexes (*arrows*). The tachycardia terminated spontaneously followed by a sinus P wave and back to back ventricular complexes. Normal sinus rhythm followed as shown on the right side of the tracing. Note that the tachycardia terminated with a ventricular complex (*block arrow*) rather than a P wave. SVT terminating with a QRS complex is usually from focal atrial tachycardia. This type of SVT may not respond to adenosine.

**Figure 17.5: Focal Atrial Tachycardia.** The origin of the tachycardia can be identified as right atrial or left atrial based on the configuration of the P waves in leads $V_1$ and aVL. If the ectopic focus is in the right atrium **(A)**, the P waves are inverted in $V_1$ or if biphasic are initially upright and terminally negative. In lead aVL, the P waves are upright or biphasic. If the ectopic focus is in the left atrium **(B)**, the P waves are positive in $V_1$. If biphasic, the P waves are initially inverted and terminally upright. In lead aVL, the P waves are isoelectric (*flat*) or inverted. AV, atrioventricular; RA, right atrium; LA, left atrium.

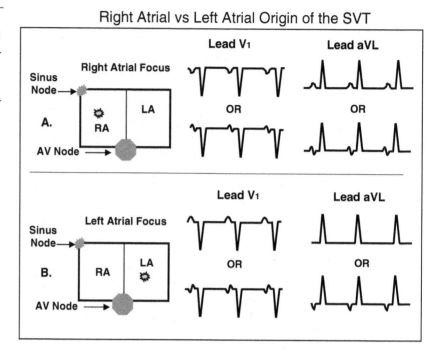

Right Atrial vs Left Atrial Origin of the SVT

## ■ Localizing the tachycardia:

### ▥ Superior versus inferior origin:

□ **Superior origin:** If the tachycardia originates superiorly in either right or left atria, the P waves are upright in II, III, and aVF. Superior origin of the atrial tachycardia includes the atrial appendages and superior pulmonary veins (Fig. 17.6A). The tachycardia may be difficult to differentiate from sinus tachycardia.

□ **Inferior origin:** If the tachycardia originates inferiorly in either right or left atria, the P waves are inverted in leads II, III, and aVF. Inferior origin of the atrial tachycardia includes the inferior vena cava and coronary sinus orifice as well as the inferior pulmonary veins (Fig. 17.6B).

▥ Examples of focal atrial tachycardia are shown in Figs. 17.7 to 17.10.

## ECG Findings of Focal Atrial Tachycardia

1. Presence of a regular narrow complex tachycardia >100 bpm.

2. The P waves are uniform in configuration but are different in morphology when compared with P waves of normal sinus origin.

3. The P waves precede the QRS complexes with a PR interval shorter than the R-P interval. This finding, however, may be reversed depending on the integrity of the AV node and presence of AV conduction abnormality. The PR interval generally measures ≥0.12 seconds.

4. Second degree or higher grades of AV block may occur because the tachycardia is not dependent on the AV node.

5. The baseline between 2 P waves is isoelectric unlike atrial flutter where the baseline is wavy and undulating.

6. The tachycardia terminates with a QRS complex rather than a P wave.

**Figure 17.6: Focal Atrial Tachycardia.** If the P waves are upright in II, III and aVF, the origin of the tachycardia is in the superior right or left atria **(A)**. If the P waves are inverted in II, III, and aVF, the origin of the tachycardia is in the inferior right or left atria **(B)**.

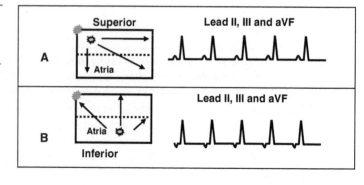

## Mechanism

- Focal atrial tachycardia is a type of SVT originating from a single focus in the atria. The impulse spreads to the atria in a circumferential manner. The mechanism of the tachycardia may be due to intraatrial reentry, enhanced automaticity, or triggered activity. These mechanisms are impossible to differentiate using the 12-lead ECG. Focal atrial tachycardia do not occur at random but originate more commonly in the right atrium as well as veins that drain directly into the atria such as the pulmonary veins, vena cava, and coronary sinus. They can also originate from the atrial appendages, mitral or tricuspid annulus, left side of the atrial septum, and crista terminalis.

- The P waves are uniform in configuration because the tachycardia originates from a single focus. The PR interval is usually ≥0.12 seconds in duration because the impulse has to travel within the atria and across the AV node before reaching the ventricles. The configuration of the P waves is different from P waves of normal sinus rhythm and is helpful in identifying the origin of the tachycardia.

  - When the tachycardia originates from the right atrium, the P waves are inverted in $V_1$. If biphasic, the P wave is initially upright and terminally inverted. The P waves are upright in lead aVL or it may be biphasic. Right atrial origin of the tachycardia includes the crista terminalis, tricuspid annulus, ostium of the coronary sinus, and right atrial appendage.

  - When the tachycardia originates from the left atrium, the P waves are upright in $V_1$. If biphasic, the P wave is initially inverted and terminally upright. The P waves are isoelectric (flat) or negative (inverted) in lead aVL. Left atrial tachycardia includes the pulmonary veins, mitral annulus, left side of the atrial septum, and left atrial appendage.

  - When the tachycardia originates inferiorly from either atria, the P waves are inverted in leads II, III, and aVF.

  - When the tachycardia originates superiorly from either atria, the P waves are upright in leads II, III, and aVF.

- The PR as well as the R-R interval may vary during the tachycardia, especially if the SVT is due to enhanced automaticity. This is in contrast to reentrant SVT, where these intervals are usually fixed and regular because the reentrant SVT follows a fixed pathway.

## Clinical Implications

- Nonsustained or short episodes of focal atrial tachycardia occur very frequently during monitoring. Sustained focal atrial tachycardia however is uncommon, occurring in <0.5% of symptomatic patients.

- Focal atrial tachycardia can be incessant (persists for more than 12 hours per day). This can result in tachycardia-mediated cardiomyopathy, which is more common in infants and young children because they are unable to communicate their symptoms when having the tachycardia. Although tachycardia-mediated cardiomyopathy from focal atrial tachycardia is not common, it is one of the few causes of dilated cardiomyopathies that can be reversed if the arrhythmia is identified and successfully treated.

- If the tachycardia originates from the right atrium close to the sinus node, or in the right superior pulmonary vein, the tachycardia may be mistaken for sinus tachycardia. Atrial tachycardia with 2:1 AV block can be mistaken for atrial flutter with 2:1 AV block. In atrial tachycardia with block, the baseline between 2 P waves is isoelectric, unlike atrial flutter where the baseline between 2 flutter waves is wavy and undulating. The treatment for these different arrhythmias is not the same.

- Focal atrial tachycardia can also be mistaken for atypical AVRT, atypical AVNRT, and junctional tachycardia. All these arrhythmias have P waves preceding the QRS complex with a shorter PR than R-P interval. In general, atypical AVRT and atypical AVNRT may be terminated with vagal maneuvers or with AV nodal blockers. When AVNRT or AVRT terminates, the last part of the tachycardia is a retrograde P wave. In focal atrial tachycardia, the SVT terminates with a QRS complex. This type of tachycardia should be recognized because this may not respond to adenosine.

- The size of the P wave may also be useful in identifying a retrograde P wave originating from the AV node. Because the AV node is in the lower mid-atria, the retrograde P waves may be narrow in AVNRT and in AV junctional tachycardia since both atria are activated simultaneously, whereas the P waves from focal atrial tachycardia or AVRT are broader.

- Focal atrial tachycardia may be due to acute myocarditis, chronic cardiomyopathy, or a local pathology in the atria such as an atrial tumor. It can also occur spontaneously in muscle sleeves of veins directly draining into the atria such as the pulmonary veins, vena cava, and coronary sinus. These cells may possess automatic properties similar to that of the sinus node and become the dominant pacemakers of the heart when their firing rate is enhanced. Focal atrial tachycardia can be due to pharmacologic agents such as dobutamine and other catecholamines, theophylline, caffeine, and nicotine. When focal atrial tachycardia is due to digitalis toxicity, the tachycardia is usually associated with 2:1 AV block.

- The atrial impulse is conducted to the ventricles through the normal AV conduction system. AV block can occur because the tachycardia is not dependent on the AV node. Vagal maneuvers and AV nodal blockers (adenosine, beta blocker, calcium channel blockers, and digitalis) can slow down the ventricular rate by causing AV block, but may not terminate the arrhythmia. However, if the mechanism of the SVT is due to micro-reentry or triggered activity, the tachycardia may be responsive to adenosine or verapamil.

## Acute Treatment

- If the tachycardia is due to digitalis toxicity, digitalis should be discontinued. Digitalis toxicity is enhanced by hypokalemia, hypomagnesemia, and hypercalcemia. These electrolyte abnormalities should be corrected. Potassium supplements are usually given to minimize the effects of digitalis toxicity. The use of digoxin binding agents should be considered if the arrhythmia is persistent and is poorly tolerated.

■ Tachycardia is also precipitated by metabolic and blood gas disorders or use of pharmacologic agents such as theophylline, albuterol, or catecholamines. These metabolic and respiratory abnormalities should be corrected and the offending agents should be discontinued.

■ Because focal atrial tachycardia is a regular narrow complex tachycardia, the tachycardia is difficult to distinguish from atypical AVNRT and atypical AVRT. Thus, the acute treatment for the tachycardia is similar to any regular narrow complex SVT. These include vagal maneuvers, AV nodal blockers such as adenosine, beta blocker, calcium channel blockers, and digitalis (if digitalis is not the cause of the tachycardia). A significant number of focal atrial tachycardia (atrial tachycardia due to microreentry or triggered activity) may respond to adenosine or verapamil. Thus, adenosine remains the drug of choice for any regular narrow complex tachycardia and should be tried before other agents are considered. If the tachycardia is not responsive to adenosine or AV block occurs without converting the SVT to normal sinus rhythm, longer acting AV nodal agents such as diltiazem, verapamil, or beta blockers can be given to slow down the ventricular rate by causing AV block.

■ Focal atrial tachycardia from enhanced automaticity generally will not respond to adenosine. Class IA (procainamide), Class IC (flecainide and propafenone), or Class III (sotalol, amiodarone) antiarrhythmic agents should be considered if adenosine and other AV nodal blocking agents are not effective.

■ Electrical cardioversion is not effective when the mechanism of the tachycardia is due to enhanced automaticity but may be effective if the tachycardia is due to intra-atrial reentry or triggered activity. Unless patient is in circulatory shock, electrical cardioversion is contraindicated when the tachycardia is known to be due to digitalis toxicity (atrial tachycardia with 2:1 AV block with history of digitalis intake) or the tachycardia is due to metabolic or electrolyte abnormalities.

■ When the tachycardia is intractable to medical therapy, electrical ablation (or if not feasible, surgical excision) of the arrhythmogenic focus should be considered.

## Prognosis

■ In infants and young children, in whom the tachycardia is more difficult to detect, the mortality is high because a tachycardia-mediated cardiomyopathy may occur. This type of cardiomyopathy is reversible if the tachycardia is recognized as the cause of the cardiomyopathy.

■ Focal atrial tachycardia is usually associated with structural cardiac diseases. The prognosis will depend on the etiology of the cardiac abnormality. The overall prognosis of focal atrial tachycardia from digitalis excess and metabolic, respiratory, or electrolyte abnormalities will depend on the underlying condition. In the absence of structural cardiac disease, the overall prognosis is generally good.

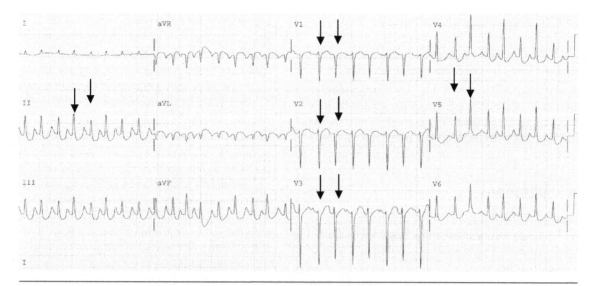

**Figure 17.7: Focal Atrial Tachycardia.** The electrocardiogram is from a patient with acute exacerbation of asthma. The P waves are inverted in aVL and are upright in leads II, III, and aVF suggesting a superior left atrial origin of the impulse. Electrical alternans is seen in leads II and in all precordial leads (*arrows*). Although electrical alternans is frequently associated with AVRT, it is also seen in other types of supraventricular tachycardia as shown here. AVRT, atrioventricular reentrant tachycardia.

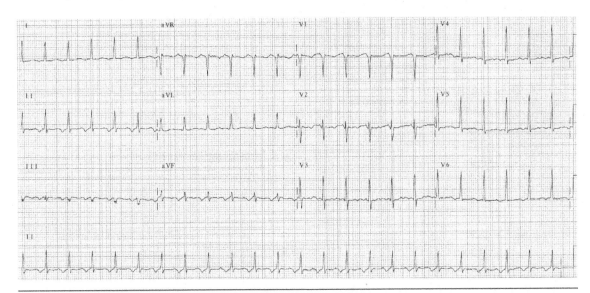

**Figure 17.8:    Focal Atrial Tachycardia.** The P waves are inverted in leads II, III, and aVF and upright in V$_1$. The PR interval is >0.12 seconds and the R-P interval is longer than the PR interval. This type of SVT is usually due to focal atrial tachycardia originating from the inferior wall of the left atrium. The above SVT, however, is difficult to differentiate from atypical AVNRT, atypical AVRT, or junctional tachycardia. Because the P waves are broad, the SVT is more likely the result of focal atrial tachycardia or AVRT rather than AVNRT or junctional tachycardia. SVT, supraventricular tachycardia; AVNRT, atrioventricular nodal reentrant tachycardia; AVRT, atrioventricular reentrant tachycardia.

Focal Atrial Tachycardia

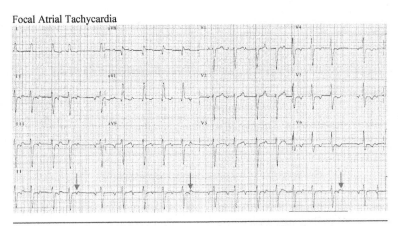

**Figure 17.9:    Focal Atrial Tachycardia with Second-Degree Atrioventricular (AV) Block.** The P waves precede the QRS complexes and are inverted in leads II, III, and aVF, negative in aVL, and upright in V$_1$. There is gradual prolongation of the PR interval until a ventricular complex is dropped (*arrows*). Because second-degree AV block is present, AVRT is not possible and AVNRT is highly unlikely. AVNRT, atrioventricular nodal reentrant tachycardia; AVRT, atrioventricular reentrant tachycardia.

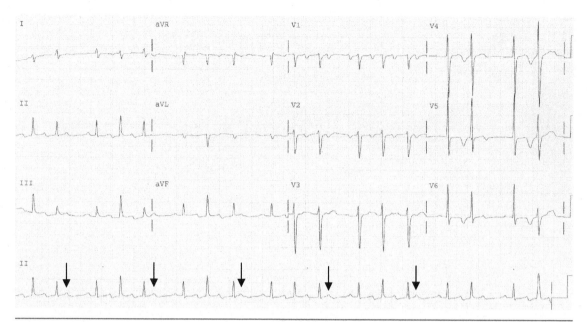

**Figure 17.10:** **Focal Atrial Tachycardia with Second-Degree Atrioventricular (AV) Block.** A 12-lead electrocardiogram showing focal atrial tachycardia with second-degree AV Wenckebach. The P waves precede the QRS complexes with a rate of 150 beats per minute. The mechanism of the focal atrial tachycardia was thought to be IART because the patient had previous atrial septal defect repair, which is a possible focus of reentry. The patient was successfully cardioverted electrically to normal sinus rhythm. Focal atrial tachycardia from enhanced automaticity generally does not respond to electrical cardioversion. The presence of AV block excludes AVRT and upright P waves in II, III, and aVF makes AVNRT unlikely. AVNRT, atrioventricular nodal reentrant tachycardia; AVRT, atrioventricular reentrant tachycardia; IART, intraatrial reentrant tachycardia. Arrows point to the nonconducted P waves.

## Multifocal Atrial Tachycardia

- **Multifocal atrial tachycardia (MAT):** MAT is characterized by the presence of atrial complexes originating from different foci in the atria. The P waves are irregular with varying sizes and shapes and varying PR and R-R intervals (Figs. 17.11–17.14). Because the R-R intervals are irregular, the arrhythmia can be mistaken for atrial fibrillation.

- The diagnosis of MAT is based on the presence of three or more consecutive P waves of different morphologies with an isoelectric baseline between P waves with a rate >100 bpm.

- Typical examples of MAT are shown in Figures 17.12 to 17.14.

### ECG Findings of MAT

1. At least three consecutive P waves with different morphologies with a rate >100 bpm should be present.
2. The PR as well as the R-R interval is variable with isoelectric baseline between P waves.

### Mechanism

- MAT is most probably due to enhanced automaticity. Multiple independent automatic foci are present in the atria, resulting in varying configurations of the P wave.

**Figure 17.11:** **Multifocal Atrial Tachycardia (MAT).** Diagrammatic representation of MAT showing at least three consecutive P waves of different sizes and shapes with a rate >100 beats per minute.

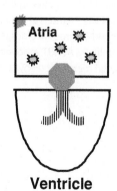

**Multifocal atrial tachycardia (MAT).**

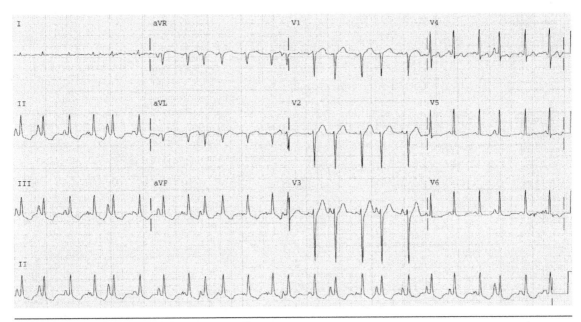

**Figure 17.12:   Multifocal Atrial Tachycardia (MAT).** The electrocardiogram shows MAT. For MAT to be present, three consecutive P waves of varying morphologies should be present with a rate >100 beats per minute. The rate is irregular, the PR intervals are variable, and the baseline between two P waves is isoelectric.

## Clinical Implications

■ MAT is also called chaotic atrial tachycardia. When the rate is <100 bpm, the arrhythmia is often called chaotic atrial rhythm or multifocal atrial rhythm. Because of the irregular heart rate, the tachycardia is often mistaken for atrial fibrillation.

■ MAT is commonly seen in elderly patients with acute exacerbations of chronic obstructive pulmonary disease (COPD) as well as those with electrolyte or metabolic abnormalities and pulmonary infection. Most of these patients with acute exacerbations of COPD are on theophylline or beta agonists. These medications are implicated as the cause of the MAT.

## Acute Treatment

■ Treatment of the tachycardia is directed toward the underlying cause, which is usually COPD. If the patient is on theophylline or beta agonist, the drug should be discontinued.

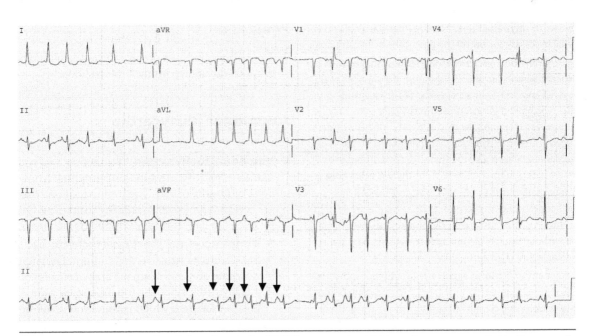

**Figure 17.13:   Multifocal Atrial Tachycardia (MAT).** In MAT, the QRS complexes are preceded by P waves of varying sizes and shapes. At least three consecutive P waves with varying morphologies are present with a rate over 100 beats per minute (*arrows*).

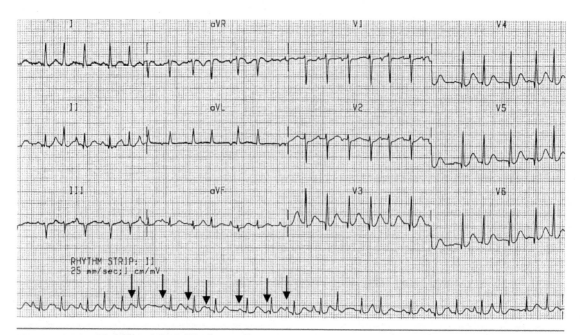

**Figure 17.14: Multifocal Atrial Tachycardia.** Note the presence of P waves of varying morphologies preceding each QRS complex (*arrows*) in the long lead rhythm strip at the bottom of the tracing. The baseline between P waves remains isoelectric.

Any electrolyte, blood gas, or metabolic abnormality should be corrected. Any associated cardiac disease or pulmonary infection should be treated.

■ MAT should be differentiated from atrial fibrillation. Patients with atrial fibrillation need to be anticoagulated, whereas patients with MAT do not need anticoagulation.

■ The rate of the tachycardia is usually not rapid and usually does not exceed 130 bpm. However, because MAT occurs more frequently in elderly individuals with COPD, the rate may not be tolerable especially when there is heart failure, ischemic heart disease, or respiratory insufficiency. Pharmacologic therapy may be necessary to control the rate of the tachycardia.

■ Nondihydropyridine calcium channel blockers may be used to control the ventricular rate and diminish the number of ectopic atrial impulses. Diltiazem (20 mg IV) or verapamil (5 to 10 mg IV) may be given intravenously. Diltiazem may be continued as an IV infusion drip at 5 to 15 mg per hour after the rate has been controlled with the initial bolus. Verapamil should not be given if there is left ventricular dysfunction (ejection fraction ≤40%) or there is heart failure.

■ Although beta blockers are also effective, these drugs are usually contraindicated because MAT is frequently seen in the setting of bronchospastic pulmonary disease. In patients without reactive airway disease, beta blockers are effective agents.

■ Although antiarrhythmic agents are usually not indicated for MAT, amiodarone may be tried for rate control and for suppression of ectopic atrial impulses if the arrhythmia has not improved with the above agents. Magnesium given intravenously has also been used with varying success when other agents have failed even in the absence of hypomagnesemia.

■ Digitalis is not effective and has a narrow margin of safety in patients with chronic pulmonary disease and should not be given.

■ MAT frequently deteriorates to atrial fibrillation. The rate in atrial fibrillation may be easier to control than the rate in MAT; however, anticoagulation may be necessary.

■ Electrical cardioversion has no place in the therapy of MAT. MAT is an example of SVT from enhanced automaticity and electrical cardioversion will not be effective.

## Prognosis

■ The arrhythmia is usually well tolerated and prognosis depends on the underlying medical condition.

## Junctional Tachycardia

■ **Junctional tachycardia:** AV junctional tachycardia is due to repetitive impulses originating from the AV node or bundle of His. The impulse follows the normal AV conduction system resulting in narrow QRS complexes. There are two types of junctional tachycardia:

■ **Nonparoxysmal junctional tachycardia:** The SVT has a slower rate of 70 to 120 bpm. Despite the very slow rate of <100 bpm, the arrhythmia is considered a tachycardia since the intrinsic rate of the AV junction is exceeded, which is usually 40 to 60 bpm (Fig. 17.15). AV junctional rhythm with a rate ≤100 bpm is more appropriately called accelerated junctional rhythm rather than junctional "tachycardia." The tachycardia is nonparoxysmal with a slow onset and

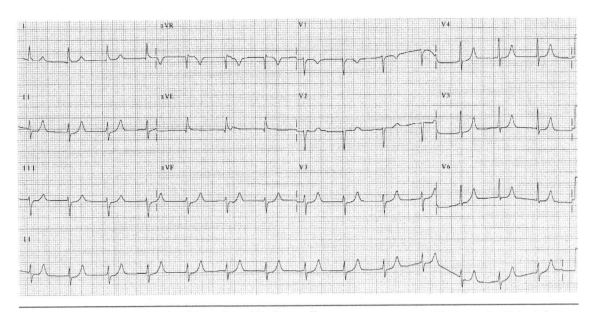

**Figure 17.15:   Nonparoxysmal Junctional Tachycardia.** No P waves are noted in the entire 12-lead electrocardiogram. Although the ventricular rate is <100 beats per minute, the arrhythmia is accepted as junctional tachycardia since the rate exceeds the intrinsic rate of the atrioventricular junction, which is 60 beats per minute.

termination. This type of tachycardia may be due to enhanced automaticity or triggered activity.

■ **Paroxysmal or focal junctional tachycardia:** This type of tachycardia is rare. The tachycardia is also called junctional ectopic tachycardia or automatic junctional tachycardia. The American College of Cardiology/American Heart Association Task Force on Practice Guidelines/European Society of Cardiology guidelines on SVT refer to this tachycardia as focal junctional tachycardia. The tachycardia varies from 110 to 250 bpm and is often paroxysmal with sudden onset and abrupt termination. The mechanism of the tachycardia is due to enhanced automaticity or triggered activity.

■ **ECG findings:** The ECG of AV junctional tachycardia overlaps those of other SVT. Because the tachycardia is not dependent on the atria or ventricles, the relationship between the P wave and the QRS complex is variable. The retrograde P waves are narrow and may occur before or after the QRS complex. It may also be synchronous with the QRS complex. When this occurs, the P waves are not visible. The diagrams in Fig. 17.16 summarize the ECG findings of junctional tachycardia.

## Nonparoxysmal Junctional Tachycardia

■ When the retrograde P wave precedes the QRS complex, the PR interval is usually <0.12 seconds. The width of the retrograde P wave is usually thinner than a normal sinus P wave, because the impulse originates from the AV node. Thus, both atria are activated

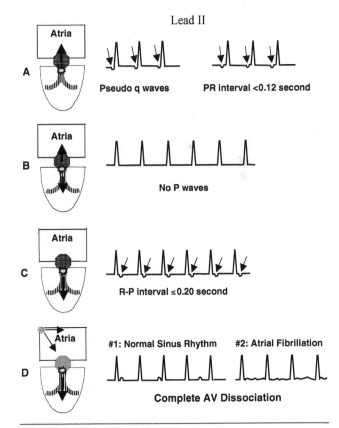

**Figure 17.16:   Junctional Tachycardia. (A)** Atrial activation occurs earlier than ventricular activation (P wave is in front of the QRS complex). **(B)** Atrial activation is synchronous with ventricular activation (no P waves are present). **(C)** Ventricular activation occurs earlier than atrial activation (P waves occur after the QRS complex). **(D)** Complete atrioventricular dissociation during normal sinus rhythm (#1) and during atrial fibrillation (#2).

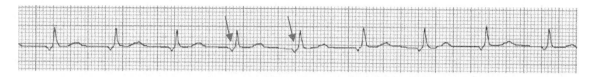

**Figure 17.17:   Nonparoxysmal Junctional Tachycardia.**  Lead II rhythm strip showing accelerated junctional rhythm at 87 beats per minute. Retrograde P waves are inscribed just before the QRS complexes (*arrows*), which can be mistaken for Q waves (pseudo-Q waves). Note that the P waves are narrow measuring less than 0.05 seconds.

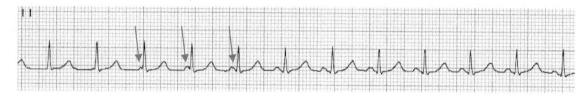

**Figure 17.18:   Nonparoxysmal Junctional Tachycardia.**  Lead II rhythm strip again showing accelerated junctional rhythm at 73 beats per minute. Note that the retrograde P waves are inscribed after the QRS complexes and are narrow (*arrows*). Because the P waves occur during ventricular systole, this can result in cannon A waves in the jugular neck veins.

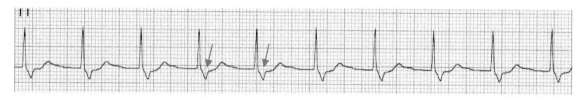

**Figure 17.19:   Nonparoxysmal Junctional Tachycardia.**  The initial half of the tracing shows nonparoxysmal junctional tachycardia of 106 beats per minute. There is isorhythmic atrioventricular dissociation (*arrows*) until the sinus P waves capture the QRS complexes at a slightly higher rate of 110 beats per minute.

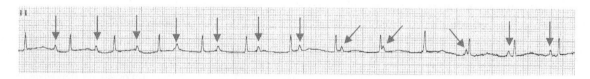

**Figure 17.20:   Accelerated Junctional Rhythm with Complete Atrioventricular Dissociation.**  The atrial and ventricular rates are almost similar at 80 beats per minute. The sinus P waves however are completely dissociated from the QRS complexes. Arrows point to the P waves.

**A.** During tachycardia

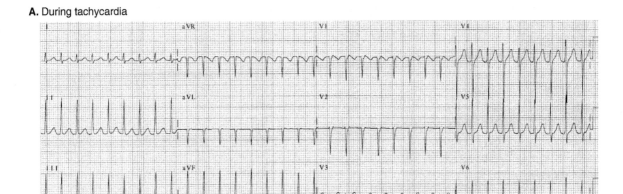

**B:** Upon conversion to normal sinus rhythm

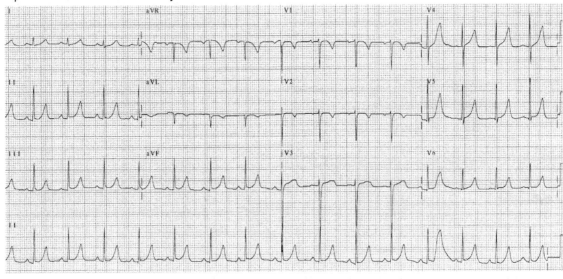

**Figure 17.21:    Paroxysmal Junctional Tachycardia. (A)** Twelve-lead electrocardiogram (ECG) of a 6-year-old boy with paroxysmal tachycardia with a rate of 206 beats per minute. There are no P waves during tachycardia and is consistent with paroxysmal junctional tachycardia. **(B)** A 12-lead ECG on conversion to normal sinus rhythm.

simultaneously. When it follows the QRS complex, the R-P interval is usually ≤0.20 seconds.

■ The rate of the tachycardia can be enhanced by sympathetic or parasympathetic manipulation. Atropine, dobutamine and other adrenergic agents can increase the rate of the tachycardia. Examples of nonparoxysmal junctional tachycardia are shown in Figures 17.17 through 17.20.

## Paroxysmal Junctional Tachycardia

■ Paroxysmal or focal junctional tachycardia is rare. The SVT is more commonly seen in children than in adults. Shown is a 12-lead ECG of a 6-year-old boy with paroxysmal tachycardia from focal junctional tachycardia. The tachycardia has no P waves making it difficult to differentiate from AV nodal reentrant tachycardia (Fig. 17.21).

## ECG Findings of Junctional Tachycardia

■ The ECG findings of nonparoxysmal and paroxysmal or focal junctional tachycardia are similar except for the difference in rate, onset, and termination of the tachycardia.

1. The QRS complexes are narrow unless there is preexistent bundle branch block or the impulse is conducted with aberration.

2. The QRS complexes are regular. In focal junctional tachycardia, the ventricular rate is 110 to 250 bpm. In nonparoxysmal junctional tachycardia, the ventricular rate is slower and varies from 70 to 130 bpm.

3. The P waves may occur synchronously with the QRS complex and may not be visible.

4. When P waves are present, they are retrograde and are inverted in leads II, III, and aVF. The retrograde P waves may occur before or after the QRS complexes. When the retrograde P waves occur before the QRS complexes, the PR interval is short and is usually <0.12 seconds. When the retrograde P waves follow the QRS complexes, the R-P interval is usually ≤0.20 seconds.

5. Complete AV dissociation may occur since the tachycardia does not need the atria (or the ventricles) for its participation. The sinus node captures the atria; however, the ventricles are separately controlled by the junctional tachycardia resulting in complete AV dissociation.

6. A junctional tachycardia can also occur in the presence of atrial fibrillation resulting in regularization of the R-R interval since the ventricles are completely dissociated from the atria.

## Mechanism

■ The AV junction includes the whole AV node down to the bifurcation of the bundle of His. The AV node consists of three parts with distinct electrophysiologic properties. The superior portion of the AV node is the atrionodal or AN region, which lies directly adjacent to the atria. The middle portion of the AV node is the main body or nodal (N) region and the distal part that is directly contiguous to the bundle of His is the nodo-His or NH region. The AV junction, excluding the middle portion of the AV node, contains cells with automatic properties that may compete with the sinus node as the pacemaker of the heart. Although cells in the AV junction have automatic properties, the intrinsic rate of these cells is slower than that of the sinus node. These cells therefore are normally depolarized by the spread of the faster sinus impulse and serve as latent or backup pacemakers. When the firing rate of the cells in the AV junction is enhanced and becomes faster than the rate of the sinus node, junctional rhythm may become the dominant rhythm.

■ The junctional rhythm may control both atria and ventricles simultaneously. The impulse is conducted anterogradely to the ventricles through the normal conduction system resulting in QRS complexes that are narrow, similar to the QRS complexes of normal sinus rhythm. The P waves are retrograde and are inverted in leads II, III, and aVF because the atrial impulse travels from below upward in the atria. The retrograde P waves are narrower (thinner) than the normal sinus P waves because the atria are activated simultaneously when the rhythm starts from the AV junction.

▪ The retrograde P waves may occur in front of the QRS complexes if retrograde conduction of the junctional impulse to the atria is faster than anterograde conduction to the ventricles.

▪ The retrograde P waves may follow the QRS complex if anterograde conduction of the impulse to the ventricles is faster than retrograde conduction to the atria.

▪ The P waves may not be visible if conduction of the impulse to the atria and ventricles are synchronous resulting in simultaneous activation of both chambers. When this occurs, the smaller P wave will be embedded within the larger QRS complexes and will not be visible.

▪ The junctional rhythm may also control the ventricles but not the atria, if retrograde conduction of the impulse is blocked at the AV node. When this occurs, the sinus node may retain control of the atria resulting in complete or incomplete AV dissociation. If there is atrial fibrillation, the ventricles are controlled independently by a junctional impulse causing the R-R intervals to become regular. This is usually the case when there is digitalis toxicity.

■ Nonparoxysmal junctional tachycardia may be due to enhanced automaticity involving cells within the AV junction or it may be due to triggered activity. Triggered activity as a mechanism for tachycardia usually occurs when conditions are abnormal, such as when there is digitalis toxicity, increased intracellular calcium, or marked adrenergic activity. Digitalis prevents the exchange of sodium and potassium during repolarization by inhibiting the enzyme $Na^+/K^+$ ATPase. The build up of $Na^+$ inside the cell causes the $Na^+/Ca^{++}$ exchange mechanism to be activated resulting in accumulation of $Ca^{++}$ inside the cell. The increased $Ca^{++}$ inside the cell is the mechanism by which digitalis exerts its positive inotropic effect. When there is digitalis toxicity, the less negative membrane potential due to calcium overload may "trigger" afterdepolarizations to occur during phase 4 of the action potential. These afterdepolarizations may reach threshold potential resulting in a series of action potentials that may become sustained. Nonparoxysmal junctional tachycardia and atrial tachycardia with 2:1 block are arrhythmias that are usually due to digitalis toxicity (see SVT due to Triggered Activity in this chapter).

## Clinical Implications

### Nonparoxysmal Junctional Tachycardia

■ Most junctional tachycardia seen in the adult is nonparoxysmal. The tachycardia is relatively common and the diagnosis can be made fairly easily. It has a rate of 70 to 120 bpm. Although the rate of the tachycardia could be <100 bpm, the arrhythmia is traditionally accepted as tachycardia because it exceeds the intrinsic rate of the AV junction, which is 40 to 60 bpm. Junctional impulses with rates <100 bpm are preferably called accelerated junctional rhythm rather than junctional tachycardia.

■ The tachycardia is nonparoxysmal because of its gradual onset and termination. The tachycardia is usually self-limiting, often lasting for a few hours to a few days even without therapy. Although the arrhythmia is benign and may not be associated with any hemodynamic abnormalities, nonparoxysmal junctional tachycardia may be a marker of a serious underlying cardiac condition because the tachycardia usually occurs in the setting of acute inferior myocardial infarction, myocarditis, congestive heart failure, hypokalemia, digitalis toxicity, and use of pharmacologic agents such as dobutamine and other sympathomimetic agents. The arrhythmia can also occur after cardiac surgery. It may be a manifestation of sick sinus syndrome. It may also occur in normal individuals.

- The rate of nonparoxysmal junctional tachycardia is relatively slow; thus, the arrhythmia is usually tolerable and may not cause any symptom. However, because the QRS complexes are not preceded by P waves, the tachycardia may result in hemodynamic deterioration because of loss of atrial contribution to left ventricular filling especially in patients with left ventricular dysfunction. This can result in low cardiac output and hypotension. When retrograde P waves follow the QRS complex, atrial contraction occurs during ventricular systole, when the AV valves are closed, resulting in cannon A waves in the neck and pulmonary veins. This can cause hypotension and low cardiac output mimicking the symptoms of pacemaker syndrome (see Chapter 26, The ECG of Cardiac Pacemakers).

- Nonparoxysmal junctional tachycardia is seldom incessant (the tachycardia seldom persists >12 hours a day). When this occurs, a tachycardia-mediated cardiomyopathy can occur. This complication is more frequently seen in focal junctional tachycardia, which has a faster rate and is more common in infants and children, most of whom are unable to complain of symptoms related to the arrhythmia.

## Focal Junctional or Paroxysmal Junctional Tachycardia

- Focal junctional tachycardia is rare in adults. It is also rare, but is more common in children. Paroxysmal junctional tachycardia has a rate of 110 to 250 bpm. The tachycardia is paroxysmal because of its sudden onset and abrupt termination. The tachycardia is also called junctional ectopic tachycardia or automatic junctional tachycardia. The tachycardia may be associated with congenital heart disease such as ventricular or atrial septal defects, although they are also seen in structurally normal hearts. They can also occur during the immediate postoperative period. When the tachycardia is incessant, meaning the tachycardia occurs more than 12 hours per day, it may cause a tachycardia-mediated cardiomyopathy especially in children.

## Acute Treatment

### Nonparoxysmal Junctional Tachycardia

- Nonparoxysmal junctional tachycardia has a relatively slow rate, is very well tolerated, and often self-limiting and generally does not need any drug therapy. It may be related to an underlying abnormality, which should be recognized and corrected. This includes electrolyte and metabolic abnormalities such as hypokalemia, blood gas disturbances, chronic obstructive pulmonary disease, myocardial ischemia, or inflammatory disorders involving the myocardium. It can also be triggered by digitalis toxicity and use of dobutamine and other sympathomimetic agents.

- The presence of nonparoxysmal junctional tachycardia or accelerated junctional rhythm with a rate of <100 bpm may be a sign of underlying sinus node disease. When sinus node dysfunction is suspected, the junctional rhythm should not be suppressed.

- Nonparoxysmal junctional tachycardia is frequently due to digitalis toxicity. Digitalis should be discontinued if the drug is the cause of the tachycardia. If digitalis is continued inappropriately, it may result in more serious, even fatal, arrhythmias. The arrhythmia can be monitored without additional therapy if the rate of the tachycardia is <100 bpm and the patient is hemodynamically stable. Any electrolyte or metabolic abnormality should be corrected. If the tachycardia is rapid or there is hypokalemia, potassium supplements should be given. Potassium should also be given if the serum level is <4 mEq/L, especially in postoperative patients. The rate of the tachycardia can be slowed with phenytoin 5 to 10 mg/kg IV given as a 250-mg bolus diluted with saline and injected IV slowly over 10 minutes, followed by 100 mg IV every 5 minutes as needed to a maximum dose of 1 g. Phenytoin is effective only if the tachycardia is digitalis induced. Side effects of hypotension, profound bradycardia, or respiratory depression can occur especially if the phenytoin is rapidly administered. Beta blockers given IV have also been used to control the ventricular rate (see Appendix, Commonly Used Injectable Pharmacologic Agents, specifically sections on intravenous dosing with metoprolol, atenolol, esmolol, or propranolol). Treatment with digoxin-immune Fab fragments should be considered if the arrhythmia is life-threatening or the patient is hemodynamically unstable and digitalis toxicity is the cause of the tachycardia. It should also be given if the digoxin level exceeds 10 ng/mL.

- The pharmacologic treatment of nonparoxysmal junctional tachycardia not due to digitalis toxicity is similar to that of focal junctional tachycardia.

- In patients with accelerated junctional rhythm (nonparoxysmal junctional tachycardia) with retrograde P waves occurring during ventricular systole associated with symptoms of hypoperfusion and low cardiac output mimicking the pacemaker syndrome, temporary atrial or AV sequential pacing is usually effective.

## Focal Junctional Tachycardia

- If the rate of the tachycardia is unusually rapid, such as the case with focal junctional tachycardia, the tachycardia should be treated like any regular narrow complex tachycardia. Although focal junctional tachycardia is rare, the ECG findings mimic those of AVNRT, AVRT, and focal atrial tachycardia, which are more common and are more responsive to adenosine. Thus, adenosine should be tried initially and if not effective, beta blockers or nondihydropyridine calcium channel blockers should be tried (see Treatment of AVNRT in this chapter).

- If AV nodal blockers are not effective, type IC (flecainide or propafenone) and type III (amiodarone or sotalol) agents may be tried to suppress the ectopic focus. The choice of antiarrhythmic agent should be based on the presence or absence of left ventricular dysfunction. When left ventricular dysfunction is present, amiodarone is the preferred agent.

- In patients who do not respond to medications or in patients in whom the tachycardia continues to become recurrent or incessant, catheter ablation may be considered. Ablative procedures may be associated with some risk of AV block because the foci involves the AV node and bundle of His.

## Prognosis

- Nonparoxysmal junctional tachycardia is usually associated with structural cardiac disease or digitalis excess but the arrhythmia itself is self limiting. Focal junctional tachycardia may also occur in structurally normal hearts and is more common in pediatric patients and young adults. If the tachycardia becomes incessant, it may result in tachycardia-mediated cardiomyopathy.
- The overall prognosis depends on the underlying cardiac disease associated with the tachycardia.

## SVT from Triggered Activity

- **Triggered activity:** Another possible mechanism of SVT is triggered activity. Triggered activity is due to the presence of afterdepolarizations. These are additional depolarizations that are triggered by the previous action potential. Afterdepolarizations may be single or repetitive and may not always reach threshold potential. However, when these afterdepolarizations reach threshold potential, repetitive firing may result in sustained arrhythmia. This is unlike enhanced automaticity, which is not dependent on the previous impulse but is caused by automatic firing of a cell because of the presence of phase 4 diastolic depolarization. Afterdepolarizations occur when conditions are abnormal, such as when there is digitalis toxicity or when there is excess calcium or catecholamines.

- Triggered automaticity may be due to early or late afterdepolarizations.
  - **Early afterdepolarizations:** These are afterdepolarizations that occur during phase 2 or phase 3 of the action potential (Fig. 17.22A).
  - **Late afterdepolarizations:** These are afterdepolarizations that occur during phase 4 of the action potential (Fig. 17.22B).
- The role of triggered activity as a cause of SVT is uncertain except in atrial tachycardia with 2:1 AV block and in nonparoxysmal junctional tachycardia. Both arrhythmias are frequently associated with digitalis toxicity (Figs 17.23 to 17.25).

## Atrial Tachycardia with 2:1 AV Block

- **Atrial tachycardia with 2:1 AV block:** Atrial tachycardia with 2:1 AV block is an arrhythmia resulting from triggered activity. This tachycardia is almost always from digitalis toxicity. Digitalis excites atrial and ventricular myocytes, which may result in atrial and ventricular tachycardia. Digitalis also blocks the AV node; thus, the combination of atrial tachycardia with AV block usually in a 2:1 ratio, is most commonly an arrhythmia related to digitalis toxicity (Fig. 17.24). The tachycardia arises from a single focus in the atria close to the sinus node, causing the P wave to be upright in leads II, III, and aVF, resembling sinus tachycardia (Figs. 17.25).
- Atrial tachycardia with varying degrees of AV block may occur in patients who are not on digitalis. In these patients, the mechanism for the tachycardia may be due to enhanced automaticity rather than triggered activity.
- Fig. 27.26 summarizes the different ECG patterns of narrow complex SVT and Fig. 27.27 is an algorithm how to diagnose narrow complex tachycardias.

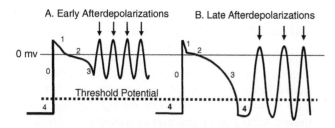

**Figure 17.22: Triggered Activity. (A)** Triggered activity from early afterdepolarizations (phase 2 or 3 of the action potential). **(B)** Triggered automaticity from late afterdepolarizations (phase 4 of the action potential). The dotted line represents threshold potential and 0, 1, 2, 3, and 4 represent the different phases of the action potential. The arrows point to afterdepolarizations.

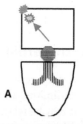 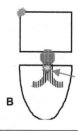

**Figure 17.23: Supraventricular Tachycardia (SVT) from Triggered Activity. (A)** Atrial tachycardia with 2:1 atrioventricular block is an example of SVT due to triggered activity. The ectopic focus (*arrow*) usually originates from the right atrium close to the sinus node (*arrow*). **(B)** Nonparoxysmal junctional tachycardia arising from the AV junction (*arrow*).

Lead II

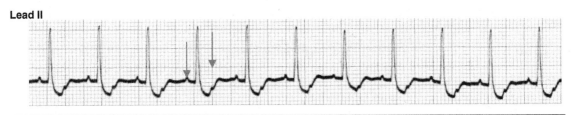

**Figure 17.24:   Atrial Tachycardia with 2:1 Atrioventricular (AV) Block.** The P waves (*arrows*) are upright in lead II with a rate of 230 beats per minute. Atrial tachycardia with 2:1 AV block is usually from digitalis toxicity. The configuration of the ST segment is typical of digitalis effect.

## Approach to a Patient with Narrow Complex Tachycardia

- When a narrow complex tachycardia with a QRS duration of <0.12 seconds is present, the ECG should first be inspected for gross irregularity of the R-R intervals.
- **Grossly irregular R-R intervals (Fig. 17.28):**
  - **Multifocal atrial tachycardia:** Distinct P waves of different configurations are present preceding each QRS complex.
  - **Atrial fibrillation:** The baseline shows fibrillatory waves. No definite P waves or flutter waves are present.
  - **Atrial flutter:** Flutter waves are present with a saw tooth or undulating baseline.
- **Regular R-R intervals with no visible P waves (Fig. 17.29):**
  - **AVNRT**
  - Junctional tachycardia (paroxysmal or nonparoxysmal)

## Narrow Complex Tachycardia with Regular R-R Intervals

- **Regular R-R intervals with upright P waves in front of the QRS complexes (Fig. 17.30):** If the P waves are upright in lead II, retrograde activation of the atria (AVNRT or AVRT) is excluded. The most likely possibilities are:
  - **Sinus tachycardia**
  - Focal atrial tachycardia
  - Sinoatrial reentrant tachycardia
- **Regular R-R intervals with retrograde P waves in front of the QRS complexes (Fig. 17.31):** The presence of retrograde P waves in front of the QRS complexes excludes sinus tachycardia and SART and favors:
  - **Focal atrial tachycardia**
  - Junctional tachycardia (paroxysmal or nonparoxysmal)
  - Atypical AVNRT
  - Atypical AVRT
- **Retrograde P waves between QRS complexes (Fig. 17.32):** Retrograde P waves between QRS complexes with R-P interval equal to PR interval. This excludes sinus tachycardia and SART and includes the following possible arrhythmias:
- **Regular R-R intervals with retrograde P waves after the QRS complexes (Fig. 17.33):** When R-P interval is shorter than PR interval, the possible arrhythmias include:
  - **AVRT:** (R-P interval ≥80 milliseconds)
  - AVNRT: (R-P interval <80 milliseconds)
  - Junctional tachycardia (paroxysmal or nonparoxysmal)
- **Complete AV dissociation with regular R-R intervals (Fig. 17.34):** When there is complete AV dissociation with regular R-R intervals, AVRT is not possible and AVNRT is highly unlikely. This is almost always

Lead V$_1$

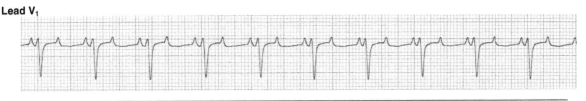

**Figure 17.25:   Atrial Tachycardia with 2:1 Atrioventricular Block.** The patient is not on digitalis. The atrial rate is approximately 180 beats per minute and the baseline between the P waves is isoelectric.

# Summary of the Different SVT and Possible Diagnoses

| Lead II | Possible Diagnoses |
|---|---|

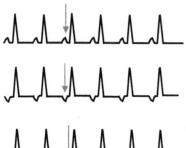

**Sinus Tachycardia**
Sinoatrial Reentrant Tachycardia
Focal Atrial Tachycardia

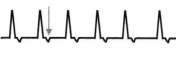

**Focal Atrial Tachycardia**
Junctional Tachycardia
Atypical AVNRT
Atypical AVRT

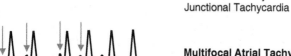

**Junctional Tachycardia**
AVNRT

**AVNRT**
Junctional Tachycardia

**AVNRT**
Junctional Tachycardia

**AVRT**
AVNRT
Junctional Tachycardia

**AVRT**
**Atrial Flutter with 2:1 AV Block**
AVNRT
Focal Atrial Tachycardia
Junctional Tachycardia

**Multifocal Atrial Tachycardia**

**Nonparoxysmal Junctional Tachycardia with Complete AV Dissociation**

**Figure 17.26: Different Electrocardiogram Patterns of Narrow Complex Supraventricular Tachycardia in Lead II.** The best possible diagnosis is highlighted in bold letters and is listed from top to bottom. The algorithm for diagnosing narrow complex tachycardia is shown in the next page. AVNRT, atrioventricular nodal reentrant tachycardia; AVRT, atrioventricular reentrant tachycardia.

due to junctional tachycardia with complete AV dissociation.

- **Junctional tachycardia with complete AV dissociation**
- **Retrograde P Waves with second-degree AV Wenckebach (Fig. 17.35):** This is almost always due to focal atrial tachycardia. This excludes AVRT and makes AVNRT highly unlikely.

## ECG of Narrow Complex Tachycardia

1. When the R-R interval is irregular, atrial fibrillation, multifocal atrial tachycardia, and atrial flutter with variable AV block are the main considerations. Focal atrial tachycardia with variable AV block is also possible although rare.

2. When the R-R interval is regular, the diagnosis of the tachycardia depends on the location and polarity of the P waves in lead II.
   - No P waves are present
     - AVNRT
     - Junctional tachycardia
   - If the P waves are upright in lead II, the primary considerations are:
     - Sinus tachycardia
     - Focal atrial tachycardia
     - SART

**Figure 17.27:    Algorithm for Diagnosing Narrow Complex Tachycardia.** AVNRT, atrioventricular nodal reentrant tachycardia; AVRT, atrioventricular reentrant tachycardia.

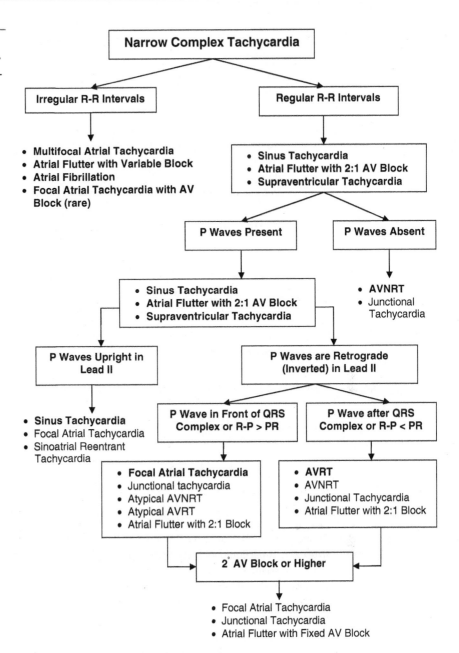

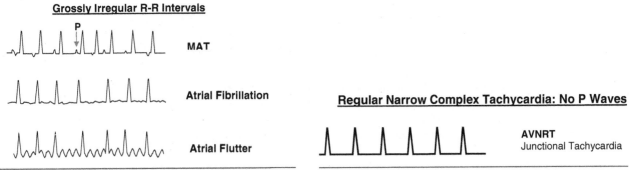

**Figure 17.28:    Narrow Complex Tachycardia with Irregular R-R Intervals.** When the R-R interval in a narrow complex tachycardia is grossly irregular, the possibilities include multifocal atrial tachycardia (MAT), atrial fibrillation, and atrial flutter with variable atrioventricular block.

**Figure 17.29:    Supraventricular Tachycardia with Regular R-R intervals and No P Waves.** This is commonly due to atrioventricular nodal reentrant tachycardia. Junctional tachycardia is another possibility, although this is not as common.

**Upright P waves in front of the QRS complexes in Lead II**

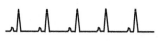

Sinus tachycardia
Focal AT
SART
(Excludes AVNRT and AVRT)

**Figure 17.30:** **Regular R-R Intervals with Upright P Waves before QRS complexes in Lead II.** This is almost always the result of sinus tachycardia. Focal atrial tachycardia and sino-atrial reentrant tachycardia are other possibilities.

## Retrograde P Waves in Front of QRS Complexes

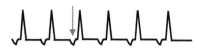

Focal Atrial Tachycardia
Atypical AVNRT
Atypical AVRT
Junctional Tachycardia
(Excludes Sinus tachycardia and SART)

**Figure 17.31:** **Retrograde P Waves in Front of the QRS Complex.** This is most commonly the result of focal atrial tachycardia. Other possibilities include atypical atrioventricular nodal reentrant tachycardia, atypical atrioventricular reentrant tachycardia, and junctional tachycardia, both paroxysmal and nonparoxysmal.

## Retrograde P Waves with R-P Interval = PR Interval

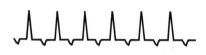

Atrial Flutter with 2:1 AV Block
AVRT
Focal Atrial Tachycardia
Atypical AVNRT
Junctional Tachycardia
(Excludes Sinus tachycardia and SART)

**Figure 17.32:** **Retrograde P Waves with R-P Interval Equal to PR Interval.** Atrial flutter with 2:1 AV block is a distinct possibility with the second flutter wave embedded within the QRS complexes. This can also be due to AVRT, focal atrial tachycardia, atypical AVNRT and junctional tachycardia both paroxysmal and nonparoxysmal. AV, atrioventricular; AVNRT, atrioventricular nodal reentrant tachycardia; AVRT, atrioventricular reentrant tachycardia.

## Retrograde P Waves after QRS Complex

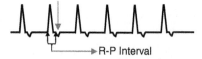

→ R-P Interval

**AVRT** (R-P ≥80 milliseconds)
AVNRT (R-P <80 milliseconds)
Junctional Tachycardia
Focal Atrial Tachycardia with $1^0$ AV Block

**Figure 17.33:** **Retrograde P Waves with R-P Interval < PR Interval.** This is typically from atrioventricular reentrant tachycardia. Other possibilities include atrioventricular nodal reentrant tachycardia and junctional tachycardia both paroxysmal and nonparoxysmal. Arrow points to the retrograde P wave.

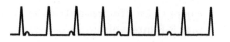

**Junctional Tachycardia** with complete AV dissociation. The P waves are sinus in origin and are independent from the QRS complex.

**Figure 17.34:** **Junctional Tachycardia with Complete AV Dissociation.** The P waves are upright in lead II and are completely dissociated from the QRS complexes. The upright P waves represent normal sinus rhythm.

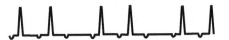

**Focal atrial tachycardia
with 2° AV Block**

**Figure 17.35: Retrograde P waves with Second-Degree Atrioventricular Wenckebach.** This is almost always from focal atrial tachycardia. Focal junctional tachycardia is also possible, but is unlikely.

■ If the P waves are retrograde (inverted), the differential diagnosis revolves around the position of the P waves in relation to the QRS complexes

　■ Retrograde P waves before the QRS complex with PR interval ≥0.12 seconds

　　☐ Focal atrial tachycardia

　　☐ Atypical AVNRT

　　☐ Atypical AVRT

　　☐ Junctional tachycardia

　　☐ Atrial flutter with 2:1 block

　■ Retrograde P waves before the QRS complex with PR interval <0.12 seconds

　　☐ Junctional tachycardia

　　☐ AVNRT (typical and atypical)

　　☐ Atypical AVRT

## Clinical Implications

■ Identification of the P wave (or its absence) is crucial to the diagnosis of narrow complex tachycardia. Several maneuvers are often helpful in identifying the P waves if they are not obvious in the surface ECG.

　■ Although the P wave should be inspected in all 12 standard leads of the ECG, leads II and $V_1$ are the most useful. Lead II is very useful, especially in determining the polarity of the P wave and therefore the origin of the tachycardia.

　■ The ECG may be magnified to 2× the standard size and the speed of the recording may be doubled so that the P waves may be better identified. This maneuver is usually not very useful unless the voltage of the ECG is small especially in the limb leads (lead II).

　■ Special leads may be taken (other than the standard 12 leads). These include:

　　☐ The left arm electrode can be used as the exploring electrode and positioned at different areas in the precordium. The rest of the extremity electrodes retain their usual position. The ECG is recorded in lead I.

　　☐ If this maneuver is not helpful, a Lewis lead can be recorded by placing the left arm electrode over the fourth right intercostal space beside the sternum ($V_1$ position) and the right arm electrode at the second right intercostal space beside the sternum. The ECG is recorded in lead I.

☐ An esophageal pill electrode can be swallowed and positioned behind the left atrium. The electrode is connected to a standard precordial lead such as $V_1$.

☐ Intracardiac recordings may be obtained by inserting an electrode transvenously into the atria and connected to a standard precordial lead such as $V_1$.

☐ If a central line is already in place, intracardiac ECG can be obtained by filling the length of the catheter with saline. The tip of the central line should be near or at the right atrium and if multiple catheter lumens are present, the port closest to the right atrium should be used. A needle is inserted and left at the injecting port of the catheter. The needle is connected to $V_1$ or any precordial lead in the ECG (usually with an alligator clamp) and recorded in $V_1$.

## Suggested Readings

2005 American Heart Association Guidelines for Cardiopulmonary Resuscitation and Emergency Cardiovascular Care. Part 7.3: management of symptomatic bradycardia and tachycardia. *Circulation.* 2005;112:IV-67–IV-77.

Bar FW, Brugada P, Dassen WRM, et al. Differential diagnosis of tachycardia with narrow QRS complex (shorter than 0.12 second). *Am J Cardiol.* 1984;54:555–560.

Blomstrom-Lunndqvist C, Scheinman MM, Aliot EM, et al. ACC/AHA/ESC guidelines for the management of patients with supraventricular arrhythmias—executive summary: a report of the American College of Cardiology/American Heart Association Task Force on Practice Guidelines, and the European Society of Cardiology Committee for Practice Guidelines (Writing Committee to Develop Guidelines for the Management of Patients With Supraventricular Arrhythmias). *J Am Coll Cardiol.* 2003;42:1493–1453.

Chauhan VS, Krahn AD, Klein GJ, et al. Supraventricular tachycardia. *Med Clin North Am.* 2001;85:193–223.

Chen S-A, Chiang C-E, Yang C-J, et al. Sustained atrial tachycardia in adult patients. Electrophysiological characteristics, pharmacological response, possible mechanisms, and effects of radiofrequency ablation. *Circulation.* 1994;90:1262–1278.

Donovan KD, Power BM, Hockings BE, et al. Usefulness of atrial electrograms recorded via central venous catheters in the diagnosis of complex cardiac arrhythmias. *Crit Care Med.* 1993;21:532–537.

Engelstein ED, Lippman N, Stein KM, et al. Mechanism-specific effects of adenosine on atrial tachycardia. *Circulation.* 1994; 89:2645–2654.

Esberger D, Jones S, Morris F. ABC of clinical electrocardiography: junctional tachycardias. *BMJ*. 2002;324: 662–665.

Farre J, Wellens HJJ. The Value of the electrocardiogram in diagnosing site of origin and mechanism of supraventricular tachycardia. In: Wellens HJJ, Kulbertus HE, eds. *What's New in Electrocardiography*. Boston: Martinus Nijhoff; 1981.

Ganz LI, Friedman PL. Supraventricular tachycardia. *N Engl J Med*. 1995;332:162–173.

Guidelines 2000 for Cardiopulmonary Resuscitation and Emergency Cardiovascular Care: 7D: the tachycardia algorithms. *Circulation*. 2000;102(Suppl I):I-158–I-165.

Haissaguerre MH, Sanders P, Hocini M, et al. Pulmonary veins in the substrate for atrial fibrillation. *J Am Coll Cardiol*. 2004;43:2290–2292.

Kastor JA. Multifocal atrial tachycardia. *N Engl J Med*. 1990;322: 1713–1717.

Kistler PM, Roberts-Thomson KC, Haqqani HM, et al. P-wave morphology in focal atrial tachycardia. Development of an algorithm to predict the anatomic site of origin. *J Am Coll Cardiol*. 2006;48:1010–1017.

Kistler PM, Sanders P, Hussin A. Focal atrial tachycardia arising from the mitral annulus. Electrocardiographic and electrophysiologic characterization. *J Am Coll Cardiol*. 2003;41: 2212–2219.

Kumagai K, Ogawa M, Noguchi H, et al. Electrophysiologic properties of pulmonary veins assessed using microelectrode basket catheter. *J Am Coll Cardiol*. 2004;43:2281–2289.

Levine JH, Michael JR, Guarnieri T. Treatment of multifocal atrial tachycardia with verapamil. *N Engl J Med*. 1985;312:21–25.

Madias JE, Bazar R, Agarwal H. Anasarca-mediated attenuation of the amplitude of ECG complexes: a description of a heretofore unrecognized phenomenon. *J Am Coll Cardiol*. 2001;38:756–764.

Madias JE, Narayan V, Attari M. Detection of P waves via a "saline-filled central venous catheter electrocardiographic lead" in patients with low electrocardiographic voltage due to anasarca. *J Am Coll Cardiol*. 2003;91:910–914.

Manolis AS, Mark Estes III NA. Supraventricular tachycardia mechanisms and therapy. *Arch Intern Med*. 1987;147: 1706–1716.

Marrouche NF, SippensGroenewegen A, Yang Y, et al. Clinical and electrophysiologic characteristics of left septal atrial tachycardia. *J Am Coll Cardiol*. 2002;40:1133–1139.

Mehta AV, Perlman PE. Ectopic automatic atrial tachycardia in children: an overview. *J Arrhythmia Manage*. 1990: 12–19.

Olgen JE, Zipes DE. Specific arrhythmias: diagnosis and treatment. In: Libby P, Bonow RO, Mann DL, et al. eds. *Braunwald's Heart Disease, A Textbook of Cardiovascular Medicine*. 8th ed., Philadelphia, PA: Elsevier Saunders; 2005: 863–931.

Reddy CP and Arnett JD. Automatic atrial tachycardia and nonparoxysmal atrioventricular junctional tachycardia. In: Horowitz LN, ed. *Current Management of Arrhythmias*. South Hamilton, Ontario: BC Decker Inc; 1991: 67–73.

Salerno JC, Kertesz NJ, Friedman RA, et al. Clinical course of atrial ectopic tachycardia is age-dependent: Results and treatment in children <3 or ≥3 years of age. *J Am Coll Cardiol*. 2004;43:438–444.

Saoudi N, Cosio F, Waldo A, et al. Classification of atrial flutter and regular atrial tachycardia according to electrophysiological mechanisms and anatomical bases. *Eur Heart J*. 2001;22:1162–1182.

Tang CW, Scheinman MM, Van Hare GF. Use of P wave configuration during atrial tachycardia to predict site of origin. *J Am Coll Cardiol*. 1995;26:1315–1324.

Wagner GS. Ventricular preexcitation. In: *Marriott's Practical Electrocardiography*. 10th ed. Philadelphia: Lippincott Williams and Wilkins; 2001:124–137.

Wagner GS. Reentrant junctional tachyarrhythmias. In: *Marriott's Practical Electrocardiography*. 10th ed. Philadelphia: Lippincott Williams and Wilkins; 2001:330–344.

Wellens HJJ. Atrial tachycardia. How important is the mechanism? *Circulation*. 1994;90:1576–1577.

Wellens HJJ, Conover MB. Narrow QRS tachycardia. In: *The ECG in Emergency Decision Making*. 2nd ed. St. Louis: W.B. Saunders/Elsevier; 2006:92–106.

Wellens HJJ, Conover MB. Digitalis-induced emergencies. In: *The ECG in Emergency Decision Making*. 2nd ed. St. Louis: W.B. Saunders/Elsevier; 2006:158–176.

Xie B, Thakur RK, Shah CP, et al. Clinical differentiation of narrow QRS complex tachycardias. *Emerg Med Clin North Am*. 1998;16:295–330.

Yamane T, Shah DC, Peng JT, et al. Morphological characteristics of P waves during selective pulmonary vein pacing. *J Am Coll Cardiol*. 2001;38:1505–1510.

# Atrial Flutter

## Electrocardiogram Findings

- Atrial flutter is a supraventricular arrhythmia with a regular atrial rate of 300 ± 50 beats per minute (Fig. 18.1). Other features include:
  - Very regular and uniform flutter waves with a saw tooth or picket fence appearance.
  - The flutter waves are typically inverted in leads II, III, and aVF and upright in $V_1$.
  - The ventricular rate is variable depending on the number of atrial impulses conducted through the atrioventricular (AV) node.
  - The QRS complexes are narrow unless there is preexistent bundle branch block or the atrial impulses are conducted aberrantly or through a bypass tract.
- Atrial flutter is due to reentry within the atria. There are two types of atrial flutter based on electrocardiogram (ECG) presentation: typical and reverse typical.
  - **Typical atrial flutter:** This is the most common ECG pattern occurring in 90% of all atrial flutter. In typical atrial flutter, the atrial impulse travels from top to bottom across the lateral wall of the right atrium and circles back from bottom to top across the atrial septum. The flutter waves are inverted in lead II and upright in $V_1$ (Fig. 18.2A).
  - **Reverse typical atrial flutter:** This type is uncommon occurring only in 10% of cases. The atrial impulse travels down the atrial septum and up the lateral wall of the right atrium, which is the reverse of typical atrial flutter. This will cause the flutter waves to become upright in lead II and inverted in $V_1$ (Fig. 18.2B).
- **Atrial rate:** The diagnosis of atrial flutter is based on the atrial rate, which is regular with a sawtooth configuration and is typically 300 ± 50 beats per minute (bpm). The

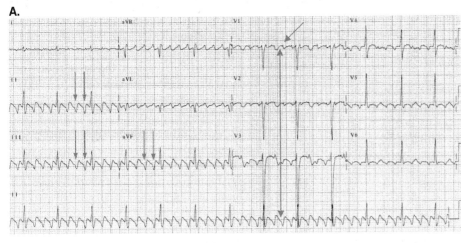

**A.**

**B.**

5 small blocks

1 2 3 4

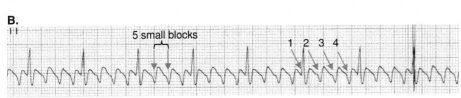

**Figure 18.1:  Atrial Flutter.**
**(A)** Twelve-lead ECG showing atrial flutter. The flutter waves are regular with saw tooth or picket fence appearance and are typically inverted in leads II, III, and aVF and upright in $V_1$ (*arrows*). **(B)** Lead II is magnified from the ECG in **(A)** to show the appearance of the flutter waves. There is 4:1 AV conduction, meaning that there are four flutter waves (*arrows*) for every QRS complex. The flutter waves are separated by five small blocks, which is equivalent to a rate of 300 beats per minute. ECG, electrocardiogram; AV, atrioventricular.

**Figure 18.2: Diagrammatic representation of Atrial Flutter. (A)** Classical atrial flutter with typically inverted flutter waves in lead II. The impulse travels down the lateral wall of the right atrium and up the atrial septum (*arrow*) in a counterclockwise direction. The reverse type travels through the same pathway, **(B)** down the atrial septum (*arrow*) and up the right atrial wall in a clockwise direction, which is the opposite of classical atrial flutter. This causes the flutter waves to be upright in lead II.

### A. Typical Atrial Flutter

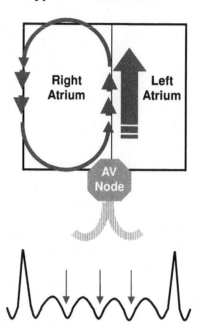

Flutter waves inverted in lead II

### B. Reverse Typical Atrial Flutter

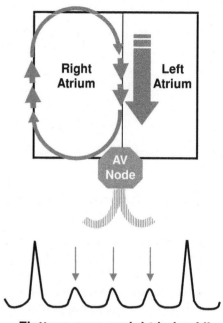

Flutter waves upright in lead II

atrial rate is the most important in differentiating atrial flutter from the other supraventricular arrhythmias.

- The atrial rate is calculated by counting the number of small boxes between two flutter waves and dividing this number from 1,500 (see Chapter 5, Heart Rate and Voltage).
- The atrial rate in atrial flutter may be <250 bpm if the patient is taking antiarrhythmic agents that can slow atrial conduction such as quinidine, sotalol, or amiodarone.
- The baseline between flutter waves is usually wavy and undulating.

- **Ventricular rate:** Atrial flutter is easy to recognize when the ventricular rate is slow as when there is 4:1 AV conduction, as shown in Figure 18.1. However, when the ventricular rate is rapid as when there is 2:1 AV conduction (Fig. 18.3A,B), especially when the QRS complexes are wide due to bundle branch block (Fig. 18.3C), the flutter waves may be obscured by the QRS complexes and ST and T waves making atrial flutter difficult or even impossible to recognize.

## Ventricular Rate in Atrial Flutter

- The ventricular rate in atrial flutter depends on the number of atrial impulses that are conducted through the AV node, thus the ventricular rate can be very rapid or very slow.

- **Atrial flutter with 1:1 AV conduction:** Atrial flutter with 1:1 AV conduction is rare but is possible (Fig. 18.4). When atrial flutter with 1:1 AV conduction occurs, every atrial impulse is followed by a QRS complex; therefore, the atrial rate and ventricular rate are the same and is 300 ± 50 bpm (250 to 350 bpm).

- **Atrial flutter with 2:1 AV conduction:** Atrial flutter with 2:1 AV conduction (or 2:1 AV block) is the most common presentation of atrial flutter in the acute setting. It is also the most difficult to recognize and is the most commonly overlooked tachycardia with a narrow QRS complex. Approximately 10% of tachycardia thought to be SVT is due to atrial flutter. Atrial flutter should always be distinguished from SVT because the acute treatment of atrial flutter is different from that of SVT.

- When atrial flutter with 2:1 AV block occurs, every other atrial impulse is followed by a QRS complex, alternating with every other impulse that is not conducted. The ventricular rate is half the atrial rate. Because the atrial rate is typically 300 bpm, the ventricular rate in atrial flutter with 2:1 conduction is approximately 150 bpm (Fig. 18.5).

- **Atrial flutter with 2:1 AV block:** When there is a regular tachycardia with narrow QRS complexes and the ventricular rate is 150 bpm, especially when inverted "P" waves are present in lead II, atrial flutter with 2:1 AV block should be the first arrhythmia to consider.

- The following examples show some of the difficulties in recognizing atrial flutter when 2:1 AV block is present (Figs. 18.6–18.8).

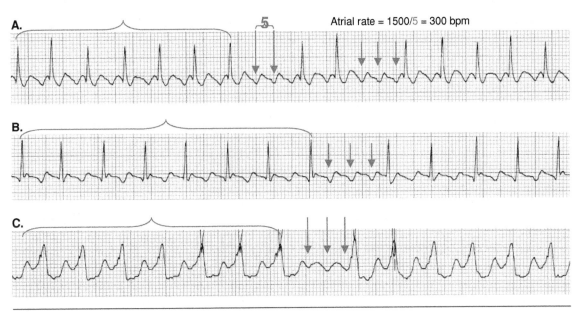

**Figure 18.3:    Atrial Flutter. (A)** The diagnosis of atrial flutter is based on the presence of flutter waves with typical saw tooth appearance with a rate of 300 ± 50 beats per minute. The atrial rate is calculated by measuring the distance between two flutter waves and dividing the number of small blocks from 1500 as shown in **(A)**. When the ventricular rate is rapid because of 2:1 atrioventricular conduction (marked by the brackets in **A** and **B**), especially when the QRS complexes are wide because of bundle branch block as shown in **(C)**, the diagnosis of atrial flutter is difficult and may not be possible unless there is slowing of the ventricular rate so that the flutter waves can be recognized (*arrows*).

## Atrial Flutter and Supraventricular Tachycardia

- **Differentiating atrial flutter from supraventricular tachycardia (SVT):** When the diagnosis of atrial flutter is uncertain, vagal maneuvers such as carotid sinus pressure, is useful in differentiating atrial flutter from other types of regular narrow complex SVT as shown (Fig. 18.9).
  - **Atrial flutter:** In atrial flutter, carotid sinus pressure or AV nodal blockers such as adenosine or verapamil will slow AV nodal conduction resulting in a slower ventricular rate but will not convert atrial flutter to normal sinus rhythm (Figs. 18.9 and 18.10).
  - **Regular narrow complex SVT:** When the narrow complex tachycardia is due to SVT, the tachycardia may convert to normal sinus rhythm with carotid stimulation. SVT from reentry but not atrial flutter (Fig. 18.10) is frequently terminated by AV nodal blockers to normal sinus rhythm (see Chapter 16, Supraventricular Tachycardia due to Reentry).
- **Atrial flutter versus atrial tachycardia:** Atrial flutter with 2:1 AV block may be mistaken for atrial tachycardia with 2:1 AV block. Atrial tachycardia with 2:1 AV block is usually from digitalis toxicity, whereas atrial flutter with 2:1 AV block is unrelated to digitalis and the

patient may in fact require digitalis or other AV nodal blocking agents to slow down the ventricular rate.
  - **Atrial rate:** The atrial rate is the most important feature in distinguishing atrial flutter from atrial tachycardia (Figs. 18.11 to 18.14). In atrial flutter with 2:1 AV block, the atrial rate is approximately 300 ± 50 bpm with the lowest rate at 240 to 250 bpm. In atrial tachycardia with 2:1 AV block, the atrial rate is approximately 200 ± 50 bpm (150 to 250 bpm) (Fig. 18.11).
  - **Morphology of the P wave:** When the atrial rate of atrial flutter and atrial tachycardia overlaps, the two arrhythmias may be differentiated by the morphology of the P wave. In atrial flutter, the flutter waves are typically inverted in leads II, III, and aVF and the baseline between the QRS complexes is wavy and undulating (Fig. 18.12). In atrial tachycardia with AV block, the P waves are typically upright in leads II, III, and aVF and the baseline between the P waves is isoelectric or flat (Fig. 18.11).
- **Atrial flutter with variable block:** As shown in Figures 18.15 through 18.17, atrial flutter is easy to recognize when the ventricular rate is slow as when AV conduction is 3:1 or higher. In atrial flutter with variable AV block, the number of flutter waves for every QRS complex varies from beat to beat (Fig. 18.17).
- **Atrial flutter with complete AV block:** The diagnosis of complete AV block during atrial flutter should be

**A.** Atrial flutter with 1:1 AV conduction

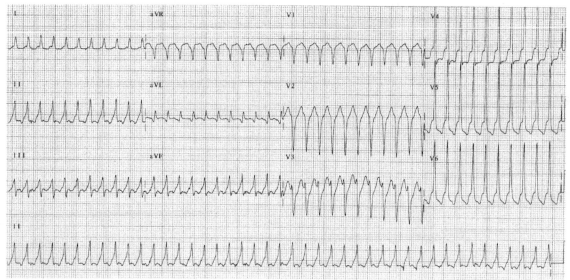

**B.** Magnified lead II rhythm strip

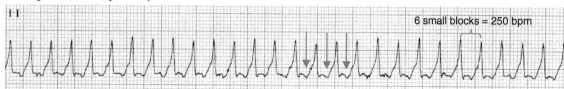

6 small blocks = 250 bpm

**C.** Same patient with 2:1 AV conduction

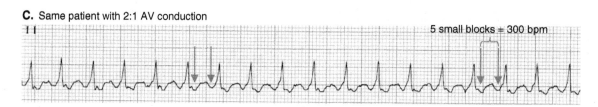

5 small blocks = 300 bpm

**Figure 18.4: Atrial Flutter with 1:1 Atrioventricular (AV) Conduction. (A–C)** From the same patient. **(A, B)** Atrial flutter with 1:1 AV conduction. **(C)** The same patient during 2:1 AV conduction. Arrows point to the flutter waves, which are typically inverted in lead II with a rate ≥250 beats per minute.

considered when the ventricular rate is regular and is in the low 40s, as shown in Figure 18.18. When complete AV block occurs, the R-R intervals become regular because of the presence of a ventricular escape rhythm, independent of the atrial rhythm.

## Common Mistakes in Atrial Flutter

■ Atrial flutter can be confused with other conditions other than SVT. Although the diagnosis of atrial flutter is straightforward when the ventricular rate is slow, the presence of motion artifacts, especially in patients with tremors such as those with Parkinson disease or pa-

tients receiving intravenous infusion from a volumetric infusion pump, can be mistaken for flutter waves (Figs. 18.19 to 18.22).

## ECG Findings of Atrial Flutter

1. Atrial rate of $300 \pm 50$ bpm with a minimum atrial rate of 240 to 250 bpm.

2. Very regular and uniform flutter waves with a saw tooth or picket fence appearance.

3. Flutter waves are typically inverted in leads II, III, and aVF and upright in $V_1$ in 90% of cases, although this may be reversed in 10% of cases, `becoming upright in leads II, III, and aVF and inverted in $V_1$.

**A.** Atrial flutter with 2:1 AV block

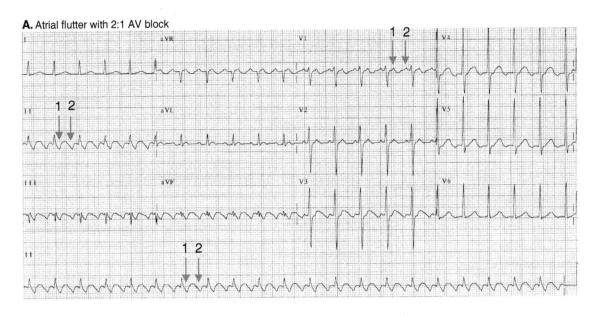

**B.** Atrial flutter with 2:1 AV block

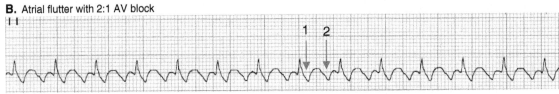

**Figure 18.5:    Atrial Flutter with 2:1 Atrioventricular (AV) Block.  (A)** A 12-lead electrocardiogram showing atrial flutter with 2:1 AV block. There are two flutter waves for every ventricular complex. The two flutter waves are identified by the arrows and are labeled 1 and 2. The first flutter wave in lead II (*arrow 1*) may be mistaken for S wave and the arrhythmia may be misdiagnosed as SVT. **(B)** Lead II rhythm strip from **(A)**, which is magnified to show the flutter waves (*arrows*).

## Lead II: Atrial flutter with 2:1 AV block

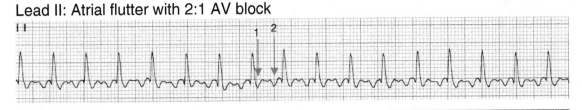

**Figure 18.6:    Atrial Flutter with 2:1 Atrioventricular Block.** The first flutter wave (*arrow 1*) deforms the terminal portion of the QRS complex and may be mistaken for an S wave. The second flutter wave (*arrow 2*) is more obvious and precedes the QRS complex but can be mistaken for an inverted P wave. Thus, the arrhythmia can be mistaken for supraventricular tachycardia.

## Lead II: Atrial flutter with 2:1 AV block

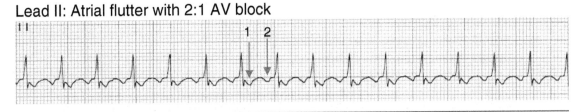

**Figure 18.7:    Atrial Flutter with 2:1 Atrioventricular Block.** The first flutter wave (*arrow 1*) may be mistaken for a depressed ST segment or inverted T wave.

**A.**

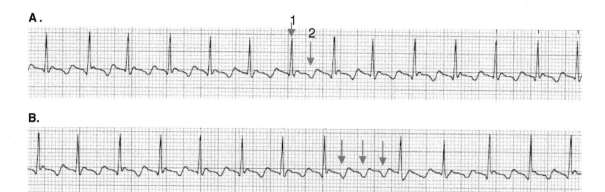

**B.**

**Figure 18.8:   Atrial Flutter with 2:1 Atrioventricular (AV) Block.** The diagnosis of atrial flutter with 2:1 AV block is not possible in rhythm strip **(A)**. The first flutter wave (*arrow 1*) is buried within the QRS complex and the second flutter wave (*arrow 2*) can be mistaken for an inverted T wave. The diagnosis became evident only after sudden spontaneous slowing of the ventricular rate **(B)** (*arrows*), revealing the classical saw tooth flutter waves between the QRS complexes.

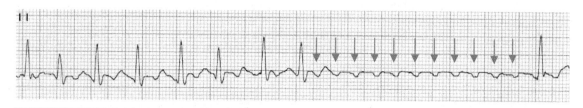

**Figure 18.9:   Atrial Flutter.** When the diagnosis is in doubt, carotid sinus stimulation may slow down the ventricular rate so that the flutter waves (*arrows*) can be identified. Atrial flutter will not convert to normal sinus rhythm with carotid sinus pressure or with atrioventricular nodal blockers.

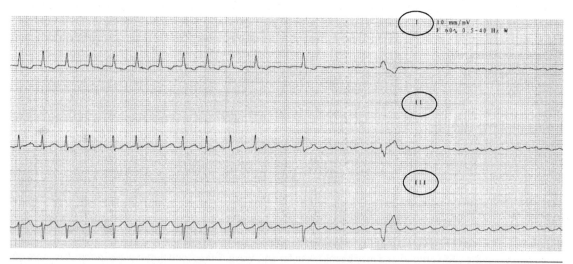

**Figure 18.10:   Atrial Flutter Resembling Atrioventricular Nodal Reentrant Tachycardia.** Leads I, II, and III are simultaneously recorded. A narrow complex tachycardia with a rate of 125 beats per minute is seen on the left half of the tracing. The tachycardia was thought to be due to AV nodal reentrant tachycardia because no obvious P waves were noted. Adenosine was given intravenously, resulting in AV block. Upright flutter waves are now obvious in leads II and III with a rate of 250 beats per minute (six small blocks). The tachycardia is due to atrial flutter with 2:1 AV block. AV, atrioventricular.

**Upright P waves, rate 200 ± 50 bpm**          **Flat or isoelectric baseline**

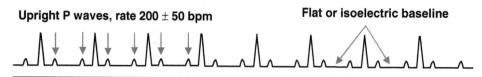

**Figure 18.11:   Atrial Tachycardia with 2:1 Atrioventricular Block.** The atrial rate is typically 200 ± 50 beats per minute and the P waves are upright and separated by an isoelectric or flat line in lead II.

**Inverted flutter waves:**
**(minimum rate 240-250 bpm)**

**Undulating or wavy baseline**

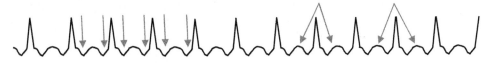

**Figure 18.12:** **Atrial Flutter with 2:1 Atrioventricular Block.** In atrial flutter, the atrial rate is 300 ± 50 beats per minute. The flutter waves are typically inverted in lead II (*arrows*) and are separated by a continuously wavy baseline.

## Atrial Flutter and Atrial Tachycardia with 2:1 AV Block

| Atrial Tachycardia with 2:1 AV Block |
| --- |
| • Atrial rate approximately 200 ± 50 bpm or 150 - 250 bpm |
| • Upright P waves in lead II |
| • Isoelectric baseline |

**Lead II**

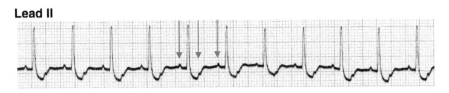

**Figure 18.13:** **Atrial Tachycardia with 2:1 Atrioventricular (AV) Block.** Lead II rhythm strip showing atrial tachycardia with 2:1 AV block with an atrial rate of 230 beats per minute (6.5 small blocks). In atrial tachycardia, the atrial rate is typically 150–250 beats per minute. Note also that the P waves are upright in lead II with an isoelectric baseline. Atrial tachycardia with 2:1 AV block is usually due to digitalis toxicity and the ST segment depression shown above is characteristic of digitalis effect.

| Atrial Flutter with 2:1 AV Block |
| --- |
| • Atrial rate approximately 300 ± 50 bpm (minimum rate 240-250 bpm) |
| • Inverted atrial complexes in lead II |
| • Undulating or wavy baseline |

**A. Before**                    Atrial rate = 1500/6 = 250 bpm

**B. After**                    Atrial rate = 1500/8 = 188 bpm

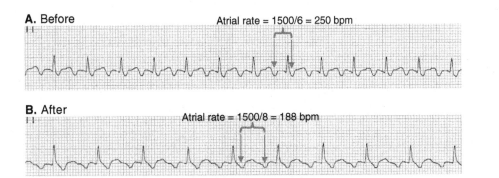

**Figure 18.14:** **Atrial Flutter (AF) Before and After Administration of Antiarrhythmic Agent.** Lead II rhythm strips from the same patient before **(A)** and after **(B)** giving sotalol orally. The atrial rate in AF can become slower than 240 to 250 beats per minute if an antiarrhythmic agent is given that can slow the atrial rate. **(A)** The atrial rate was 250 beats per minute before receiving sotalol. **(B)** The atrial rate had decreased to 188 beats per minute after therapy. The flutter waves retain their typically inverted pattern in lead II, an important feature in differentiating atrial tachycardia from atrial flutter with 2:1 atrioventricular block.

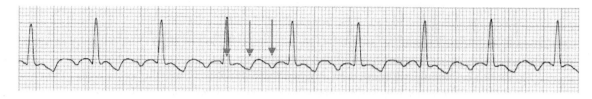

**Figure 18.15:    Atrial Flutter with 3:1 Atrioventricular Block.** Rhythm strip showing three flutter waves (*arrows*) for each QRS complex. The first flutter wave (*first arrow*) is buried within the QRS complex.

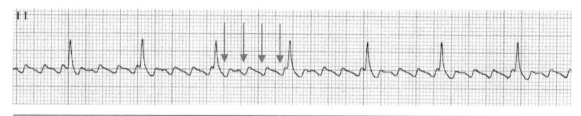

**Figure 18.16:    Atrial Flutter with 4:1 Atrioventricular Block.** There are four flutter waves (*arrows*) for each QRS complex.

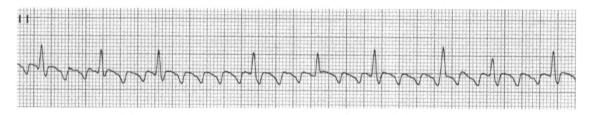

**Figure 18.17:    Atrial Flutter with Variable Atrioventricular (AV) Block.** The R-R intervals are irregular because conduction of the atrial impulse across the AV node is variable.

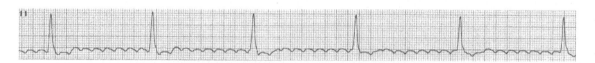

**Figure 18.18:    Atrial Flutter and Complete Atrioventricular (AV) Block.** Lead II rhythm strip showing atrial flutter with complete AV block. The R-R intervals are regular with a ventricular rate of 33 beats per minute. The atrial rate is 300 beats per minute.

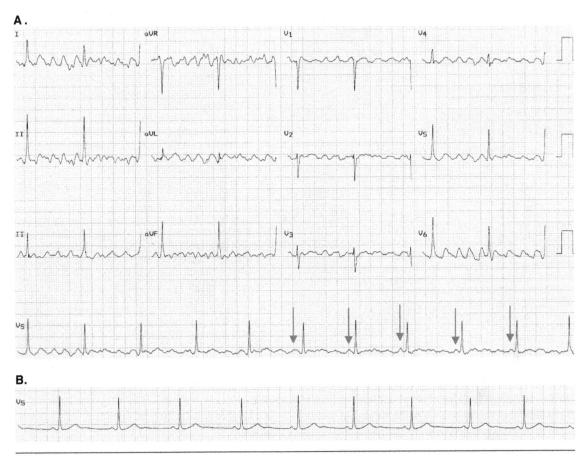

**Figure 18.19: Motion Artifacts Resembling Atrial Flutter. (A, B)** From the same patient. **(A)** Suspicious atrial flutter although distinct P waves are recognizable before each QRS complex in long lead V₅ (*arrows*). The repeat electrocardiogram after the electrodes were stabilized **(B)** distinctly shows that the rhythm is normal sinus and not atrial flutter.

4. The ventricular rate is variable depending on the number of atrial impulses conducted through the AV node.
5. The QRS complexes are narrow unless preexistent bundle branch block is present; the atrial impulses are conducted with aberration or are conducted through a bypass tract.

## Mechanism

■ Atrial flutter is a reentrant arrhythmia within the atria. It is usually precipitated by premature atrial complexes or repeti-

tive impulses originating from other areas contiguous to the atria such as the pulmonary veins.

■ **Typical atrial flutter:** The typical form of atrial flutter, which is the most common presentation, has a reentrant pathway located within the right atrium. The impulse travels down the lateral wall and up the atrial septum in a counterclockwise direction, resulting in negative or inverted flutter waves in leads II, III, and aVF and upright flutter waves in V₁. The reentrant circuit involves an area of slow conduction between the tricuspid orifice and

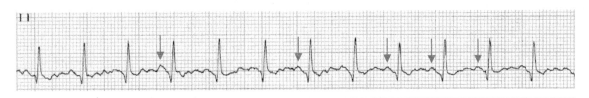

**Figure 18.20: "Atrial Flutter" due to Motion Artifacts.** Another example of "atrial flutter" due to motion artifacts is shown. P waves can still be identified preceding each QRS complex (*arrows*).

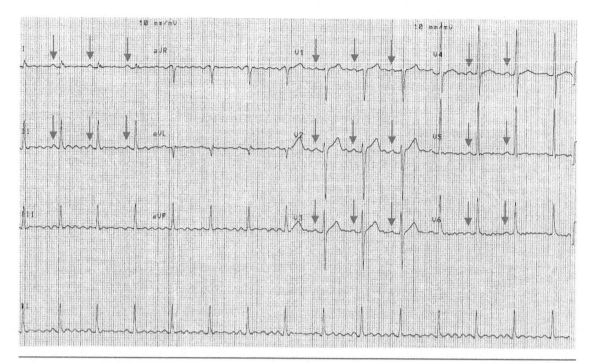

**Figure 18.21:    Artifacts Resembling Atrial Flutter.**  The patient was referred with a diagnosis of atrial flutter based on the electrocardiogram obtained from a doctor's office. The tracing shows that there are definite sinus P waves preceding the QRS complexes especially in leads I, II, and also in $V_1$ to $V_6$ (*arrows*). The rhythm therefore is not atrial flutter but normal sinus and the flutter-like undulations seen in leads II, III, and aVF are due to artifacts. Normal sinus rhythm was verified when the patient arrived for the consultation.

mouth of the inferior vena cava called the cavotricuspid isthmus. This is the usual site of radiofrequency ablation.

■ **Reverse typical atrial flutter:** The other form of atrial flutter, which is less common, has the same reentrant circuit but is reversed in direction. The atrial impulse travels down the atrial septum and up the lateral wall in a clock-

wise direction, resulting in flutter waves that are upright in leads II, III, and aVF and inverted in $V_1$.

■ The reentrant circuit in atrial flutter can also occur in other locations other than the right atrium and includes the left atrium, in the area of the pulmonary veins, or around a scar or surgical lesion within the atria. Atrial flutter within the

**A.** Lead II rhythm strip

**B.** Lead II rhythm strip

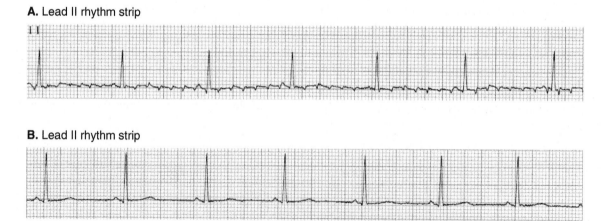

**Figure 18.22:    "Atrial Flutter" Caused by Infusion Pump.  (A, B)** From the same patient. The rhythm strip in **(A)** shows artifacts caused by infusion of intravenous fluids using an IVAC volumetric infusion pump. The artifacts can be mistaken for atrial flutter. The lead II rhythm strip in **(B)** was taken after the IV infusion pump was discontinued. IV, intravenous.

left atrium is more difficult to map because of its left atrial location.

## Clinical Significance

■ The incidence of atrial flutter is variable. It is more common in men than in women. Although atrial flutter may occasionally become persistent lasting for days or months, it seldom occurs as a chronic rhythm, very often converting to normal sinus rhythm or deteriorating to atrial fibrillation. Atrial flutter and atrial fibrillation are frequently associated arrhythmias.

■ Atrial flutter is usually associated with organic or structural cardiac disease or it may be precipitated by an acute condition.

  ■ An acute precipitating cause, usually surgery (cardiac or noncardiac), pneumonia, acute myocardial infarction, or congestive heart failure can be identified in 60% of cases.

  ■ The remaining cases are associated with chronic cardiac or pulmonary diseases or hypertension.

  ■ Atrial flutter not accompanied by structural cardiac disease or any precipitating condition is called lone atrial flutter. Lone atrial flutter is rare occurring only in 1.7% of all cases.

■ Atrial flutter with a rapid ventricular rate of 150 bpm with 2:1 AV conduction is the most frequent presentation in the acute setting. Less frequently, it may occur at a slower rate with a conduction ratio of 4:1. Atrial flutter with an odd conduction ratio of 1:1, 3:1, or 5:1 are much less common.

■ The rapid ventricular rate associated with atrial flutter may occur in patients with accessory pathways. It can also occur when there is increased adrenergic activity or when there is thyrotoxicosis. In patients with atrial fibrillation or atrial flutter who are being converted to normal sinus with Class IA (quinidine, procainamide, and disopyramide) and Class IC (propafenone or flecainide) agents, atrial flutter with 1:1 AV conduction can occur. Atrial flutter with fast ventricular rate may cause hemodynamic collapse and symptoms of low cardiac output, resulting in dizziness or frank syncope especially when there is left ventricular dysfunction or obstructive valvular disease.

■ Because atrial flutter follows a fixed pathway within the atria, the atrial rate is regular and is one of the most regular among all supraventricular tachyarrhythmias. Atrial flutter with 2:1 AV block may be confused with SVT, especially when one flutter wave is buried within the QRS complex and the other flutter wave is inscribed midway between two QRS complexes. The flutter waves can be identified by slowing the ventricular rate with vagal maneuvers or, if unsuccessful, with AV nodal blocking agents. Adenosine, however, should not be injected when the tachycardia has wide QRS complexes because hypotension or ventricular fibrillation may occur if the tachycardia turns out to be ventricular.

■ Atrial flutter with 2:1 AV block should be differentiated from atrial tachycardia with 2:1 AV block. Atrial tachycardia with 2:1 AV block is commonly associated with digitalis toxicity, whereas atrial flutter with 2:1 block may require more digitalis to slow the ventricular rate.

■ **Atrial rate:** In atrial flutter, the minimum atrial rate is 240 to 250 bpm. In atrial tachycardia with 2:1 AV block, the atrial rate is usually 200 ± 50 bpm.

■ **Morphology of the P waves:** In atrial flutter, the flutter waves are inverted in II, III, and aVF and the baseline between the flutter waves is usually wavy and undulating. In atrial tachycardia with 2:1 AV block, the P waves are upright in II, III, and aVF and the baseline between the P waves is usually isoelectric or flat.

■ Similar to atrial fibrillation, atrial flutter can cause systemic thromboembolism and the incidence of stroke approaches that of atrial fibrillation.

■ Because atrial flutter is associated with mechanical atrial contraction, the physical findings of atrial flutter often show jugular neck vein pulsations coincident with each flutter wave in the ECG. Thus, the number of atrial pulsations (A waves) will be faster than the ventricular rate because atrial flutter is usually associated with AV block. When there is variable AV block, an irregular heart rate will be present, which can be mistaken for atrial fibrillation. The intensity of the first heart sound is constant when the AV block is fixed but is variable when there is varying AV conduction.

## Therapy

■ In patients who are hemodynamically unstable and are hypotensive with low cardiac output, immediate direct current cardioversion is indicated and receives a Class I recommendation according to the 2003 American College of Cardiology/American Heart Association Task Force on Practice Guidelines, and the European Society of Cardiology practice guidelines for the management of patients with supraventricular arrhythmias. Immediate cardioversion is also indicated among stable patients and also carries a Class I recommendation since atrial flutter can be easily converted to normal sinus rhythm with low energy settings of 50 joules or less using monophasic shocks. Therapy of atrial flutter is similar to that of atrial fibrillation and includes three considerations:

  ■ Anticoagulation to prevent thromboembolism

  ■ Control of ventricular rate

  ■ Conversion of atrial flutter to normal sinus rhythm

■ **Anticoagulation to prevent thromboembolism:** Anticoagulation should always be considered in all patients if the duration of atrial flutter is ≥48 hours or the duration is not definitely known. Atrial flutter, similar to atrial fibrillation, is associated with increased incidence of thromboembolism. This is further discussed in Chapter 19, Atrial Fibrillation.

■ **Control of ventricular rate:** Control of ventricular rate in atrial flutter is frequently more difficult than control of ventricular rate in atrial fibrillation. The pharmacologic agents that are commonly used include AV nodal blocking agents such as calcium channel blockers (verapamil or diltiazem), beta blockers, digitalis, and amiodarone. The agent of choice depends on the clinical status of the patient. The following are the recommendations for control of ventricular rate in patients with atrial flutter according to the 2003 American College of Cardiology/American Heart Association Task Force on Practice Guidelines, and the European Society of Cardiology practice guidelines for supraventricular arrhythmias.

- **Poorly tolerated:** If the arrhythmia is poorly tolerated, direct current cardioversion to convert atrial flutter to normal sinus rhythm is a Class I recommendation. The use of nondihydropyridine calcium channel blockers (verapamil, diltiazem) or beta blockers (metoprolol, propranolol, or esmolol) are the most useful and effective agents in controlling ventricular rate in atrial flutter and receive a Class IIa recommendation. The beta blockers and calcium channel blockers have the same efficacy in slowing the ventricular rate. These agents are more effective than digitalis or amiodarone. Calcium blockers and beta blockers should not be used when there is acute decompensated heart failure or when the patient is hypotensive. Intravenous digoxin or amiodarone are the preferred agents and receive a Class IIb recommendation.

- **Stable patients:** Conversion of atrial flutter to normal sinus rhythm with direct current cardioversion or with the use of atrial or transesophageal pacing both receive Class I recommendation even among stable patients. Calcium channel blockers and beta blockers are the most effective agents and receive Class I recommendation for control of ventricular rate in atrial flutter. Digitalis and amiodarone are less effective and receive a Class IIb recommendation.

- **Conversion of atrial flutter to normal sinus rhythm:** AV nodal blockers, such as calcium channel blockers, beta blockers, and digoxin can slow AV conduction and control the ventricular rate, but are not effective in converting atrial flutter to normal sinus rhythm. Conversion of atrial flutter to normal sinus rhythm can be accomplished by the following:
  - Antiarrhythmic agents
  - Rapid atrial pacing
  - Electrical cardioversion
  - Catheter ablation
  - Antitachycardia devices
  - Surgery

- **Antiarrhythmic agents:** The use of antiarrhythmic agents in converting atrial flutter to normal sinus rhythm is reserved for stable patients. The following antiarrhythmic agents are effective in converting atrial flutter to normal sinus rhythm: Class IA antiarrhythmic agents (procainamide), Class IC (flecainide and propafenone), and Class III agents (amiodarone, ibutilide and sotalol). Among the antiarrhythmic agents mentioned, the only intravenous agents available in the United States are ibutilide, amiodarone, and procainamide.

  - **Ibutilide:** Ibutilide, a Class III antiarrhythmic agent, is the most effective in acutely converting atrial flutter to normal sinus rhythm. This agent receives a Class IIa recommendation in converting stable patients with atrial flutter to normal sinus rhythm. Up to 78% of atrial flutter will convert to normal sinus rhythm within 90 minutes of infusion. The drug is less effective in converting atrial fibrillation to normal sinus rhythm. For patients weighing >60 kg, an initial 1 mg dose is injected intravenously for 10 minutes. The same dose may be repeated after 10 minutes if the initial 1 mg bolus is not effective. Torsades de pointes can occur in 2% to 4% of cases. The drug should not be given if the QTc is prolonged, there is sick sinus syndrome, or left ventricular dysfunction.

  - **Procainamide:** Procainamide, a Class IA antiarrhythmic agent, is given intravenously with a loading dose of 10 to 14 mg/kg for 30 minutes. This is followed by a maintenance infusion of 1 to 4 mg/minute. Procainamide should be combined with AV nodal blocking agents because 1:1 AV conduction can occur during infusion. This agent receives a Class IIb recommendation for converting stable patients with atrial flutter to normal sinus rhythm.

  - **Amiodarone:** Amiodarone, a Class III antiarrhythmic agent, is effective in converting atrial flutter to normal sinus rhythm. It is also effective in controlling the ventricular rate of atrial flutter. The agent is not as effective as ibutilide, but is the least proarrhythmic and the drug of choice when left ventricular dysfunction is present. The dose of amiodarone for terminating atrial flutter is 5 mg/kg given intravenously in 10 minutes. This drug receives a Class IIb recommendation for both rate control and for conversion of atrial flutter to normal sinus rhythm.

  - **Other agents:** Propafenone and flecainide (Class IC agents) and sotalol (Class III agent) are not available as intravenous agents in the United States. Dosing is discussed in Chapter 19, Atrial Fibrillation. These agents receive a Class IIb recommendation for conversion of atrial flutter to normal sinus rhythm. Class IC agents should be combined with AV nodal blocking agents to prevent 1:1 AV conduction.

- **Rapid atrial pacing:** Although electrical cardioversion is very effective in converting atrial flutter to normal sinus rhythm, rapid atrial pacing may be preferable to electrical cardioversion since rapid atrial pacing does not require intravenous sedation. Among stable patients, atrial or transesophageal pacing carries a Class I recommendation for converting atrial flutter to normal sinus rhythm. Rapid atrial pacing is performed by introducing an electrode catheter transvenously into the right atrium. It can also be performed transesophageally by swallowing a pill electrode positioned behind the left atrium. The pacemaker impulse may be able to block the reentrant circuit causing the arrhythmia to terminate. Atrial fibrillation may develop during rapid atrial pacing, which is much easier to control with AV nodal blocking agents and is a more acceptable arrhythmia than atrial flutter. Conversion of atrial flutter to atrial fibrillation is considered a favorable outcome of atrial pacing. Atrial fibrillation may initially occur during transition from atrial flutter to normal sinus rhythm. There are two types of atrial flutter based on response to rapid atrial pacing:

- **Type I.** Atrial flutter is called type I if it can be converted to normal sinus rhythm with rapid atrial pacing. The atrial rate in type I atrial flutter is classically >240 bpm and includes both typical and reverse typical atrial flutter as well as atrial flutter associated with reentry around surgical lesions within the atria.
- **Type II.** Atrial flutter is called type II when it can not be interrupted by rapid atrial pacing. The atrial rate is more rapid than type I atrial flutter and exceeds 340 beats per minute.

- **Electrical cardioversion.** Atrial flutter is one of the most responsive arrhythmias that can be terminated successfully with very low energy settings. Approximately 25 to 50 joules or less may be enough to terminate atrial flutter especially if biphasic current is used. Fifty to 100 joules is usually needed during elective cardioversion and is effective in >95% of patients. Direct current cardioversion is the treatment of choice when rapid conversion to normal sinus rhythm is desired and receives a Class I recommendation for both stable and unstable patients.

- **Catheter ablation of the reentrant pathway:** Long-term therapy of atrial flutter especially when recurrent includes ablation of the reentrant pathway with an endocardial catheter. In typical atrial flutter, the reentry is confined to the right atrium and part of the pathway involves an area between the tricuspid orifice and mouth of the inferior vena cava called the cavotricuspid isthmus. This is the area where the reentrant circuit is usually interrupted by radiofrequency ablation.

- **Antitachycardia devices:** Permanent pacemakers are capable of delivering rapid atrial pacing and can be implanted in patients who are responsive to rapid atrial pacing. Devices capable of delivering shocks within the atrium are also capable of converting atrial flutter to normal sinus rhythm. These devices, however, are currently not available for clinical use.

- **Surgery:** This is similar to radiofrequency ablation except that surgery is performed to ablate the reentrant circuit. This approach is feasible in patients who are also scheduled to undergo coronary bypass surgery or open heart surgery for valvular disease.

## Prognosis

- Unlike atrial fibrillation, atrial flutter does not continue indefinitely and usually lasts only for a few days or a few weeks, although atrial flutter have been documented to last for several years. Atrial flutter usually degenerates to atrial fibrillation. It can result in tachycardia-mediated cardiomyopathy if the ventricular rate is not controlled. It may also cause thromboembolic events similar to atrial fibrillation.

- Atrial flutter is usually associated with cardiac or pulmonary disease or an acute precipitating event. Unlike lone atrial fibrillation where 10% to 30% of patients do not have associated cardiac or pulmonary disease, lone atrial flutter is rare. The prognosis of atrial flutter therefore depends on the underlying condition.

## Suggested Readings

Blomstrom-Lundqvist C, Scheinman MM, Aliot EM, et al. ACC/AHA/ESC guidelines for the management of patients with supraventricular arrhythmias—executive summary. A report of the American College of Cardiology/American Heart Association Task Force on Practice Guidelines, and the European Society of Cardiology Committee for Practice Guidelines (Writing Committee to Develop Guidelines for the Management of Patients with Supraventricular Arrhythmias). *J Am Coll Cardiol.* 2003;42:1493–1531.

Fuster V, Ryden LE, Cannom DS, et al. ACC/AHA/ESC 2006 Guidelines for the management of patients with atrial fibrillation: A report of the American College of Cardiology/American Heart Association Task Force on Practice Guidelines and the European Society of Cardiology Committee for Practice Guidelines (Writing Committee to Revise 2001 Guidelines for the Management of Patients with Atrial Fibrillation). *J Am Coll Cardiol.* 2006;48:e149–e246.

Ghali WA, Wasil BI, Brant R, et al. Atrial flutter and the risk of thromboembolism: a systematic review and meta-analysis. *Am J Med.* 2005;118:101–107.

Saoudi N, Cosio F, Waldo A, et al. A classification of atrial flutter and regular atrial tachycardia according to electrophysiological mechanisms and anatomical basis. A statement from a joint expert group from the working group of arrhythmias of the European Society of Cardiology and the North American Society of Pacing and Electrophysiology. *Eur Heart J.* 2001; 22:1162–1182.

Waldo AL, Biblo LA. Atrioventricular nodal-independent supraventricular tachycardias. In: Topol E, ed. *Textbook in Cardiovascular Medicine.* 2nd ed. Philadelphia: Lippincott Williams & Wilkins; 2002:1429–1451.

Wellens HJJ. Contemporary management of atrial flutter. *Circulation.* 2002:106:649–652.

# 19

# Atrial Fibrillation

## Electrocardiogram Findings

- **Prevalence:** Atrial fibrillation (AF) is the most common sustained arrhythmia that one encounters in clinical practice. It accounts for approximately one third of all hospitalizations from cardiac arrhythmias. In the general population, approximately 2.2 million Americans or <1% have AF; however, the prevalence varies according to the age group and is higher in the elderly.
  - AF is rare in children and young adults.
  - It is also rare in individuals younger than age 60 years because <1% of the population in this age group has AF.
  - It increases to more than 8% among patients older than 80 years of age.
  - The median age of patients with AF is approximately 75 years.
- **Electrocardiogram (ECG) findings:** AF is a common cause of stroke in the elderly. AF therefore should be recognized because the risk of stroke can be minimized if the arrhythmia is treated appropriately. The following are the ECG features of AF.
  - Presence of very irregular and disorganized atrial activity represented in the ECG as fibrillatory waves. These fibrillatory waves, also called "F" waves, are due to several independent reentrant wavelets within the atria (Fig. 19.1).
  - The fibrillatory waves may be fine or coarse and have varying morphologies, which can be mistaken for P waves.

- Fibrillatory waves may not be present. Instead, a flat line with irregularly irregular R-R intervals may be present.
- The atrial rate in AF is ≥350 beats per minute (bpm).
- The ventricular rate is irregularly irregular and depends on the number of atrial impulses conducted through the atrioventricular (AV) node.
- The QRS complexes are narrow unless there is bundle branch block, aberrant conduction, or preexcitation.

## Atrial Fibrillation

- **Atrial rate:** There are no distinct P waves in AF. Instead, fibrillatory or F waves are present with a rate that exceeds 350 bpm. The F waves vary in size and shape and may be coarse or fine or, in some instances, it may not be visible in any lead of a complete 12-lead ECG. When fibrillatory waves are not visible, the diagnosis of AF is based on the presence of irregularly irregular R-R intervals as shown (Fig. 19.2B).

### Ventricular Rate

- **Ventricular rate:** The ventricular response during AF is irregularly irregular and the rate will depend on the state of the AV node. When there is heightened parasympathetic activity or AV nodal disease, the ventricular rate may be very slow. Conversely, when there increased sympathetic activity, the ventricular rate may be very

## Lead II

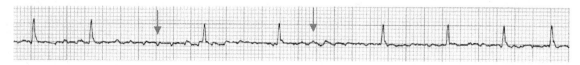

**Figure 19.1:    Atrial Fibrillation.** Rhythm strip showing atrial fibrillation. Note the presence of fibrillatory waves (*arrows*) between irregularly irregular R-R intervals.

**A.**

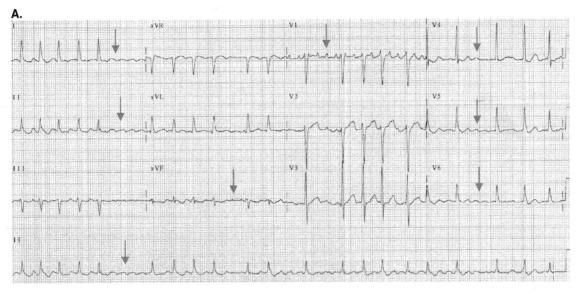

**B.**

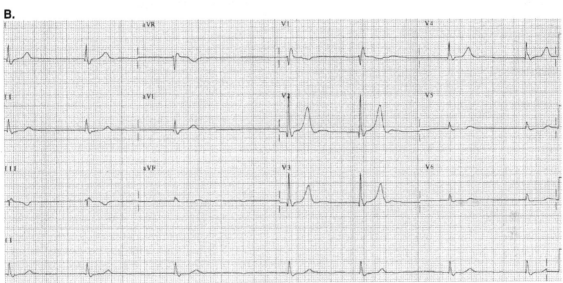

**Figure 19.2:    Atrial Fibrillation.** Two different ECGs are shown. **(A)** AF with fibrillatory waves in V₁ and in several other leads marked by the arrows. **(B)** Twelve-lead ECG from another patient with AF showing absence of atrial activity with virtually no fibrillatory waves in the whole tracing. The diagnosis of AF is based on the presence of irregularly irregular R-R intervals. AF, atrial fibrillation; ECG, electrocardiogram.

rapid. Because the ventricular rate in AF is irregularly irregular, the heart rate should be calculated using a long lead rhythm strip rather than using only the distance between two QRS complexes, as shown in the following section.

- **Six second time lines:** If 3-second time lines are present in the ECG monitor strip, 6 seconds can be easily measured. This is equivalent to 30 large blocks in the ECG paper (Fig. 19.3). The number of QRS complexes are counted inside the 6-second time line and multiplied by 10 to give the heart rate per minute. The first QRS complex is not counted because this serves as baseline.

- **Ten seconds:** If the heart rate is very slow, a longer interval such as 10 seconds is measured. This is equivalent to 50 large blocks (Fig. 19.4). The number of QRS complexes counted within the 10-second interval multiplied by 6 is the heart rate per minute. Again, the first QRS complex is not counted.

## The Ventricular Rate in AF

- The ventricular rate during AF can be slow or rapid as shown in Figs. 19.5A-E. When the ventricular rate is

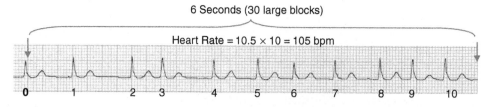

**Figure 19.3: Six-Second Markers.** Thirty large blocks is equivalent to 6 seconds. In this example, there are 10.5 QRS complexes within the 6-second time markers, thus the heart rate is 10.5 × 10 = 105 beats per minute.

slow (Figs. 19.5A–C), AF can be easily recognized. However, when the ventricular rate is faster (Fig. 19.5D,E), AF is more difficult to diagnose because the QRS complexes are clustered together and the undulating baseline and irregularly irregular R-R intervals become more difficult to evaluate.

## Clinical Classification of AF

- **Classification:** AF may be classified according to its clinical rather than its electrocardiographic presentation. The American College of Cardiology/American Heart Association Task Force on Practice Guidelines, and the European Society of Cardiology Committee (ACC/AHA/ESC) 2006 guidelines for the management of AF identify several types of AF.
  - **Nonvalvular AF:** AF is considered nonvalvular when it occurs in the absence of rheumatic mitral valve disease, prosthetic heart valve, or mitral valve repair.
  - **Valvular AF:** AF is considered valvular when it is associated with rheumatic mitral stenosis, prosthetic heart valve, or the patient has previously undergone valve repair.
  - **Lone AF:** AF occurring in individuals <60 years of age with structurally normal hearts and no evidence of pulmonary disease. These individuals are not hypertensive and have no clinical or echocardiographic evidence of cardiac or pulmonary disease. These patients are important to identify because they are low risk for thromboembolism.

- **First detected:** As the name implies, AF is detected for the first time, regardless of duration or previous episodes. A number of patients with first-detected AF have the potential to revert to normal sinus rhythm spontaneously.
- **Recurrent:** AF is recurrent if two or more episodes have occurred. The AF may be paroxysmal or persistent.
- **Paroxysmal:** When recurrent AF has sudden onset and abrupt termination. The episodes are usually self terminating lasting for <7 days with most episodes lasting <2 hours.
- **Persistent:** AF is persistent if the arrhythmia is more than 7 days in duration. This also includes AF of much longer duration, including those lasting for more than 1 year. In persistent AF, the episodes are no longer self terminating, although the AF can be terminated with pharmacologic agents or with electrical cardioversion.
- **Permanent:** AF is permanent if the arrhythmia can no longer be converted to normal sinus rhythm with electrical cardioversion or pharmacologic agents. The arrhythmia is usually persistent, lasting >1 year, or a previous electrical cardioversion has failed.

- **Associated diseases:** The most common diseases associated with AF include hypertension, ischemic heart disease, heart failure, valvular diseases, and diabetes mellitus.
- **Mechanism:** AF is a reentrant arrhythmia characterized by the presence of multiple independent reentrant wavelets within the atria (Fig. 19.6). The fibrillatory waves have a rate of >350 bpm. These fibrillatory waves are often precipitated by premature atrial complexes

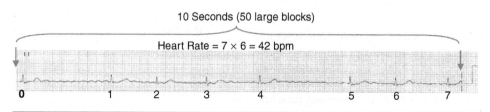

**Figure 19.4: Ten-Second Markers.** When the heart rate is very slow, 10 seconds is a more accurate marker. This is equivalent to 50 large blocks. In the above example, there are seven QRS complexes within the 10-second time marks. The heart rate is 7 × 6 = 42 beats per minute.

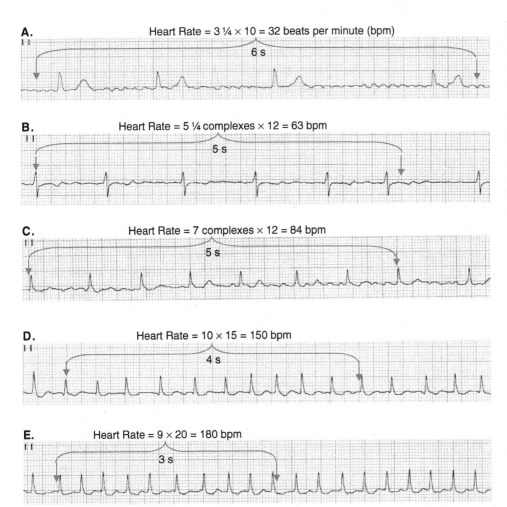

**A.** Heart Rate = 3 ¼ × 10 = 32 beats per minute (bpm)
6 s

**B.** Heart Rate = 5 ¼ complexes × 12 = 63 bpm
5 s

**C.** Heart Rate = 7 complexes × 12 = 84 bpm
5 s

**D.** Heart Rate = 10 × 15 = 150 bpm
4 s

**E.** Heart Rate = 9 × 20 = 180 bpm
3 s

**Figure 19.5: Atrial Fibrillation (AF).** AF is usually recognized by the irregularly irregular R-R intervals and undulating baseline. As the ventricular rate becomes faster **(A–E)**, the R-R intervals become less irregular. The ventricular rate in rhythm strip **(E)** is so rapid that the R-R interval almost looks regular and can be mistaken for supraventricular tachycardia instead of AF.

originating from the atrial wall or crista terminalis (Fig. 19.7). More recently, it has been shown that AF can also be initiated by repetitive firing of automatic foci within the pulmonary veins. These rapidly firing automatic foci may occur in one or more pulmonary veins. They cannot be recorded in the surface ECG, but can be recorded with intracardiac techniques. These ectopic impulses can also originate from large veins draining into the atria, including the superior vena cava and coronary sinus, and can precipitate AF when there is appropriate substrate for reentry.

## Common Mistakes in AF

- **Atrial fibrillation can be mistaken for supraventricular tachycardia:** As previously mentioned, when the ventricular rate is unusually rapid, the R-R interval may look regular because the QRS complexes are clustered very close together. Thus, AF with a very rapid ventricular rate can be mistaken for supraventricular tachycardia (Fig. 19.8). The diagnosis of AF can be ascertained by slowing the ventricular rate with vagal

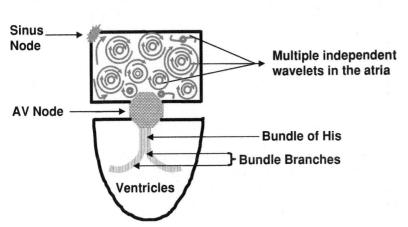

Sinus Node

AV Node

Multiple independent wavelets in the atria

Bundle of His
Bundle Branches

Ventricles

**Figure 19.6: Diagrammatic Representation of Atrial Fibrillation (AF).** AF is a reentrant arrhythmia characterized by the presence of multiple independent wavelets within the atria with an atrial rate of >350 beats per minute. These reentrant wavelets can be precipitated by ectopic impulses originating from the pulmonary veins as well as other large veins draining into the atria.

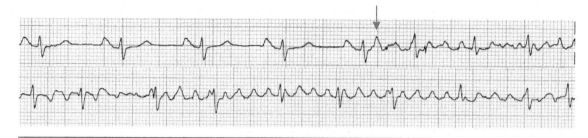

**Figure 19.7:** **Premature Atrial Complex (PAC) Precipitating Atrial Fibrillation.** Rhythm strip showing a single PAC (*arrow*) precipitating atrial fibrillation. The rhythm strips are continuous.

maneuvers such as carotid sinus pressure. When carotid sinus pressure is applied, an irregularly irregular R-R interval with fibrillatory or undulating baseline can be demonstrated between the QRS complexes (Fig. 19.9).

■ **AF can be mistaken for multifocal atrial tachycardia:** The fibrillatory waves, especially when they are coarse, may be mistaken for P waves. Some of these fibrillatory or "F" waves may be inscribed before the QRS complexes. When this occurs, AF may be mistaken for multifocal atrial tachycardia (Fig. 19.10). In multifocal atrial tachycardia, anticoagulation is not necessary because this arrhythmia is not associated with increased risk of thromboembolic events, whereas in AF, anticoagulation is standard therapy for the prevention of stroke, especially in high-risk patients.

■ AF may be diagnosed even when fibrillatory waves are absent by the irregularly irregular R-R intervals (Fig. 19.11). However, in patients with permanently implanted ventricular pacemakers (Fig. 19.12), patients

with complete AV dissociation (Fig. 19.13), or complete AV block (Fig. 19.14), the R-R intervals may become completely regular. If there are no fibrillatory waves present, the diagnosis of AF may be missed completely. Patients with unrecognized AF are at risk for stroke as these patients will not be treated appropriately.

■ **AF with regular R-R intervals:** The ventricular rate in AF is irregularly irregular. The ventricular rate can become regular when there is complete AV dissociation or complete AV block.

■ **Complete AV dissociation:** AF with complete AV dissociation is frequently due to digitalis toxicity. Digitalis blocks the AV node and excites the AV junction and ventricles resulting in junctional or ventricular ectopic rhythms. AF with an irregularly irregular R-R interval that suddenly becomes regular may be due to digitalis toxicity (Fig. 19.13). In complete AV dissociation, the ventricles are no longer controlled by the AF, but rather by a separate

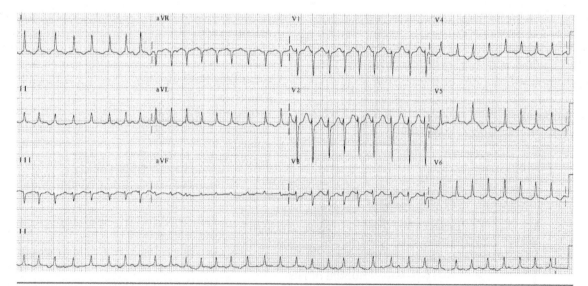

**Figure 19.8:** **Atrial Fibrillation with Rapid Ventricular Response.** When the ventricular rate is very rapid, the irregularity in the R-R intervals may not be obvious. The arrhythmia can be mistaken for supraventricular tachycardia especially when F waves are not grossly apparent. Note, however, that the R-R intervals are not regular. Carotid sinus stimulation may be helpful in establishing the diagnosis.

Carotid Sinus Stimulation

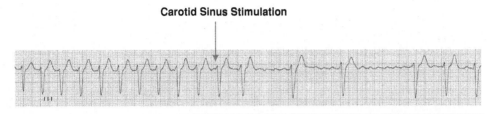

**Figure 19.9:    Carotid Sinus Stimulation.**  The rhythm looks regular and can be mistaken for supraventricular tachycardia. When the diagnosis of AF is in doubt, carotid sinus stimulation may be helpful in differentiating AF from other narrow complex supraventricular arrhythmias. Carotid sinus stimulation (*arrow*) causes slowing of the ventricular rate resulting in prolongation of the R-R interval. This will allow identification of a wavy baseline representing the fibrillating atria. AF, atrial fibrillation.

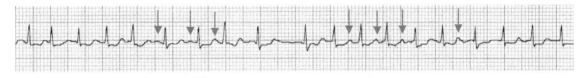

**Figure 19.10:    Atrial Fibrillation (AF).**  The coarse F waves may be mistaken for P waves (*arrows*) and AF may be misdiagnosed as multifocal atrial tachycardia.

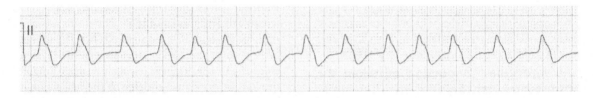

**Figure 19.11:    Atrial Fibrillation (AF).**  Even in the absence of fibrillatory waves between QRS complexes, AF may be diagnosed by the irregularly irregular R-R intervals as shown (*above*). However, when the R-R intervals are regular (*below*) the diagnosis of AF may be difficult.

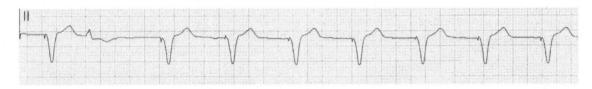

**Figure 19.12:    Atrial Fibrillation.**  The presence of atrial fibrillation may be difficult to diagnose in a patient with a ventricular pacemaker if there are no fibrillatory waves in baseline electrocardiogram as shown. The presence of atrial fibrillation was suspected only after the patient sustained a transient ischemic attack.

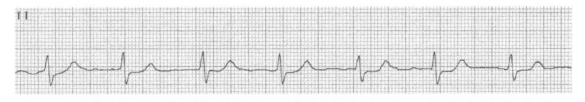

**Figure 19.13:    Atrial Fibrillation (AF) with Complete Atrioventricular (AV) Dissociation.**  This patient with known chronic AF suddenly developed regular R-R intervals because of AV dissociation. When the ventricular rate in atrial fibrillation suddenly regularizes, the etiology is usually digitalis toxicity.

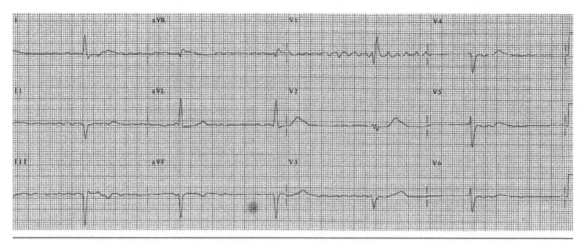

**Figure 19.14: Atrial Fibrillation (AF) and Complete Atrioventricular (AV) Block.** The rhythm is AF although the R-R intervals are regular. The QRS complexes are wide with a very slow rate of approximately 33 beats per minute. The rhythm is AF with complete AV block.

pacemaker, usually the AV junction with a regular rate that exceeds 60 bpm.

- **Complete AV Block:** When there is complete AV block, the atrial fibrillatory impulses will not be able to conduct to the ventricles. An AV junctional or ventricular escape rhythm usually comes to the rescue; otherwise, the ventricles will become asystolic. In complete AV block, the ventricular rate is slow and regular usually in the mid to low 40s (Fig. 19.14).

- **Aberrant ventricular conduction mistaken for premature ventricular complex:** Premature atrial impulses are normally conducted to the ventricles with narrow QRS complexes very similar to a normal sinus impulse. If the impulse is too premature, it may find one of the bundle branches still refractory from the previous impulse and will be conducted with a wide QRS complex. These premature atrial impulses that are followed by wide QRS complexes are aberrantly conducted impulses, which can be mistaken for premature

ventricular complex. Aberrantly conducted atrial impulses usually have right bundle branch block configuration with rSR' pattern in $V_1$ because the right bundle branch has a longer refractory period than the left bundle branch in most individuals.

- **Ashman phenomenon:** In AF, the R-R intervals are irregularly irregular. Some R-R intervals are longer and other R-R intervals are shorter. When the R-R intervals are longer or the heart rate is slower, the refractory period of the conduction tissues becomes longer. When the R-R intervals are shorter or the heart rate is faster, the refractory period is shorter. If a long R-R interval is followed by a short R-R interval (long/short cycle), the atrial impulse may find the right bundle branch still refractory from the previous impulse and will be conducted with a wide QRS complex. This aberrantly conducted complex is the second complex (the complex with a short cycle following a long cycle), as shown in Figure 19.15. This variability in the refractory period of

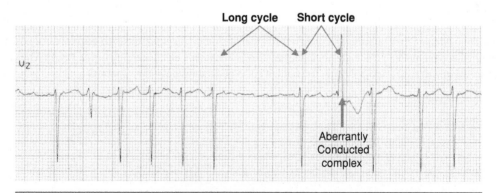

**Figure 19.15: Ventricular Aberration.** Arrow pointing up shows an aberrantly conducted supraventricular impulse, which is the second QRS complex after a long R-R interval. Aberrantly conducted complexes are wide usually with a right bundle branch block pattern. The wide QRS complex can be easily mistaken for a premature ventricular complex.

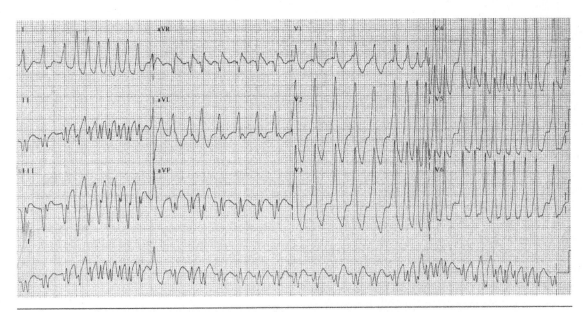

**Figure 19.16:   Atrial Fibrillation (AF) and Wolff-Parkinson-White (WPW) Syndrome.** Note the presence of irregularly irregular R-R intervals with very bizarre QRS complexes because of AF with varying degrees of ventricular fusion. AF occurring in the presence of WPW syndrome may result in hemodynamic instability and sudden cardiac death due to ventricular fibrillation.

the conduction system during long/short cycles in AF is called the Ashman phenomenon.

## Atrial Fibrillation and Wolff-Parkinson-White Syndrome

- **Atrial fibrillation and Wolff-Parkinson-White (WPW) syndrome:** The most dreadful complication of AF can occur in patients with WPW syndrome (see Chapter 20, Wolff-Parkinson-White Syndrome). In WPW syndrome, an accessory pathway connects the atrium directly to the ventricles; thus, the atrial impulse can reach the ventricles not only through the AV node but also through the bypass tract. AF associated with a bypass tract can deteriorate to ventricular fibrillation and can cause sudden cardiac death (Fig. 19.16).
  - Unlike the AV node, which consists of special cells with long refractory periods, the bypass tract consists of ordinary working myocardium with much shorter refractory period. Thus, during atrial flutter (atrial rate ≥250 bpm) or AF (atrial rate ≥350 bpm), the rapid atrial impulses which are normally delayed or blocked at the AV node due to its longer refractory period, may be conducted directly to the ventricles through the bypass tract resulting in very rapid ventricular rate.
  - AV nodal blocking agents are standard drugs for controlling the ventricular rate in AF. These drugs

are contraindicated when there is WPW syndrome because they enhance conduction across the bypass tract resulting in rapid ventricular rate and hemodynamic collapse (see Chapter 20, Wolff-Parkinson-White Syndrome).

## ECG Findings

1. Fibrillatory waves are present in baseline ECG representing disorganized atrial activity.
2. The R-R intervals are irregularly irregular.
3. The ventricular rate is variable and depends on the number of atrial impulses conducted through the AV node. In younger individuals, the ventricular rate is faster and usually varies from 120 to 150 bpm, but is slower in older individuals.
4. The QRS complexes are narrow unless there is preexistent bundle branch block, ventricular aberration, or preexcitation.

## Mechanism

- In AF, multiple independent reentrant wavelets are present within the atria. These reentrant wavelets may be precipitated by premature atrial complexes or spontaneous depolarizations originating from pulmonary veins as well as other large veins draining into the atria.
- For AF to become sustained, the atria is usually enlarged and structural changes such as scarring and fibrosis are usually present. These structural changes in the atria provide a substrate for reentry.

## Clinical Significance

■ The prevalence of AF increases with age. At age 50, approximately 0.5% have AF. This increases to more than 8% by age 80 years. The median age of a patient with AF is 75 years. The incidence of AF is higher among patients with congestive heart failure and high blood pressure, which can be reduced with angiotensin-converting enzyme inhibitors or with angiotensin receptor blockers.

■ AF and atrial flutter are the only two arrhythmias that increase the risk for stroke and thromboembolism. The thrombus is usually located in the left atrial appendage. Thrombus confined to the left atrial appendage can not be diagnosed by transthoracic echocardiography. Transesophageal echo is the best imaging modality that can detect a left atrial appendage thrombus.

■ **Valvular AF:** Valvular AF includes patients with AF associated with rheumatic mitral valve disease, especially those with mitral stenosis and patients with prosthetic mitral valve or previous mitral valve repair. These patients are high risk for stroke and should be adequately anticoagulated with warfarin.

■ **Nonvalvular AF:** Patients with AF who do not have any of these features have nonvalvular AF. The risk of stroke for patients with nonvalvular AF is low unless they have markers that increase their risk for thromboembolism. These markers come under the eponym of $CHADS_2$ (Cardiac failure, Hypertension, Age >75 years, Diabetes, and Stroke). History of stroke or previous transient ischemic attack carries a risk that is twice that of the other risks features, thus a factor of 2 is added under Stroke.

■ **Lone AF:** When AF is not associated with any known cause or any evidence of cardiopulmonary disease in a patient younger than 60 years of age, lone AF is present. This is seen in up to 20% to 25% of all patients with persistent AF. Patients with lone AF should be identified because these patients are low risk for thromboembolism.

■ AF may be reversible and transient when it occurs acutely in the setting of pneumonia or other acute respiratory infections, acute myocarditis, pericarditis, thyrotoxicosis, pulmonary embolism, acute myocardial infarction, or after cardiac or noncardiac surgery. It may also be precipitated by excess intake of alcohol often called "holiday heart syndrome" and other metabolic abnormalities. AF may spontaneously convert to normal sinus rhythm if the cause is reversible and may not recur when these conditions are corrected or stabilized.

■ Symptoms of AF may vary from a completely asymptomatic patient to one with frank syncope. When the ventricular rate is unusually rapid exceeding 150 bpm, symptoms of hypotension, dizziness, even frank syncope, congestive heart failure, or myocardial ischemia may occur because of decreased cardiac output. The decreased cardiac output is due to loss of atrial contribution to left ventricular (LV) filling. The rapid ventricular rate also shortens diastole further decreasing ventricular filling.

■ AF can cause tachycardia mediated cardiomyopathy. It may precipitate heart failure and pulmonary edema in patients with LV dysfunction and stenotic valves including mitral stenosis especially when the ventricular rate is not controlled.

■ When AF is present, the most common underlying abnormality is usually hypertension or coronary artery disease. Other frequent underlying conditions associated with AF include cardiomyopathy, hyperthyroidism, valvular heart disease (especially mitral stenosis or insufficiency), chronic obstructive pulmonary disease, and pericarditis.

■ Congestive heart failure, regardless of etiology, is now increasingly recognized as a cause of AF. The use of angiotensin-converting enzyme inhibitors and blockers of the renin-angiotensin aldosterone system has been shown to decrease the incidence of AF in patients with heart failure as well as in patients with high blood pressure, especially those with LV hypertrophy.

■ The physical findings in AF include:

  ■ Disappearance of the jugular "A" waves in the neck because of the loss of normal sinus rhythm

  ■ Absence of fourth heart sound

  ■ Varying intensity of the first heart sound because of the varying R-R intervals. When the R-R interval is prolonged, the intensity of the first heart sound is softer. When the R-R interval is short, the intensity of the first heart sound is louder.

  ■ When a systolic murmur is present, AF may be useful in differentiating whether the heart murmur is outflow (aortic stenosis or functional murmur) or inflow (mitral regurgitation) in origin. If the intensity of the murmur increases after a long R-R interval, the murmur is outflow in origin. If the intensity of the murmur does not change following a long R-R interval, the murmur is due to mitral regurgitation.

## Treatment

■ Treatment of AF is similar to that of atrial flutter and revolves around three conditions:

  ■ **Rate control:** The ventricular rate should be adequately controlled in *all* patients with AF.

  ■ **Rhythm control:** AF should be converted to normal sinus rhythm with electrical cardioversion or pharmacologic therapy in *selected* patients with AF.

  ■ **Prevention of thromboembolism:** Anticoagulation is one of the cornerstones in the therapy of AF. It should be considered in *all* patients who are high risk for stroke.

## Rate Control

■ The ventricular rate should always be adequately controlled in all patients with AF. ABCD are the drugs of choice for controlling the ventricular rate in AF as well as in atrial flutter (Amiodarone, Beta blockers, Calcium channel blockers, Digoxin). The drugs of choice are not necessarily in alphabetical order. Beta blockers, nondihydropyridine calcium channel blockers, and digoxin are effective for rate control. They are not effective in converting AF to normal sinus rhythm. They should not be given when there is preexcitation. Amiodarone is effective both for rate control and for rhythm control (conversion of AF to normal sinus rhythm) but has several side effects and is not approved by the Food and Drug Administration for rate control or for rhythm control in AF. This agent nevertheless is included as a therapeutic agent based on recommended guidelines and clinical efficacy reported in the literature.

- The choice of the most appropriate agent for controlling the ventricular rate in AF in the acute setting depends on the clinical presentation.
  - **Normal systolic function:** In stable patients with normal systolic function, intravenous nondihydropyridine calcium channel blockers and beta blockers receive Class I recommendation for control of ventricular rate in AF. Intravenous digoxin or amiodarone also receive Class I recommendation when there is LV dysfunction and heart failure or when the use of other AV nodal blocking agents are inappropriate.
    - **Nondihydropyridine calcium channel blockers:**
      - **Diltiazem:** Diltiazem is a nondihydropyridine calcium channel blocker. The initial dose is 0.25 mg/kg (or 15 to 20 mg) given IV over 2 minutes. The heart rate and blood pressure should be monitored carefully. The drug has a rapid onset of action and should control the ventricular rate within 5 to 10 minutes of administration. If the heart rate remains tachycardic 10 minutes after the initial bolus, a higher dose of 0.35 mg/kg (or 20 to 25 mg) is given IV similar to the first dose. The second dose may be more hypotensive than the initial dose and should be given more slowly. This will allow the blood pressure and heart rate to be monitored more carefully while the drug is being administered. When the heart rate is controlled, usually below 100 bpm, a maintenance dose of 5 to 15 mg/hour (usually 10 mg/hr) is infused. Diltiazem has a short half life of 3 to 4 hours, but becomes more prolonged when maintenance infusion is added. The IV maintenance dose is titrated according to the desired heart rate. An oral maintenance dose of diltiazem is started within 3 hours after the initial IV dose so that the IV infusion can be discontinued within 24 hours. The total oral dose is usually 1.5 times the expected 24-hour cumulative IV dose. A total of 120 to 360 mg of short-acting diltiazem is given orally in three to four divided doses. A long-acting preparation can be given once or twice daily.
      - **Verapamil:** Verapamil is another nondihydropyridine calcium channel blocker. The initial dose is 0.075 to 0.15 mg/kg (or 5 to 10 mg) given IV over 2 minutes. The same dose can be repeated after 15 to 30 minutes if needed. Verapamil has a longer duration of action of 4 to 12 hours and, unlike diltiazem, does not need a continuous maintenance IV infusion. It is more hypotensive and more negatively inotropic than diltiazem; thus, the patient should be carefully monitored especially if the patient is already on a beta blocker. The hypotension may respond to calcium gluconate given 1 gram IV. Oral maintenance dose is 120 to 360 mg daily in divided doses. A long-acting preparation can be given once daily.
  - **Beta blockers:** Beta blockers are preferred in patients with myocardial ischemia or thyrotoxicosis and also receive Class I recommendation for rate control.
    - **Metoprolol:** Metoprolol is a selective $\beta_1$ blocker. The initial dose is 2.5 to 5 mg IV over 2 minutes up to three doses (maximum dose of 15 mg given within 15 minutes). This is followed by an oral maintenance dose of 25 to 100 mg (usually 50 mg) given twice daily. The oral dose is titrated according to the desired heart rate.
    - **Atenolol:** Atenolol is also a selective $\beta_1$ blocker. It does not carry indication for controlling the ventricular rate of AF, but is approved for use in hypertension and acute myocardial infarction. The initial dose is 5 mg IV over 5 minutes. A second dose may be given 10 minutes later if needed, for a total intravenous dose of 10 mg. This is followed by an oral dose of 50 mg 10 minutes after the last intravenous dose and another 50 mg 12 hours later. A maintenance oral dose of 50 mg is given once daily. The oral dose is titrated according to the desired heart rate.
    - **Propranolol:** This is a nonselective $\beta_1$ $\beta_2$ blocker. The initial dose is 0.15 mg/kg IV. Up to 10 mg is given slowly IV at 1 mg per minute. The IV dose is followed by an oral dose of 80 to 240 mg daily given in divided doses. The oral dose is titrated according to the heart rate. A long-acting preparation is also available and is given once daily.
    - **Esmolol:** This agent is ultra–short-acting with a half-life of 9 minutes. A loading dose is needed, which is 0.5 mg/kg (500 mcg/kg) infused over a minute. This is followed by an initial maintenance dose of 0.05 mg/kg/min (50 mcg/kg/minute) infused for 4 minutes. The patient is evaluated after 5 minutes if a higher maintenance dose is needed. The patient should be carefully monitored during infusion so that the appropriate maintenance dose can be adjusted, which can vary up to 60 to 200 mcg/kg/minute. See Appendix: Commonly Used Injectable Pharmacologic Agents for further dosing.
  - **Digoxin:** This agent is not the preferred agent when LV function is preserved. However, when there is hypotension (preventing the use of calcium channel blockers or beta blockers) or the patient has bronchospastic pulmonary disease (preventing the use of beta blockers)

or patient has LV dysfunction or heart failure, this agent receives a Class I recommendation. It is not effective as monotherapy and is generally combined with other AV nodal blocking agents for rate control. Dosing is described under LV dysfunction.

- **Amiodarone:** In patients with normal systolic function, amiodarone given intravenously receives a Class IIa recommendation for rate control when other AV nodal blocking agents are ineffective or inappropriate. It receives a Class IIb recommendation when given orally to control heart rate when other agents have been tried and are unsuccessful in controlling the ventricular rate at rest or during exercise. Dosing is described under LV dysfunction.

■ **Patients with LV systolic dysfunction:** In patients with heart failure, digoxin and amiodarone are the preferred agents.

- **Digoxin:** Digoxin receives a Class I recommendation when given orally or intravenously when there is heart failure from LV systolic dysfunction. A loading dose is necessary and may vary. For rapid control of ventricular rate in the acute setting, the initial dose recommended by the ACC/AHA/ESC 2006 guidelines on the management of AF is 0.25 mg IV over 2 minutes every 2 hours. The dose should not exceed 1.5 mg IV within 24 hours. Maintenance dose is 0.125 to 0.375 mg daily given intravenously or orally. For heart rate control in a nonacute setting, an oral dose of 0.5 mg daily may be given for 2 to 4 days followed by an oral maintenance dose of 0.125 to 0.375 mg daily. Digoxin has a very slow onset of action (1 hour or more) and its maximal effect is not until after 6 hours. It is usually not a very effective agent in controlling the ventricular rate in AF when used as monotherapy and receives a Class III recommendation when given as the sole agent in patients with paroxysmal AF. It may be effective in controlling heart rates at rest as well as in individuals who are sedentary but control of the rate of atrial fibrillation is lost during physical activity or in conditions associated with adrenergic stress such as febrile illnesses, hyperthyroidism, or exacerbations of chronic obstructive pulmonary disease.

- **Amiodarone:** Intravenous amiodarone receives a Class I recommendation to control the ventricular rate in patients with AF with heart failure. In the acute setting when rate control is necessary, 150 mg is given IV over 10 minutes followed by a maintenance infusion of 1 mg/minute IV for 6 hours and 0.5 mg/minute IV for the next 18 hours. The oral dose has a very slow onset of action and is more appropriate to use in nonacute setting. The oral dose is 800 mg daily in divided doses for 1 week. Another option is to give a lower dose of 600 mg daily in divided doses for 1 week or 400 mg daily in divided doses for 4 to 6 weeks. Any of these regimens is followed by long-term oral maintenance dose of 200 mg daily. Amiodarone affects the pharmacokinetics of warfarin, verapamil, and digoxin. The dose of these pharmacologic agents should be reduced when amiodarone is started.

- **Other agents:** Intravenous injection of nondihydropyridine calcium channel blockers and beta blockers may be given cautiously for rate control when there is LV dysfunction. These agents however are contraindicated (Class III) when the patient is acutely decompensated. Diltiazem has a shorter half-life and is less negatively inotropic than verapamil and may be more tolerable.

■ **WPW syndrome:** In patients with WPW syndrome, the use of AV nodal blocking agents to control ventricular rate during AF is inappropriate and may be dangerous. Inhibition of the AV node with any AV nodal blocking agents such as calcium channel blockers, beta blockers, or digitalis will allow atrial fibrillatory impulses to pass more efficiently through the bypass tract, which may result in ventricular fibrillation. Instead of AV nodal blockers, antiarrhythmic agents that increase the refractory period of the bypass tract such as type IA agents (procainamide) or drugs that can inhibit both AV node and bypass tract such as type IC and type III agents (ibutilide or amiodarone), may be given intravenously to hemodynamically stable patients to control the ventricular rate. Otherwise, the AF should be converted to normal sinus with electrical cardioversion. The treatment of AF in patients with WPW syndrome is further discussed in Chapter 20, Wolff-Parkinson-White Syndrome.

■ **Nonpharmacologic control of ventricular rate in AF:** The following are used only when pharmacologic agents are not effective in controlling the ventricular rate, especially when there is tachycardia-mediated cardiomyopathy.

- ■ **AV nodal ablation:** If the ventricular rate in AF can not be controlled with AV nodal blocking agents or other antiarrhythmic agents, radiofrequency ablation of the AV node combined with insertion of a permanent ventricular pacemaker is an option. Before AV nodal ablation is considered, the patient should be tried on medications and performed as a last resort especially in patients with tachycardia-mediated cardiomyopathy.

- ■ **Pulmonary vein isolation:** Isolation of the pulmonary veins may be performed either surgically or with radiofrequency ablation to maintain normal sinus rhythm (see Rhythm Control in this chapter) rather that for control of ventricular rate during AF.

■ **Rate control:** The following is a summary of pharmacologic agents recommended by the ACC/AHA/ESC guidelines for rate control in AF (Table 19.1).

## Rhythm Control

■ Rhythm control or conversion of AF to normal sinus rhythm is not necessary in all patients with AF. In the AFFIRM (Atrial Fibrillation Follow-up Investigation of Rhythm Management) and RACE (Rate Control vs. Electrical Cardioversion

**TABLE 19.1**

### Doses of Pharmacologic Agents for Rate Control in AF

| Pharmacologic Agents | Initial and Maintenance Doses |
|---|---|
| Diltiazem | 0.25 mg/kg IV over 2 min followed by IV maintenance dose of 5–15 mg/hr |
| Verapamil | 0.075–0.15 mg/kg IV over 2 min |
| Metoprolol | 2.5–5.0 mg IV over 2 min up to 3 doses |
| Propranolol | 0.15 mg/kg IV |
| Esmolol | 500 mcg/kg IV over 1 min loading dose; maintenance dose is 60–200 mcg/kg/min IV |
| Digoxin | 0.25 mg IV each 2 hr up to 1.5 mg and maintenance dose is 0.125 to 0.375 mg daily IV or orally |
| Amiodarone | 150 mg over 10 min IV loading dose and maintenance dose of 0.5 to 1.0 mg/min IV |

The table summarizes the doses of pharmacologic agents recommended by the American College of Cardiology/American Heart Association/European Society of Cardiology 2006 practice guidelines for control of ventricular rate in AF. Any of these agents may be given to patients with normal systolic function although in patients with left ventricular dysfunction, especially in patients with acute decompensated heart failure, only digoxin or amiodarone are the preferred agents.

AF, atrial fibrillation; IV, intravenous.

for Persistent Atrial Fibrillation) trials, there was no difference in mortality or incidence of stroke among patients with AF who were treated aggressively with electrical cardioversion and maintenance of the AF to normal sinus rhythm with antiarrhythmic agents when compared with patients with AF who were not cardioverted and were given only AV nodal blocking agents to control the ventricular rate. Both groups were anticoagulated. Thus, rhythm control in patients with AF should be individualized and should be reserved for patients who are symptomatic because quality of life can be improved, especially among patients with low cardiac output from LV dysfunction.

■ **Methods of converting AF to normal sinus rhythm:** Rhythm control or conversion of AF to normal sinus rhythm can be achieved with pharmacologic therapy or electrical cardioversion. Conversion of AF to normal sinus rhythm carries the risk of thromboembolization whether the conversion is spontaneous, electrical, or pharmacologic. The risk is increased if the duration of the AF is >48 hours. The longer the duration of AF, the higher the risk of thromboembolization because the atria will remain paralyzed even after the rhythm has converted to normal sinus. This risk is highest immediately after cardioversion, when AF has converted to normal sinus rhythm. Even among patients with negative transesophageal echocardiogram, atrial thrombi may develop

after cardioversion from atrial stunning resulting in stagnant flow in the atria and left atrial appendage.

■ **Spontaneous conversion:** Spontaneous conversion of AF to normal sinus rhythm can occur in a large number of patients with acute onset AF. Spontaneous conversion occurs most frequently during the first 24 to 48 hours. The chance of spontaneous conversion to normal sinus rhythm becomes less and less as the duration of AF becomes longer. The chance of spontaneous conversion is significantly less when the duration of AF is more than 7 days. Additionally, the efficacy of antiarrhythmic agents in converting AF to normal sinus rhythm also becomes markedly diminished if the patient is in AF for more than 7 days.

■ **Pharmacologic therapy:** The use of drugs to convert patients with AF to normal sinus rhythm is simpler when compared with electrical cardioversion because it does not require IV sedation. They are most effective when given within 7 days of AF onset. Pharmacologic cardioversion however is less effective than electrical cardioversion. The toxic effect of these agents is also a major issue since most of these agents are proarrhythmic. Among the pharmacologic agents that have been shown to be effective in converting AF to normal sinus rhythm are type IA agents (procainamide, quinidine, and disopyramide), type IC agents (propafenone and flecainide), and type III agents (ibutilide, dofetilide, and amiodarone). When any of these agents are given to convert AF to normal sinus rhythm, the patient should be hospitalized. The only exception is amiodarone, which is the least proarrhythmic and can be initiated orally in the outpatient setting. Types IA and IC agents can potentially cause AF to convert to atrial flutter with one to one conduction across the AV node. An AV nodal blocker such as a beta blocker or a nondihydropyridine calcium channel blocker therefore should be given at least 30 minutes before these agents are administered. The pharmacologic agent of choice to terminate AF to normal sinus rhythm will depend on the duration of the AF as well as the presence or absence of LV systolic dysfunction.

  □ **AF of <7 days' duration:** According to the ACC/AHA/ESC 2006 guidelines for the management of patients with AF, the following agents have been proven effective for pharmacological conversion of AF to normal sinus rhythm when the AF is <7 days' duration. These agents can be given orally or intravenously. Agents that are most effective include Class IC agents (flecainide or propafenone) and Class III agents (dofetilide or ibutilide). These agents carry a Class I recommendation for pharmacologic conversion of AF to normal sinus rhythm. Less effective is amiodarone, which carries a Class IIa recommendation. Other antiarrhythmic agents such as Class IA agents (quinidine, procainamide, and disopyramide) are less effective and carry a Class IIb recommendation. The use of sotalol and digoxin is not recommended and should not be administered for conversion of AF to normal sinus rhythm (Class III recommendation).

- **Preserved systolic function:** There are several agents that can be used to convert AF to normal sinus rhythm when LV systolic function is preserved.

- **Flecainide:** This agent receives Class I recommendation and can be given orally or intravenously. The oral dose for flecainide is 200 to 300 mg given once. The oral dose should not be given out of hospital for the patient to self administer as a "pill in the pocket strategy" unless the drug has been tried and proven to be safe and effective during initial hospitalization. An AV nodal blocker such as a calcium channel blocker or a beta blocker should be given at least 30 minutes before flecainide is given to prevent rapid ventricular rates from occurring should the rhythm convert to atrial flutter. The IV dose is 1.5 to 3.0 mg/kg given over 10 to 20 minutes. The intravenous preparation is not available in the United States.

- **Propafenone:** The drug also receives a Class I recommendation and can be given orally or intravenously. The oral dose is 600 mg given once. The IV dose is 1.5 to 2.0 mg/kg given over 10 to 20 minutes. The intravenous preparation is not available in the United States. The success rate varies from 56% to 83%. Similar to flecainide, the agent can be prescribed for self-administration by the patient as a "pill in the pocket strategy" only after initial therapy in the hospital has shown that the drug is safe and effective and the patient does not have any evidence of sick sinus syndrome or structural cardiac disease. AV nodal blockers are routinely given as background therapy in AF. Otherwise, if the patient is not on AV nodal blocker, it should be given at least 30 minutes before taking a type IC agent to prevent one to one conduction across the AV node should the patient develop atrial flutter.

- **Ibutilide:** The drug is available only intravenously and receives a Class I recommendation. The drug is given over 10 minutes as a 1 mg dose, diluted or undiluted. The dose is repeated after 10 minutes if the rhythm has not converted.

- **Dofetilide:** The drug is given only orally and receives a Class I recommendation. Its use is restricted to cardiologists who are allowed access to this agent. Initial dosing is based on kidney function and is contraindicated in patients with severe renal dysfunction (creatinine clearance of <20 mL/minute). In patients with normal renal function (creatinine clearance >60 mL/minute), the dose is 500 mcg twice daily. Maintenance dose is 500 to 1,000 mcg daily. The QT interval should be carefully monitored during therapy.

- **Amiodarone:** The drug can be given intravenously or orally and receives a Class IIa recommendation. The IV dose is 5 to 7 mg/kg over 30 to 60 minutes followed by 1.2 to 1.8 g per day of continuous infusion or in divided oral doses until a total dose of 10 g is given. The maintenance dose is 200 to 400 mg per day. The oral dose is given only

if immediate conversion of AF to normal sinus rhythm is not essential. The oral in-hospital dose is 1.2 to 1.8 g/day in divided doses until 10 g is given. Maintenance dose is 200 is 400 mg/day. Another option is to give 30 mg/kg as single dose. Amiodarone is the only antiarrhythmic agent that can be initiated without hospitalizing the patient. In outpatients, a smaller dose of 600 to 800 mg is given orally daily in divided doses until a total of 10 g is given. This is followed by a lower maintenance dose of 200 to 400 mg a day. Amiodarone enhances the effect of warfarin and digoxin. The doses of both agents should be reduced when amiodarone is initiated.

- **Quinidine:** Quinidine is given only orally and receives a Class IIb recommendation. The dose is 0.75 to 1.5 g in divided doses over 6 to 12 hours. The drug is combined with an AV nodal blocker to prevent increase in ventricular rate before AF converts to normal sinus. The drug can prolong the QT interval and can cause torsades de pointes. If patient is on digoxin, serum levels should be carefully monitored because quinidine increases the levels of digoxin, which can result in digitalis toxicity.

- **Left ventricular (LV) dysfunction:** When LV dysfunction (LV ejection fraction ≤40%) or congestive heart failure is present, only amiodarone and dofetilide (both type III agents) are the preferred agents for conversion of AF to normal sinus rhythm. These are the least negatively inotropic antiarrhythmic agents.

- **Amiodarone:** Loading dose is described above. The maintenance dose is 100 to 400 mg daily.

- **Dofetilide:** The drug is given orally and its use is restricted to cardiologists who are familiar with the use of this agent. Dosing is described previously.

- **AF of more than 7 days' duration:** When AF is more than 7 days' duration, only Class III agents (amiodarone, ibutilide, and dofetilide) are effective and are the only antiarrhythmic agents recommended. Most patients with AF of more than 7 days' duration have persistent AF. Class IA and Class IC agents are less effective and carry a Class IIb recommendation. According to the ACC/AHA/ESC 2006 guidelines for the management of patients with AF, sotalol and digoxin may be harmful and are not recommended for pharmacologic conversion of AF to normal sinus rhythm regardless of the duration of AF.

- **Rhythm control:** The following is a summary of pharmacologic agents for rhythm control according to the ACC/AHA/ESC practice guidelines for management of patients with AF (Table 19.2).

- **Electrical or direct current cardioversion:** This procedure is performed under intravenous sedation. If the AF is more than 48 hours' duration, DC cardioversion should not be performed until after the patient is adequately anticoagulated for a minimum of 3 weeks. If the need for conversion to normal sinus rhythm is more immediate, electrical cardioversion can be carried out if a transesophageal echocardiogram can be performed and

**TABLE 19.2**

## Pharmacologic Agents for Conversion of AF to Normal Sinus Rhythm

| Pharmacologic Agents | Recommended Doses |
| --- | --- |
| Amiodarone (Class III agent) | Oral: 1.2–1.8 g daily in divided doses until 10 g total then maintain dose to 200–400 mg daily or 30 mg/kg as a single dose<br>IV/oral: 5–7 mg/kg over 30–60 min IV, then 1.2–1.8 g daily continuous IV or orally in divided doses until a total of 10 g, then 200–400 mg daily |
| Dofetilide (Class III) | Oral only: Normal kidney function (creatinine clearance >60 mL/min, 500 mcg BID. The dose is adjusted in patients with renal dysfunction |
| Ibutilide (Class III) | IV only: 1 mg over 10 min. Repeat after 10 min with the same dose if necessary |
| Flecainide (Class IC) | Oral: 200–300 mg one dose<br>IV: 1.5 to 3.0 mg/kg over 10–20 min (the IV dose is not available in the United States) |
| Propafenone (Class IC) | Oral: 600 mg one dose<br>IV: 1.5 to 2.0 mg/kg over 10–20 min (the IV dose is not available in the United States) |
| Quinidine (Class IA) | Oral only: 0.75 to 1.5 g in divided doses over 6–12 h usually with another agent that will slow ventricular rate |

The table summarizes the doses of pharmacologic agents recommended by the American College of Cardiology/American Heart Association/European Society of Cardiology practice guidelines for conversion of AF to normal sinus rhythm. In patients with left ventricular dysfunction, only amiodarone and dofetilide are the preferred agents.
AF, atrial fibrillation; IV, intravenous.

no evidence of intracardiac thrombi can be demonstrated.

☐ Electrical cardioversion is the most effective in converting AF to normal sinus rhythm. Most patients will need an initial energy setting of 200 joules for conversion. The energy setting is increased gradually if the initial shock is unsuccessful. The shock is synchronized with the QRS complex to prevent the delivery of the shock during the vulnerable phase of the cardiac cycle, which can result in ventricular fibrillation. Devices that deliver direct current cardioversion with biphasic waveform have been shown to be more effective than devices that deliver the monophasic waveform.

☐ The patient should be adequately anticoagulated and should preferably be on antiarrhythmic agent before electrical cardioversion is performed.

■ **Nonpharmacologic therapy:** This is another option in converting patients with AF especially in symptomatic patients with recurrent AF who are not responsive to medical therapy.

☐ **Surgical ablation:** Maze procedure is performed by making atrial incisions at certain critical geographic location in the atria so that AF will not become sustained. This is usually performed in patients with AF in conjunction with other cardiac surgical procedures such as replacement or repair of mitral valve or during coronary bypass surgery.

☐ **Catheter ablation:** This procedure involves isolation of the pulmonary veins similar to a surgical maze procedure but is performed with catheterization techniques. The pulmonary veins are usually the site of ectopic foci that can precipitate AF.

## Prevention of Stroke

■ AF is a common cause of stroke in the elderly. The use of antithrombotic agents therefore is one of the cornerstones in the therapy of AF and is the standard of care in preventing strokes in patients with AF. Patients with AF who are high risk for stroke should be identified so that they can be protected with adequate anticoagulation. This is regardless whether the AF is paroxysmal, persistent, or permanent. Similarly, patients with AF who are low risk for stroke should also be identified so that they do not have to be exposed to the side effects of anticoagulation.

■ **Highest risk of stroke:** Patients with AF who are highest risk of stroke (≥6% per year) needs to be fully anticoagulated with warfarin. The following patients with AF are highest risk for stroke:

☐ **Valvular AF:** Patients with valvular AF are very high risk for developing stroke. Valvular AF includes patients with rheumatic mitral stenosis as well as patients with prosthetic mitral valve or previous mitral valve repair. Their risk for thromboembolism is approximately 15 to 20 times that of patients with AF but without these cardiac abnormalities. Patients with mitral prosthetic valves should be anticoagulated with warfarin to an International Normalized Ratio (INR) of 2.5 to 3.5. Patients with mitral stenosis and previous mitral valve repair should be anticoagulated to an INR of 2.0 to 3.0.

☐ **Previous history of thromboembolism:** Patients with AF with previous history of stroke, transient ischemic accident (TIA), or other forms of thromboembolism are also at high risk for developing stroke. Their risk is increased 2.5 times those with AF but without previous history of thromboembolism. These patients should also be anticoagulated with warfarin to an INR of 2.0 to 3.0.

■ **Lowest risk of stroke:** Patients with AF who are lowest risk for stroke ($\leq$2% per year) are patients with lone AF. The ACC/AHA/ESC 2006 guidelines on AF defines lone AF as patients who are <60 years of age and have no evidence of cardiac or pulmonary disease. These patients are not hypertensive and have normal echocardiograms and are low risk for thromboembolism. The guidelines recommend that these patients should be on aspirin, 81 to 325 mg daily although they also have the option of receiving no therapy. Among patients <60 years of age with heart disease but none of the risk features for thromboembolism, these patients are also low risk for stroke but should be on aspirin 81 to 325 mg daily. These patients do not need to be anticoagulated with warfarin.

■ **Intermediate or moderate risk for stroke:** Some patients with nonvalvular AF (no prosthetic mitral valve or rheumatic mitral stenosis) may have risk features for stroke that are intermediate (3% to 5% per year) when compared with patients in AF, but without these risk features. These intermediate risk markers come under the eponym of CHADS$_2$.

☐ **C** = Cardiac failure or left ventricular dysfunction (ejection fraction $\leq$35%)

☐ **H** = Hypertension

☐ **A** = Advanced age (>75 years)

☐ **D** = Diabetes mellitus

☐ **S$_2$** = Stroke, TIA, or previous history of thromboembolism.

☐ In nonvalvular AF, each of the above risk features increases the incidence of stroke and receives a weight of one except stroke/TIA or previous history of thromboembolism, which gives the patient two times the risk of the other risk features and is thus equivalent to a weight of 2, thus **S$_2$**.

☐ CHADS$_2$ serves as a useful guide in determining the intensity of antithrombotic therapy in patients with nonvalvular AF.

■ **One intermediate risk feature:** Any one of the above risk features: cardiac failure, hypertension, advanced age, and diabetes (CHAD) but not stroke or TIA, is an intermediate risk for thromboembolism. These patients have the option of either taking aspirin 81 to 325 mg daily or warfarin monitored to an INR of 2 to 3.

■ **Previous history of stroke or two or more risk factors:** Patients with history of stroke or TIA or with 2 or more intermediate risk features should receive warfarin and should be anticoagulated to an INR of 2.0 to 3.0.

■ **Anticoagulation during electrical or pharmacologic cardioversion:** If cardioversion is planned in patients with AF of more than 48 hours' duration or the duration of AF is not known, these patients should be anticoagulated for at least 3 to 4 weeks before electrical or pharmacologic cardioversion is attempted. If immediate cardioversion is planned, the patient should undergo transesophageal echocardiography to exclude thrombus in the left atrial appendage. If a thrombus is present, cardioversion is delayed and the patient is fully anticoagulated for at least 3 to 4 weeks before electrical cardioversion can be performed. If a thrombus is not present, intravenous heparin is given and electrical cardioversion is performed under intravenous anesthesia. Anticoagulation is continued after successful cardioversion for at least 3 to 4 weeks preferably 12 weeks. This includes patients with lone AF who undergo cardioversion. In many patients who are successfully cardioverted, the normal sinus rhythm in the ECG is often not accompanied by effective atrial contraction. This electromechanical dissociation may persist for several days or weeks. Thus, anticoagulation should be continued. The risk of stroke is similar among patients undergoing pharmacologic or electrical cardioversion and is highest within 3 days after the procedure. Among patients developing strokes after cardioversion, all episodes occurred within 10 days after the procedure.

■ Warfarin is the standard treatment for anticoagulating patients with AF. Aspirin does not equal the protection given by warfarin except in patients with lone AF or those with a 0 to 1 risk factor for stroke.

■ Table 19.3 summarizes the use of antithrombotic agents in patients with AF.

## Prognosis

■ AF is more common in the elderly and is an independent risk factor for death. The mortality in patients with AF is twice that of patients in normal sinus rhythm. This increase in mortality is associated with the severity of the underlying heart disease.

■ AF is associated with increased risk of stroke and heart failure. It is a common cause of morbidity in elderly patients with approximately 15% of all thromboembolic strokes from AF.

■ In patients younger than 60 years of age without clinical or echocardiographic evidence of structural heart disease or

**TABLE 19.3**

### Antithrombotic Agents for Prevention of Stroke in AF

| Low Risk | Moderate Risk | High Risk |
|---|---|---|
| • Lone atrial fibrillation<br><br>Aspirin<br>81–325 mg daily<br>or no therapy<br><br>• Age <60 years, has heart disease but no risk features<br><br>Aspirin<br>81–325 mg daily | • Any one of the following intermediate risk features:<br>Congestive heart failure or ejection fraction ≤35%, hypertension, age ≥75 years or diabetes<br><br>Aspirin 81–325 mg daily<br>or<br>Warfarin (INR 2.0–3.0) | • Valvular AF or previous history of stroke or transient ischemic attack or 2 or more intermediate risk features<br><br>Warfarin (INR of 2.0–3.0)<br><br>• For mechanical mitral valve<br><br>Warfarin (INR 2.5–.5) |

The table summarizes the antithrombotic agents recommended by the 2006 American College of Cardiology/American Heart Association/European Society of Cardiology guidelines for prevention of stroke in patients with AF.
AF, atrial fibrillation; IV, intravenous; INR, International Normalized Ratio.

chronic pulmonary disease, AF is generally benign. The risk of stroke, however, increases above this age or when associated with conditions that are known to increase the risk for stroke.

## Suggested Readings

The Atrial Fibrillation Follow-up Investigation of Rhythm Management (AFFIRM) Investigators. A comparison of rate control and rhythm control in patients with atrial fibrillation. *N Engl J Med*. 2002;347:1825–1833.

Blomstrom-Lundqvist C, Scheinman MM, Aliot EM, et al. ACC/AHA/ESC Guidelines for the management of patients with supraventricular arrhythmias—executive summary. A report of the American College of Cardiology/American Heart Association Task Force on Practice Guidelines, and the European Society of Cardiology Committee for Practice Guidelines (Writing Committee to Develop Guidelines for the Management of Patients with Supraventricular Arrhythmias). *J Am Coll Cardiol*. 2003;42: 1493–1531.

Botteron GW, Smith JM. Cardiac arrhythmias. In: Carey CF, Lee HH, Woeltje KF, eds. *The Washington Manual of Medical Therapeutics*. 29th ed. Philadelphia: Lippincott Williams & Wilkins; 1998:130–156.

Capucci A, Villani GQ, Piepoli MF. Reproducible efficacy of loading oral propafenone in restoring sinus rhythm in patients with paroxysmal atrial fibrillation. *Am J Cardiol*. 2003; 92:1345–1347.

Fuster V, Ryden LE, Cannom DS, et al. ACC/AHA/ESC 2006 guidelines for the management of patients with atrial fibrillation—executive summary; a report of the American College of Cardiology/American Heart Association Task Force and the European Society of Cardiology Committee on Practice Guidelines and the European Society of Cardiology Committee for Practice Guidelines (Writing Committee to Revise the 2001 Guidelines for the Management of Patients with Atrial Fibrillation). *J Am Coll Cardiol*. 2006;48:854–906.

Gage BF, Waterman AD, Shannon W, et al. Validation of clinical classification schemes for predicting stroke: results from the National Registry of Atrial Fibrillation. *JAMA*. 2001;285: 2864–2870.

Rockson SG, Albers GW. Comparing the guidelines: anticoagulation therapy to optimize stroke prevention in patients with atrial fibrillation. *J Am Coll Cardiol*. 2004;43:929–935.

Roy D, Talajic M, Nattel S, et al. Rhythm control versus rate control for atrial fibrillation and heart failure. *N Engl J Med*. 2008;358:2667–2677.

Sherman DG, Kim SG, Boop BS, et al. Occurrence and characteristics of stroke events in the atrial fibrillation follow-up investigation of sinus rhythm management (AFFIRM) study. *Arch Intern Med*. 2005;165;1185–1198.

Singh BN, Singh SN, Reda DJ, et al. Amiodarone versus sotalol for atrial fibrillation. *N Engl J Med*. 2005;352:1861–1872.

Van Gelder IC, Hagens VE, Bosker HA, et al. A comparison of rate control and rhythm control in patients with recurrent persistent atrial fibrillation. *N Engl J Med*. 2002;92:1834–1840.

van Walraven WC, Hart RG, Wells GA, et al. A clinical prediction rule to identify patients with atrial fibrillation and a low risk for stroke while taking aspirin. *Arch Intern Med*. 2003;163: 936–943.

# Wolff-Parkinson-White Syndrome

## Anatomy of the Conduction System

- **Wolff-Parkinson-White (WPW) syndrome:** WPW syndrome is a clinical entity characterized by preexcitation of the ventricles with symptoms of paroxysmal tachycardia.
  - **Normal atrioventricular (AV) conduction:** In normal individuals, the atria and ventricles are separated by a dense mass of fibrous tissues that prevent the spread of electrical impulses from atria to ventricles. The only pathway by which the atrial impulse can reach the ventricles is through the AV node and normal intraventricular conduction system (Fig. 20.1A).
  - **WPW syndrome:** In WPW syndrome, a bypass tract is present, which connects the atrium directly to the ventricle. The atrial impulse therefore is able to reach the ventricles not only through the AV node, but also through the bypass tract (Fig. 20.1B).

This accessory pathway can cause premature activation of the ventricles. It can also serve as a pathway for reentry, which may result in clinical symptoms of paroxysmal tachycardia.

## Preexcitation of the Ventricles

- **Ventricular preexcitation:** When a bypass tract is present, conduction of the sinus impulse to the ventricles is altered as shown in Figure 20.2.
  - **Atrial activation:** During normal sinus rhythm, activation of the atria is not altered. The sinus P wave remains normal.
  - **Ventricular activation:** When a bypass tract is present, the ventricles are activated through two separate pathways: the AV node and bypass tract. The QRS complex represents a fusion complex.

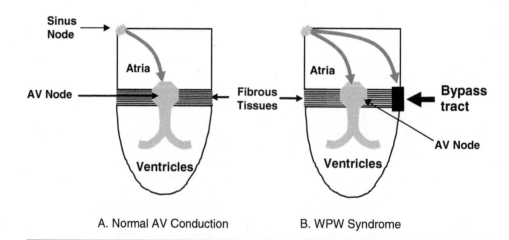

A. Normal AV Conduction          B. WPW Syndrome

**Figure 20.1:   The Conduction System in Normal Individuals and in Patients with the WPW Syndrome. (A)** The normal AV conduction system. The atrial impulse can enter the ventricles only through the AV node (*arrow*). **(B)** A bypass tract connecting the atrium directly to the ventricle across the AV groove. When a bypass tract is present, an atrial impulse can enter the ventricles not only through the AV node but also through the bypass tract (*arrows*). AV, atrioventricular.

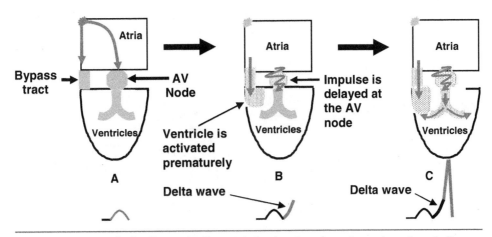

**Figure 20.2: Ventricular Preexcitation. (A)** The sinus impulse activates the atria and a P wave is normally recorded. **(B)** The sinus impulse is normally delayed at the AV node but is conducted directly through the bypass tract causing the ventricles to be prematurely activated. This causes the PR interval to shorten and the initial portion of the QRS complex to be slurred. **(C)** The impulse finally emerges from the atrioventricular node and activates the rest of the ventricles normally.

☐ **Bypass tract:** Unlike in normal individuals in whom the sinus impulse can reach the ventricles only through the AV node, the presence of a bypass tract allows the atrial impulse to be conducted directly to the ventricles thus activating the ventricles prematurely. This causes the PR interval to be shorter than normal (Fig. 20.2B). The impulse spreads by muscle cell to muscle cell conduction causing the initial portion of the QRS complex to be inscribed slowly. This slow initial upstroke of the QRS complex is called the delta wave.

☐ **AV node:** The sinus impulse is normally delayed at the AV node. As the impulse emerges from the AV node, it activates the ventricles rapidly through the normal conduction system causing the rest of the QRS complex to be inscribed normally (Fig. 20.2C).

## Electrocardiogram Findings

■ **Electrocardiogram (ECG) findings:** The classical ECG findings in WPW syndrome include a short PR interval, a delta wave, and secondary ST and T wave abnormalities.

   ■ **Short PR interval:** The PR interval is short since the bypass tract conducts more rapidly than the AV node causing the ventricles to be excited prematurely. The PR interval is shorter than normal, but does not have to measure <0.12 seconds.

   ■ **Delta wave:** The delta wave is the initial portion of the QRS complex with a slow upstroke, as shown in Figure 20.3. It represents premature activation of the ventricles at the area of insertion of the bypass

tract. Because conduction of the impulse is by direct muscle spread, which is slow and inefficient, this causes the initial portion of the QRS complex to be inscribed sluggishly. This initial portion with the slurred upstroke is called the delta wave.

■ **ST and T wave abnormalities:** The ST and T wave changes are secondary to the abnormal activation of the ventricles. The direction of the ST segment and T wave is opposite that of the delta wave.

## The Bypass Tract

■ **Bypass tract:** Unlike the His-Purkinje system, the bypass tract consists of ordinary heart muscle and does not contain cells that are specialized for conduction.

■ The bypass tract may be left sided or right sided.

■ It may be single or multiple.

■ Conduction may be constant or intermittent (Figs. 20.4 and 20.5).

■ The bypass tracts may be active or inactive.

■ The bypass tract may conduct only anterogradely (from atrium to ventricle), only retrogradely (from ventricle to atrium) or both.

   ☐ **Manifest or overt bypass tract:** The bypass tract is manifest or overt if it is capable of conducting anterogradely from atrium to ventricle resulting in the classical pattern of preexcitation.

   ☐ **Concealed bypass tract:** The bypass tract is concealed if it is capable of conducting only retrogradely from ventricle to atrium. The baseline ECG will not show any evidence of preexcitation during normal sinus rhythm, but the presence of

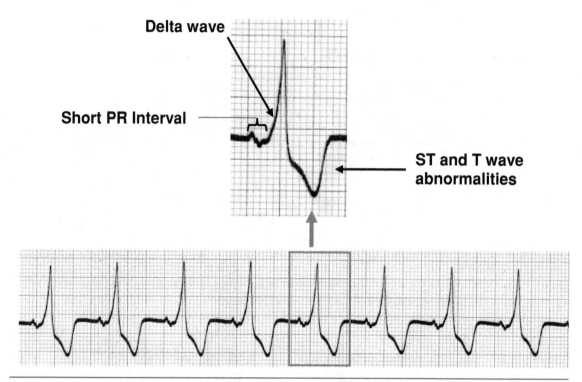

**Figure 20.3: Ventricular Preexcitation.** A QRS complex is magnified from the rhythm strip to show the short PR interval measuring 0.11 seconds, delta wave, and ST-T abnormalities.

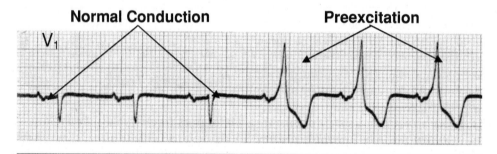

**Figure 20.4: Intermittent Preexcitation.** The rhythm strip is recorded in V$_1$. The first three complexes show no evidence of preexcitation. The PR interval is prolonged and the QRS complexes are narrow. The last three complexes show ventricular preexcitation. The PR interval is short, the QRS complexes are wide and delta waves are present. The ST segments are also depressed with inverted T waves pointing away from the direction of the delta wave.

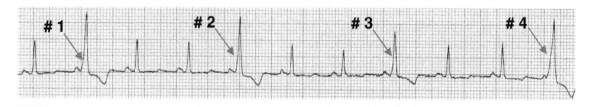

**Figure 20.5: Intermittent Preexcitation.** Intermittent preexcitation is shown by arrows #1–#4. The other complexes are conducted normally without preexcitation.

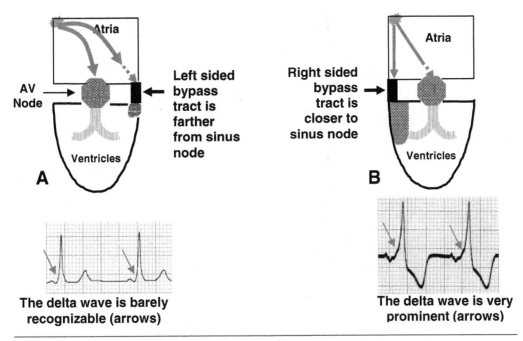

**Figure 20.6:  Size of the Delta Wave.  (A)** The delta wave is barely recognizable because of a smaller amount of myocardium activated from the bypass tract. This occurs when the bypass tract is left sided or conduction through the AV node is enhanced. **(B)** The delta wave is more prominent because a larger amount of myocardium is activated from the bypass tract. This is often seen in right sided bypass tracts or when there is delay in the conduction of the impulse at the AV node. AV, atrioventricular.

a bypass tract can potentially cause a reentrant tachycardia to occur.

## The Delta Wave

- **Size of the delta wave:** The delta wave may be very conspicuous or it may be barely recognizable in the baseline ECG, depending on the amount of ventricular myocardium activated from the bypass tract.
  - **Small delta wave:** The delta wave may be barely recognizable if only a small amount of ventricular myocardium is activated from the bypass tract. This occurs if the bypass tract is left sided because a left-sided bypass tract is farther from the sinus node compared with a right-sided bypass tract. The farther the distance from the sinus node, the longer it takes for the sinus impulse to reach the bypass tract (Fig. 20.6A). This may result in normal or near normal PR interval. The delta wave is also small and inconspicuous if the atrial impulse is efficiently conducted through the AV node.
  - **Large or prominent delta wave:** The delta wave is prominent if a larger portion of the myocardium is activated from the bypass tract (Fig. 20.6B). This occurs when the bypass tract is right sided bringing it closer to the sinus node. The delta wave is also prominent if the sinus impulse is delayed at the AV node.

## Localizing the Bypass Tract

- An ECG is helpful in predicting the location of the bypass tract during normal sinus rhythm, during narrow complex tachycardia, and during wide complex tachycardia.
- After preexcitation is diagnosed in the 12-lead ECG, the bypass tract can be localized during sinus rhythm by the following observations.
  - **Left-sided bypass tract:** When the bypass tract is left sided, the left ventricle is activated earlier than the right ventricle. The impulse will travel from left ventricle to right ventricle in the direction of $V_1$, which is located on the right side of the sternum (Fig. 20.7). Thus, during normal sinus rhythm, a positive delta wave or tall R or Rs complex will be recorded in $V_1$. This pattern of preexcitation is also called type A. Tall R waves in $V_1$ can be mistaken for right bundle branch block, right ventricular hypertrophy or posterior infarction.
  - **Right-sided bypass tract:** When the bypass tract is right sided, the right ventricle is activated earlier than the left ventricle. The impulse spreads from right ventricle to left ventricle away from lead $V_1$. This results in a negative delta wave with deep S or rS complex in $V_1$ (Fig. 20.8). This pattern of preexcitation is also called type B. Because the S waves are deeper than the R waves in $V_1$, the ECG may be

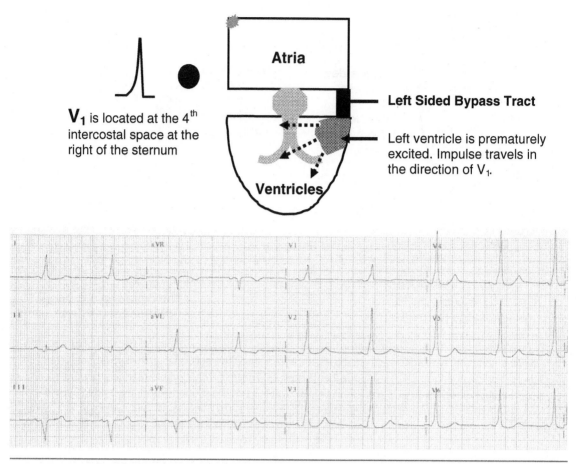

**$V_1$ is located at the 4<sup>th</sup> intercostal space at the right of the sternum**

**Left Sided Bypass Tract**

Left ventricle is prematurely excited. Impulse travels in the direction of $V_1$.

**Figure 20.7: Left-Sided Bypass Tract.** When the bypass tract is left sided, the initial impulse spreads from left ventricle to right ventricle during normal sinus rhythm as shown in the above diagram (*arrows*). This will result in tall R waves in $V_1$. In this example, the bypass tract was localized at the posterior wall of the left ventricle and was successfully ablated.

mistaken for left bundle branch block, left ventricular hypertrophy, or anteroseptal myocardial infarction.

- **Location:** Approximately 50% to 60% of all bypass tracts are located at the free wall of the left ventricle, 20% to 30% at the posteroseptal area (left or right), 10% to 20% at the free wall of the right ventricle and the remaining 5% are located in the anteroseptal area (mostly right sided).

- **Left sided versus right sided:** The morphology of the QRS complex in $V_1$ is useful in differentiating a left-sided from a right-sided bypass tract.

  - **Right-sided bypass tracts:** As previously discussed, the bypass tract is right sided if the QRS complex is predominantly negative (QS or rS) in $V_1$. Right-sided bypass tracts may be located at the posteroseptal area, right ventricular free wall or anteroseptal area (Figs. 20.9 and 20.10).

  - **Left-sided bypass tracts:** If the QRS complex is predominantly upright (tall R or Rs) in $V_1$, the bypass tract is left sided. Left-sided bypass tracts may be located at the left ventricular free wall or the pos-

teroseptal area. Anterior or anteroseptal bypass tracts rarely exist because the aortic annulus and mitral annulus are contiguous structures (Fig. 20.9).

- Several methods of predicting the location of the bypass tract during normal sinus rhythm have been described. The bypass tract can be more accurately localized if the delta wave contributes significantly to the QRS complex. Although there are limitations in using the 12-lead ECG for localizing the bypass tract, the algorithm of Olgin and Zipes, shown below, is the simplest and most practical.

  - **Step 1. Configuration of the QRS complex in $V_1$:**
    - ☐ A tall R wave in $V_1$ indicates that the bypass tract is left sided.
    - ☐ A deep S wave in $V_1$ indicates that the bypass tract is right sided.

  - **Step 2A. Right-sided bypass tract:** If the bypass tract is right sided, it may be posteroseptal, anteroseptal, or free wall in location.
    - ☐ **Posteroseptal:** QS complexes in the leads II, III, and aVF indicate that the bypass tract is posteroseptal in location.

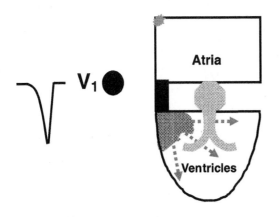

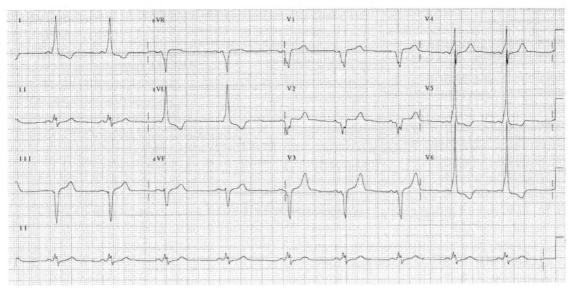

**Figure 20.8:  Right-Sided Bypass Tract.**  When the bypass tract is right sided, the right ventricle is activated earlier than the left ventricle. This causes the initial impulse to spread from right ventricle to left ventricle away from lead $V_1$ resulting in QS or rS complexes in $V_1$. This electrocardiogram can be mistaken for left bundle branch block, left ventricular hypertrophy, or anteroseptal myocardial infarction.

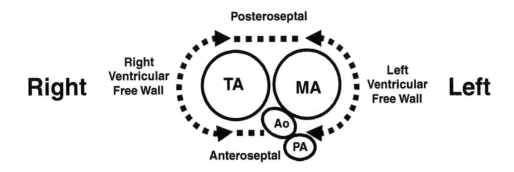

**Figure 20.9:  Location of the Bypass Tract.**  The position of the bypass tract at the level of the AV grove is shown by the diagram. Right-sided bypass tracts are located at the right ventricular free wall, posteroseptal, or anteroseptal areas, whereas left-sided bypass tracts are located at the left ventricular free wall or posteroseptal area. The left anteroseptal area is occupied by the aortic root and the presence of a left sided anteroseptal bypass tract is rare. Ao, aorta; AV, atrioventricular; MA, mitral annulus; PA, pulmonary artery; TA, tricuspid annulus.

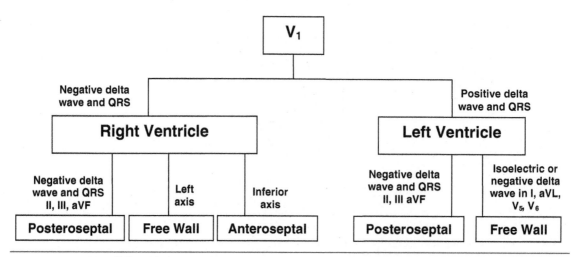

**Figure 20.10:** **Localizing the Bypass Tract.** Adapted from Olgin and Zipes.

- ☐ **Anteroseptal:** An inferior axis indicates that the bypass tract is anteroseptal in location.
- ☐ **Free wall:** The presence of left axis indicates that the bypass tract is located at the right ventricular free wall.
- ■ **Step 2B. Left-sided bypass tract:** This may be posteroseptal or free wall.
  - ☐ **Posteroseptal:** QS complexes in leads II, III, and aVF indicate that the bypass tract is posteroseptal in location.
  - ☐ **Left ventricular free wall:** An isoelectric or negative delta wave in I, aVL, $V_5$, and $V_6$ indicates free wall bypass tract.

## Left-Sided Bypass Tract

- ■ **Left ventricular free wall:** Figure 20.11 is an example of a bypass tract at the free wall of the left ventricle. Tall

R waves or Rs complexes in $V_1$ suggest that the bypass tract is left sided. Negative delta waves or QS complexes in leads I and aVL suggest that the bypass tract is at the free wall since the impulse is traveling away from these leads.

- ■ **Left-sided posteroseptal bypass tract:** Example of left-sided posteroseptal bypass tract is shown in Figure 20.12. Tall R waves are present in $V_1$ consistent with a left-sided bypass tract. Deep Q waves are present in II, III, and aVF suggest that the bypass tract is posteroseptal because the electrical impulse is traveling away from these leads.

## Right-Sided Bypass Tract

- ■ **Right-sided posteroseptal bypass tract:** Example of a right-sided posteroseptal bypass tract is shown in Figure 20.13. $V_1$ shows QS complexes consistent with a

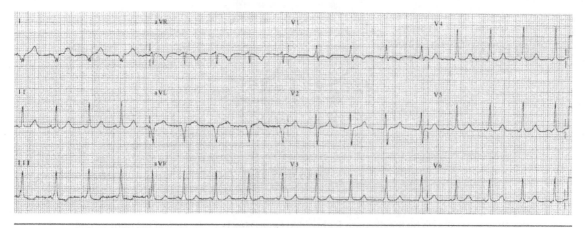

**Figure 20.11:** **Left Ventricular Free Wall.** Tall R waves are present in $V_1$ consistent with a left sided bypass tract. QS complexes are present in I and aVL resembling a lateral infarct. This suggests that the impulse is traveling away from the positive sides of leads I and aVL consistent with a bypass tract at the lateral free wall of the left ventricle.

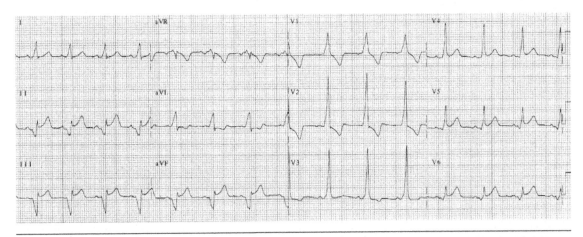

**Figure 20.12:   Left-Sided Posteroseptal Bypass Tract.** Deep Q waves are present in leads II, III, and aVF resembling an inferior infarct. This is consistent with a posteroseptal bypass tract. The bypass tract is left sided because tall R waves are present in $V_1$.

right-sided bypass tract. QS complexes are also present in leads II, III, and aVF, suggesting that the bypass tract is posteroseptal in location.

■ **Anteroseptal bypass tract:** Anteroseptal bypass tracts are usually right sided. Right-sided anteroseptal bypass tract has QS or rS in $V_1$ with the axis directed inferiorly toward +30° to +120°. Q wave is present in aVL but not in $V_6$ (Fig. 20.14).

■ **Right ventricular free wall:** Figure 20.15 shows a bypass tract at the right ventricular free wall. The QRS complex has a left bundle branch block pattern with left axis deviation. QS or rS complexes are present in $V_1$ and the QRS complex in the frontal plane is usually directed to the left with an axis of +30° to –60°, resulting in tall R waves in I and aVL.

## The WPW Syndrome

### ECG Findings

1. Short PR interval
2. Delta wave
3. ST and T wave abnormalities

### Mechanism

■ The main abnormality in WPW syndrome is the presence of a bypass tract that is separate from the normal AV conduction system. This anomalous pathway is also called accessory pathway or bundle of Kent. The bypass tract consists of

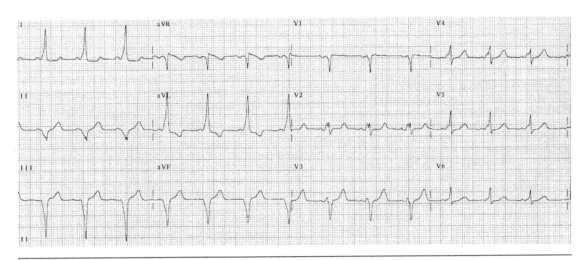

**Figure 20.13:   Right-Sided Posteroseptal Bypass Tract.** QS complexes are present in leads II, III, and a VF consistent with a posteroseptal bypass tract. $V_1$ shows a QS complex consistent with a right-sided posteroseptal bypass tract.

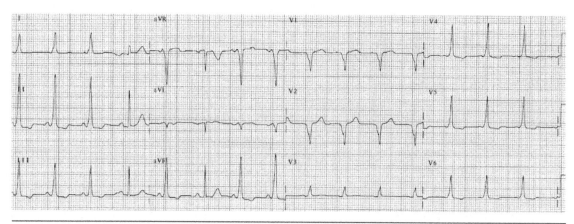

**Figure 20.14:** **Right-Sided Anteroseptal Bypass Tract.** QS complexes are present in $V_1$ and $V_2$ consistent with a right sided bypass tract. The axis of the QRS complex in the frontal plane is inferior ($>+60°$). This is consistent with an anteroseptal bypass tract.

ordinary myocardium that bridges the atrium directly to the ventricle across the AV groove.

- During normal sinus rhythm, the only pathway by which the sinus impulse can reach the ventricles is through the AV node. The impulse is normally delayed at the AV node, resulting in a PR interval of 0.12 to 0.20 seconds. If a bypass tract is present, a second pathway is created by which the ventricles can be activated. Thus, during normal sinus rhythm, the impulse is normally delayed at the AV node but is conducted directly to the ventricle through the bypass tract. This causes the ventricle to be prematurely activated resulting in a shorter than normal PR interval usually measuring <0.12 seconds. As the impulse finally emerges from

the AV node, it is conducted rapidly through the His-Purkinje system allowing the rest of the ventricles to be activated normally and more efficiently.

- Preexcitation of the ventricle is seen in the ECG as a short PR interval with a delta wave.

  - **Shortened PR interval:** The PR interval is short because the atrial impulse reaches the ventricle faster through the bypass tract than through the AV node. The PR interval usually measures <0.12 seconds when there is preexcitation. However, the PR interval does not always have to be <0.12 seconds for preexcitation to occur. A normal PR interval ≥0.12 seconds is seen in approximately 25% of patients with preexcitation.

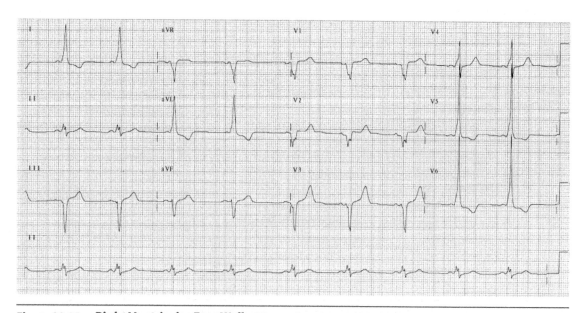

**Figure 20.15:** **Right Ventricular Free Wall.** QS complexes are present in $V_1$ consistent with a right-sided bypass tract. There is also left axis deviation of the QRS complexes of approximately $-30°$ consistent with a bypass tract at the right ventricular free wall.

- **Delta wave:** The delta wave is the slow, slurred initial deflection of the QRS complex. It represents myocardial conduction of the impulse through the ventricle at the area of insertion of the bypass tract. The delta wave is inscribed sluggishly because the impulse is propagated by direct myocardial spread. This causes the QRS complex to be inscribed slowly and is widened.
- **ST-T changes:** The ST and T wave abnormalities are secondary to the abnormal activation of the ventricles and are directed away from the delta wave.
- The size of the delta wave depends on the amount of myocardium activated by the accessory pathway. If there is significant delay of the impulse at the AV node, a larger portion of myocardium will be activated through the bypass tract resulting in a longer, larger, and more conspicuous delta wave. This causes a more bizarre and wider QRS complex. If the impulse is quickly and efficiently conducted across the AV node, the amount of myocardium activated by the bypass tract will be small and the delta wave may be barely noticeable because most of the ventricles will be activated through the normal His-Purkinje system. The size of the delta wave also depends on the location of the bypass tract. A right-sided bypass tract is closer to the sinus node than a left-sided bypass tract causing the ventricles to be activated earlier. A right-sided bypass tract therefore is expected to have a shorter PR interval and a more prominent delta wave than a left-sided bypass tract.
- When there is preexcitation, the QRS complex is actually a fusion complex. The initial portion of the QRS complex is due to activation of the ventricles from the accessory pathway. The delta wave therefore represents the impulse that is contributed by the bypass tract. The remaining QRS complex represents activation of the ventricles through the normal AV conduction system.

## Clinical Significance

- Preexcitation of the ventricles is an electrocardiographic diagnosis characterized by the presence of a short PR interval and a delta wave. This specific pattern of preexcitation is also called the WPW ECG. Not all patients with the WPW ECG will develop symptoms of tachycardia. When preexcitation of the ventricles is associated with symptoms of tachycardia, the clinical entity is called WPW syndrome.
- The bypass tract can be right sided (connecting the right atrium to the right ventricle anywhere within the tricuspid ring) or left sided (connecting the left atrium to the left ventricle anywhere within the mitral ring). It may be located anteroseptally, posteroseptally, or laterally at the free wall of the left or right ventricle. More than half of bypass tracts are located at the left lateral free wall connecting the left atrium to the left ventricle, about 20% to 30% are posteroseptal in location, 10% to 20% are at the right lateral wall connecting the right atrium to the right ventricle, and the remaining 5% are anteroseptal in location. Anteroseptal bypass tracts are mainly right sided.

- The bypass tract may be single or multiple. Conduction may be fixed or intermittent and may be anterograde only (atrium to ventricle), retrograde only (ventricle to atrium) or both. Ventricular preexcitation therefore can manifest in different patterns and can be mistaken for other abnormalities not only during normal sinus rhythm, but also during tachycardia. Accordingly, preexcitation of the ventricle can be mistaken for left or right bundle branch block; left or right ventricular hypertrophy; posterior, inferior, anterior, and lateral Q wave myocardial infarction; non-Q wave myocardial infarction; myocardial ischemia; or other repolarization abnormalities. It can also be mistaken for ectopic beats or intermittent bundle branch block. The WPW ECG therefore is a great masquerader of several ECG abnormalities.
- The 12-lead ECG is helpful in localizing the bypass tract during normal sinus rhythm. The more prominent the delta wave (or the greater the ventricular preexcitation), the more accurate is the localization. The location of the bypass tract during normal sinus rhythm should be compared with the location of the bypass tract during tachycardia. This may help identify if more than one bypass tract is present.
- Approximately 10% to 20% of patients with Ebstein's anomaly has WPW syndrome with more than one bypass tract commonly present. In Ebstein's anomaly, the right ventricle is atrialized because of a downward displacement of the tricuspid leaflets into the right ventricle; thus, Ebstein's anomaly should always be suspected when a bypass tract is right sided. Other cardiac diseases associated with preexcitation include hypertrophic cardiomyopathies and mitral valve prolapse.
- The presence of preexcitation can cause auscultatory changes in the heart.
  - **Right-sided bypass tract:** If the bypass tract is right sided, the right ventricle is activated earlier than the left ventricle. Delay in activation of the left ventricle will cause a softer first heart sound. Earlier activation of the right ventricle will cause earlier closure of the pulmonic component of the second sound, which can result in a single or paradoxically split second heart sound.
  - **Left-sided bypass tract:** If the bypass tract is left sided, the left ventricle is activated earlier than the right ventricle. This can cause the first heart sound to be accentuated. Delay in activation of the right ventricle will cause the pulmonic second sound to be further delayed resulting in wide splitting of the second heart sound. These auscultatory findings become audible only when a significant portion of the QRS complex is contributed by the bypass tract.

## Treatment and Prognosis

- **Asymptomatic patients:** The presence of preexcitation in the baseline ECG may not be associated with symptoms and may be discovered unexpectedly during a routine ECG for reasons unrelated to symptoms of tachycardia.

**Figure 20.16: Conduction across the Bypass Tract. (A)** The bypass tract can conduct only anterogradely from atrium to ventricle (*dotted arrow*); **(B)** only retrogradely, from ventricle to atrium; and **(C)**, both anterogradely and retrogradely, from atrium to ventricle and from ventricle to atrium.

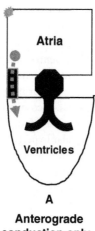

**A**

**Anterograde conduction only**

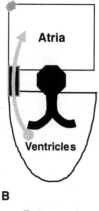

**B**

**Retrograde conduction only**

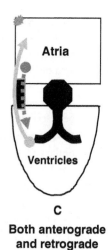

**C**

**Both anterograde and retrograde conduction**

- Among asymptomatic patients with intermittent preexcitation, without structural or congenital heart disease who continue to remain completely asymptomatic, the preexcitation may disappear, with a good prognosis. Routine electrophysiologic testing is not recommended.

- Among asymptomatic patients with ECG pattern of preexcitation that is fixed or constant, the prognosis will depend on the physiologic characteristics and refractory period of the accessory pathway. The American College of Cardiology/American Heart Association (ACC/AHA) Task Force on Practice Guidelines for Clinical Intracardiac Electrophysiologic and Catheter Ablation Procedures does not recommend routine electrophysiologic testing in asymptomatic patients with preexcitation except those with a family history of sudden death or patients who are engaged in high-risk occupations or activities.

- **Symptomatic patients:** In patients with classical preexcitation manifested by short PR interval and delta wave associated with clinical symptoms of tachycardia, the overall prognosis remains good except that there is an approximate 0.15% to 0.39% chance of sudden cardiac death occurring over a 3- to 10-year follow-up. The ACC/AHA/European Society of Cardiology (ESC) guidelines for the management of patients with supraventricular arrhythmias consider ablation therapy as Class I indication for patients with accessory pathways that are symptomatic. Antiarrhythmic therapy in these patients receives a Class IIa recommendation.

## Arrhythmias Associated with the WPW Syndrome

- One of the clinical features of the WPW syndrome is its predisposition to develop arrhythmias. The following are the most important arrhythmias associated with the WPW syndrome:

- AV reciprocating tachycardia or AVRT
  - □ Orthodromic or narrow complex AVRT
  - □ Antidromic or wide complex AVRT
- Atrial fibrillation
- The electrophysiologic characteristics of the bypass tracts are highly variable. Some bypass tracts can conduct only anterogradely from atrium to ventricle (Fig. 20.16A), some only retrogradely from ventricle to atrium (Fig. 20.16B), and others can conduct both anterogradely from atrium to ventricle and retrogradely from ventricle to atrium (Fig. 20.16C). This may influence the type of arrhythmia associated with the WPW syndrome.

## Narrow Complex and Wide Complex AV Reciprocating Tachycardia

- **AV reciprocating tachycardia (AVRT):** AVRT is the most common arrhythmia associated with the WPW syndrome. AVRT is a supraventricular tachycardia that may have narrow or wide QRS complexes. The QRS complexes may be narrow or wide depending on how the ventricles are activated during the tachycardia.

  - **Narrow complex AVRT:** This type of AVRT has narrow QRS complexes because the atrial impulse enters the ventricles anterogradely through the AV node during tachycardia (Fig. 20.17A). The impulse follows the intraventricular conduction system and activates the ventricles, normally resulting in QRS complexes that are identical to that during normal sinus rhythm. This type of AVRT is also called orthodromic or narrow complex AVRT and was discussed in Chapter 16, Supraventricular Tachycardia due to Reentry.

  - **Wide Complex AVRT:** This type of AVRT has wide QRS complexes because the atrial impulse enters the ventricles through the bypass tract during the

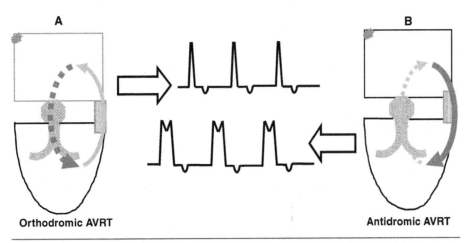

**Figure 20.17:   Orthodromic and Antidromic AVRT.  (A)** Orthodromic AVRT. During tachycardia, the impulse is conducted from atrium to ventricle across the AV node resulting in narrow QRS complexes. **(B)** Antidromic AVRT. During tachycardia, the atrial impulse is conducted from atrium to ventricle across the bypass tract resulting in wide QRS complexes, which can be mistaken for ventricular tachycardia. AVRT, atrioventricular reciprocating tachycardia.

tachycardia (Fig. 20.17B). The impulse activates the ventricles outside the normal conduction system resulting in wide QRS complexes, which can be mistaken for ventricular tachycardia. Wide complex AVRT is also called antidromic AVRT and is further discussed in this chapter.

## Narrow Complex or Orthodromic AVRT

- **Mechanism of narrow complex AVRT.** Narrow complex AVRT is discussed in more detail in Chapter 16. The

tachycardia is triggered by a premature atrial or ventricular impulse. Figure 20.18 illustrates how a premature atrial impulse can precipitate a narrow complex AVRT.

- The premature atrial impulse should be perfectly timed to occur when the AV node has fully recovered from the previous impulse while the bypass tract is still refractory. Because the AV node has a shorter refractory period, the premature atrial impulse is able to conduct through the AV node, but is blocked at the bypass tract (Fig. 20.18A).

- The ventricles are activated through the normal AV conduction system, resulting in a narrow QRS

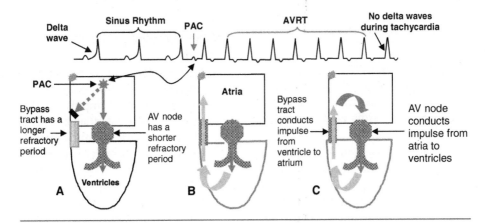

**Figure 20.18:   Orthodromic or Narrow Complex AVRT.  (A)** A premature atrial complex (PAC) is conducted through the AV node but not through the bypass tract. **(B)** The ventricles are activated exclusively through the normal conduction system causing the QRS complex to be narrow. **(C)** The impulse is conducted from ventricles to atria across the bypass tract. The atria are activated retrogradely allowing the impulse to be conducted back to the ventricles through the AV node. Note that delta waves are present only during normal sinus rhythm but not during tachycardia. AV, atrioventricular; AVRT, atrioventricular reciprocating tachycardia.

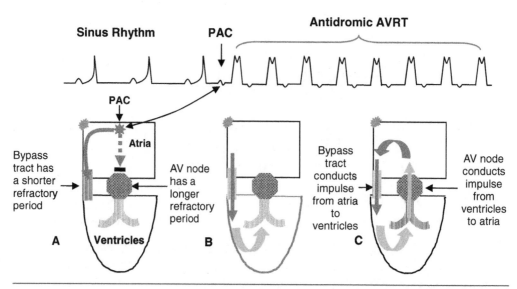

**Figure 20.19: Antidromic or Wide Complex AVRT. (A)** A premature atrial complex (PAC) is conducted through the bypass tract but not through the AV node. **(B)** The QRS complex is wide because the ventricles are activated outside the normal conduction system. **(C)** The impulse is conducted retrogradely from ventricles to atria through the atrioventricular conduction system. The atria are activated retrogradely allowing the impulse to be conducted back to the bypass tract. AVRT, atrioventricular reciprocating tachycardia.

complex (Fig. 20.18B). After the ventricles are activated, the impulse is conducted retrogradely from ventricle to atrium across the bypass tract. After the atria are activated, the impulse can reenter the AV node resulting in a narrow complex tachycardia called orthodromic AVRT (Fig. 20.18C). Delta waves are not present during tachycardia because activation of the ventricles occurs exclusively through the AV node.

## Wide Complex or Antidromic AVRT

- **Mechanism of wide complex AVRT:** Antidromic or wide complex AVRT is triggered by a premature impulse originating from the atria or ventricles. The diagram illustrates how the tachycardia is initiated (Fig. 20.19).
  - The premature atrial impulse should be perfectly timed to occur when the bypass tract has fully recovered from the previous impulse while the AV node is still refractory. Because the bypass tract has a shorter refractory period, the premature atrial impulse will enter the bypass tract but is blocked at the AV node (Fig. 20.19A).
  - The atrial impulse activates the ventricles through the bypass tract (Fig. 20.19B). The impulse spreads from one ventricle to the other by muscle cell to muscle cell conduction, causing a wide QRS com-

plex. The impulse is conducted retrogradely to the atria across the AV conduction system. The atria are activated retrogradely, thus completing the circuit. The atrial impulse can again reenter the bypass tract and the circuit starts all over again (Fig. 20.19C).

## Conduction Pathways in Antidromic AVRT

- **Wide complex AVRT:** There are two types of wide complex AVRT:
  - **Ventriculoatrial conduction across the AV node:** In wide complex AVRT, anterograde conduction of the atrial impulse to the ventricles occurs through the bypass tract and retrograde conduction of the impulse from ventricles to atria occurs through the AV node (Fig. 20.20A). This wide complex AVRT is called type I antidromic AVRT. This type of wide complex tachycardia may be terminated by vagal maneuvers and AV nodal blockers because the AV node is part of the reentrant circuit.
  - **Ventriculoatrial conduction across another bypass tract:** Retrograde conduction of the ventricular impulse to the atria may occur through a second bypass tract instead of the AV node, although this is extremely rare (Fig. 20.20B). This wide complex AVRT is called type II. Type II wide complex AVRT

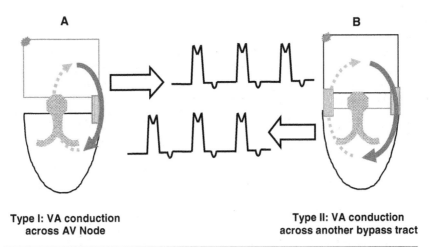

**Type I: VA conduction across AV Node**

**Type II: VA conduction across another bypass tract**

**Figure 20.20: VA Conduction in Antidromic AVRT. (A)** In type I antidromic AVRT, the atrial impulse enters the ventricles through the bypass tract and returns to the atria through the AV node. This type of antidromic AVRT can be terminated by AV nodal blockers. **(B)** In type II antidromic AVRT, the impulse enters the ventricles through the bypass tract and returns to the atria through a second bypass tract. This type of antidromic AVRT cannot be terminated by AV nodal blockers. Both wide complex tachycardia look identical and can be mistaken for ventricular tachycardia. AV, atrioventricular; VA, ventriculoatrial; AVRT, atrioventricular reciprocating tachycardia.

can not be terminated by vagal maneuvers or AV nodal blockers because the AV node is not part of the reentrant circuit. The ECG of type I and type II wide complex AVRT are identical showing wide QRS complexes.

- **Localizing the bypass tract during wide complex AVRT:** The ventricular insertion of the bypass tract can be localized during a wide complex tachycardia.

- **Right bundle branch block configuration:** If the wide complex AVRT has a right bundle branch block configuration (R waves are taller than S waves in $V_1$), the bypass tract is left sided. During tachycardia, the left ventricle is activated earlier than the right ventricle. Thus, the impulse spreads from left ventricle to right ventricle causing a tall QRS complex in $V_1$ (Fig. 20.21A).

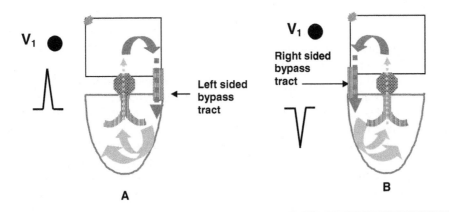

$V_1$

Left sided bypass tract

$V_1$

Right sided bypass tract

**A**

**B**

**Figure 20.21: Localizing the Bypass Tract during Wide Complex AVRT. (A)** When the bypass tract is left sided (bypass tract connects left atrium to left ventricle), tall R waves are recorded in $V_1$ during wide complex tachycardia. Because the left ventricle is activated first, the impulse will travel from left ventricle to right ventricle toward $V_1$. **(B)** If the bypass tract is right sided, the right ventricle is activated first and the impulse is conducted from right ventricle to left ventricle causing deep S waves in $V_1$. AVRT, atrioventricular reciprocating tachycardia.

- **Left bundle branch block configuration:** If the wide complex AVRT has a left bundle branch block configuration (S waves are deeper than the R waves in V$_1$), the bypass tract is right sided. During wide complex AVRT, the right ventricle is activated earlier that the left ventricle. Thus, the ventricular impulse spreads from right ventricle to left ventricle causing a negative complex in V$_1$ (Fig. 20.21B).

- Figure 20.22 is from a patient with right-sided bypass tract. During wide complex AVRT (Fig. 20.22B), the QRS complexes have a left bundle branch block configuration consistent with a right-sided bypass tract. During narrow complex AVRT (Fig. 20.22C,D), the retrograde P waves are upright in leads I and aVL, which is also consistent with a right-sided bypass tract. The location of the bypass tract during narrow complex AVRT matches the location of the bypass tract during wide complex AVRT and during normal sinus rhythm. If the location of the bypass tract during tachycardia and during normal sinus rhythm does not match, more than one bypass tract may be present.

- Figures 20.22C,D are from the same patient as Figures 20.22A, B. Retrograde P waves (arrows) are upright in leads I and aVL during narrow complex AVRT consistent with right-sided bypass tract.

## Antidromic or Wide Complex AVRT

- Another example of wide complex AVRT is shown in Fig. 20.23. The QRS complexes are tall in V$_1$ consistent with a left-sided bypass tract.

## Wide Complex AVRT

- **Treatment:** The reentrant pathway during wide complex AVRT generally involves the same structures as that during narrow complex AVRT. Thus, vagal maneuvers and AV nodal blockers are usually effective in terminating the tachycardia (Fig. 20.24A). Before AV nodal blocking agents are given, it should be ascertained that the wide complex tachycardia is not ventricular tachycardia because catastrophic results may occur if the tachycardia turns out to be ventricular rather than supraventricular. Furthermore, adenosine, which is a very effective agent in converting AVRT to normal sinus rhythm, can cause atrial fibrillation in up to 10% of patients. This may be catastrophic if the patient has preexcitation. Additionally, if the wide complex AVRT uses a second bypass tract for ventriculoatrial conduction (type II wide complex AVRT), AV nodal blockers will not be effective in terminating the tachycardia because the AV node is not part of the reentrant path-

way. Thus, ibutilide, procainamide, or flecainide, which are capable of blocking the reentrant circuit at the level of the bypass tract (Fig. 20.24B), are the preferred agents according to the ACC/AHA/ESC guidelines in the management of patients with supraventricular arrhythmias.

## ECG Findings of Antidromic or Wide Complex AVRT

1. The QRS complexes are wide measuring ≥120 milliseconds. The tachycardia is difficult to distinguish from ventricular tachycardia.

2. The tachycardia is very regular because the tachycardia uses a fixed reentrant circuit.

3. AV block is not possible because the atria and ventricles are part of the reentrant pathway.

4. Although retrograde P waves are present, similar to orthodromic AVRT, the P waves can not be identified because they are obscured by the ST segment.

## Mechanism

- AVRT is possible only when a bypass tract is present. For tachycardia to occur, the AV node and bypass tract should have different electrophysiologic properties. The tachycardia can be triggered by a premature atrial or ventricular impulse and can be narrow complex (orthodromic) or wide complex (antidromic).

  - **Orthodromic or narrow complex AVRT:** If the bypass tract has a longer refractory period than the AV node, a perfectly timed premature atrial impulse is blocked at the bypass tract, but is conducted to the AV node and His-Purkinje system, resulting in a narrow complex or orthodromic AVRT. Unlike the baseline ECG in which delta waves are present due to preexcitation, there are no delta waves during the tachycardia because the ventricles are activated exclusively from the AV node. This tachycardia was already discussed in Chapter 16, Supraventricular Tachycardia due to Reentry.

  - **Antidromic or wide complex AVRT:** If the AV node has a longer refractory period than the bypass tract, a premature atrial impulse can enter the bypass tract but not the AV node, resulting in wide complex or antidromic AVRT. In antidromic AVRT, the premature atrial impulse is conducted through the bypass tract and activates the ventricles by direct myocardial spread resulting in a wide QRS complex. The ventricular impulse is conducted retrogradely to the atria across the AV node and reenters the ventricles through the bypass tract. The reentrant tachycardia involves a large circuit consisting of the bypass tract, ventricles, bundle branches, bundle of His, AV node, and atria before circling back to the bypass tract to activate the ventricles. Because the ventricles are activated exclusively from the bypass tract, the whole QRS complex is not a fusion complex and is essentially a delta wave.

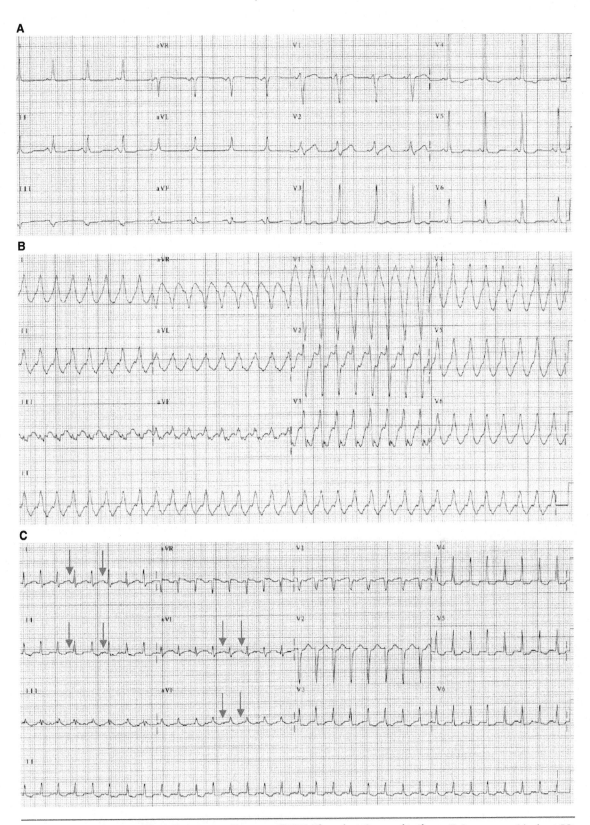

**Figure 20.22:** **(A) Baseline Electrocardiogram (ECG) Showing Preexcitation.** Delta waves with short PR intervals are present in leads I, aVL, $V_2$, and $V_3$ consistent with preexcitation. The QRS complex is negative in $V_1$ with deep S waves consistent with a right sided bypass tract. **(B) Wide Complex AVRT.** The 12-lead ECG is from the same patient as **(A)**. It shows a wide complex tachycardia with deep S wave in $V_1$ suggesting that the bypass tract is right sided. This wide complex tachycardia can be mistaken for VT. **(C)** Narrow complex tachycardia. The ECG shows narrow complex AVRT. The frontal leads are magnified in **(D)** to show that the retrograde P waves (*arrows*) are upright in I and aVL consistent with a right-sided bypass tract. *(continued)*

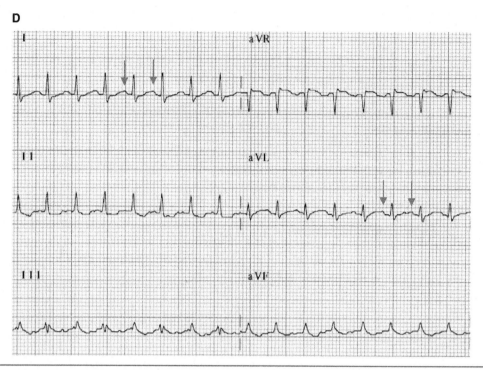

**Figure 20.22:** (Continued) **(D)** Narrow complex AVRT. The ECG is from **(C)**. Only the frontal leads are magnified to show that the P waves are upright in leads I and aVL during SVT. AVRT, atrioventricular reciprocating tachycardia; SVT, supraventricular tachycardia.

## Clinical Significance

- Narrow complex AVRT is the most common arrhythmia in patients with the WPW syndrome occurring in approximately 85% to 95% of patients who have symptoms of tachycardia. Wide complex AVRT is rare, occurring only in 5% to 10% of patients with WPW syndrome. Antidromic or wide complex AVRT is a classic example of wide complex tachycardia of supraventricular origin.

- Wide complex AVRT is difficult to differentiate from ventricular tachycardia because both arrhythmias have wide QRS complexes. Ventricular tachycardia usually occurs in patients with history of myocardial infarction or left ventricular systolic dysfunction. Wide complex AVRT occurs in patients who are younger with known preexcitation and generally preserved left ventricular systolic function. The ECG algorithm for diagnosing wide complex tachycardia of ventricular origin is further discussed in Chapter 22, Wide Complex Tachycardia.

- The ventricular insertion of the bypass tract can be localized during wide complex tachycardia. The bypass tract is left sided if the QRS complexes have a right bundle branch block configuration (R waves are taller than S waves in $V_1$). If the QRS complexes have a left bundle branch block configuration (S waves are deeper than the height of the R waves in $V_1$), the bypass tract is right sided.

- Although it can be assumed that patients with preexcitation who develop narrow complex tachycardia have AVRT as the cause of the tachycardia, in more than 5% of patients with preexcitation, the narrow complex tachycardia is due to AV nodal reentrant tachycardia rather than AVRT. The exact mechanism of the tachycardia is important if radiofrequency ablation is being considered.

- Patients with Ebstein anomaly may have more than one bypass tract. These patients may not respond to AV nodal blockers during wide complex AVRT because the AV node may not be part of the reentrant pathway. Similarly, ablation therapy may not be as effective because several bypass tracts may be present.

- Wide or narrow complex AVRT is paroxysmal with abrupt onset and sudden termination. During tachycardia, prominent jugular venous pulsations from cannon A waves are usually seen in the neck. These jugular pulsations are due to synchronous contraction of both atria and ventricles.

## Treatment

- **Wide complex tachycardia of uncertain diagnosis:** Wide complex AVRT may be difficult to differentiate from ventricular tachycardia. If the diagnosis of the wide complex tachycardia is uncertain and there is possibility that the tachycardia is ventricular rather than supraventricular, AV nodal blockers, especially verapamil, should be avoided. Verapamil is negatively inotropic and a potent vasodilator. If verapamil is inadvertently given to a patient with ventricular tachycardia,

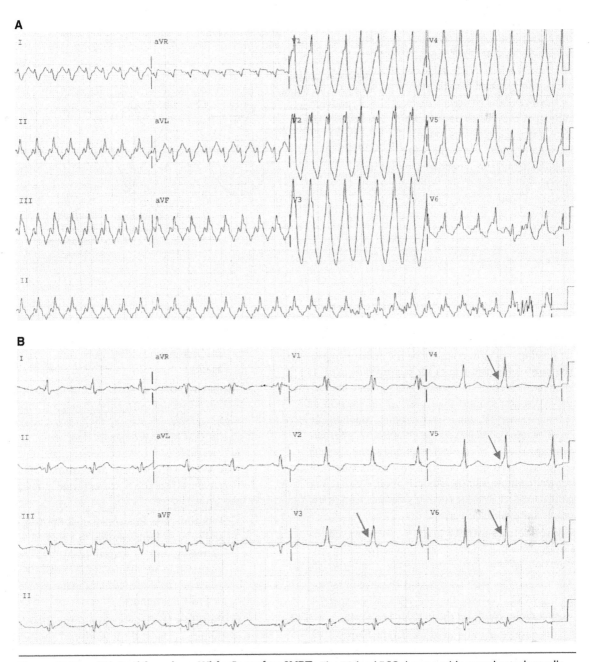

**Figure 20.23:    (A) Antidromic or Wide Complex AVRT.** The 12-lead ECG shows a wide complex tachycardia from antidromic AVRT. The QRS complexes show tall R waves in $V_1$ consistent with a left-sided bypass tract. The tachycardia can be mistaken for ventricular tachycardia. **(B) After Conversion to Normal Sinus Rhythm**. The 12-lead ECG is from the same patient as **(A)**. The rhythm is normal sinus. There are multiple leads showing short PR interval and delta waves (*arrows*) consistent with ventricular preexcitation. Negative delta waves are present in III and aVF with tall R waves in $V_1$ consistent with a left-sided posteroseptal bypass tract. The location of the bypass tract during wide complex AVRT matches that during normal sinus rhythm. AVRT, atrioventricular reciprocating tachycardia; ECG, electrocardiogram.

the patient may become hemodynamically unstable because most patients with ventricular tachycardia have left ventricular systolic dysfunction. Additionally, AV nodal blockers should not be given if there is irregularity in the R-R interval, which may indicate atrial fibrillation with preexcitation. Finally, patients with preexcitation who develop wide complex tachycardia may not be due to AVRT but may be due to focal atrial tachycardia or atrial flutter conducting across a bypass tract. This type of wide complex tachycardia will not respond to AV nodal blockers. Agents that will slow conduction across the bypass tract such as ibutilide, procainamide, or flecainide given intravenously are preferred agents according to the

**Figure 20.24:    Effect of AV Nodal Blockers in Wide Complex AVRT.** If the retrograde pathway involves the AV node as shown in **(A)**, vagal maneuvers and AV nodal blockers will be effective in terminating the tachycardia. However, if the AV node is not part of the reentrant pathway **(B)**, AV nodal blockers will not be effective in terminating the tachycardia. Antiarrhythmic agents that can block the impulse at the bypass tract are the preferred agents for terminating the tachycardia. The asterisks indicate that the drugs are available as intravenous preparations. VA, ventriculoatrial; AV, atrioventricular.

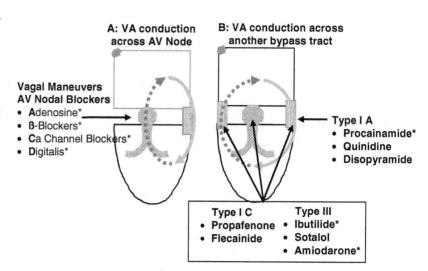

ACC/AHA/ESC guidelines for the management of patients with supraventricular arrhythmias.

- **Wide complex AVRT:** Wide complex AVRT can be terminated by slowing conduction across the AV node or bypass tract. The most vulnerable arm of the tachycardia circuit is the AV node, which can be inhibited with vagotonic maneuvers such as Valsalva, carotid sinus pressure, immersion of the face in cold water (diving reflex), gagging, coughing, or straining. If vagotonic maneuvers are not effective, pharmacologic therapy should be considered among stable patients and electrical cardioversion among patients who are not stable. Electrical cardioversion is also an option even among stable patients, especially if the etiology or mechanism of the wide complex tachycardia is uncertain.
  - **Pharmacologic agents:** AV nodal blockers and antiarrhythmic agents that inhibit conduction across the bypass tract are both effective in terminating wide complex AVRT.
    - **Adenosine:** Although adenosine is effective in terminating AVRT, it is not the best agent when there is wide complex AVRT for the following reasons:
      - Adenosine can cause atrial fibrillation in up to 10% of patients, which may be catastrophic in patients with preexcitation. Thus, resuscitative equipment should be available if adenosine is being given to a patient with known WPW syndrome.
      - There is a subset of antidromic AVRT in which AV conduction of the impulse occurs through one bypass tract and ventriculoatrial conduction occurs through another bypass tract. AV nodal blockers such as adenosine will not be effective because this type of AVRT does not use the AV node as part of the reentrant circuit.
      - Finally, there are other supraventricular arrhythmias such as focal atrial tachycardia and atrial flutter that can result in wide complex tachycardia when a bypass tract is present. These arrhythmias will conduct to the ventricles across the by-

pass tract and will not respond to adenosine because the AV node is not involved with the tachycardia. Thus, antiarrhythmic agents that can slow the impulse at the bypass tract are preferred agents.

- **Antiarrhythmic agents:** According to the ACC/AHA/ESC guidelines for the management of patients with supraventricular arrhythmias, antiarrhythmic agents that block the bypass tract are more effective and are preferred in the acute treatment of wide complex AVRT. This includes procainamide, ibutilide, or flecainide. Flecainide is not available intravenously in the United States.
  - **Procainamide:** Procainamide is the drug of choice and is given intravenously to a total dose of 10 to 12 mg/kg, not to exceed 1,000 mg. The dose is given within 30 minutes at the rate of 100 mg every 2 to 3 minutes followed by a maintenance infusion of 1 to 4 mg/minute.
  - **Ibutilide:** One mg is given intravenously over 10 minutes. The 10-mL solution can be injected slowly IV or diluted with $D_5W$ to a total volume of 100 mL and infused over 10 minutes. If the wide complex AVRT has not converted to normal sinus rhythm after 10 minutes, the same dose is repeated. Experience with ibutilide is not as extensive as that with procainamide although the drug may be as effective.
  - **Other antiarrhythmic agents:** Other Class IA (quinidine and disopyramide) IC (propafenone) and Class III agents (sotalol) are not available as intravenous preparations, but are effective for long-term therapy by inhibiting the bypass tract. These agents are negatively inotropic and should not be given when there is left ventricular dysfunction or heart failure. If the patient has left ventricular systolic dysfunction, amiodarone is the preferred agent. Amiodarone, however,

has not been shown to be more effective than other agents and has several long-term toxic effects and is reserved in the treatment of patients with structural cardiac disease.

- **Electrical cardioversion:** Electrical cardioversion is reserved for patients who are hemodynamically unstable with hypotension, congestive heart failure, or with symptoms of ischemia from tachycardia. It is also an initial option to patients who are hemodynamically stable. It should also be considered if the patient does not respond to initial pharmacologic therapy or when the diagnosis of the wide complex tachycardia remains uncertain. In stable patients, a low energy setting is generally adequate in terminating the tachycardia (50 joules).

- **Intracardiac pacing:** The tachycardia can also be terminated by a perfectly timed premature atrial complex or premature ventricular complex because the atria and ventricles are part of the reentrant circuit. Before the era of radiofrequency ablation, insertion of permanent pacemakers with antitachycardia properties has been used in the treatment of both antidromic and orthodromic AVRT. The device can detect the tachycardia and paces the atria or ventricles to interrupt the arrhythmia.

- **Radiofrequency ablation:** Radiofrequency ablation of the bypass tract using catheter techniques is now the preferred therapy and receives a Class I recommendation in symptomatic patients with preexcitation especially in younger individuals to obviate the need for long-term antiarrhythmic therapy. The procedure is usually very effective with more than 95% chance of cure. If radiofrequency ablation is not technically feasible, ablation surgery should be considered.

## Prognosis

- Patients with preexcitation who develop symptoms from tachycardia, overall prognosis remains good. These patients should be referred to an electrophysiologist for further evaluation with a chance for complete cure.

## Atrial Fibrillation

- Atrial fibrillation is one of the most dreadful arrhythmias associated with WPW syndrome. This arrhythmia has the potential of degenerating to ventricular fibrillation, which can result in sudden cardiac death. The ECG findings of atrial fibrillation in the presence of preexcitation are:
  - Irregularly irregular R-R intervals.
  - Varying morphologies of the QRS complexes.
  - The ventricular rate is usually rapid.

- During atrial fibrillation, the atrial impulses can reach the ventricles through both AV node and bypass tract resulting in varying degrees of ventricular fusion. Because the bypass tract consists of ordinary myocardium, it can allow atrial complexes to enter the ventricles resulting in very rapid ventricular rates (Fig. 20.25).

- Atrial fibrillation degenerating to ventricular fibrillation is rare, even among symptomatic patients with WPW syndrome. Atrial fibrillation however carries the potential for sudden death. Patients with WPW syndrome with bypass tracts that are capable of conducting at rates >240 beats per minute (R-R interval between two preexcited complexes ≤250 milliseconds or ≤6 small blocks) are at risk for sudden death as shown in Figures 20.25 and 20.26.

## Atrial Fibrillation in Patients with WPW Syndrome

- **Treatment:** The standard treatment of atrial fibrillation is to slow the ventricular rate with AV nodal blocking agents such as calcium channel blockers, beta blockers, and digoxin. In patients with preexcitation, the use of these agents is not only contraindicated, but also may be catastrophic. AV nodal blockers slow down conduction and decrease the number of impulses entering the ventricles anterogradely through the AV node. This will reduce the number of impulses bombarding the ventricular end of the bypass tract, rendering the bypass tract less refractory (Fig. 20.27). Calcium channel blockers can also cause peripheral vasodilatation, which may result in reflex increase in sympathetic tone. This may increase conduction through the bypass tract. The use of digitalis is particularly dangerous because digitalis does not only block the AV node, but also enhances conduction through the bypass tract.

- Electrical cardioversion is the treatment of choice in patients with atrial fibrillation who are unstable. In stable patients, procainamide is the pharmacologic agent of choice. Ibutilide, amiodarone, propafenone, and sotalol are also effective. These agents can slow the ventricular rate but can also convert atrial fibrillation to sinus rhythm.

## Atrial Fibrillation and WPW Syndrome

### ECG Findings of Atrial Fibrillation and WPW Syndrome

1. The R-R intervals are irregularly irregular.
2. The ventricular rate is unusually rapid.

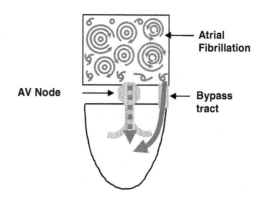

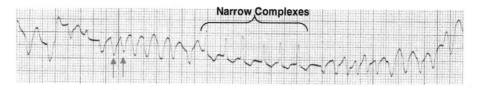

**Figure 20.25: Atrial Fibrillation and the WPW Syndrome.** In patients with WPW syndrome with atrial fibrillation, atrial impulses can enter the ventricles through both bypass tract and AV node. Note that in the middle of the rhythm strip, narrow QRS complexes are present (*bracket*). These impulses are conducted through the AV node. The wide QRS complexes (*arrows*) are preexcited and are conducted through the bypass tract. Some QRS complexes are fusion complexes due to activation of the ventricles from both bypass tract and AV node. The R-R interval between two wide QRS complexes measure <250 milliseconds (distance between the two arrows) making the patient high risk for ventricular fibrillation. WPW, Wolff-Parkinson-White; AV, atrioventricular.

3. The QRS complexes have different configurations, some narrow, some wide, and others in between.

## Mechanism

■ When atrial fibrillation occurs in a patient without a bypass tract, atrial impulses can reach the ventricles only through the AV node because this is the only pathway that connects the atria to the ventricles. Accordingly, the ventricular rate is usually controlled because the capacity of the AV node to transmit atrial fibrillatory impulses to the ventricles is limited.

■ When atrial fibrillation occurs in a patient with WPW syndrome, the bypass tract serves as a second pathway, in addition to the AV node, for atrial impulses to reach the ventricles. Because the bypass tract consists of ordinary myocardium, it is capable of conducting atrial impulses more rapidly to the ventricles than the AV node, resulting in very rapid ventricular rates, which can degenerate to ventricular fibrillation and sudden death.

■ The QRS complexes have varying configurations because two separate pathways are involved in conducting atrial impulses to the ventricles. Wide QRS complexes occur when atrial impulses are conducted through the bypass tract and narrow complexes are present when the AV node and conduction system transmit atrial impulses to the ventricles. In addition, fusion complexes of varying configurations are present when the AV node and bypass tract simultaneously contribute to ventricular activation.

## Clinical Implications

■ Atrial fibrillation is the most serious arrhythmia associated with WPW syndrome. The arrhythmia can result in very rapid ventricular responses, which can lead to hypotension, diminished coronary perfusion, and ventricular fibrillation. This may cause sudden death even in healthy individuals.

■ Approximately 30% to 40% of patients with preexcitation with symptoms of tachycardia will develop atrial fibrillation. The presence of AVRT increases the incidence or predisposition to develop atrial fibrillation, which (in the presence of preexcitation) may degenerate to ventricular fibrillation. Conversely, in patients with AVRT, successful ablation of the accessory pathway will diminish the incidence of atrial fibrillation.

■ It is possible that completely asymptomatic patients with preexcitation may suddenly develop atrial fibrillation as the

**A.**

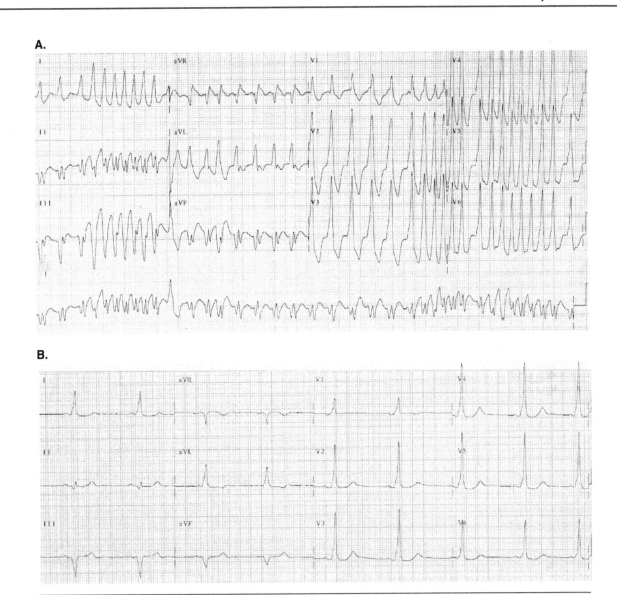

**B.**

**Figure 20.26:    Atrial Fibrillation and WPW Syndrome.** ECG **(A)** shows atrial fibrillation in a patient with known WPW syndrome. Note the irregularly irregular R-R intervals and the presence of bizarre QRS complexes of varying morphologies. The R-R interval between both preexcited complexes measures ≤250 milliseconds, making patient high risk for ventricular fibrillation. **(B)** From the same patient upon conversion to normal sinus rhythm. ECG **(B)** shows preexcitation. The patient underwent successful ablation of a left-sided posteroseptal bypass tract. ECG, electrocardiogram; WPW, Wolff-Parkinson-White.

initial symptom degenerating to ventricular fibrillation, although this is exceedingly rare. Electrophysiologic testing in patients who are asymptomatic is not necessary, as previously discussed.

■ Patients with preexcitation who are symptomatic have a higher chance of developing atrial fibrillation, although the chance that the atrial fibrillation can degenerate to ventricular fibrillation is also rare. Patients with preexcitation who are symptomatic should be risk stratified so that those who are high risk for cardiac sudden death can be identified.

■ The following markers suggest that the patient is low risk for sudden death.

□ Patients with preexcitation in the resting ECG, but are completely asymptomatic.

□ The preexcitation is noted only intermittently during routine ECG.

□ There is immediate disappearance of preexcitation during stress testing.

□ The delta waves disappear when procainamide is given intravenously.

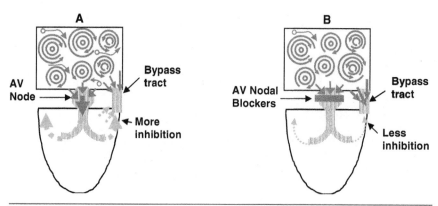

**Figure 20.27: Atrial Fibrillation and the WPW Syndrome. (A)** During atrial fibrillation, atrial impulses can enter the ventricles through the AV node and bypass tract. Atrial impulses entering the AV node can activate the ventricles and at the same time depolarize the ventricular end of the bypass tract retrogradely (*arrows*). This can render the bypass tract refractory, thus slowing down the number of atrial impulses entering the ventricles through the bypass tract. **(B)** When AV nodal agents are given, the number of atrial impulses entering the AV node is decreased. This will also decrease the number of impulses depolarizing the ventricular end of the bypass tract. Because there is less inhibition of the ventricular end of the bypass tract, the bypass tract is less refractory and will allow more atrial impulses to enter the ventricles through the bypass tract anterogradely. AV, atrioventricular; WPW, Wolff-Parkinson-White.

■ The following are markers of a high-risk patient. These observations suggest that the bypass tract has a short refractory period and is capable of conducting atrial impulses rapidly.

□ The delta wave persists during stress testing.

□ The refractory period of the bypass tract is short measuring ≤250 milliseconds between preexcited complexes. This can be measured during spontaneously occurring atrial fibrillation or it can be induced in the electrophysiology lab during electrophysiologic testing.

□ History of cardiac arrest from ventricular fibrillation.

□ Presence of multiple accessory pathways.

□ Presence of Ebstein anomaly.

## Treatment

■ Treatment of atrial fibrillation in patients with WPW syndrome associated with wide QRS complexes includes direct current cardioversion, use of antiarrhythmic agents, and radiofrequency ablation.

■ **Direct current cardioversion:** In hemodynamically unstable patients associated with rapid ventricular rates, direct current cardioversion receives a Class I recommendation. It carries a Class II a recommendation among patients who are stable according to the 2006 ACC/AHA/ESC guidelines in the management of patients with atrial fibrillation.

■ **Antiarrhythmic agents:** In patients with atrial fibrillation who are not hemodynamically unstable and do not need to be cardioverted, pharmacologic agents that block the bypass tract can be given as initial therapy.

■ **Procainamide:** Procainamide is the drug of choice and is given intravenously at a dose of 10 to 12 mg/kg within 30 minutes at the rate of 100 mg every 2 to 3 minutes, not to exceed 1,000 mg. This is followed by a maintenance infusion of 1 to 4 mg/minute. This is effective not only in slowing the ventricular rate, but also in converting atrial fibrillation to normal sinus rhythm in more than 50% of patients with atrial fibrillation. This drug carries a Class I indication according to the 2006 ACC/AHA/ESC practice guidelines.

■ **Ibutilide:** One mg of ibutilide is given IV slowly over 10 minutes and repeated if needed after an interval of 10 minutes. Ibutilide can block both bypass tract and AV node. This is effective in converting atrial fibrillation to normal sinus rhythm and also carries a Class I recommendation.

■ **Flecainide:** Intravenous flecainide receives a Class IIa recommendation in stable patients with atrial fibrillation with rapid ventricular rates with wide QRS complexes. The intravenous dose is 1.5 to 3.0 mg/kg over 10 to 20 minutes. This agent is not available intravenously in the United States.

■ **Other antiarrhythmic agents:** Amiodarone, quinidine, and disopyramide can also inhibit the bypass tract and carry a Class IIb recommendation. Only amiodarone is available intravenously. The other agents are not available as IV preparations in the United States.

In patients with preexcitation, AV nodal blocking agents are contraindicated and may be fatal when there is atrial fibrillation. AV nodal blocking agents decrease the number of impulses entering the ventricles through the AV node, making the bypass tract less refractory. It can also enhance conduction across the bypass tract. This will allow more fibrillatory impulses to pass through the bypass tract from atrium to ventricle, thus increasing the ventricular rate during atrial fibrillation. Digoxin is particularly a dangerous pharmacologic agent to use in patients with WPW syndrome with atrial fibrillation. Digoxin not only blocks the AV node, but also enhances conduction through the bypass tract, further increasing the ventricular rate during atrial fibrillation. Verapamil also inhibits the AV node and is a potent vasodilator. It may enhance conduction through the bypass tract by reflex increase in sympathetic tone. These agents receive a Class III recommendation.

- In patients with concealed bypass tracts (no evidence of preexcitation in baseline ECG) who develop atrial fibrillation, the treatment of atrial fibrillation is similar to a patient without a bypass tract. AV nodal blocking agents such as beta blockers, calcium channel blockers, and digitalis can be given safely in controlling the ventricular rate during atrial fibrillation. The use of digitalis as long-term maintenance therapy, however, should be discouraged unless other AV nodal blocking agents are ineffective or are poorly tolerated.

- Some patients may be mistakenly identified as having concealed bypass tracts because they do not manifest any evidence of preexcitation in baseline ECG. These patients may not have any preexcitation because the bypass tract is not given the chance to become manifest—either from its distal location

from the sinus node (left-sided bypass tracts) or efficient conduction of the sinus impulse across the AV node. Anterograde conduction of the atrial impulse to the ventricles may occur during atrial fibrillation. These patients are difficult to identify unless electrophysiologic testing is performed.

## Prognosis

- Prognosis is good even among patients with history of atrial fibrillation because electrical ablation is curative. If radiofrequency ablation is not feasible, surgical ablation should be considered.

## Other Causes of Ventricular Preexcitation

- Ventricular preexcitation may be due to pathways other than direct connection between the atrium and the ventricle. The following summarizes the different pathways that can cause preexcitation.
  - **Bundle of Kent:** The bypass tract connects the atrium directly to the ventricle (Fig. 20.28A). This is the most common cause of preexcitation.
  - **Mahaim fibers:** Mahaim fibers may have different connections:
    - **Nodoventricular connection:** A bypass tract connecting the AV node directly to the ventricle (Fig. 20.28B).

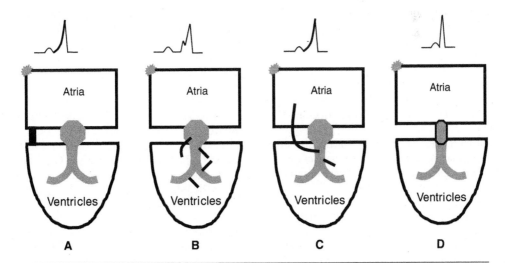

**Figure 20.28: Other Causes of Preexcitation. (A)** Preexcitation with a bypass tract connecting the atrium directly to the ventricles. This is associated with the classic ECG of WPW syndrome. **(B)** Mahaim fibers connecting the AV node directly to the ventricle (nodo-ventricular fiber), bundle of His directly to ventricle (Hisioventricular fiber) and bundle branches or fascicles directly to the ventricles (fasciculoventricular fiber). **(C)** A bypass tract connecting the atrium directly to the bundle of His. This is often associated with a Hisioventricular fiber resulting in a pattern similar to the WPW ECG **(A)**. **(D)** A small AV node resulting in a short PR interval and a normal QRS complex. ECG, electrocardiogram; WPW, Wolff-Parkinson-White.

□ **Hisioventricular connection:** A bypass tract connecting the His bundle directly to the ventricle (Fig. 20.28B,C).

□ **Fasciculoventricular connection:** A bypass tract connecting the right bundle, left bundle, or fascicles directly to the ventricles (Fig. 20.28B)

□ **Atrio-Hisian connection:** Connects the atria directly to the His bundle, thus bypassing the AV node (Fig. 20.28C).

■ **Superconducting AV node:** Small AV node resulting in a short PR interval with normal QRS complex (Fig. 20.28D).

## Suggested Readings

Blomstrom-Lundqvist C, Scheinman MM, Aliot EM, et al. ACC/AHA/ESC guidelines for the management of patients with supraventricular arrhythmias—executive summary: a report of the American College of Cardiology/American Heart Association Task Force on Practice Guidelines, and the European Society of Cardiology Committee for Practice Guidelines (Writing Committee to Develop Guidelines for the Management of Patients With Supraventricular Arrhythmias). *J Am Coll Cardiol.* 2003;42:1493–1531.

Boahene KA, Klein GJ, Yee R, et al. Atrial fibrillation in the Wolff-Parkinson-White syndrome. Diagnostic and management strategies. In: Horowitz LN, ed. *Current Management of Arrhythmias.* Philadelphia: BC Decker; 1991:123–129.

Cain ME, Lindsay BD. Preexcitation syndromes: diagnostic and management strategies. In: Horowitz LN, ed. *Current Management of Arrhythmias.* Philadelphia: BC Decker; 1991:91–103.

Calkins H, Langberg J, Sousa J, et al. Radiofrequency catheter ablation of accessory atrioventricular connections in 250 patients. *Circulation.* 1992;85:1337–1346.

Castellanos A, Interian Jr A, Myerburg RJ. The resting electrocardiogram. In: Fuster V, Alexander RW, O'Rourke RA, eds. *Hurst's The Heart.* 11th ed. New York: McGraw-Hill; 2004:295–324.

Dresing TJ, Schweikert RA, Packer DL. Atrioventricular nodal-dependent tachycardias. In: Topol EJ, ed. *Textbook of Cardiovascular Medicine.* 2nd ed. Philadelphia: Lippincott; 2002:1453–1478.

Fuster V, Ryden LE, Cannom DS, et al. ACC/AHA/ESC 2006 guidelines for the management of patients with atrial fibrillation—executive summary; a report of the American College of Cardiology/American Heart Association Task Force and the European Society of Cardiology Committee on Practice Guidelines and the European Society of Cardiology Committee for Practice Guidelines (Writing Committee to Revise the 2001 Guidelines for the Management of Patients with Atrial Fibrillation). *J Am Coll Cardiol.* 2006;48:854–906.

Gallagher JJ, Pritchett ELC, Sealy WC, et al. The preexcitation syndromes. *Progr Cardiovasc Dis.* 1978;20:285–327.

Guidelines 2000 for Cardiopulmonary Resuscitation and Emergency Cardiovascular Care: 7D: the tachycardia algorithms. *Circulation.* 2000;102 (Suppl I):I-158–I-165.

Klein GJ, Bashore TM, Sellers TD, et al. Ventricular fibrillation in the Wolff-Parkinson-White syndrome. *N Engl J Med.* 1979;301:1078–1079.

Krahn AD, Manfreda J, Tate RB, et al. The natural history of electrocardiographic preexcitation in men. The Manitoba Follow-up Study. *Ann Intern Med.* 1992;456–460.

Lindsay BD, Crossen KJ, Cain ME. Concordance of distinguishing electrocardiographic features during sinus rhythm with the location of accessory pathways in Wolff-Parkinson-White syndrome. *Am J Cardiol.* 1987;59:1093–1102.

March HW, Selzer A, Hultgren HN. The mechanical consequences of anomalous atrioventricular excitation (WPW syndrome). *Circulation.* 1961;23:582–592.

Michelson EL. Clinical perspectives in management of Wolff-Parkinson-White syndrome, Part 1: recognition, diagnosis, and arrhythmias. *Mod Concepts Cardiovasc Dis.* 1989;58:43–48.

Michelson EL. Clinical perspectives in management of Wolff-Parkinson-White syndrome, Part 2: diagnostic evaluation and treatment strategies. *Modern Concepts Cardiovasc Dis.* 1989;58:49–54.

Olgin JE, Zipes DP. Specific arrhythmia: diagnosis and treatment. In: Libby P, Bonow RO, Mann DL, et al., eds. *Braunwald's Heart Disease, A Textbook of Cardiovascular Medicine.* 8th ed. Philadelphia: Elsevier Saunders; 2008:863–931.

Pappone C, Manguso F, Santinelli R, et al. Radiofrequency ablation in children with asymptomatic Wolf-Parkinson-White syndrome. *N Engl J Med.* 2004;351:1197–1205.

Reddy GV, Schamroth L. The localization of bypass tracts in the Wolff-Parkinson-White syndrome from the surface electrocardiogram. *Am Heart J.* 1987;113:984–993.

Wellens HJJ. Wolff-Parkinson-White syndrome Part I. Diagnosis, arrhythmias, and identification of the high risk patient. *Mod Concepts Cardiovasc Dis.* 1983;52:53–56.

Wellens HJJ. Wolff-Parkinson-White syndrome Part II. Treatment. *Mod Concepts Cardiovasc Dis.* 1983;52:57–59.

Wellens HJJ, Conover MB. Narrow QRS tachycardia. *The ECG in Emergency Decision Making.* Philadelphia: WB Saunders; 1992:73–103.

Wellens HJJ, Gorgels AP. The electrocardiogram 102 years after Einthoven. *Circulation.* 2004;109:562–564.

Zuberbuhler JR, Bauersfeld SR. Paradoxical splitting of the second heart sound in the Wolff-Parkinson-White syndrome. *Am Heart J.* 1965;70:595–602.

# Ventricular Arrhythmias

## Premature Ventricular Complexes

- **Ventricular complexes:** Premature impulses originating from the ventricles that occur earlier than the next expected normal sinus impulse are called premature ventricular complexes (PVCs) (Fig. 21.1).
  - PVCs are not preceded by P waves.
  - They are wide measuring ≥0.12 seconds because they originate from the ventricles below the bifurcation of the bundle of His. The impulse does not follow the normal intraventricular conduction system and is conducted from one ventricle to the other by direct muscle cell to muscle cell transmission.
  - The ST segment and T waves are opposite in direction (discordant) to the QRS complex.
  - The QRS complex is followed by a pause that is usually fully compensatory.
- PVCs are often called ventricular extrasystoles. They occur very frequently in individuals with normal or abnormal hearts and are one of the most commonly encountered complexes in electrocardiography.
- PVCs can be unifocal or multifocal.
  - **Unifocal:** Premature ventricular impulses that originate from a single location in the ventricle are unifocal PVCs. The PVCs are uniform and have identical configuration (Fig. 21.2).
- **Multifocal:** Ventricular complexes that originate from two or more locations in the ventricle are multifocal PVCs. These PVCs have different configurations (Fig. 21.3).
- **Interpolated PVC:** The PVC is interpolated when it is inserted between two sinus impulses without altering the basic sinus rate. An interpolated PVC is not followed by a pause (Fig. 21.4).
- The PVC may or may not be followed by a fully compensatory pause.
  - **Fully compensatory pause:** The pause after a PVC is usually fully compensatory because the PVC does not discharge the sinus node prematurely; thus, the regularity of the sinus impulse is not interrupted (Fig. 21.5). The presence of a fully compensatory pause often differentiates a PVC from a premature atrial complex.
  - **Less than fully compensatory pause:** The pause after a PVC may be less than fully compensatory if the PVC is conducted retrogradely to the atria (ventriculoatrial conduction; Fig. 21.6) and discharges the sinus node prematurely. Because the sinus node is discharged earlier, its rate is reset causing the pause to be less than fully compensatory. The impulse may often suppress the sinus node, which may result in a much longer than fully compensatory pause.

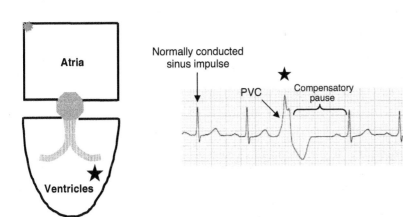

**Figure 21.1: Premature Ventricular Complex (PVC).** The diagram on the left shows an impulse (*star*) originating from the ventricle below the bifurcation of the bundle of His. The rhythm strip on the right shows two sinus complexes followed by a wide, bizarre looking complex called PVC (*marked by a star*). This complex is premature occurring before the next sinus impulse. The QRS deflection is wide and the ST segment and T wave are discordant followed by a compensatory pause.

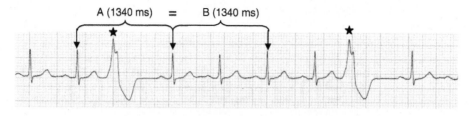

**Figure 21.2:   Unifocal Premature Ventricular Complexes (PVCs).** The two PVCs noted in the rhythm strip, marked by stars, are identical in configuration and are unifocal in origin. Note also that the pause following the PVC is fully compensatory, meaning that distance A, which straddles the PVC, measures the same as distance B, which straddles a normal sinus impulse. ms, milliseconds.

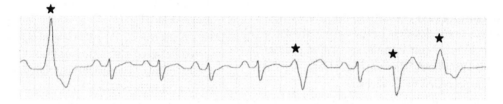

**Figure 21.3:   Multifocal Premature Ventricular Complexes (PVCs).** The PVCs marked by the stars have different configurations and are multiformed. These PVCs originate from different locations in the ventricles and are multifocal in origin.

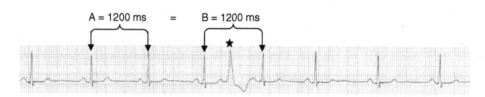

**Figure 21.4:   Interpolated Premature Ventricular Complex (PVC).** The PVC (*star*) is interpolated if it is sandwiched between two sinus complexes and is not followed by a pause. Note that the basic rate is not altered by the PVC (distance A, which represents the basic sinus rate is the same as distance B, which straddles a PVC). ms, milliseconds.

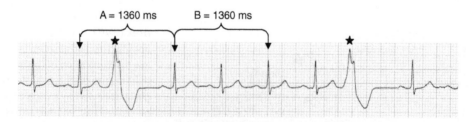

**Figure 21.5:   Fully Compensatory Pause.** Rhythm strip shows a premature ventricular complex (PVC) with a fully compensatory pause. The pause after a PVC is fully compensatory if the PVC does not reset the sinus node; thus, distance **A**, which straddles a PVC, measures the same as distance **B**, which straddles a normal sinus impulse.

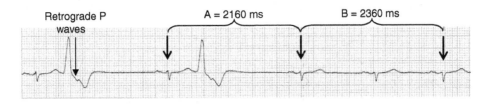

**Figure 21.6:    Less Than Fully Compensatory Pause.** Rhythm strip shows two premature ventricular complexes (PVCs) with retrograde conduction to the atria. When this occurs, the PVC may reset the sinus node. Note that the distance between two sinus impulses straddling a PVC (distance **A**) is shorter than the distance between two impulses straddling a sinus impulse (distance **B**). ms, milliseconds.

- **Ventriculoatrial conduction:** The ventricular impulse may conduct retrogradely across the atrioventricular (AV) node to activate the atria (Fig. 21.6). Although retrograde conduction to the atria may occur after a PVC, the retrograde P waves are not always visible because they are buried within the ST-T complex.
- **R on T phenomenon:** This refers to an early PVC striking the terminal portion of the T wave of the previous complex (Fig. 21.7). A PVC manifesting the R on T phenomenon has a short coupling interval.
- **End-diastolic PVC:** The PVC is end-diastolic if it occurs very late in diastole, so late that the next sinus P wave is already inscribed (Fig. 21.8). This usually results in a fusion complex. An end-diastolic PVC has a long coupling interval.
- **Coupling interval:** The coupling interval is the distance between the PVC and the preceding QRS complex. The coupling interval of most PVCs is usually constant. End-diastolic PVCs have long coupling intervals because they occur very late during diastole after the sinus P wave is inscribed (Fig. 21.8). Conversely, PVCs manifesting the R on T phenomenon have short coupling intervals, usually measuring ≤0.40 seconds. Because the coupling interval is short, the PVCs occur at the downslope of the T wave of the previous complex (Fig. 21.7), which corresponds to the vulnerable period of the ventricles. This may potentially trigger a ventricular arrhythmia.

- PVCs can occur as single beats but can be repetitive, occurring in bigeminy, trigeminy, quadrigeminy, etc.
  - **PVCs in bigeminy:** PVCs are bigeminal if every other complex is a PVC (Fig. 21.9).
  - **PVCs in trigeminy:** PVCs are trigeminal if every third complex is a PVC (Fig. 21.10). It is also trigeminal if there are two consecutive PVCs and the third complex is a sinus impulse (Fig. 21.11).
  - **PVCs in quadrigeminy:** The PVCs are quadrigeminal if every fourth complex is a PVC (Fig. 21.12).
  - **Paired PVCs:** PVCs occur in pairs or in couplets when two PVCs occur consecutively (Fig. 21.11).
- PVCs may originate from the right ventricle or left ventricle. The electrocardiogram (ECG) is helpful in differentiating one from the other.

## PVCs from the Right Ventricle

- **Right ventricular PVC:** PVC that originates from the right ventricle has a left bundle branch block (LBBB) configuration. Right ventricular PVCs may originate from any of the following locations (Fig. 21.13):
  - **Right ventricular apex:** The PVC has LBBB configuration and the axis in the frontal plane is deviated to the left (Fig. 21.14).

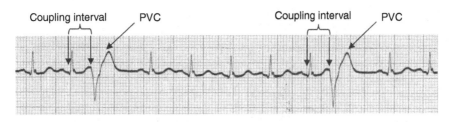

**Figure 21.7:    R on T Phenomenon.** The premature ventricular complexes (PVCs) occur early, hitting the T wave of the previous complex. These PVCs have short coupling intervals of ≤0.40 seconds. The down slope of the T wave corresponds to the vulnerable period of the ventricle when the ventricular myocytes are in the process of repolarization. This can result in reentry within the ventricles when a stimulus like a PVC occurs.

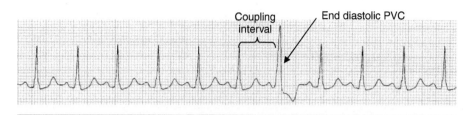

**Figure 21.8:** **End-Diastolic Premature Ventricular Complex (PVC).** The PVC is end-diastolic when it occurs very late, after the sinus P wave has been inscribed.

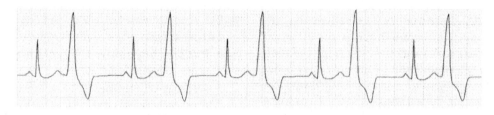

**Figure 21.9:** **Premature Ventricular Complexes (PVCs) in Bigeminy.** The PVCs alternate with normal sinus complexes.

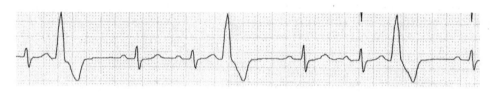

**Figure 21.10:** **Premature Ventricular Complexes (PVCs) in Trigeminy.** There are two sinus complexes and the third complex is a PVC.

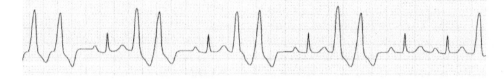

**Figure 21.11:** **Trigeminy, also Ventricular Couplets or Paired Premature Ventricular Complexes (PVCs).** One sinus complex and two consecutive PVCs also constitute trigeminy. These PVCs can also be described as occurring in pairs or in couplets.

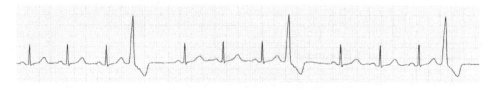

**Figure 21.12:** **Premature Ventricular Complexes (PVCs) in Quadrigeminy.** Every fourth complex is a PVC.

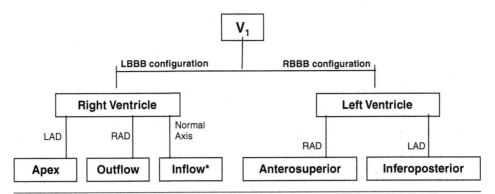

**Figure 21.13:   Localizing the Origin of the Premature Ventricular Complex (PVC).**  See text for explanation. LAD, left axis deviation; LBBB, left bundle branch block; RAD, right axis deviation; RBBB, right bundle branch block. *When the PVC has a normal axis, the PVC could originate from the right ventricular inflow or the area between the right ventricular apex and right ventricular outflow.

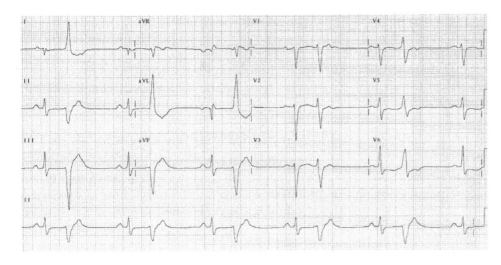

**Figure 21.14:   Premature Ventricular Complexes (PVCs) of Right Ventricular Origin.**  PVCs originating from the right ventricular apex have left bundle branch block (LBBB) configuration (rS complex in $V_1$ and tall R in $V_6$) with left axis deviation. The pattern is very similar to a pacemaker induced ventricular rhythm with the endocardial electrode positioned at the apex of the right ventricle.

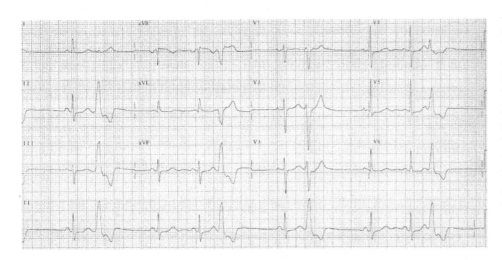

**Figure 21.15:   Premature Ventricular Complexes (PVCs) Originating from the Right Ventricular Outflow.**  The PVCs have left bundle branch block (LBBB) configuration with rS in $V_1$ and tall R waves in $V_6$. There is right axis deviation of the PVC in the frontal plane. These PVCs originate below the pulmonic valve in the right ventricular outflow area.

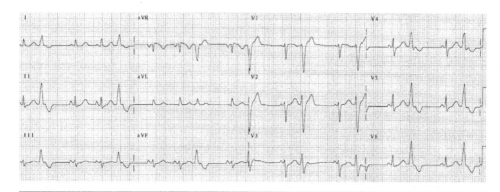

**Figure 21.16: Premature Ventricular Complexes (PVCs) from Right Ventricular Inflow.** PVCs from right ventricular inflow (tricuspid area) have left bundle branch block (LBBB) configuration with rS complex in $V_1$ and tall R in $V_6$. The axis of the PVC is normal in the frontal plane. This type of PVC may also originate between right ventricular apex and right ventricular outflow.

- **Right ventricular outflow:** The PVC has a LBBB configuration and the axis in the frontal plane is deviated to the right (Fig. 21.15).
- **Right ventricular inflow:** The PVC has LBBB configuration and the axis of the PVC in the frontal plane is normal. A PVC with this configuration can originate from the right ventricular inflow (tricuspid area), although it could also originate from the area between the right ventricular apex and right ventricular outflow (Fig. 21.16).

## PVCs from the Left Ventricle

- **Left ventricular PVC:** PVC that originates from the left ventricle have right bundle branch block (RBBB) configuration. Left ventricular PVCs may originate from the anterosuperior or inferoposterior areas (Fig. 21.13):
  - **Anterosuperior area:** This area is supplied by the left anterior fascicular branch of the left bundle branch. The PVC has a RBBB configuration and the axis is deviated to the right (Fig. 21.17).
  - **Inferoposterior area:** This area is supplied by the left posterior fascicular branch of the left bundle branch. The PVC has a RBBB configuration and the axis is deviated to the left (Fig. 21.18).
- Figure 21.14 shows PVCs originating from right ventricular apex; Figure 21.15 shows PVCs originating from the right ventricular outflow.

## Ventricular Parasystole

- **Parasystole:** Parasystole refers to an independent ectopic impulse that competes with the sinus node as the pacemaker of the heart. This ectopic impulse may be located in the atria, AV junction, or ventricles. The most commonly recognized location of a parasystole is in the ventricles.
- **Ventricular parasystole:** Regular automatic cells from the AV junction and ventricles can not discharge independently because they are constantly depolarized and reset by the propagated sinus impulse. These automatic cells serve as backup pacemakers and become

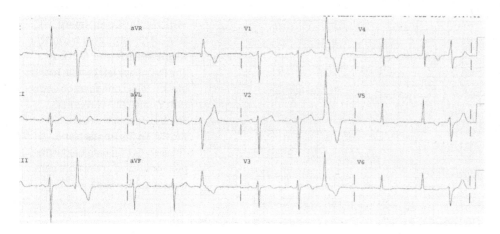

**Figure 21.17: Premature Ventricular Complexes (PVCs) from Left Ventricle.** PVCs originating from the left ventricle in the area supplied by the left anterior fascicle have right bundle branch block (RBBB) configuration and right axis deviation.

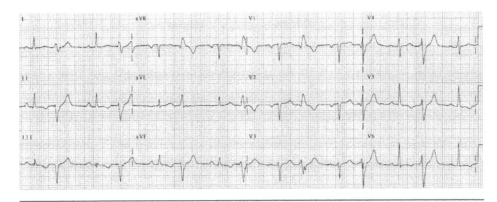

**Figure 21.18: Premature Ventricular Complexes (PVCs) from the Left Ventricle.**
PVCs originating from the left ventricle in the area supplied by the left posterior fascicle have right bundle branch block (RBBB) configuration and left axis deviation.

manifest only when the sinus node fails. Parasystole is different in that the cells are protected and cannot be discharged or reset by the sinus impulse. The parasystolic focus therefore can compete independently with the sinus impulse for control of the ventricles. The ventricular parasystole may or may not be able to capture the ventricles depending on the state of refractoriness of the ventricles. Thus, when the ventricles are not refractory from the previous sinus impulse, the parasystole may be able to capture the ventricles. Similarly, when the ventricles are still refractory from the previous impulse, the parasystole will not be able to capture the ventricles. Additionally, the sinus impulse and the ventricular parasystole may be able to capture the ventricles simultaneously resulting in fusion beats.

- A premature ventricular impulse is therefore considered parasystolic when all of the following features are present (Fig. 21.19).
  - The coupling intervals of the ventricular complexes are variable.
  - Fusion complexes are present.
  - The ventricular complexes are mathematically related. Because the parasystolic focus is firing continuously, the longer interectopic intervals are multiples of the shorter interectopic intervals.

## Classification of Ventricular Arrhythmias

- **Classification of ventricular arrhythmias:** According to the American College of Cardiology/American Heart Association/European Society of Cardiology (ACC/AHA/ESC) 2006 guidelines, ventricular arrhythmias can be classified according to clinical presentation, ECG presentation, and disease entity.
- **Clinical presentation:**
  - Hemodynamically stable
    - Asymptomatic
    - Minimally symptomatic (palpitations)
  - Hemodynamically unstable
    - Presyncope (dizziness, lightheadedness, feeling faint or "graying out")
    - Syncope (sudden loss of consciousness with spontaneous recovery)

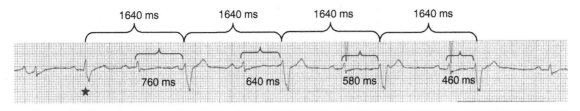

**Figure 21.19: Ventricular Parasystole.** The rhythm is normal sinus interrupted by ectopic ventricular complexes with coupling intervals that vary from 460 to 760 milliseconds. The intervals between the ectopic ventricular complexes are constant measuring 1,640 milliseconds. The first ventricular complex marked by a star is a fusion complex. The presence of variable coupling intervals, fusion complex, and the constant intervals between the ectopic ventricular complexes suggest that the ventricular impulse is parasystolic.

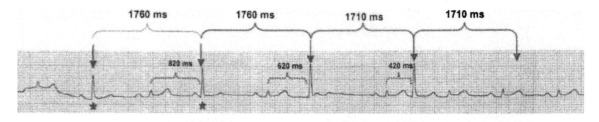

**Figure 21.20:   Ventricular Parasystole.** The rhythm is normal sinus. Parasystolic impulses compete with the sinus rhythm resulting in ventricular complexes (*arrows*) with variable coupling intervals (*dotted brackets*). Fusion complexes (*marked by stars*) are also present. The last parasystolic impulse occurred during the refractory period of the ventricles and was not captured (*last arrow*).

□ Sudden cardiac death (death from unexpected circulatory arrest occurring within an hour after onset of symptoms).

□ Sudden cardiac arrest (death from unexpected circulatory arrest usually from cardiac arrhythmia occurring within an hour after onset of symptoms in which medical intervention such as defibrillation reverses the event).

■ **Electrocardiographic presentation:**
  ▪ Nonsustained ventricular tachycardia (VT)
    □ Monomorphic (Fig. 21.21)
    □ Polymorphic
  ▪ Sustained VT
    □ Monomorphic (Fig. 21.22)
    □ Polymorphic
  ▪ Bundle branch reentrant tachycardia
  ▪ Bidirectional VT (Fig. 21.23)
  ▪ Torsades de pointes (Figs. 21.24 to 21.29)
  ▪ Ventricular flutter (Fig. 21.30)
  ▪ Ventricular fibrillation (Fig. 21.31)

■ **Disease entity:** The clinical and disease entities in which ventricular arrhythmias may occur include coronary disease, heart failure, congenital heart disease, neurological disorders, structurally normal hearts, sudden infant death syndrome, and cardiomyopathies (dilated, hypertrophic, and arrhythmogenic right ventricular cardiomyopathy).

## Ventricular Tachycardia

■ **VT:** Three PVCs in a row is a triplet. Three or more consecutive PVCs with a rate that exceeds 100 beats per minute (bpm) is VT. VT can be classified as sustained or nonsustained, monomorphic or polymorphic.

  ▪ **Nonsustained VT:** VT is nonsustained if the tachycardia terminates spontaneously within 30 seconds (Fig. 21.21).

  ▪ **Sustained VT:** VT is sustained if the tachycardia lasts more than 30 seconds (Fig. 21.22). It is also sustained if the tachycardia is associated with hemodynamic compromise, such as dizziness, hypotension, or near syncope, even if the duration of the VT is <30 seconds.

  ▪ **Monomorphic VT:** VT is monomorphic if the ventricular complexes have a single or uniform configuration and may be nonsustained (Fig. 21.21) or sustained (Fig. 21.22).

  ▪ **Polymorphic VT:** VT is polymorphic if the QRS complexes are multiformed or have different configurations and may be nonsustained (Fig. 21.24) or sustained (Fig. 21.25 and Figs. 21.27-21.28).

■ **Bundle branch reentrant tachycardia:** This type of VT is due to reentry. The pathway usually involves the left bundle branch, bundle of His, right bundle branch, ventricular septum, and back to the left bundle branch and

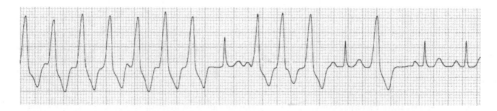

**Figure 21.21:   Nonsustained Monomorphic Ventricular Tachycardia (VT).** Three or more consecutive premature ventricular complexes (PVCs) with a rate of >100 complexes per minute is VT. The VT is monomorphic because the ventricular complexes have the same configuration. The VT is nonsustained because the duration of the tachycardia is <30 seconds.

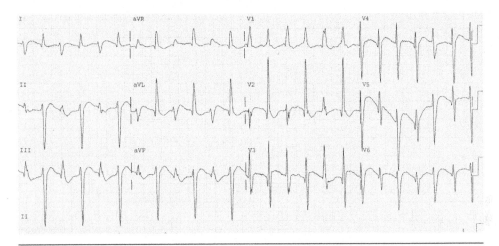

**Figure 21.22:** **Sustained Monomorphic Ventricular Tachycardia (VT).** The VT is monomorphic because the QRS complexes are uniform. VT is sustained if the duration is >30 seconds or the tachycardia is associated with hemodynamic symptoms of hypotension, dizziness or near syncope even if the tachycardia terminates spontaneously within 30 seconds.

**Figure 21.23:** **Bidirectional Ventricular Tachycardia.** The QRS complexes have right bundle branch block (RBBB) configuration with tall R waves in $V_1$. The axis of the QRS complex in the frontal leads alternates from left axis to right axis indicating that the origin of the tachycardia alternates between left anterior and left posterior fascicles.

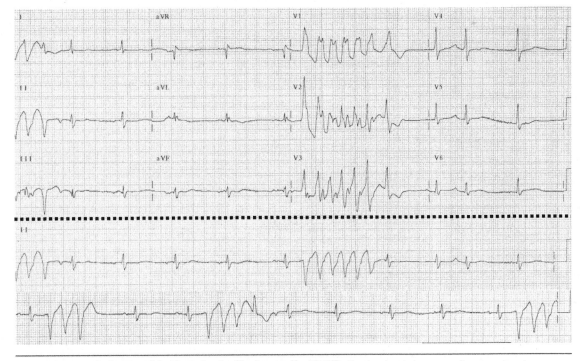

**Figure 21.24:** **Polymorphic Ventricular Tachycardia (PVT).** Twelve-lead electrocardiogram showing non-sustained PVT. The rate of the PVT is very rapid and irregular and the QRS complexes have varying morphologies. The QTc is >0.46 seconds and is prolonged. When the QTc is prolonged, the PVT is called torsades de pointes. Lead II rhythm strips are recorded at the bottom of the tracing.

**A.**

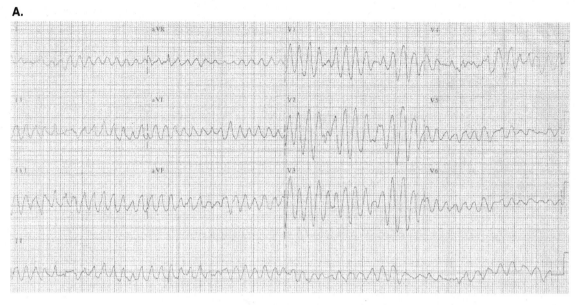

**B.**

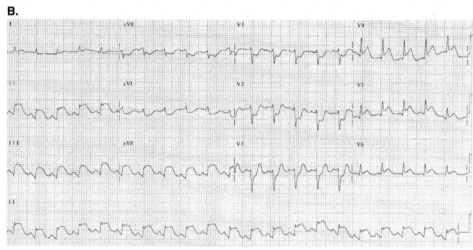

**Figure 21.25:  Polymorphic Ventricular Tachycardia (PVT).** **(A)** Twelve-lead electrocardiogram (ECG) showing PVT. The QRS complexes have different sizes and shapes and the rate is very rapid and irregular at almost 300 beats per minute. **(B)** The ECG immediately after successful cardioversion showed acute inferior myocardial infarction with a QTc of <0.44 seconds.

**Figure 21.26:  Torsades de Pointes.** Electrocardiogram (ECG) **(A)**: Baseline 12-lead ECG showing unusually prolonged QTc of >0.70 seconds. Rhythm strip **(B)** is from the same patient showing nonsustained torsades de pointes. There are pauses (long cycles) on termination of the tachycardia. These pauses prolong the QT interval of the next complex. The compensatory pauses of single PVCs also result in long cycles, which also prolong the QTc of the next complex and facilitates the onset of torsades de pointes.

**A.**

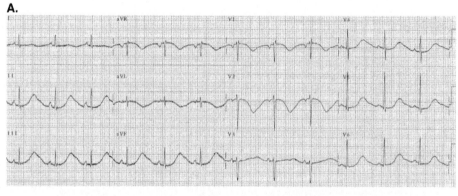

**B.**

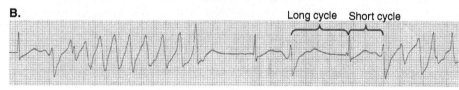

Long cycle    Short cycle

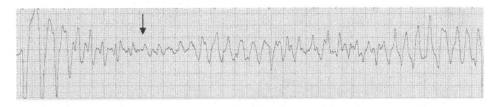

**Figure 21.27:    Torsades de Pointes.** The classical pattern of torsades de pointes is seen in the rhythm strip. The polarity of the QRS complexes keeps changing. Some QRS complexes seem to point up and others down. An isoelectric zone is marked by the arrow, which represents the "node." The taller complexes represent the "spindle."

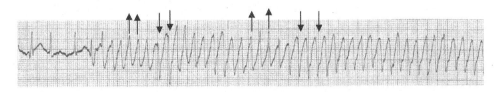

**Figure 21.28:    Polymorphic Ventricular Tachycardia.** The ventricular tachycardia starts with the fourth complex and continues to the end of the rhythm strip. Note that the rate of the tachycardia is unusually rapid and the ventricular complexes are polymorphic with some complexes pointing downward and other complexes pointing upward as shown by the arrows.

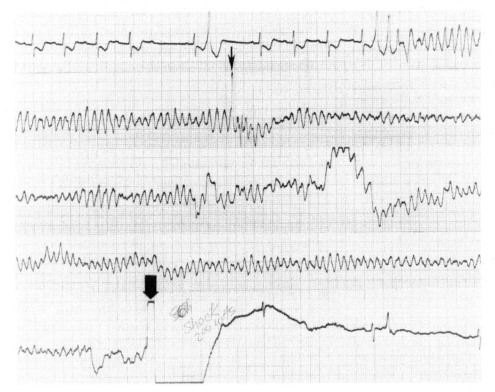

**Figure 21.29:    Polymorphic Ventricular Tachycardia (PVT).** Continuous rhythm strip showing sustained PVT deteriorating to ventricular fibrillation terminated by DC shock of 200 joules. The small arrow at the second rhythm strip is a precordial thump that was not successful in terminating the tachycardia. The QTc is not prolonged.

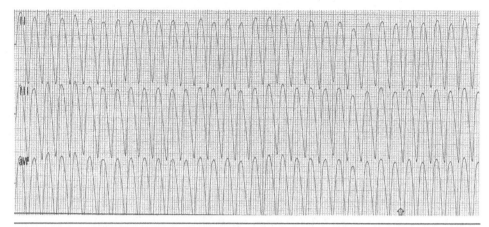

**Figure 21.30: Ventricular Flutter.** The QRS complexes are wide and uniform with a rate of approximately 300 beats per minute. The QRS complexes are monomorphic and there are no iso-electric intervals between the QRS complexes. Ventricular flutter is similar to monomorphic ventricular tachycardia (VT) except for the higher heart rate and has the same clinical significance.

left ventricle. During tachycardia, the right ventricle is activated anterogradely through the right bundle branch and the left ventricle through the ventricular septum. Thus, the QRS complexes are wide measuring ≥0.14 seconds with a LBBB pattern. During normal sinus rhythm, the baseline ECG usually shows evidence of His-Purkinje system disease with complete or incomplete LBBB often with a slightly prolonged PR interval. This type of VT should be identified because if sustained and recurrent, the VT may respond to radiofrequency ablation.

- **Bidirectional tachycardia:** In bidirectional tachycardia, the VT originates from two separate locations, the left anterior and left posterior fascicles of the left ventricle. Thus, the VT has RBBB configuration and the axis of the ectopic impulse alternates between right and left axis in the frontal plane (Fig. 21.23). When the ectopic impulse originates from the left anterior fascicle, the QRS complex is deviated to the right. When the ectopic impulse originates from the left posterior fascicle, the QRS complex is deviated to the left (see origin of PVCs, Fig. 21.13). This type of VT is frequently associated with digitalis toxicity.

## Polymorphic Ventricular Tachycardia

- **Polymorphic VT:** Polymorphic VT or PVT refers to a wide complex tachycardia with varying morphology of the QRS complexes (Fig. 21.24). The tachycardia is very unique in that the QRS complexes keep changing in size, shape, and direction. The rate of the tachycardia is usually rapid and irregular causing the patient to become hemodynamically unstable even when the VT is only of short duration. The configuration of the QRS complex may fluctuate and appear upright and then twists itself to become inverted with an isoelectric transition point, thus resembling a "spindle and node." The PVT may occur in short bursts and may be self-terminating. If the arrhythmia becomes sustained (>30 seconds), the tachycardia may degenerate to ventricular fibrillation and can cause sudden death.

## Torsades de Pointes

- **Torsades de pointes:** PVT may or may not be associated with prolonged QT interval. When the PVT is associated with prolonged QT interval, the VT is called torsades de pointes. When the PVT is associated with normal QT interval, the VT is a regular form of PVT. Torsades de pointes should be differentiated from regular PVT because the treatment of torsades de pointes is different from that of regular PVT.
- **Regular PVT:** The 12-lead ECG of a patient with sustained PVT is shown (Fig. 21.25A). The 12-lead ECG immediately after she was successfully cardioverted to normal sinus rhythm showed acute inferior myocardial infarction (Fig. 21.25B) with normal QTc of <0.44 seconds.

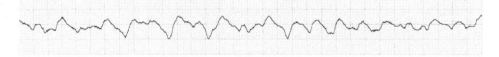

**Figure 21.31: Ventricular Fibrillation.** In ventricular fibrillation, the rhythm is very disorganized and ineffective with an undulating baseline. The QRS complexes are very irregular and are not well defined. This rhythm is fatal unless the patient is successfully resuscitated.

- **Torsades de pointes:** The presence of prolonged QTc differentiates torsades de pointes from regular PVT. The QT interval is measured during normal sinus rhythm before or immediately on termination of the tachycardia. The QT interval should be corrected for heart rate because the QT interval measures longer with slower heart rates and shorter with faster heart rates. The QT interval corrected for heart rate is the QTc. The QTc is prolonged when it measures >0.44 seconds in men and >0.46 seconds in women and in children. Prolonged QTc should always be recognized because it predisposes to torsades de pointes even among patients without cardiac disease, which can be fatal. The step by step calculation of the QTc is shown in Chapter 2, Basic Electrocardiography.
- Prolongation of the QTc may be inherited or it may be acquired.
  - **Inherited prolongation of the QTc:** These patients are usually young and have family history of sudden death, often occurring at a young age. In some patients with congenitally prolonged QTc, the QTc does not stay prolonged, but may vary. Thus, screening of asymptomatic patients with family history of prolonged QTc may not show QT prolongation in the initial ECG examination. Additionally, about a third of patients who are known carriers of long QT syndrome confirmed by genetic testing will not show QTc prolongation. The duration of the QTc parallels the risk of developing torsades de pointes and sudden death. A long QTc of ≥0.50 seconds in patients with congenitally prolonged QT syndrome is a marker of increased cardiovascular risk. Because the QT duration exhibits marked variability, the longest QTc measured at any time during follow-up of a patient with congenital long QT syndrome provides important prognostic information.
  - **Acquired prolongation of the QTc:** In normal individuals, QTc prolongation can occur during acute myocardial ischemia, electrolyte abnormalities (hypokalemia, hypocalcemia, and hypomagnesemia), use of antiarrhythmic agents (Class IA and Class III), antihistaminics, antifungals, antimicrobials, tricyclic antidepressants, and nutritional causes resulting from alcohol, liquid protein diet, anorexia, and starvation. A long list of agents that can cause prolonged QTc can be accessed through Web sites at www.torsades.org or www.qtdrugs.org.
- During tachycardia, the QRS complexes of torsades de pointes and regular PVT are similar and are both polymorphic. During normal sinus rhythm, the QTc of torsades de pointes is prolonged, whereas the QTc of regular PVT is not. Torsades de pointes is pause dependent, occurring when there is bradycardia, which is known to prolong the QTc. The arrhythmia is frequently seen in the setting of long/short cycles as shown in Figure 21.26B.

- PVT with or without prolongation of the QTc is a serious arrhythmia that can become sustained and can cause sudden death. Even when the tachycardia is short and self-terminating, it is associated with symptoms and is usually not tolerable because of the very rapid ventricular rate as shown in the examples (Figs. 21.28 and 21.29).
- **Ventricular flutter:** Ventricular flutter is similar to monomorphic VT except for a higher heart rate of approximately 300 bpm. There is no isoelectric interval between the QRS complexes. Because of the unusually rapid ventricular rate, the arrhythmia is seldom tolerated (Fig. 21.30). Ventricular flutter and VT are treated similarly.
- **Ventricular fibrillation:** Ventricular fibrillation is a disorganized ventricular rhythm with poorly defined QRS complexes. The baseline is undulating and the QRS complexes are very irregular with varying sizes and shapes (Fig. 21.31). Monomorphic and polymorphic VT and ventricular fibrillation are frequently seen in patients with cardiac disease and severe left ventricular dysfunction. It can also occur in patients with structurally normal hearts such as patients with prolonged QT syndrome or patients with the Brugada syndrome.
- Figure 21.32 summarizes diagrammatically the different ventricular arrhythmias.

## Summary of ECG Findings

1. A PVC is a premature complex that is wide with an ST segment and T wave that are opposite in direction to the QRS complex. This is followed by a pause that is fully compensatory. PVCs are often called ventricular extrasystoles with coupling intervals that are fixed.

2. A ventricular parasystole is a ventricular ectopic impulse that is protected. It is identified by the presence of fusion complexes, variable coupling intervals, and longer interectopic intervals that are mathematically related to the shorter interectopic intervals.

3. VT is present when three or more PVCs occur consecutively with a rate >100 bpm. VT can be sustained or nonsustained, monomorphic, or polymorphic.
   - The VT is nonsustained if the duration of the tachycardia is ≤30 seconds.
   - The VT is sustained if the duration is >30 seconds or if the tachycardia is associated with hemodynamic symptoms such as hypotension, dizziness, or syncope even if the tachycardia is self-terminating with a duration of ≤30 seconds.
   - VT is monomorphic if the QRS complexes are uniform in configuration.
   - VT is polymorphic if the QRS complexes have varying morphologies.
     - Torsades de pointes is a special form of polymorphic VT associated with prolonged QTc.
     - Regular polymorphic VT is similar to torsades de pointes except that the baseline QT interval is not prolonged.

## Summary of the Different Types of Ventricular Complexes

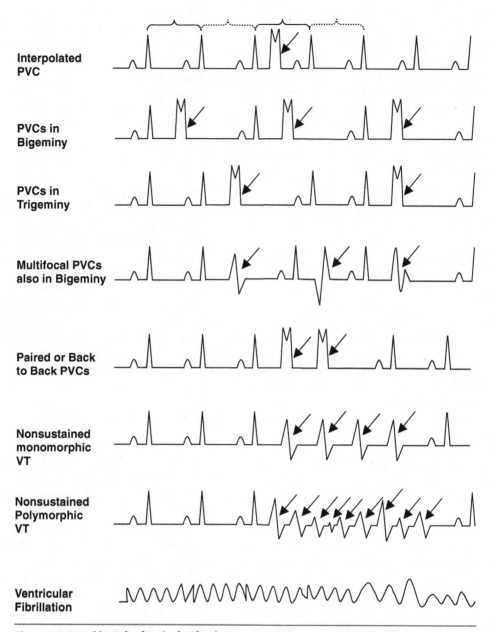

**Figure 21.32:  Ventricular Arrhythmias.** Diagram shows examples of different ventricular arrhythmias. Arrows point to the ventricular ectopic complexes.

4. Ventricular flutter has monomorphic ventricular complexes with a rate of approximately ≥250 bpm. The QRS complexes are not separated by isoelectric intervals.

5. Ventricular fibrillation has very disorganized rhythm with poorly defined QRS complexes with a rate of >300 bpm and is fatal if not emergently cardioverted.

## Mechanism

- PVCs look different from normally conducted sinus impulses because PVCs originate from the ventricles below the bifurcation of the bundle of His. The impulse activates the ventricles sequentially by spreading from one ventricle to

the other. This is in contrast to a supraventricular impulse, which originates above the bifurcation of the bundle of His, resulting in activation of both ventricles synchronously causing the QRS complexes to be narrow.

- PVCs are commonly extrasystolic and are usually related to the preceding impulse most probably because of reentry of the impulse within the ventricles. Thus, the coupling intervals of extrasystoles are constant or fixed.

- A ventricular parasystole is an independent pacemaker that is protected and is not depolarized by the propagated sinus impulse. It can therefore compete with the sinus node independently for control of the ventricles. Unlike ventricular extrasystoles, it bears no relationship to the preceding ventricular complex; thus, the coupling interval is not fixed. The impulse can capture the ventricles only when the ventricles are not refractory from the previous sinus impulse. Fusion beats are therefore present and the intervals between parasystolic impulses are mathematically related.

- The origin of the ventricular impulse can be predicted by examining the morphology of the QRS complex in the 12-lead ECG. Briefly, ectopic ventricular complexes originating from the left ventricle will show positive or tall R waves in $V_1$ (RBBB pattern) because the impulse has to travel from left ventricle to right ventricle toward lead $V_1$. Ventricular complexes originating from the right ventricle will show negative or deep S waves in $V_1$ (LBBB pattern) because the impulse has to travel from right ventricle to left ventricle away from $V_1$.

- VT both sustained and nonsustained may be due to enhanced automaticity of cells within the myocardium or His-Purkinje system. It could also be due to triggered activity, as in digitalis toxicity. It can also be due to reentry requiring the presence of two separate pathways with different electrophysiologic properties within the ventricles.

- Repolarization of the millions of individual myocardial cells in the ventricles is not homogeneous because there are intrinsic differences in the action potential duration among the various cells composing the myocardium. This inhomogeneity or dispersion in ventricular repolarization will cause some cells to become excitable, whereas others continue to be refractory. This period may be extended when phase 3 is delayed or when there is prolongation of the action potential duration and QT interval. An ectopic impulse presented to the ventricles during this vulnerable period, which corresponds to the mid and terminal portion of phase 3 of the action potential, represented by the downslope of the T wave in the ECG (R on T phenomenon) may cause a reentrant tachycardia within the ventricles. Thus, QT dispersion >100 milliseconds, representing the difference between the longest and shortest QT interval in the 12-lead ECG, may be helpful in predicting those who are high risk for ventricular arrhythmias.

- When acute myocardial ischemia and injury are present, the triggering impulse may not have to occur during the vulnerable phase of ventricular repolarization to cause ventricular arrhythmias because the presence of injured myocardium can further increase QT dispersion. Thus, in the setting of acute myocardial infarction, early and late PVCs are as likely to trigger VT.

## Clinical Significance

- **Simple PVCs:** Single and frequent PVCs including multiformed complexes are commonly seen in patients with cardiac disease, although they are also present in healthy individuals with structurally normal hearts. In normal individuals, the frequency of ectopic ventricular complexes increases with increasing age.
  - **During infancy:** PVCs are rare during infancy. In a 24-hour Holter study of 134 healthy, full-term newborn infants, 19 had premature complexes, all supraventricular.

  - **During childhood:** Among healthy children, ages 7 to 11 years, 24-hour Holter monitor showed premature complexes only in 20 of 92 children. The premature complexes were supraventricular in 19 children and only 1 had a PVC.
  - **Medical students:** Among 50 healthy male medical students, 24-hour Holter study showed isolated PVCs in 25 (50%) and were multifocal in 6 (12%). One (2%) had couplets and another (2%) had nonsustained VT defined as three or more PVCs in a row with a rate >100 bpm.
  - **Elderly population:** Among 98 healthy elderly patients aged 60 to 85, 78 (80%) had ventricular arrhythmias. Ventricular couplets were present in 11 (11%) and nonsustained VT in 4 (4%). Multiformed PVCs were present in 34 (35%), 12 (12%) had ≥30 PVCs any hour, 7 (7%) have ≥60 PVCs any hour, and 17 (17%) had total of ≥100 PVCs in 24 hours.

- **Frequent and complex PVCs:** Complex PVCs consisting of frequent multiformed ventricular complexes and nonsustained monomorphic VT are generally benign in completely asymptomatic individuals if there is no demonstrable cardiac disease and left ventricular systolic function is preserved. However, in patients with structural cardiac diseases, especially those with left ventricular dysfunction, these ventricular arrhythmias need further evaluation.
  - **Healthy population:** Long-term follow-up (3 to 9.5 years, mean 6.5 years) of 73 asymptomatic and healthy individuals, age 18 to 72 years, with frequent complex ventricular ectopy including those with nonsustained VT by 24-hour Holter (mean PVCs per hour 566, multiformed PVCs 63%, ventricular couplets 60%, nonsustained VT 26%), showed no increased mortality and a long-term prognosis similar to that of the general healthy population.
  - **Patients with left ventricular dysfunction:** Although these ventricular arrhythmias are not targets for pharmacologic therapy in the hospital or outpatient setting, patients with left ventricular dysfunction (ejection fraction of ≤40%) with frequent and complex ventricular ectopy should be referred for further evaluation because they may be at risk for more serious arrhythmias.

- **Ventricular parasystole:** Ventricular arrhythmias that are known to be parasystolic are considered benign and require no therapy. A ventricular parasystole should always be suspected when the coupling intervals of the PVCs are not fixed. They are also recognized by fusion beats and the intervals between complexes are mathematically related.

- **Sustained VT and ventricular fibrillation:** Sustained VT and ventricular fibrillation are malignant arrhythmias that can cause sudden death. They commonly occur as a complication of acute myocardial infarction. They are also seen in patients with structural cardiac diseases especially ischemic, nonischemic, and hypertrophic cardiomyopathies. It is rare in patients with structurally normal hearts unless there is:
  - **Long QT syndrome, acquired or congenital**
  - **Brugada syndrome**
  - **Wolff-Parkinson-White syndrome**

- **The long QT syndrome:** The QT interval is prolonged when the QTc measures >0.44 seconds (or >440 milliseconds) in men and >0.46 seconds (or >460 milliseconds) in women. A long QT interval predisposes to torsades de pointes, which is a special type of polymorphic VT. The following is a simplified review of the ionic changes that occur in the ventricular myocyte that can result in prolongation of the QT interval (see Chapter 1, Basic Anatomy and Electrophysiology).

  - **Mechanism of the prolongation of the QT interval:** During depolarization or phase 0 of the action potential, the fast sodium channels open briefly allowing sodium ions to enter the cell. The entry of positive ions into the cell causes the polarity of the cell to change abruptly from −90 to +10 to +20 mV. Depolarization is immediately followed by repolarization consisting of phases 1 through 3 of the action potential. This corresponds to the J point extending to the end of the T wave in the surface ECG. During phase 2, which corresponds to the plateau phase of the action potential, the polarity of the cell is maintained at approximately 0 mV for a sustained duration. This is due to entry of calcium into the cell because of activation of the slow or "L-type" calcium channels during depolarization. This slow but sustained flow of positive ions into the cell is counterbalanced by the flow of potassium out of the cell because the cell membrane is more permeable to potassium than other ions. This loss of potassium makes the inside of the cell more negative as positive ions are lost. Thus, the entry of calcium into the cell (entry of positive ions) combined with flow of potassium out of the cell (loss of positive ions) results in an equilibrium that is sustained for a prolonged duration corresponding to the plateau or phase 2 of the action potential. When the calcium channels are inactivated, the entry of calcium into the cell is suddenly prevented although the outward flow of potassium continues. This inequity in calcium entry and potassium outflow advances the action potential to phase 3. Phase 3 or rapid repolarization is due to continuous efflux of potassium from the cell causing the cell to become more negative until the resting potential of –90 mV is reached. This marks the end of phase 3 of the action potential, which corresponds to the end of the T wave in the surface ECG.

  - As long as the potential of the ventricular myocyte is prevented from reaching –90 mV, which is the normal resting potential, the cell is not fully repolarized. Thus, any mechanism that will prolong or increase the entry of sodium or calcium into the cell will make the inside of the cell more positive and will delay or prolong the duration of the action potential. Similarly, any mechanism that will inhibit or delay the exit of potassium out of the cell will make the cell less negative. This will also prolong the duration of the action potential.

  - Phases 0 through 3 of the transmembrane action potential correspond to the duration of the action potential of individual myocardial cells. This is equivalent to the QT interval in the surface ECG. Prolongation of phases 1 through 3 will result in prolongation of the QT interval.

- **Causes of prolonged QT interval:** Prolongation of the QT interval may be acquired or it may be congenital.

  - **Acquired long QT:** In normal individuals with normal QTc, several pharmacologic agents can prolong the QT interval. These include type IA antiarrhythmic agents (quinidine, disopyramide, and procainamide), type III antiarrhythmic drugs (dofetilide, ibutilide, sotalol, and amiodarone), antipsychotic agents (chlorpromazine, thioridazine, and haloperidol), macrolide antibiotics (erythromycin, clarithromycin), antifungal agents (ketonazole and itraconazole), electrolyte disturbances notably hypomagnesemia and hypokalemia, and other agents such as pentamidine and methadone. A long list of pharmacologic agents that can prolong the QT interval can be accessed at www.torsades.org. Although the use of a single pharmacologic agent (quinidine or ibutilide) may cause QT prolongation and torsades de pointes almost immediately, occasionally, a combination of two agents may be needed to prolong the QT interval such as the concurrent use of erythromycin and ketonazole. Erythromycin, a macrolide antibiotic, and ketonazole, an antifungal agent, are both metabolized by the liver through the cytochrome P-450 3A4 (CYP 3A4) metabolic pathway. Either agent can potentially prolong the QT interval although prolongation of the QT interval is more significant when both agents are taken concurrently because they compete for the same metabolic pathway resulting in increased plasma concentration of both agents. Similarly, an agent that does not prolong the QT interval but depends on the CYP 3A4 metabolic pathway for clearance such as a calcium channel blocker (verapamil) when combined with a drug that prolongs the QT interval such as erythromycin can result in further prolongation of the QT interval since verapamil also depends on the same pathway as that of erythromycin for clearance. The effect on QT prolongation and potential for torsades de pointes may be more delayed, however.

  - **Congenital long QT:** Congenital or inherited prolongation of the QT interval affects young individuals especially the first 2 decades of life and is a common cause of sudden death in this age group. Two types of long QT syndrome have been clinically described.

    - The first familial long QT syndrome described by Jervell and Lange-Nielsen is associated with sensorineural deafness. This type of long QT syndrome is inherited as autosomal recessive. The second familial long QT syndrome is the Romano-Ward syndrome and is inherited as autosomal dominant but is not associated with congenital deafness.

    - With the advent of genetic testing, seven long QT syndromes have been described thus far and are labeled LQT1 to LQT7 according to the sequence in which the abnormal locus of the genetic defect have been discovered. The first three entities—LQT1, LQT2, and LQT3—are the most common and comprise almost 95% of all identified cases of congenital long QT syndromes. The prolongation of the QT is due to a genetic defect involving the potassium channel in most cases except LQT3 and LQT4, which are due to a defect in sodium transport. The genetic abnormality involves the ion channel in almost all cases except LQT4, which does not affect the ion channel directly, but only its supporting structure.

☐ Patients with long QT syndrome can be confirmed by genetic testing, although a negative genetic test will not exclude the presence of congenital long QT syndrome because up to 40% of patients with congenital long QT have not been linked to any genetic abnormality. Additionally, the use of genetic testing remains very expensive and may not be affordable when screening several family members with history of long QT syndrome or known sudden death in the family. It also takes several weeks before the results are known. Thus, the diagnosis of long QT syndrome is more commonly based on phenotypic ECG abnormalities.

☐ When the ECG is used in the diagnosis of patients with congenital long QT syndrome, marked variability in the duration of the QTc in serial ECGs can occur. Even in normal individuals, the QT interval can vary by as much as 50 to 75 milliseconds over a 24-hour period. Thus, screening of individuals with family history of long QT syndrome and sudden death may not show any initial QT prolongation. Additionally, almost a third of patients who are confirmed carriers have normal or borderline QTc of 0.40 to 0.46 seconds. The longest QTc, including those measured before age 10 years, provides important prognostic information during adolescence in patients with congenital long QT syndrome. Thus, a long QTc measuring ≥0.50 seconds identifies a patient who has increased risk of cardiovascular events and shorter QT intervals of <0.50 seconds decreases the risk of cardiovascular events. In these patients, however, there is no clear cut QT interval that is considered safe because QTc of ≤0.46 seconds are also at risk for syncope and sudden death.

☐ The following is a summary of the known long QT syndromes:

■ **LQT1:** Long QT1 is the first mutation to be identified. It is one of the most common, accounting for approximately 50% of known long QT abnormalities. The abnormality involves the short arm of chromosome 11. The gene was identified using cloning techniques and was named KvLQT1 because it encodes a potassium channel, but was eventually renamed KCNQ1. Homozygous mutation of the gene causes the Jervell and Lange-Nielsen syndrome. The syndrome is associated with congenital deafness, which is also due to the abnormality

in the same potassium channels involved with the production of potassium-rich endolymph in the inner ear. It is a much more common cause of sudden death younger than age 10 years when compared with the other long QT syndromes. Prolongation of the QT is due to delay in phase 3 of the action potential because of delay in the transport of potassium (α-subunit of the slow potassium rectifier or IKs). In addition to the prolonged QT, the T wave in the ECG has a slow indistinct onset, but is otherwise normal. Patients with LQT1 are most symptomatic during exertion because the QT interval becomes longer with exercise in contrast to patients with LQT3 who are most symptomatic during rest or sleep. The QT interval can be prolonged by intravenous injection of epinephrine. Thus, in symptomatic individuals, if the initial QT is not prolonged, the long QT can be unmasked with epinephrine.

■ **LQT2:** Long QT2 is also one of the most common long QT abnormalities with up to 40% of all congenital cases of long QT syndrome. The defect resides in chromosome 7 and the identified gene is called HERG (human ether a-go-go related gene) or KCNH2. Similar to LQT1, this gene is also involved with the potassium current. Unlike LQT1 that affects the slow potassium currents (called slow K rectifier or IKs), the gene is involved with the fast potassium currents (called rapid K rectifier or IKr), which is the most important in determining the duration of the action potential. Most pharmacologic agents that prolong the QT interval also inhibit the same potassium channel. In LQT2, the shape of the T wave in the ECG is bifid or split. Mutation of the HERG gene causes another abnormality characterized by an unusually short QT interval of ≤0.30 seconds called congenital short QT syndrome, which is also associated with sudden death.

■ **LQT3:** Unlike LQT1 and LQT2, which are involved with potassium transport, LQT3 involves mutation of the gene encoding a sodium channel. The abnormality is located in chromosome 3 and the gene is called SCN5A. LQT3 is less common than the first two long QT syndromes. The abnormality in the sodium channel causes prolongation of phase 2 of the action potential. This is due to delayed closure of the fast sodium channels on completion of rapid depolarization resulting in continuous entry of sodium ions into the cell, thus prolonging the duration of the action potential. The baseline ECG will show asymmetric T waves with a steep downslope. Most patients are symptomatic at rest or sleep, which causes the QT interval to prolong because of bradycardia. Mutation of the gene SCN5A has been implicated as the cause of the Brugada syndrome, where most of the arrhythmic events occur during sleep (see Brugada Syndrome).

■ **LQT4:** Long QT4 is the only other long QT syndrome associated with abnormality in sodium transport. It is the only long QT syndrome that is not a "channelopathy" because the abnormality does not directly involve an ion channel but its supporting structure. The abnormality resides in chromosome 4 and the gene is called ankyrin-B. The abnormality affects the sinus node and the clinical manifestations include symptoms of sinus node dysfunction. This is manifested as bradyarrhythmias as well as tachyarrhythmias including the tachycardia bradycardia syndrome.

- **LQT5:** This abnormality involves mutation of gene KCNE1 in chromosome 21. The gene is also called minK. This type of long QT syndrome is rare. Homozygous mutation of this gene can also cause the Jervell and Lange-Nielsen syndrome. The abnormality involves the transport of potassium (β-subunit of the slow K rectifier or IKs) similar to LQT1. Prolongation of the action potential is due to delay in phase 3. The surface ECG usually shows T wave with a wide base.

- **LQT6:** The abnormality also resides in chromosome 21 and involves the KCNE2 gene. This type of long QT syndrome is rare. The abnormality affects the rapid outward potassium transport (outward rapid K rectifier or IKr) resulting in decreased potassium efflux with prolongation of phase 3 of the action potential. The T wave has low amplitude.

- **LQT7:** The abnormality resides in chromosome 17 and the gene involved is called KCNJ2. This abnormality prolongs the action potential duration through its effect on the inward rectifying currents involved with potassium transport, thus delaying phase 3. Both cardiac and skeletal muscle cells can be affected resulting in prolongation of the QT and hypokalemia induced periodic paralysis with a large U wave looking component in the ECG. This disorder is very rare and is often referred to as the Andersen syndrome.

- **Timothy syndrome often identified as LQT8:** Timothy syndrome involves mutation of the L-type calcium channel. The defect involves chromosome 12 and the identified gene is CACNA1C. Calcium channel dysfunction causes multisystem involvement with osseous deformities including dysmorphic features and syndactyly in addition to autism, cognitive defects, and malignant ventricular arrhythmias. This very rare syndrome has also been referred to as LQT8.

- **Brugada syndrome:** Another example in which malignant ventricular arrhythmias can occur in individuals with structurally normal hearts is the Brugada syndrome. Patients with this syndrome can be identified by the presence of a peculiar electrocardiographic pattern in baseline ECG characterized by RBBB with rSR′ configuration confined to $V_1$ to $V_3$. In $V_1$ or $V_2$, the J point and ST segment are elevated with a coved or upward convexity terminating into an inverted T wave (type I). In some patients, the elevated ST segment may assume a saddle back configuration (type II) or often a triangular pattern instead of a coved appearance (type III). Types II and III terminate in upright T waves. The ST elevation is confined to the right-sided precordial leads and is not accompanied by reciprocal ST depression. It may be permanent in some individuals, although, in others, it may vary from time to time. When these ECG changes are not present, the ST segment abnormalities can be unmasked by administration of sodium channel blocker such as procainamide, flecainide, or ajmaline. The QTc is not prolonged. Examples of the Brugada ECG are shown in Chapter 23, Acute Coronary Syndrome: ST Elevation Myocardial Infarction, differential diagnosis of ST segment elevation. Approximately 90% of patients with the Brugada ECG are males.

- **Mechanism:** The abnormality has been identified to be a mutation in chromosome 3 involving gene SCN5A. Only the epicardial cells of the right ventricle are affected. These epicardial cells have abnormal sodium channels, which causes premature repolarization. The premature repolarization causes shortening of the duration of the action potential only of the abnormal cells. Repolarization of normal endocardial cells is not affected. The shortened duration of repolarization of the epicardial cells will cause these cells to repolarize earlier when compared with endocardial cells. Thus, during repolarization, a gradient between the abnormal epicardial and the normally repolarizing endocardial cells is created during phase 2 of the action potential resulting in elevation of the ST segment, only in the right precordial leads $V_1$ to $V_3$. This difference in repolarization between normal and abnormal cells can facilitate a reentrant arrhythmia.

- This syndrome is a genetic defect without associated structural cardiac disease and can cause sudden death from polymorphic VT. Thus, the syndrome is primarily an electrical abnormality because it has no other clinical manifestations other than the ventricular arrhythmia. This clinical entity is endemic in Southeast Asia including Thailand, Japan, and the Philippines and affects mostly males in their mid to late 30s. The ECG abnormalities as well as the ventricular arrhythmias are enhanced by vagal activity; thus, the ventricular arrhythmias are commonly manifested during sleep. Because of its nocturnal frequency, it is often called sudden unexpected nocturnal death syndrome or SUNDS. Fever has also been shown to be a predisposing factor. The syndrome is inherited as autosomal dominant with variable expression similar to arrhythmogenic right ventricular cardiomyopathy.

- In patients with the Brugada ECG who are symptomatic with syncope because of polymorphic VT or ventricular fibrillation, mortality is high. The incidence of VT and fibrillation is similar whether the patient is on a beta blocker, taking an antiarrhythmic agent (amiodarone) or the patient has an implanted automatic defibrillator. Only an implanted defibrillator is effective in preventing sudden death and therefore the only known effective therapy in reducing mortality. According to the ACC/AHA/ESC 2006 guidelines on ventricular arrhythmias, the implantable defibrillator receives Class I recommendation in patients with previous cardiac arrest and Class IIa recommendation in patients with history of syncope or documented VT. There are only few agents that are useful during an arrhythmic event. This includes isoproterenol, which receives a Class IIa recommendation and quinidine, a Class IIb recommendation.

- Although symptomatic patients with the Brugada ECG are high risk for sudden death, the significance of the

Brugada ECG in the general asymptomatic population is uncertain because not all patients with the Brugada ECG will develop VT or ventricular fibrillation.

☐ Among 63 patients with the Brugada ECG reported by Brugada et al. in 1998, 41 were diagnosed after resuscitated cardiac arrest or syncope and 22 were asymptomatic, detected incidentally because of family history of sudden death. Of the 22 asymptomatic individuals, 6 (27%) developed ventricular arrhythmias during a mean follow-up of 27 months, whereas among the 41 symptomatic patients, 14 (34%) had a recurrence of the ventricular arrhythmia during a mean follow-up of 37 months. They concluded that asymptomatic patients with the Brugada ECG have the same risk of developing a cardiac arrhythmia when compared with patients who had previous history of aborted sudden death.

☐ However, among 32 cases with the Brugada ECG detected in a population-based study of 4,788 asymptomatic Japanese individuals younger than 50 years of age who had biennial examinations and were followed for 41 years, there were 7 (26%) unexpected deaths in patients with the Brugada ECG compared with 20 (74%) in the control group. In most cases, the ECG finding was intermittent and was nine times higher in men than in women.

☐ In another community-based study of 13,929 subjects also in Japan, the Brugada ECG was found in 98. There was one death during a follow-up of 2.6 years compared with 139 deaths among those without the Brugada ECG. The total mortality of patients with the Brugada ECG was not different from those without the abnormality.

■ **Wolff-Parkinson-White (WPW) syndrome:** The WPW syndrome is another clinical entity in which malignant ventricular arrhythmias can occur in the absence of structural cardiac disease that can result in sudden death. The ECG recognition, mechanism and the different arrhythmias associated with the syndrome, is further discussed in Chapter 20, Wolff-Parkinson-White Syndrome.

## Acute Therapy

■ **Ventricular fibrillation:** The emergency treatment of patients with ventricular fibrillation is direct current electrical defibrillation.

■ **Direct current defibrillation:** Direct current unsynchronized shocks set at 360 joules if monophasic (or 200 joules if biphasic) should be delivered immediately. The ACC/AHA/ESC 2006 guidelines for management of ventricular arrhythmias, recommends that if the initial shock is unsuccessful, five cycles of cardiopulmonary resuscitation should be provided before delivering the second shock and if the second shock is also not effective, another five cycles of cardiopulmonary resuscitation is provided before delivering the third shock. The previous

recommendation was to deliver three shocks in a row followed by cardiopulmonary resuscitation.

■ **Precordial thump:** An initial option, which is a Class IIb recommendation, is that a single precordial thump can be delivered by the responder. This can be tried if the patient cannot be immediately defibrillated. (Class IIb means that the usefulness or efficacy of the procedure/therapy is less well established by evidence/opinion.)

■ **Cardiopulmonary resuscitation:** If the patient has been in cardiac arrest for more than 5 minutes, a brief period of cardiopulmonary resuscitation is initially recommended before the patient is electrically defibrillated.

■ **Pharmacologic agents:**

☐ **Epinephrine:** If the arrhythmia is refractory to electrical defibrillation, epinephrine 1 mg is given IV and repeated every 3 to 5 minutes while providing continuous cardiopulmonary resuscitation.

☐ **Vasopressin:** An alternative is to give vasopressin 40 U IV given once to substitute for the first or second dose of epinephrine.

☐ **Amiodarone:** If ventricular fibrillation is refractory to electrical defibrillation, amiodarone is also given IV with a loading dose of 300 mg or 5 mg/kg and electrical defibrillation repeated. An additional dose of 150 mg of amiodarone may be given once only. Amiodarone is continued at 1.0 mg/minute for 6 hours followed by 0.5 mg/minute for the next 18 hours when the patient has stabilized. It is not necessary to give amiodarone routinely if the patient responds to the initial shock followed by a stable rhythm.

☐ **Electrolytes:** After ventricular fibrillation is stabilized, all electrolyte and acid base abnormalities should be corrected. Serum potassium should be >4 mEq/L and magnesium >2.0 mg/dL.

☐ **Beta blockers:** Beta blockers, unless contraindicated, should also be given as prophylactic therapy.

■ **Other measures:** There are conditions that may have precipitated or contributed to the arrhythmia. According to the ACC/AHA/ESC 2006 practice guidelines on ventricular arrhythmias, the contributing conditions include 6 Hs and 5 Ts. They are Hypovolemia, Hypoxia, Hydrogen ion (acidosis), Hypo- or hyperkalemia, Hypoglycemia, Hypothermia, Toxins, Tamponade, Tension pneumothorax, Thrombosis (coronary or pulmonary), and Trauma. These conditions should be identified and corrected.

■ **Sustained monomorphic VT:** The acute treatment of sustained monomorphic VT depends on whether or not the patient is hemodynamically stable. However, because electrical cardioversion is so effective in terminating monomorphic VT, cardioversion should be considered as initial therapy regardless of symptoms. Among stable patients with monomorphic VT, pharmacologic therapy can be an option. If the patient does not respond to the initial pharmacologic agent, the VT should be terminated with electrical cardioversion.

■ **Hemodynamically unstable patients with sustained monomorphic VT:** Unstable patients with monomorphic VT who are hypotensive (blood pressure <90 mm Hg), in pulmonary edema or have symptoms of myocardial ischemia from the tachycardia, the ACC/AHA/ESC 2006 guidelines for ventricular arrhythmias and the ACC/AHA guidelines for the management of ST elevation myocardial infarction recommend synchronized cardioversion with appropriate sedation starting at 100 joules of monophasic shock followed by escalating energy levels of 200 to 300 and finally 360 joules, if the initial shocks are unsuccessful.

■ **Hemodynamically stable:** In hemodynamically stable patients with sustained monomorphic VT, electrical cardioversion remains an option. Antiarrhythmic agents, however, may be considered instead of electrical cardioversion. The preferred antiarrhythmic agent will depend on the presence or absence of left ventricular systolic dysfunction.

☐ **Hemodynamically stable patients with preserved left ventricular function:** The acute pharmacologic treatment of sustained VT for patients who are stable with good left ventricular systolic function includes procainamide, amiodarone, lidocaine, or sotalol. Only one antiarrhythmic agent should be given to minimize the proarrhythmic effect of multiple drugs. If the chosen antiarrhythmic agent is not effective, electrical cardioversion should be performed to terminate the VT.

☐ **Procainamide:** The ACC/AHA/ESC 2006 guidelines for management of patients with ventricular arrhythmias recommend procainamide as the initial agent in patients with monomorphic VT who are hemodynamically stable with good left ventricular function. This agent receives a Class IIa recommendation. Procainamide is more effective than amiodarone in the early termination of stable monomorphic VT. The maximum loading dose of procainamide should not exceed 17 mg/kg. The loading dose is given as an intravenous infusion until the tachycardia is suppressed. The infusion should not exceed 50 mg/minute or a total loading dose of 1 g over 30 minutes. This is followed by a maintenance dose of 1 to 4 mg/minute. This drug is preferred among all other drugs in sustained monomorphic VT if the patient is stable and has preserved systolic function. It should not be given when there is systolic left ventricular dysfunction or there is evidence of heart failure.

☐ **Amiodarone:** Amiodarone is one of the few agents that can be given to patients with good LV function or with LV dysfunction. Although amiodarone is the recommended antiarrhythmic agent (Class I) for stable patients with sustained monomorphic VT according to the ACC/AHA 2004 practice guidelines for ST elevation myocardial infarction, it is not as effective as procainamide for early termination of stable monomorphic VT according to the ACC/AHA/ESC 2006 guidelines for ventricular arrhythmias and receives a Class IIa recommendation when the VT is refractory to electrical cardioversion or if the VT is unstable or recurrent in spite of therapy with intravenous procainamide or other drugs. The dose of amiodarone is 150 mg IV given as a bolus within 10 minutes and may be repeated every 10 to 15 minutes as needed. This is followed by an IV infusion of 1 mg/minute for the next 6 hours and 0.5 mg/minute for the next 18 hours. The total intravenous dose should not exceed 2.2 g during the first 24 hours.

☐ **Lidocaine:** If the monomorphic VT is known to be due to acute myocardial ischemia or a complication of acute myocardial infarction, lidocaine may be given as initial therapy. This agent receives a Class IIb recommendation according to the ACC/AHA/ESC 2006 practice guidelines for the management of patients with ventricular arrhythmias. Lidocaine is given IV at an initial bolus of 1 mg per kg body weight. The initial bolus should not exceed 100 mg. If the first bolus is unsuccessful, a second bolus of 0.5 to 0.75 mg/kg IV is given and a third and final bolus may be necessary. The total IV dose within the first 3 hours should not exceed 3 mg/kg body weight. The infusion is followed by a maintenance dose of 1 to 4 mg/minute.

☐ **Sotalol:** This agent is not available in the United States as an IV preparation. Similar to procainamide, it should not be given when there is LV dysfunction. Dosing is discussed in the Appendix: Commonly Used Injectable Pharmacologic Agents.

☐ **Other options:**

☐ **Electrical cardioversion:** Even among stable patients, electrical cardioversion may be considered as initial therapy instead of giving antiarrhythmic agents. If antiarrhythmic therapy was decided and was not effective, the patient should be electrically cardioverted. In stable patients, low monophasic energy settings starting at 50 joules can be given under adequate sedation.

☐ **Temporary pacing:** Temporary pacing receives a Class IIa recommendation for overdrive suppression in patients refractory to cardioversion or in patients with recurrent VT in spite of antiarrhythmic therapy.

☐ **Hemodynamically stable patients with impaired left ventricular function:** The acute therapy of patients with monomorphic VT who are hemodynamically stable but have systolic LV dysfunction (ejection fraction ≤40 % or evidence of congestive heart failure) is limited to amiodarone and lidocaine. Agents that can further depress systolic function such as sotalol and procainamide are proarrhythmic and negatively inotropic and should not be given.

- □ **Amiodarone:** Dosing is the same as in patients with normal systolic function.
- □ **Lidocaine:** Dosing is the same as in patients with normal systolic function.

- ■ **Sustained polymorphic VT:** Most patients with polymorphic VT are generally unstable because the VT has a rapid rate and electrical defibrillation is usually necessary unless the VT is self-terminating. The ACC/AHA guidelines on ST elevation myocardial infarction recommend 200 joules of monophasic shock under adequate sedation. This is followed by another shock of 200 to 300 joules if the initial shock is ineffective and a third shock of 360 joules if necessary. The more recent ACC/AHA/ESC 2006 guidelines for the management of ventricular arrhythmias suggest that any unsynchronized shock should be set to the maximum energy setting, which is 360 joules of monophasic shock, to minimize the risk of ventricular fibrillation with low level settings. After the tachycardia is terminated, pharmacologic therapy is also recommended. The type of pharmacologic agent will depend on whether the polymorphic VT is associated with normal QTc (regular polymorphic VT) or prolonged QTc (torsades de pointes).

  - ▪ **Regular PVT:** Regular PVT (normal QTc) is usually associated with myocardial ischemia and should be considered as the cause of the VT in all patients.

    - □ **Reverse myocardial ischemia:** Urgent coronary angiography, insertion of intraaortic balloon pump, and emergency myocardial revascularization should be considered as part of the overall treatment of regular polymorphic VT when there is ischemic heart disease. Anti-ischemic agents such as beta blockers should be given intravenously especially if the polymorphic VT is recurrent.

    - □ **Antiarrhythmic agents:** Therapy is similar to monomorphic VT and includes procainamide, amiodarone, lidocaine, or sotalol (see treatment of monomorphic VT). Dosing is similar to monomorphic VT. Intravenous amiodarone receives a Class I recommendation if the PVT is recurrent without QT prolongation. Lidocaine receives a Class IIb recommendation in patients with acute myocardial infarction or myocardial ischemia.

  - ▪ **Torsades de pointes:** Although the tachycardia of torsades de pointes and regular polymorphic VT look identical, treatment of these two arrhythmias are different because one is associated with prolonged QTc, whereas the other is not. In patients with torsades de pointes with acquired prolongation of the QT interval, the long QT interval is reversible and the cause should be identified and eliminated. This is in contrast to congenital long QT syndrome where prolongation of the QT may not be reversible. Nevertheless, in both congenital and acquired long QT syndrome, any identifiable cause of QT prolongation should be corrected.

    - □ **Reverse myocardial ischemia:** Myocardial ischemia can prolong the QTc and cause polymorphic VT and should be reversed with the use of anti-ischemic agents. In congenital prolonged QTc, the tachycardia

is often induced by adrenergic stimulation. Thus, beta blockers are the agents of choice and should be included as baseline therapy in patients with torsades de pointes unless the drug is contraindicated.

- □ **Correct electrolyte abnormalities:** Electrolyte abnormalities especially hypokalemia and hypomagnesemia can prolong the QT interval. If the potassium level is below 4.0 mEq/L, potassium repletion to 4.5 to 5.0 mEq/L should be considered.

- □ **Antiarrhythmic agents:** In torsades de pointes, antiarrhythmic agents that prolong the QT interval such as Class IA and Class III agents are not only ineffective but may be fatal. The following are recommended for torsades de pointes.

  - □ **Magnesium:** This agent receives a Class IIb recommendation. It may not be effective if the QT is not prolonged. One to 2 g of magnesium is diluted with 50 to 100 mL $D_5W$ and given IV as a loading dose. The solution is injected within 1 hour (5 to 60 minutes). The infusion is given more rapidly for unstable patients. This is followed by 10 to 20 g within the next 24 hours, even in patients without hypomagnesemia.

  - □ **Lidocaine:** This antiarrhythmic agent does not prolong the QT interval. The dose of lidocaine is the same as for monomorphic VT.

  - □ **Isoproterenol:** This usually serves as a bridge before a temporary pacemaker can be inserted. This is usually effective as temporary treatment in patients with acquired long QT syndrome when there is significant bradycardia, AV block, or when there are pause-dependent torsades de pointes. Because isoproterenol can cause tachycardia, it should not be given when the torsades de pointes are not pause dependent or the basic heart rate is not bradycardic. When the tachycardia is pause dependent, the VT can be prevented by increasing the heart rate resulting in overdrive suppression similar to that of an artificial pacemaker. The drug is given IV at 2 to 10 mcg/minute. The infusion is titrated according to the desired heart rate that can suppress the tachycardia.

  - □ **Phenytoin:** Phenytoin is given with a loading dose of 250 mg diluted in normal saline. The solution is infused IV over 10 minutes. Additional boluses of 100 mg are given every 5 minutes as necessary under constant blood pressure and ECG monitoring until a maximum dose of 1,000 mg is given. Dextrose should not be used as a diluent since crystallization can occur. The drug should not be given as a continuous IV infusion.

  - □ **Temporary pacemaker:** A temporary pacemaker is inserted transvenously for overdrive pacing. This is usually effective when torsades de pointes is pause dependent or the VT occur in the setting of bradycardia of <60 bpm.

**TABLE 21.1**

**Recommended Settings for External Defibrillation According to the ACC/AHA Guidelines for ST-Elevation Myocardial Infarction**

|  | Initial Shock | Second | Third |
|---|---|---|---|
| Ventricular fibrillation or pulseless VT | 200 Joules* (unsynchronized) | 200–300 Joules* (unsynchronized) | 360 Joules (unsynchronized) |
| Unstable polymorphic VT | 200 Joules* (unsynchronized) | 200–300 Joules* (unsynchronized) | 360 Joules (unsynchronized) |
| Sustained unstable monomorphic VT | 100 Joules (synchronized) | Escalating energy levels (synchronized) | |
| Sustained stable monomorphic VT | 50 Joules (Synchronized) | Escalating energy levels (Synchronized) | |

*The more recent American College of Cardiology/American Heart Association/European Society of Cardiology 2006 guidelines for management of ventricular arrhythmias recommend maximal defibrillator settings (360 joules of monophasic shock) if unsynchronized shock is delivered to minimize the risk of ventricular fibrillation with low settings.
VT, ventricular tachycardia.

- The following (Table 21.1) is a summary of the recommended initial and subsequent shocks during electrical cardioversion in patients with sustained ventricular arrhythmias according to the 2004 ACC/AHA guidelines on ST elevation myocardial infarction. All shocks are monophasic.

## Long-Term Therapy

- **Ventricular fibrillation and sustained VT:** Patients who have survived an episode of sustained VT or ventricular fibrillation are high risk for sudden death and should be referred to an electrophysiologist. These patients usually have structural cardiac disease with severe LV dysfunction. Any reversible condition that can cause arrhythmia such as electrolyte abnormalities, myocardial ischemia, severe blood gas abnormalities, or the use of agents that are proarrhythmic should be identified and corrected. Beta blockers and anticongestive agents that prolong survival in patients with left ventricular systolic dysfunction such as angiotensin-converting enzyme inhibitors, angiotensin receptor blockers, aldosterone antagonists, and, among African Americans, a hydralazine/nitrate combination should be given unless these drugs are contraindicated. In patients with poor LV systolic function, implantation of an automatic defibrillator for secondary prevention is recommended. In these patients, the use of antiarrhythmic agents does not match the efficacy of the automatic defibrillator in reducing mortality.

- **Nonsustained VT:** Patients who are completely asymptomatic but have frequent multiformed PVCs with nonsustained monomorphic VT need to be referred for further cardiac evaluation. The arrhythmia is most probably benign in asymptomatic patients with structurally normal hearts. However, in patients with impaired LV function, especially those who have survived an acute myocardial infarction, the patient has to be referred for further evaluation and therapy. Similarly, in pa-

tients with PVT, even when nonsustained, treatment and further evaluation is warranted. Treatment of systolic dysfunction with beta blockers, angiotensin-converting enzyme inhibitors, or angiotensin receptor blockers and aldosterone antagonists should be considered in addition to correction of myocardial ischemia or other metabolic, electrolyte, and blood gas abnormalities that may be present. No antiarrhythmic therapy is necessary in asymptomatic patients with nonsustained VT who have been evaluated to have structurally normal hearts.

- **PVCs:** PVCs from ventricular parasystole is considered a benign finding. Similarly, simple, benign ventricular extrasystoles are commonly seen in normal healthy individuals. These ectopic impulses may be associated with smoking; excessive coffee, tea, or alcohol; use of diet pills, sympathetic agents, thyroid hormones, diuretics; and medications for common colds or asthma, antipsychotic agents and electrolyte abnormalities. A previously asymptomatic and presumably healthy individual with a structurally normal heart who develops palpitations from simple, benign PVCs should be evaluated for these possible causes. Treatment is simply reassurance that the arrhythmia is benign and the possible cause eliminated.

## Prognosis

- Prognosis will depend on the type of ventricular arrhythmia and the underlying cardiac abnormality.

  - Sustained VT or ventricular fibrillation are serious and life-threatening arrhythmias. Most of these arrhythmias are frequently seen in patients with severe left ventricular dysfunction and has high mortality. Prognosis is improved with appropriate therapy.

  - Patients with structurally normal hearts who develop malignant ventricular arrhythmias are also at risk for sudden death. These include patients with prolonged QTc,

Brugada syndrome, and arrhythmogenic right ventricular cardiomyopathy. Prognosis is improved with medical therapy. In properly selected patients, implantation of an automatic defibrillator may be indicated.

■ In the general population, VT or ventricular fibrillation can occur as a complication of acute myocardial infarction and is a common cause of sudden death.

■ PVCs that are parasystolic are considered benign. Although acute treatment of frequent parasystolic and extrasystolic PVCs and nonsustained VT is not indicated, long-term prognosis will depend on the presence or absence of cardiac disease.

■ PVT with or without QTc prolongation, even when self-terminating and of short duration, may incur an immediate risk of morbidity and mortality. The long-term prognosis will depend on the cause of the PVT and underlying cardiac abnormality.

## Suggested Readings

2005 American Heart Association guidelines for cardiopulmonary resuscitation and emergency cardiovascular care. Part 7.3: management of symptomatic bradycardia and tachycardia. *Circulation.* 2005;112:67–77.

Ackerman MJ. The long QT syndrome: ion channel diseases of the heart. *Mayo Clin Proc.* 1998;73:250–269.

Antman EM, Anbe DT, Armstrong PW, et al. ACC/AHA guidelines for the management of patients with ST elevation myocardial infarction: executive summary: a report of the ACC/AHA Task Force on Practice Guidelines (Committee to Revise the 1999 Guidelines on the management of patients with acute myocardial infarction). *J Am Coll Cardiol.* 2004;44:671–719.

Arizona Center for Education and Research on Therapeutics. QT drug lists. www.torsades.org

Bigger JT Jr. Ventricular arrhythmias: classification and general principles of therapy. In: Horowitz LN, ed. *Current Management of Arrhythmias.* Philadelphia: BC Decker Inc; 1991:130–137.

Botteron GW, Smith JM. Cardiac arrhythmias. In: Carey CF, Lee HH, Woeltje KF, eds. *The Washington Manual of Medical Therapeutics.* 29th ed. Philadelphia: Lippincott Williams & Wilkins; 1998:130–156.

Brodsky M, Wu D, Denes P, et al. Arrhythmias documented by 24 hour continuous electrocardiographic monitoring in 50 male medical students without apparent heart disease. *Am J Cardiol.* 1977;39:390–395.

Brugada J, Brugada R, Brugada P. Right bundle-branch block and ST-segment elevation in leads $V_1$ through $V_3$. A marker for sudden death in patients without demonstrable structural heart disease. *Circulation.* 1998;97:457–460.

Castellanos Jr A, Ortiz JM, Pastis N, et al. The electrocardiogram in patients with pacemakers. *Progr Cardiovasc Dis.* 1970;13:190–209.

Conover MB. Monomorphic ventricular rhythms. In: *Understanding Electrocardiography.* 8th ed. St. Louis: CV Mosby Co.; 2003:151–170.

Conover MB. Congenital long QT syndrome. In: *Understanding Electrocardiography.* 8th ed. St. Louis: CV Mosby Co.; 2003: 369–380.

Fleg JL, Kennedy HL. Cardiac arrhythmias in a healthy elderly population: detection by 24-hour ambulatory electrocardiography. *Chest.* 1982;81:302–307.

Goldenberg I, Mathew J, Moss AJ, et al. Corrected QT variability in serial electrocardiograms in long QT syndrome. The importance of the maximum corrected QT for risk stratification. *J Am Coll Cardiol.* 2006;48:1047–1052.

Guidelines 2000 for cardiopulmonary resuscitation and emergency cardiovascular care, an international consensus on science. The American Heart Association in Collaboration with the International Liaison Committee on Resuscitation. 7D: the tachycardia algorithms. *Circulation.* 2000;102: I-158–I-165.

Gussak I, Antzelevitch C, Bjerregaard P, et al. The Brugada syndrome: clinical, electrophysiologic and genetic aspects. *J Am Coll Cardiol.* 1999;33:5–15.

Kennedy HL, Whitlock JA, Sprague MK, et al. Long-term follow-up of asymptomatic healthy subjects with frequent and complex ventricular ectopy. *N Engl J Med.* 1985;312:193–197.

Locati ET. QT interval duration remains a major risk factor in long QT syndrome patients. *J Am Coll Cardiol.* 2006;48: 1053–1055.

Matsuo K, Akahoshi M, Nakashima E, et al. The prevalence, incidence and prognostic value of the Brugada-type electrocardiogram. A population-based study. *J Am Coll Cardiol.* 2001;38:765–770.

Miyasaka Y, Tsuji H, Yamada K, et al. Prevalence and mortality of the Brugada-type electrocardiogram in one city in Japan. *J Am Coll Cardiol.* 2001;38:771–774.

Moss AJ. Long QT syndrome. *JAMA.* 2003;289:2041–2044.

Priori SG, Napolitano C, Gasparini M, et al. Natural history of Brugada syndrome. Insights for risk stratification and management. *Circulation.* 2002;105:1342–1347.

Priori SG, Schwartz PJ, Napolitano C, et al. Risk stratification in the long-QT syndrome. *N Engl J Med.* 2003;348: 1866–1874.

Southall DP, Johnston F, Shinebourne EA, et al. 24-hour electrocardiographic study of heart rate and rhythm patterns in population of healthy children. *Br Heart J.* 1981;45: 281–291.

Southall DP, Richards J, Mitchell P, et al. Study of cardiac rhythm in healthy newborn infants. *Br Heart J.* 1980;43:14–20.

Wellens HJJ, Conover M. Drug-induced arrhythmic emergencies. In: *The ECG in Emergency Decision Making.* 2nd edition. St. Louis: Saunders/Elsevier; 2006:177–186.

Zimetbaum PJ, Josephson ME, Kwaku KF. Genetics of congenital and acquired long QT syndrome. 2007 UpToDate.

Zipes DP, Camm AJ, Borggrefe M, et al. ACC/AHA/ESC 2006 guidelines for management of patients with ventricular arrhythmias and the prevention of sudden cardiac death: a report of the American College of Cardiology/American Heart Association Task Force and the European Society of Cardiology Committee for Practice Guidelines (Writing Committee to Develop Guidelines for management of patients with ventricular arrhythmias and the prevention of sudden cardiac death). *J Am Coll Cardiol.* 2006,48:e247–e346.

# Wide Complex Tachycardia

## Causes of Wide Complex Tachycardia

■ Wide complex tachycardia indicates the presence of fast and regular heart rate of >100 beats per minute (bpm) associated with wide QRS complexes measuring at least 120 milliseconds.

■ A wide complex tachycardia can be ventricular or supraventricular.

  ▪ **Ventricular tachycardia** (VT) has a wide QRS complex because the arrhythmia originates below the bifurcation of the bundle of His. The impulse does not follow the normal atrioventricular (AV) conduction system and activation of the ventricles does not occur simultaneously (Fig. 22.1A).

  ▪ **Supraventricular tachycardia** (SVT) has narrow QRS complexes because the impulse originates above the bifurcation of the bundle of His. The impulse follows the normal AV conduction system and activation of both ventricles is simultaneous. SVT can have wide QRS complexes when there is:

    □ Preexistent bundle branch block (B).

    □ AV reciprocating tachycardia (AVRT) due to the presence of a bypass tract. This wide complex tachycardia is also called antidromic AVRT (C).

    □ Ventricular aberration or rate related bundle branch block (D).

## Wide QRS Complex from Ventricular Tachycardia

■ Distinguishing VT from wide complex SVT is always a diagnostic challenge. Unless the patient is unstable, a 12-lead electrocardiogram (ECG) should always be recorded when there is wide complex tachycardia because it provides much more diagnostic information than a single-lead rhythm strip.

■ **Single-lead rhythm strip:** Very often, the tachycardia is recorded only on a rhythm strip obtained from a cardiac monitor. When only a single-lead ECG is available for interpretation, any of the following findings is diagnostic of VT:

  ▪ Unusually wide QRS complexes (Fig. 22.2).
  ▪ Complete AV dissociation (Fig. 22.3).
  ▪ Ventricular fusion complex (Figs. 22.4 to 22.6).
  ▪ Sinus captured complex or Dressler beat (Fig. 22.7).
  ▪ Ventriculoatrial conduction with block (Figs. 22.8 and 22.9).

■ **Unusually wide QRS complexes:**

  ▪ When the tachycardia has a right bundle branch block (RBBB) configuration, the tachycardia is ventricular if the width of the QRS complex exceeds 0.14 seconds. If the tachycardia has a left bundle

**Figure 22.1: Wide Complex Tachycardia. (A)** Ventricular tachycardia. **(B–D)** Examples of supraventricular (SVT) with wide QRS complexes. **(B)** SVT with preexistent bundle branch block. **(C)** Antidromic atrioventricular reciprocating tachycardia from the presence of a bypass tract. **(D)** SVT is conducted with aberration. (⟷) indicates the origin of the impulse; (*arrows*) the direction of the spread of the electrical impulse.

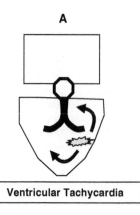
**A**
Ventricular Tachycardia

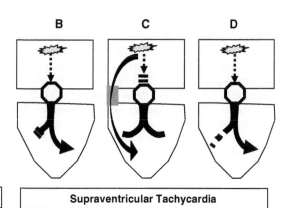
**B    C    D**
Supraventricular Tachycardia

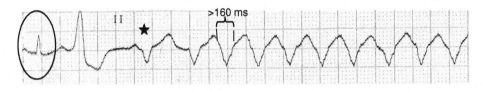

**Figure 22.2:   Tachycardia with Unusually Wide QRS Complexes.**  The QRS complexes are unusually wide measuring >160 milliseconds. This run of tachycardia with unusually wide QRS complexes is due to ventricular tachycardia (VT). The first complex (*circled*) shows no evidence of preexcitation or preexistent bundle branch block. The star indicates a fusion complex, which is also diagnostic of VT.

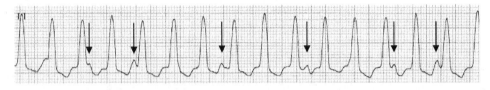

**Figure 22.3:   Complete Atrioventricular (AV) Dissociation.**  When complete AV dissociation is present, the diagnosis of the wide complex tachycardia is ventricular tachycardia. Arrows point to P waves that are completely dissociated from the QRS complexes.

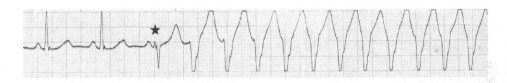

**Figure 22.4:   Ventricular Fusion Complex.**  The QRS complex marked by the star is a ventricular fusion complex. Ventricular fusion complexes are usually seen at the beginning or end of ventricular tachycardia (VT). When a ventricular fusion complex is present, the wide complex tachycardia is VT.

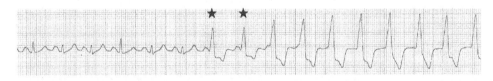

**Figure 22.5:   Ventricular Fusion Complexes.**  A rhythm strip shows fusion complexes that are marked by stars. The ventricular fusion complexes can assume any configuration other than the configuration of the QRS complexes during normal sinus rhythm or during tachycardia. The presence of a ventricular fusion complex during wide complex tachycardia is diagnostic of ventricular tachycardia.

**Figure 22.6: Ventricular Fusion Complex. (A)** Two separate impulses, ventricular and supraventricular, simultaneously activate the ventricles to cause a ventricular fusion complex. **(B)** A fusion complex occurs when two separate ventricular impulses activate the ventricles simultaneously. **(C)** A ventricular fusion complex is not possible with two separate supraventricular impulses because both are obligated to follow the same pathway to the ventricles.

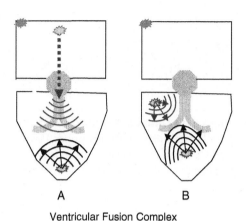
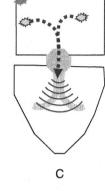

Ventricular Fusion Complex

Two supraventricular impulses can not cause a ventricular fusion complex because they have to follow the same pathway to the ventricles

**Figure 22.7: Sinus Captured and Ventricular Fusion Complexes. (A)** 12-lead electrocardiogram during wide complex tachycardia. Ventricular fusion complexes are marked by the letter F. The fusion complexes are preceded by sinus P waves (*arrowheads*). A sinus captured complex, also called Dressler's beat, is circled. **(B)** Lead II rhythm strip from the same patient recorded separately during normal sinus rhythm. The sinus-captured complex recorded in lead II is identical to the QRS complex during sinus rhythm and are both circled for comparison.

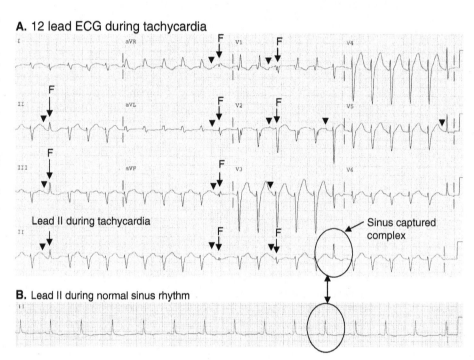

**A.** 12 lead ECG during tachycardia

Lead II during tachycardia

Sinus captured complex

**B.** Lead II during normal sinus rhythm

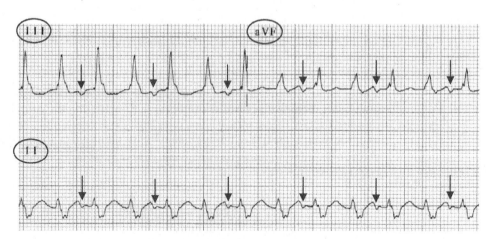

**Figure 22.8: Wide Complex Tachycardia with 2:1 Ventriculoatrial (V-A) Block.** V-A conduction is shown in leads II, III, and aVF. The retrogradely conducted P waves (*arrows*) occur after every other QRS complex representing 2:1 second-degree V-A block. V-A conduction with intermittent V-A block is diagnostic of ventricular tachycardia.

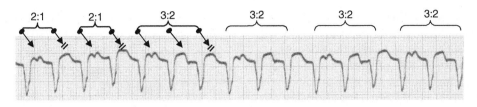

**Figure 22.9:    Ventriculoatrial (V-A) Wenckebach.** Lead II rhythm strip shows 2:1 V-A block and 3:2 V-A Wenckebach (*arrows on the left half of the rhythm strip*) with gradual prolongation of the R-P interval until a ventricular impulse is not followed by an atrial complex. The presence of intermittent V-A conduction suggests that the origin of the tachycardia is ventricular.

branch block (LBBB) configuration, the tachycardia is ventricular if the QRS complex exceeds 0.16 seconds. There should be no preexistent bundle branch block or preexcitation in baseline ECG and the patient should not be taking any antiarrhythmic medication that prolongs intraventricular conduction.

- Differentiating a wide complex tachycardia as having a RBBB or LBBB configuration may be difficult if only a single-lead monitor strip is available for interpretation (Fig. 22.2). However, an unusually wide QRS complex measuring >0.16 seconds is usually VT, regardless of the configuration of the QRS complex.

## Ventricular Tachycardia

- **Complete AV dissociation:** When sinus P waves are present and there is no relationship between the P waves and the QRS complexes, complete AV dissociation is present (Fig. 22.3). Complete AV dissociation occurs when two separate pacemakers are present: one capturing the atria and the other the ventricles. During VT, the rate of the ventricles is faster than the rate of the atria; thus, the slower atrial impulse will usually find the ventricles refractory. Complete AV dissociation occurring during a wide complex tachycardia is diagnostic of VT.

- **Ventricular fusion complex:** In VT, the sinus impulse may be able to capture the ventricles if the sinus impulse is perfectly timed to occur when the ventricles are not refractory. A ventricular fusion complex may occur if the ventricles are partly activated by the sinus impulse and partly by the VT (Figs. 22.4–22.6).

## Ventricular Fusion Complex

- **Ventricular fusion complex:** A ventricular fusion complex results when the ventricles are simultaneously

activated by two separate impulses, causing a change in the pattern of ventricular activation. At least one of the impulses should originate from the ventricles. A ventricular fusion complex therefore can occur if one impulse is ventricular and the other supraventricular (Fig. 22.6A). It can also occur if both impulses originate from two different locations in the ventricles (Fig. 22.6B). Two separate supraventricular impulses cannot produce a ventricular fusion complex because both supraventricular impulses are obligated to follow the same conduction pathway on their way to the ventricles and will not alter the pattern of ventricular activation (Fig. 22.6C). Thus, when a ventricular fusion complex occurs during a wide complex tachycardia, the diagnosis is VT. The fusion complex can assume any configuration other than the configuration of the QRS complex during sinus rhythm or during the wide complex tachycardia. Examples of ventricular fusion complexes are shown in Figures 22.2, 22.4, and 22.5.

## Sinus Captured Complex

- **Sinus captured complex:** In VT, the atrium and ventricles are completely dissociated with the ventricular rate faster than the sinus rate. The sinus impulse is, therefore, unable to capture the ventricles, because the ventricles are almost always refractory on arrival of the sinus impulse to the ventricles. If a properly timed sinus impulse arrives at the ventricles when the ventricles are not refractory, the sinus impulse may be able to capture the ventricles partially (resulting in a fusion complex) or completely (resulting in sinus captured complex). A sinus-captured complex during VT is a narrow QRS complex identical to a normally conducted sinus impulse (Fig. 22.7). Very often, sinus P waves are visible preceding fusion or sinus captured complexes. The presence of a sinus-captured complex during wide complex tachycardia is diagnostic of VT.

■ **Ventriculoatrial conduction:** Ventriculoatrial (V-A) conduction or conduction of an impulse from ventricles to atria is not commonly seen in the ECG, but has been shown to occur in 50% of patients with VT during electrophysiologic testing. One-to-one V-A conduction can occur during VT, but it can also occur during antidromic or wide complex AVRT. Not generally known as a marker of VT is V-A conduction with block.

■ **V-A conduction with block:** V-A conduction is better appreciated when recorded in a 12-lead ECG rather than a rhythm strip. The retrograde P waves are best recognized in leads II, III, and aVF. Figure 22.8 shows 2:1 V-A block and Figure 22.9 shows V-A Wenckebach. V-A block is not possible when there is antidromic AVRT because the tachycardia will not be able to sustain itself and will terminate if the impulse is blocked (see Chapter 16, Supraventricular Tachycardia due to Reentry). The presence of V-A conduction with intermittent block points to the ventricles as the origin of the arrhythmia and is diagnostic of VT.

■ The diagrams in Fig. 22.10 summarize the ECG findings of VT when only a rhythm strip is recorded.

## The 12-Lead ECG

■ **Twelve-lead ECG:** A full 12-lead ECG provides more useful information than a single-lead rhythm strip in differentiating VT from wide complex SVT and should always be recorded unless the patient is hemodynamically unstable requiring immediate electrical cardioversion. When a wide complex tachycardia is recorded in a 12-lead ECG, it does not only provide more information; a more organized approach to distinguish VT from wide complex SVT can be used (Fig. 22.11).

■ If a 12-lead ECG is recorded during a wide complex tachycardia, the following algorithm proposed by Brugada et al. attempts to diagnose VT in four simple steps (Fig. 22.11).

**Figure 22.10: Wide Complex Tachycardia.** When only a rhythm strip is recorded, the following electrocardiogram findings are diagnostic of ventricular tachycardia. **(1)** Unusually wide QRS complexes measuring >0.16 seconds. **(2)** Complete atrioventricular dissociation. **(3)** Ventricular fusion complex (*arrow*). **(4)** Sinus captured complex (*arrow*). **(5)** V-A Wenckebach **(6)** Two to one V-A block. The stars mark the sinus P waves. V-A, Ventriculoatrial.

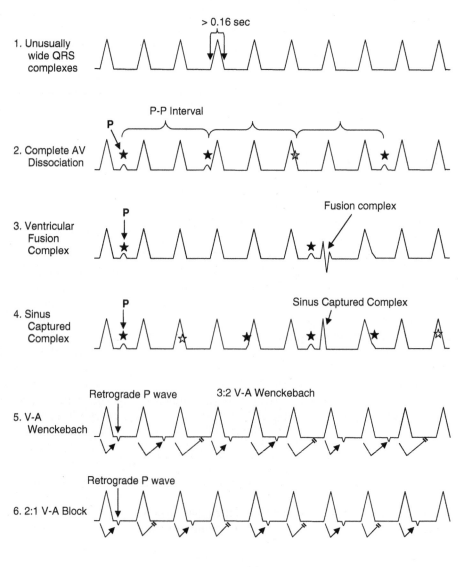

Algorithm for the Diagnosis of VT

**Figure 22.11:** **Algorithm for Wide Complex Tachycardia.** (Modified from Brugada et al.)

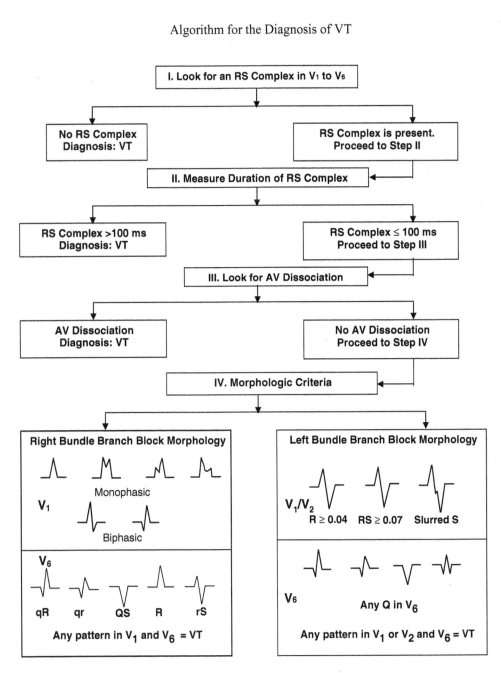

- **Step 1:** Look for an RS complex in $V_1$ to $V_6$. If there is no RS complex, the diagnosis is VT and no further analysis is needed. If an RS complex is present, proceed to step 2.

- **Step 2:** Measure the RS duration. If the RS duration is >100 milliseconds, the diagnosis is VT and no further analysis is needed. If the RS duration is ≤100 milliseconds, proceed to step 3.

- **Step 3:** Look for AV dissociation. If there is AV dissociation, the diagnosis is VT and no further analysis is needed. If AV dissociation is not present, proceed to step 4.

- **Step 4:** The morphologic criteria are used to diagnose VT (Figure 22.11)

  □ If the QRS complex is positive in $V_1$, the morphologic criteria for RBBB are used to diagnose VT.

  □ If the QRS complex is negative in $V_1$, the morphologic criteria for LBBB are used to diagnose VT.

- The full algorithm is shown in Figure 22.11. If the diagnosis of VT is not possible after going through these four simple steps, the patient should be further evaluated for other signs of VT using all possible diagnostic modalities including history, physical examination, previous ECG if available, response to vagal maneuvers, and certain pharmacologic agents.

- If the diagnosis of VT cannot be confirmed, the ECG should be evaluated for wide complex SVT. If the diagnosis remains uncertain after careful evaluation of the wide complex tachycardia, practice guidelines recommend that the tachycardia should be managed as VT.

## Step I: Absence of RS Complex in the Precordial Leads is VT

- The following illustrations will demonstrate step by step how to diagnose VT using the algorithm.
- **Step I: Look for an RS complex in the precordial leads.** The first step is to look for RS complex in $V_1$ to $V_6$. Examples of RS complexes are shown in Figure 22.12.
  - If RS complex is not present in any precordial lead $V_1$ to $V_6$, the diagnosis is VT and no further analysis is necessary (Fig. 22.13).
  - If RS complex is present in any of the precordial leads, the diagnosis of VT cannot be confirmed, proceed to step II.

## Step II: RS Duration >100 Milliseconds is VT

- **Step II: Measure the RS duration.** If an RS complex is present in any precordial lead, the diagnosis of VT is not possible. The next step is to measure the duration of the RS complex. If several RS complexes are present, the RS complex with the widest duration is selected.
  - The duration of the RS complex is measured from the beginning of the R wave to the nadir or lowest point of the S wave as shown in Figure 22.14.
  - If the duration of the RS complex is >100 milliseconds as shown in Figure 22.15, the diagnosis is VT and no further analysis is necessary.
  - If the duration of the RS complex is <100 milliseconds, the diagnosis of VT cannot be confirmed, proceed to step III.
- A wide complex tachycardia is shown in Figure 22.16. The algorithm is applied to look for VT.
  - **Step I:** Look for an RS complex. RS complexes are present in $V_2$ to $V_5$. The diagnosis of VT cannot be confirmed.
  - **Step II:** Measure the duration of the RS complex. $V_2$ is selected because it has the widest RS duration. The duration of the RS complex is >100 milliseconds. The diagnosis is VT and no further analysis is needed.

## Step III: AV Dissociation is Diagnostic of VT

- **Step III: Look for AV dissociation.** If VT is not diagnosed after steps I and II, the algorithm continues to step III. Step III of the algorithm is to look for AV dissociation.
  - Any of the 12 leads can be used when looking for AV dissociation. If AV dissociation is present, as shown in Figure 22.17, the diagnosis is VT and no further analysis is needed.
  - If AV dissociation is not present, the diagnosis of VT cannot be confirmed, proceed to step IV.

## Step IV: Morphologic Criteria

- **Step IV: Morphologic criteria.** In the fourth and final step, the QRS complex is classified as having either RBBB or LBBB morphology.
  - The morphology is RBBB if in $V_1$: the QRS complex is positive or the R wave is taller than the S wave.
  - The morphology is LBBB if in $V_1$: the QRS complex is negative or the S wave is deeper than the height of the R wave.
- **RBBB morphology:** If the tachycardia has a RBBB morphology, $V_1$ and $V_6$ should be examined for VT.
  - **$V_1$:** The following findings in $V_1$ favor VT. Monophasic or biphasic QRS complex. Examples of monophasic and biphasic QRS complexes in $V_1$ are shown in Figure 22.18.
  - **$V_6$:** The following findings in $V_6$ favor VT. Any q wave (except "qrs"), monophasic R wave, r/S ratio <1 (r wave smaller than S wave). These changes are shown in Figure 22.18.
- If a monophasic or biphasic QRS pattern is present in $V_1$ + any of the described QRS pattern is present in $V_6$, the diagnosis is VT. If the pattern is present only in $V_1$, but not in $V_6$, or the pattern is present only in $V_6$, but not $V_1$, the diagnosis of VT is not possible.

## Step IV: Wide Complex Tachycardia with RBBB Morphology

- The following example (Fig. 22.19) shows how to use the algorithm when there is a wide complex tachycardia with a RBBB configuration.
  - Step I, step II, and step III of the algorithm are unable to make a diagnosis of VT.

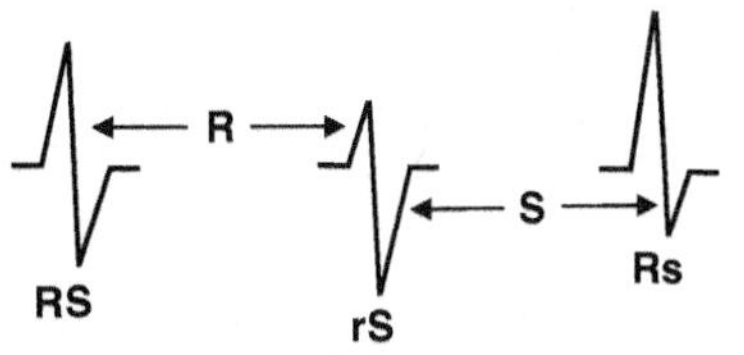

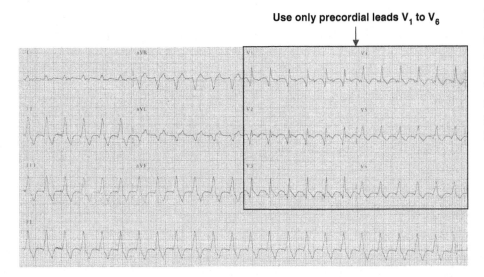

**Figure 22.12: RS Complexes.** Examples of RS complexes are shown diagrammatically. Any complex starting with a q wave or a complex with RSR′ configuration is not an RS complex.

Use only precordial leads V₁ to V₆

**Figure 22.13: Applying the Algorithm.** Step I: Look for an RS complex in V₁ to V₆ only. A qR configuration is seen in V₁, V₂, V₃, V₄, V₅, and V₆. Because there is no RS complex in any of the precordial leads, the diagnosis is ventricular tachycardia. No further analysis is necessary.

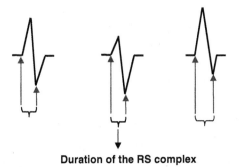

Duration of the RS complex

**Figure 22.14: RS Complexes.** Examples of RS complexes are shown. The duration of the RS complex is measured from the beginning of the R wave to the nadir of the S wave.

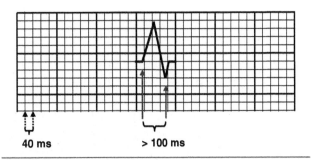

40 ms    > 100 ms

**Figure 22.15: Duration of the RS Complex.** The duration of the RS complex is measured from the beginning of the R wave to the lowest portion of the S wave as shown by the arrows. One small block in the electrocardiogram is equivalent to 40 milliseconds and 2.5 small blocks is equivalent to 100 milliseconds. If the RS duration is >100 milliseconds, the diagnosis is ventricular tachycardia and no further analysis is needed. ms, milliseconds.

**Figure 22.16:    Step II: Measure the Duration of the RS Complex.    Step I:** Look for an RS complex in the precordial leads. RS complexes are seen in $V_2, V_3, V_4, V_5,$ and probably $V_6$. Because RS complexes are present, the diagnosis of ventricular tachycardia (VT) cannot be confirmed. **Step II:** The duration of the RS complex is measured. $V_2$ has the widest RS duration and is magnified to show how the RS is measured. The RS measures 120 milliseconds. The diagnosis is VT and no further analysis is needed. ms, milliseconds.

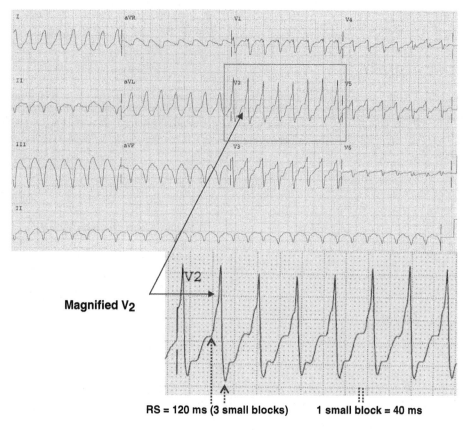

**Magnified V2**

RS = 120 ms (3 small blocks)          1 small block = 40 ms

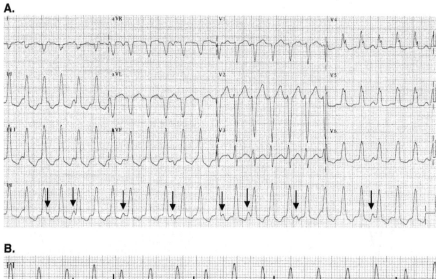

**A.**

**B.**

**Figure 22.17:    Step III: Look for Atrioventricular (AV) Dissociation.    Step I:** Look for an RS complex. Because an RS complex is present in $V_1, V_2,$ and $V_3$, the diagnosis of ventricular tachycardia (VT) can not be confirmed. **Step II:** Measure the duration of the RS complex. The RS duration in $V_2$ and in $V_3$ is <100 milliseconds. Because the duration of the RS complex is <100 milliseconds, diagnosis of VT can not be confirmed. **Step III:** Look for AV dissociation. **(B)** This is the same lead II rhythm strip shown in **(A)** and is magnified to show the AV dissociation. The P waves (*arrows*) are completely dissociated from the QRS complexes. When complete AV dissociation is present, the diagnosis is VT and no further analysis is necessary. ms, milliseconds.

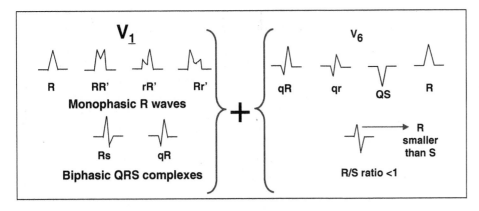

**Any pattern in $V_1$+ any pattern in $V_6$ = VT**

**Figure 22.18: Morphologic Criteria for Right Bundle Branch Block Pattern.** The morphology of the QRS complexes that favor ventricular tachycardia (VT) is shown for $V_1$ and for $V_6$. If a monophasic or biphasic complex is present in $V_1$ and any of these QRS patterns is also present in $V_6$, the diagnosis is VT.

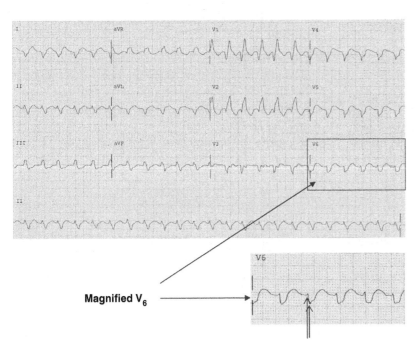

Magnified $V_6$

**Figure 22.19: Wide Complex Tachycardia with Right Bundle Branch Block (RBBB) Morphology. Step 1:** Look for an RS complex. RS is present in $V_6$. **Step 2:** Measure the RS duration. $V_6$ is magnified to show that the RS duration is <100 milliseconds. **Step 3:** Look for atrioventricular (AV) dissociation. AV dissociation is not present. **Step 4:** Morphologic criteria. Because $V_1$ is positive with a tall R wave, the morphologic criteria for RBBB are used. In $V_1$, the QRS morphology is biphasic (QR pattern), which favors ventricular tachycardia (VT). In V6, the RS ratio is <1 (r smaller than S). This also favors VT. $V_1$ and $V_6$ match the morphologic criteria for VT; therefore, the diagnosis is VT. ms, milliseconds.

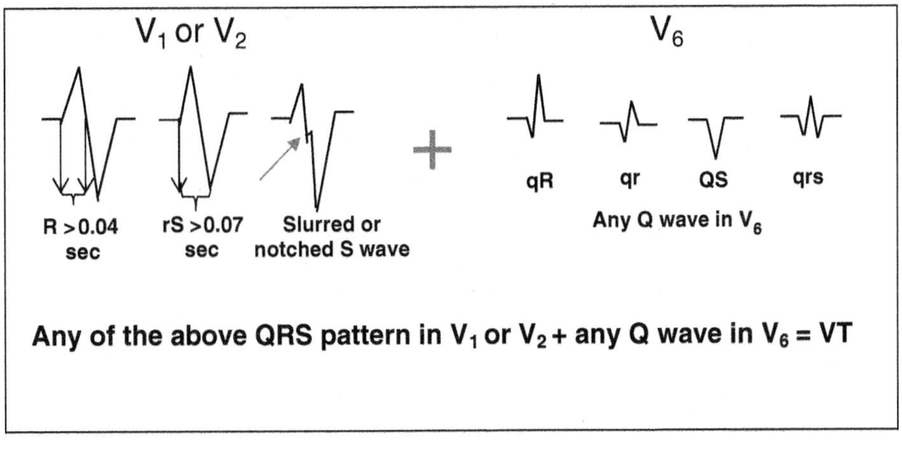

**Any of the above QRS pattern in $V_1$ or $V_2$ + any Q wave in $V_6$ = VT**

**Figure 22.20: Morphologic Criteria for Left Bundle Branch Block (LBBB) Configuration.** The diagnosis is ventricular tachycardia if any of the above QRS morphology is present in $V_1$ or $V_2$ and any Q wave is present in $V_6$. When the tachycardia has a LBBB morphology, it is faster and simpler to check $V_6$ first for any Q wave before matching the finding in $V_1$ because the only criterion in $V_6$ is to look for a Q wave.

■ Step IV of the algorithm shows RBBB configuration; thus, the RBBB morphologic criteria are used as shown in Figure 22.18.

## Step IV: Wide Complex Tachycardia with LBBB Morphology

■ **LBBB Morphology:** When the wide complex tachycardia has a LBBB configuration, $V_1$ or $V_2$ can be used. This is unlike wide complex tachycardia with RBBB configuration, where only lead $V_1$ is used. The diagnosis is VT if any of the following findings is present in $V_1$ or $V_2$ and also in $V_6$ (Fig. 22.20):

  ■ **$V_1$ or $V_2$:**

    ☐ R wave duration in $V_1$ or $V_2$ is ≥0.04 seconds or 40 milliseconds

    ☐ RS duration in $V_1$ or $V_2$ is ≥0.07 seconds or 70 milliseconds

    ☐ Slurring or notching of the downslope of the S wave.

  ■ **$V_6$:** Any q wave in $V_6$ will favor VT (Fig. 22.20). This may be a qR, qr, QS, or QRS.

■ If any of these QRS morphologies is present in $V_1$ or $V_2$ + any of the QRS morphologies is present in $V_6$, the diagnosis is VT. If the QRS morphology is present only in $V_1$ or $V_2$, but not in $V_6$, or the QRS morphology is present only in $V_6$, but not in $V_1$ or $V_2$, the diagnosis of VT is not possible.

■ When the tachycardia has LBBB morphology, it is simpler to evaluate $V_6$ before $V_1$ because the only criterion in $V_6$ is simply to look for any "q" wave. If a q wave is not present, the diagnosis of VT is not possible. If the tachycardia has RBBB morphology, $V_1$ should be inspected first because the only criterion in $V_1$ is to look for a monophasic or biphasic complex.

■ The ECG in Figure 22.21 shows a wide complex tachycardia with LBBB morphology (rS complex is present in $V_1$). Steps I to III of the algorithm are unable to make a diagnosis of VT. Using step IV of the algorithm, the QRS complex has a LBBB configuration; thus, the morphologic criteria for LBBB are used (see Figure 22.21).

## Other Findings Diagnostic of VT

■ **Other findings:** If VT cannot be diagnosed after going through the algorithm, there are other ECG findings not included in the algorithm that may suggest VT.

  ■ RBBB morphology with left axis deviation >−30° (Fig. 22.22).

  ■ LBBB morphology with right axis deviation >+90° (Fig. 22.23).

**Figure 22.21:    Applying the Algorithm.**
**Step IV: Steps I, II,** and **III** of the algorithm are unable to diagnose ventricular tachycardia (VT).
**Step IV:** Because the QRS complex in $V_1$ is negative or the S wave is deeper than the R wave, the morphologic criteria for left bundle branch block are used. $V_6$ starts with a q wave. This favors VT. $V_1$ has RS duration of 0.07 seconds. There is also notching of the downslope of the S wave in $V_2$ (*bold arrow*). Either of these findings favors VT. $V_{1-2}$ and $V_6$ match the morphologic criteria for VT; therefore, the diagnosis is VT.

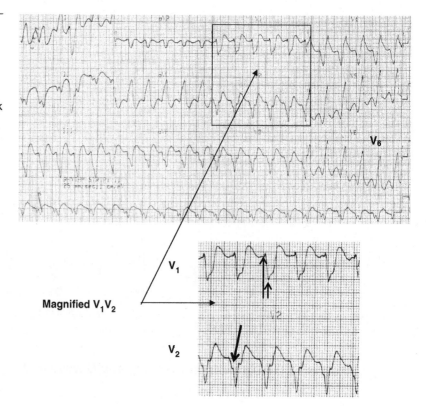

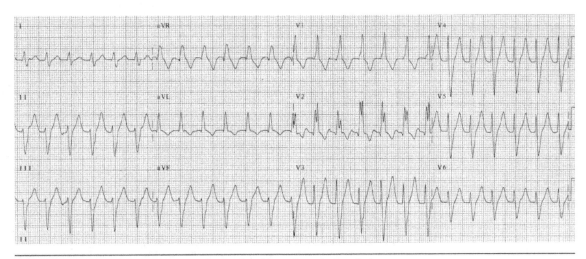

**Figure 22.22: Right Bundle Branch Block with Left Axis Deviation.** This finding favors ventricular tachycardia.

- Northwest axis: The QRS axis is between −90° to −180° (Fig. 22.24).
- Concordant QRS complexes: All QRS complexes in $V_1$ to $V_6$ are similar and are all pointing upward (positive concordance) or downward (negative concordance), as shown in Figures 22.24 and 22.25.
- Previous ECG: A previous ECG shows myocardial infarction (Fig. 22.26) or previous ECG shows that during sinus rhythm, bifascicular block is present, which changes in configuration during tachycardia (Fig. 22.27).
- **Concordance:** Negative concordance implies that all QRS complexes in the chest leads are pointing downward. Positive concordance implies that all the QRS complexes are pointing upward (Figs. 22.24 and 22.25).
- **Previous ECG:** If myocardial infarction is present in a previous ECG, the wide complex tachycardia is VT. This is based on the observation that VT is frequently associated with structural cardiac disease especially when there is left ventricular dysfunction (Fig. 22.26).
- **Previous ECG:** If LBBB or a preexistent bifascicular block such as RBBB plus a fascicular block is present in a previous ECG and the morphology of the QRS complex changes during the tachycardia, the diagnosis is VT (Fig. 22.27). This is based on the assumption that ventricular aberration cannot occur when only one fascicle is intact.

## Findings Favoring SVT

- **Wide complex SVT:** After evaluating the ECG for VT and the diagnosis of VT cannot be confirmed, the following findings in the 12-lead ECG suggest that the wide complex tachycardia is supraventricular.
  - **Triphasic pattern in $V_1$ and in $V_6$:** SVT with RBBB configuration has a triphasic rSR′ pattern in $V_1$ and

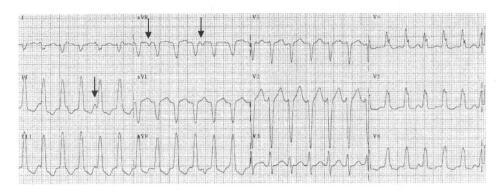

**Figure 22.23: Left Bundle Branch Block with Right Axis >90°.** This finding usually indicates ventricular tachycardia (VT). Note also the presence of complete AV dissociation (*arrows*), which also indicates VT.

**Figure 22.24: Concordance and Northwest Axis.** There is negative concordance of the QRS complexes in the precordial leads (all QRS complexes in $V_1$-$V_6$ are pointing downward with a left bundle branch block configuration). Additionally, the axis of the QRS complex is between $-90°$ and $-180°$ (northwest axis). Any of these findings indicates ventricular tachycardia.

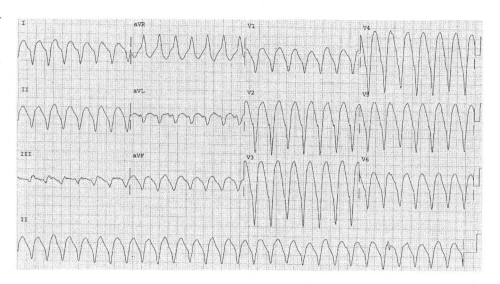

a triphasic qRS pattern in $V_6$ as shown in Figure 22.28. This is diagnostic of SVT.

- **Rabbit's ear:** In $V_1$, if the QRS complex has rabbit ear sign (left ear taller than right ear) or Rr' configuration, the diagnosis is usually VT (Fig. 22.29). If the configuration is rR' (right ear taller than left), the finding is not helpful but could be SVT if $V_6$ is triphasic (qRs) or R/S ratio is >1 (R wave taller than S wave).
- **Previous ECG:** The diagnosis is SVT if a previous ECG shows preexistent bundle branch block and the QRS complexes are identical during tachycardia and during normal sinus rhythm (Figs. 22.30 and 22.31). The presence of preexcitation in baseline ECG also suggests that the wide complex tachycardia is supraventricular (Fig. 22.32).
- **Preexistent RBBB.** If a previous ECG shows preexistent RBBB and the QRS pattern during sinus rhythm is identical to the QRS complexes during tachycardia, the tachycardia is supraventricular (Fig. 22.30).

- **Preexistent LBBB:** A similar example of wide complex SVT from preexistent LBBB is shown (Fig. 22.31). The configuration of the QRS complexes is the same during tachycardia and during normal sinus rhythm.
- **Preexcitation:** When preexcitation is present during normal sinus rhythm, the wide complex tachycardia is almost always the result of antidromic AVRT. Very often, the QRS complex during tachycardia is similar to the QRS complex during normal sinus rhythm (Fig. 22.32).

## Other Useful Modalities

- In addition to the 12-lead ECG, the following modalities are helpful in the diagnosis of wide complex tachycardia.
  - **History:** The history is often more important than the ECG in differentiating VT from SVT. The most

**Figure 22.25: Concordant Pattern.** There is positive concordance of all QRS complexes from $V_1$ to $V_6$ (all QRS complexes are pointing up in $V_1$-$V_6$). Positive concordance with a right bundle branch block configuration during a wide complex tachycardia is usually ventricular tachycardia although a wide complex SVT due to antidromic AVRT is also possible (see Fig. 22.32).

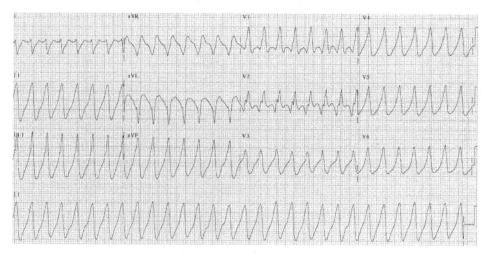

A. During tachycardia

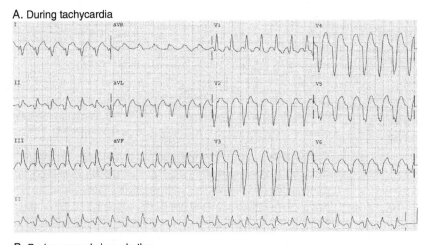

B. During normal sinus rhythm

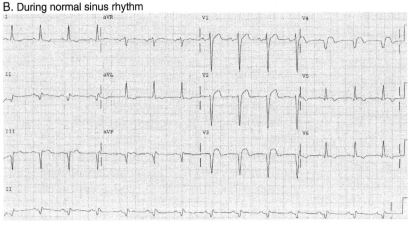

**A.** Normal sinus rhythm and preexistent LBBB

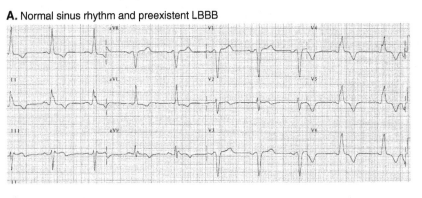

**B.** During tachycardia

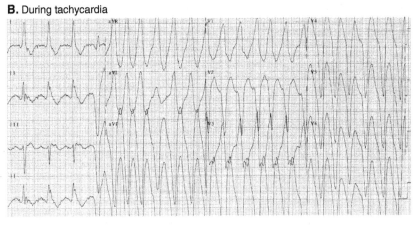

**Figure 22.26:    Previous Myocardial Infarction.** **(A)** A wide complex tachycardia. **(B)** A 12-lead electrocardiogram (ECG) obtained from the same patient during normal sinus rhythm. QS complexes with elevated ST segments are present in $V_{2-4}$. There are also pathologic Q waves in leads II, III, and aVF consistent with anterior and inferior myocardial infarctions (MI). When a previous MI is present by history or by ECG, a wide complex tachycardia occurring after the MI favors ventricular tachycardia.

**Figure 22.27:    Previous Left Bundle Branch Block (LBBB).** **(A)** Normal sinus rhythm with LBBB. When a wide complex tachycardia occurs in a patient with preexistent LBBB and the configuration of the QRS complex changes during tachycardia **(B)**, the diagnosis is ventricular tachycardia. This is based on the assumption that when there is bifascicular block, the impulse is obligated to follow the only remaining fascicle, thus ventricular aberration as a cause of the tachycardia is not possible.

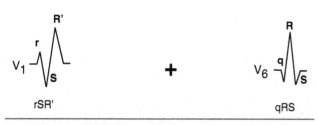

**Figure 22.28: Wide Complex Supraventricular Tachycardia (SVT).** Triphasic rSR' pattern in V₁ combined with triphasic qRS pattern in V₆ favor the diagnosis of SVT.

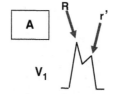
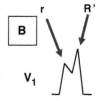

Rr' "rabbit ear sign" favors VT       rR' is not helpful but is SVT if V₆ is triphasic or R>S

**Figure 22.29: Wide Complex Supraventricular Tachycardia (SVT). (A)** When lead V₁ shows Rr' (left rabbit's ear taller than right rabbit's ear), the pattern favors ventricular tachycardia. **(B)** If lead V₁ shows rR' (also called right rabbit ear taller than left rabbit ear), the finding is not specific but could be SVT if V₆ is triphasic (qRS) or the R wave is taller than S wave (R/S ratio >1).

important feature in the history that will favor VT is the presence of a previous MI.

☐ If the patient had a previous MI and the tachycardia occurred after the MI, the diagnosis is VT.
☐ If the patient has history of tachycardia and has preexcitation, the diagnosis is SVT.

■ **Physical examination:** The presence of hemodynamic instability does not differentiate ventricular from supraventricular tachycardia with a wide QRS complex. The following physical findings however are diagnostic of VT.

☐ Cannon "A" waves
☐ Varying intensity of the first heart sound
☐ Varying volume of the arterial pulse

■ **Vagal stimulation:** If the wide complex tachycardia is due to SVT, vagal stimulation may terminate the arrhythmia or may cause significant slowing of the heart rate. This will allow the arrhythmia to be diagnosed more appropriately (Fig. 22.33). The rhythm should be recorded during vagal stimulation.

■ **Pharmacologic agents:** Adenosine, a short-acting AV nodal blocker, is useful in terminating wide complex SVT that are AV nodal–dependent. The

**Figure 22.30: Wide Complex Supraventricular Tachycardia (SVT) from Preexistent Right Bundle Branch Block (RBBB).** Electrocardiogram **(A)** and **(B)** are from the same patient. Note that the configuration of the QRS complexes during normal sinus rhythm **(A)** is identical to the QRS complexes during tachycardia **(B)** because of preexistent RBBB.

**A.** During normal sinus rhythm
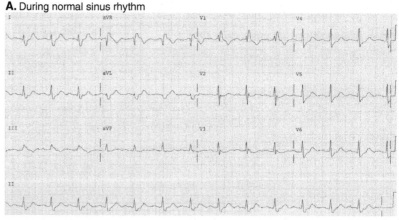

**B.** During tachycardia
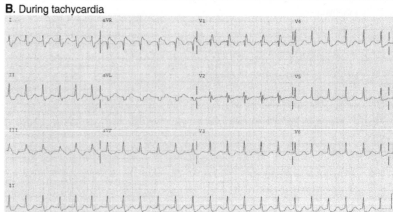

**A.** During normal sinus rhythm

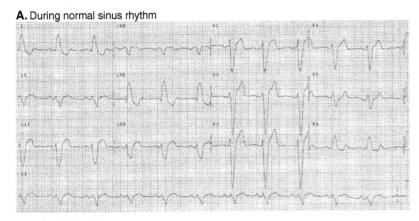

**B.** During tachycardia

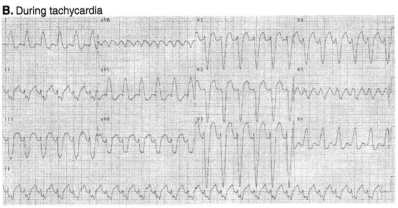

**Figure 22.31:    Wide Complex Supraventricular Tachycardia (SVT) from Preexistent Left Bundle Branch Block (LBBB).** Electrocardiogram **(A)** and **(B)** are from the same patient. Figure **(A)** shows the patient during normal sinus rhythm and **(B)** during tachycardia. Note that the configuration of the QRS complexes during the tachycardia **(B)** is the same as during normal sinus rhythm **(A)** consistent with SVT with preexistent LBBB.

**A.** During normal sinus rhythm

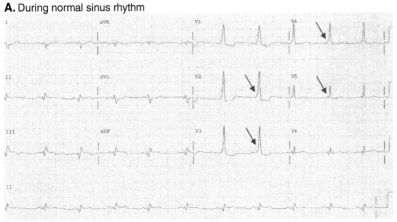

**B.** During tachycardia

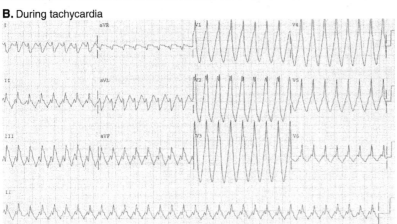

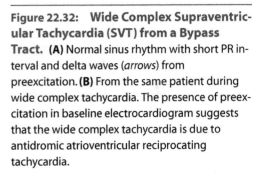

**Figure 22.32:    Wide Complex Supraventricular Tachycardia (SVT) from a Bypass Tract.** **(A)** Normal sinus rhythm with short PR interval and delta waves (*arrows*) from preexcitation. **(B)** From the same patient during wide complex tachycardia. The presence of preexcitation in baseline electrocardiogram suggests that the wide complex tachycardia is due to antidromic atrioventricular reciprocating tachycardia.

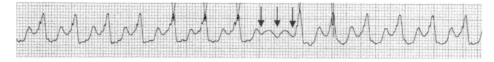

**Figure 22.33: Wide Complex Tachycardia from Atrial Flutter.** Carotid sinus stimulation can slow the ventricular rate transiently resulting in lengthening of the R-R intervals. This will allow the baseline to be inspected for atrial activity. Atrial flutter waves can be demonstrated during transient lengthening of the R-R interval (*arrows*). The tachycardia is due to atrial flutter and the wide QRS complexes are due to preexistent bundle branch block.

tachycardia should be recorded while adenosine is being injected. The cause of the tachycardia may be identified even if the tachycardia does not respond to adenosine (Fig. 22.34).

■ If the diagnosis of the wide complex tachycardia remains uncertain after careful evaluation of all available clinical information, practice guidelines recommend that the patient should be treated as VT.

## Pharmacologic Agents

■ Figure 22.34 shows a wide complex tachycardia from SVT diagnosed with injection of adenosine, a short-acting AV nodal blocker. It should be given only if the wide complex SVT is known to be supraventricular in origin. It should not be given if the diagnosis

is uncertain. It is also helpful in identifying the mechanisms of other types of wide complex tachycardia by slowing the heart rate, as shown in Figure 22.34B.

## Wide Complex Tachycardia

### Summary of ECG Findings

■ **VT:** Any of the following ECG findings suggests VT:
  ▪ Complete AV dissociation
  ▪ Ventricular fusion complex
  ▪ Sinus captured complex
  ▪ Ventriculoatrial conduction with second degree block
  ▪ Wide QRS complexes measuring >140 milliseconds when the tachycardia has a RBBB pattern or >160 milliseconds

**Figure 22.34: Wide Complex Tachycardia and Intravenous Adenosine. (A)** Twelve-lead electrocardiogram showing a wide complex tachycardia. **(B)** Leads I, II, and III were recorded while adenosine was being injected intravenously. Although the ventricular rate slowed significantly, the configuration of the QRS complexes remained unchanged because of pre-existent bundle branch block. Arrows point to the presence of atrial tachycardia with a rate of 167 beats per minute. The atrial rate is the same as the rate of the wide complex tachycardia.

**A.** Wide complex tachycardia

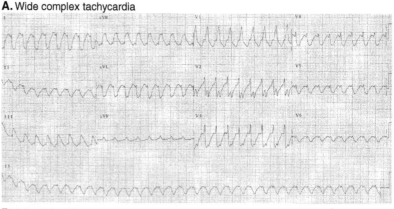

**B.** Adenosine IV

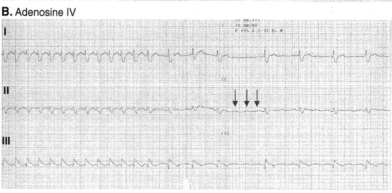

when the tachycardia has a LBBB pattern. This observation is not helpful if there is preexistent bundle branch block, preexcitation, or the patient is taking antiarrhythmic medications that prolong intraventricular conduction such as type IA or IC agents.

- If there is no RS complex in the precordial leads.
- If RS complex is present in the precordial leads and the RS duration measures >100 milliseconds.
- If the QRS complex in $V_1$ has RBBB configuration that is monophasic or biphasic and the configuration in $V_6$ is qR, QS, monophasic R wave or rS (R/S <1).
- When there is LBBB morphology with right axis deviation >+90° or >–60°.
- When there is RBBB morphology with left axis deviation >–30°.
- If the axis of the QRS complex is between –90° and –180° also called northwest axis.
- When QRS complexes are concordant in the precordial leads:
  - □ **LBBB morphology:** When the QRS complexes in the precordial leads are negatively concordant with LBBB morphology, this is almost always from VT.
  - □ **RBBB morphology:** When the QRS complexes are positively concordant with RBBB morphology, this is usually VT although wide complex SVT from antidromic AVRT is also possible.
- If a previous 12-lead ECG is available, the diagnosis is VT if:
  - □ A previous myocardial infarction (MI) is present.
  - □ Bifascicular block is present during normal sinus rhythm (LBBB or RBBB + a fascicular block) and the QRS morphology becomes different during the tachycardia.
- **SVT:** Any of the following ECG findings is consistent with SVT:
  - The tachycardia has RBBB configuration with a triphasic rSR′ pattern in $V_1$ and a triphasic qRS pattern in $V_6$.
  - In $V_1$, right rabbit ear is taller than left. In $V_6$, there is a triphasic QRS complex or R wave is taller than S wave (R/S ratio >1).
  - When a previous 12-lead ECG is available, the diagnosis is SVT if:
    - □ Bundle branch block is present during normal sinus rhythm and the QRS configuration is identical during tachycardia (wide complex SVT from preexistent bundle branch block).
    - □ Preexcitation or Wolff-Parkinson-White (WPW) ECG is present during normal sinus rhythm (antidromic AVRT).

## Mechanism

- **Complete AV dissociation:** In VT, the ventricles are driven by an impulse that is faster and separate from that of the atria. Generally, the atria continue to be controlled by normal sinus rhythm, which has a slower rate and is independent from the ectopic activity occurring in the ventricles. The presence of two independent pacemakers, one controlling the atria and the other the ventricles, will result in complete AV dissociation.
- **Wide QRS complexes:** Ventricular tachycardia has wide QRS complex because the ventricles are driven by an impulse occurring below the bifurcation of the bundle of His. Thus, the ventricles are not activated simultaneously because the impulse has to spread from one ventricle to the other ventricle outside the normal conduction system. This causes the QRS complexes to be wide measuring ≥120 milliseconds.
- **Absence of RS complex in the precordial leads:** Absence of RS complex in the precordial leads indicates VT. When this occurs, the QRS complex usually starts with a q wave. The q waves indicate that the ectopic ventricular impulse originates from the epicardium and spreads from epicardium to endocardium, causing q waves in the precordial leads. This is in contrast to SVT, which usually activates the ventricles through the His-Purkinje system and therefore the spread of the ventricular impulse is from endocardium to epicardium, causing an RS complex to be inscribed in at least one of the precordial leads.
- **Wide RS interval:** The RS interval, measured from the beginning of the R wave to the lowest point of the S wave is equivalent to the spread of the impulse across the thickness of the myocardium. If the RS interval exceeds 100 milliseconds, the diagnosis is VT. This is based on the assumption that in VT, activation of the ventricles will be less efficient and will take longer because the impulse is propagated by muscle cell to muscle cell conduction, as opposed to SVT where activation of the myocardium will be faster because the impulse is conducted through the more efficient His-Purkinje system.
- **Fusion and sinus captured complexes:** Although the atrial rate or the rate of the sinus impulse is slower than the rate of the ventricles during VT, a properly timed sinus impulse may arrive at the ventricles when the ventricles are not refractory and may be able to capture the ventricles partially (resulting in fusion complexes) or completely (resulting in sinus captured beats). Thus, when fusion or sinus captured complexes are present, the diagnosis is VT.
- **V-A conduction:** When there is VT, the ventricular impulse may be conducted to the atria retrogradely across the AV node, causing the atria to be activated from below upward. This will result in inverted P waves in leads II, III, and aVF. V-A conduction is not uncommon during VT. Wellens et al. showed that in 70 patients with VT, approximately 50% had V-A conduction during electrophysiologic testing, with 23 having 1:1 V-A conduction, 7 having 2:1 V-A, conduction, and 2 having V-A Wenckebach. V-A block may occur spontaneously. It could also be induced by carotid sinus pressure. One to one V-A conduction is not diagnostic of VT because this can also occur in wide complex AVRT. However, intermittent V-A conduction from V-A block is diagnostic of VT. V-A block is not generally known as a marker of VT because V-A conduction is not commonly seen in the surface ECG.

## Clinical Findings

- **Other modalities that are useful in differentiating VT from wide complex SVT:** Although the 12-lead ECG serves as the foundation for differentiating VT from wide complex SVT, there are other modalities that are also useful. These include the history, physical examination, response to carotid sinus pressure, and other vagal maneuvers.

  - **Clinical presentation:** The hemodynamic condition of the patient is not reliable in distinguishing VT from SVT. A patient presenting with hypotension, dizziness, or syncope does not necessarily imply that the tachycardia is ventricular. Conversely, a patient who is hemodynamically stable during the tachycardia does not necessarily indicate that the tachycardia is supraventricular. When the heart rate is very rapid (usually ≥150 beats per minute), patients usually become symptomatic and even patients with SVT may become hemodynamically unstable when there is associated left ventricular systolic or diastolic dysfunction.

  - **History:** The history is often more important than the ECG in differentiating VT from wide complex SVT.
    - ☐ History of previous MI favors VT. The tachycardia should occur after (not before) the onset of the MI.
    - ☐ History of preexcitation (WPW syndrome) indicates wide complex SVT.

  - **Physical examination:** The following physical findings suggest VT. The findings are based on the presence of AV dissociation, which is very specific for VT.
    - ☐ **Cannon "A" waves in the neck veins:** When atrial and ventricular contractions are completely dissociated, simultaneous contraction of the atria and ventricles may occur intermittently. When atrial contraction is simultaneous with ventricular contraction, cannon "A" waves will appear in the neck representing contraction of the atria against a closed tricuspid valve. This is manifested as intermittent prominent pulsations in the neck veins.
    - ☐ **Varying intensity of the first heart sound.** Another sign of AV dissociation is varying intensity of the first heart sound. The mechanism for the varying intensity of the first heart sound has been previously discussed in Chapter 8, Atrioventricular Block. The first heart sound is due to closure of the AV valves and the intensity depends on the position of the valves at the onset of systole. If the AV valves are widely open when systole occurs, the first heart sound will be loud. If the AV valves are almost closed at the onset of systole, the first heart sound will be very soft. Because the atrial kick (P wave) pushes the AV valves away from their coaptation points, a short PR interval will cause the ventricles to contract immediately when the AV valves are widely open, which will result in a loud first heart sound. If the PR interval is unusually prolonged, the AV valves will float back to a semiclosed position before the onset of ventricular contraction; thus, the first heart sound will be softer. Because AV dissociation is associated with varying PR intervals, the position of the AV valves at the onset of systole will be variable; hence, the intensity of the first heart sound will also be variable.
    - ☐ **Varying pulse volume:** If atrial contraction is perfectly timed to occur just before ventricular contraction, ventricular filling is augmented and a larger volume is ejected. Because the PR interval is variable when there is AV dissociation, atrial contribution to left ventricular filling will vary resulting in varying pulse volume.

  - **Carotid sinus pressure and other vagal maneuvers:** Another method of distinguishing VT from SVT is to perform vagal maneuvers including carotid sinus pressure. These procedures may terminate wide complex SVT, but not VT.

## Acute Therapy

- Immediate therapy depends on the clinical presentation of the patient.

  - **Unstable patient:** If the patient is unstable with hypotension or gross heart failure or the patient is having symptoms of severe ischemia related to the tachycardia, electrical cardioversion is indicated whether the wide complex tachycardia is ventricular or supraventricular.

  - **Stable patient:** If the patient is stable, pharmacologic therapy can be used. Elective cardioversion is also an option in stable patients if the tachycardia is due to VT or there is uncertainty about the etiology of the wide complex tachycardia. Carotid sinus stimulation and other vagal maneuvers are also helpful and should be tried initially to terminate SVT. It is also helpful in distinguishing VT from wide complex SVT.

- **Pharmacologic therapy:** Among stable patients, the type of pharmacologic agent will depend on whether the tachycardia is known to be ventricular, supraventricular, or the etiology of the wide complex tachycardia remains uncertain.

  - **Wide complex tachycardia due to SVT:** The treatment for wide complex SVT is similar to the treatment of narrow complex SVT. Carotid sinus pressure may terminate the arrhythmia and should be attempted before intravenous medications are given. If the arrhythmia cannot be terminated with vagal maneuvers, the drug of choice is adenosine given intravenously. If adenosine is not effective, another AV nodal blocker may be given. The choice of the AV nodal blocking agent will depend on the presence or absence of LV dysfunction as described under the treatment of narrow complex SVT.
    - ☐ **Wide complex tachycardia due to antidromic AVRT:** If the wide complex SVT is due to antidromic AVRT (WPW syndrome), the AV node may not be part of the reentrant circuit (see the Wide Complex or

Antidromic AVRT section in Chapter 20, Wolff-Parkinson-White Syndrome). In antidromic AVRT, anterograde conduction of the atrial impulse occurs at the bypass tract and retrograde conduction from ventricle to atrium may occur through another bypass tract instead of the AV node especially when there is Ebstein's anomaly. Thus, the use of AV nodal blockers will not be effective because the AV node is not part of the reentrant circuit. Type IA, type IC, and type III antiarrhythmic agents that will block conduction through the bypass tract are effective agents in terminating the tachycardia. Procainamide, ibutilide, and flecainide are the preferred agents.

- ☐ The intravenous administration of calcium channel blockers, beta blockers, or adenosine may not be appropriate unless the tachycardia is definitely SVT because these pharmacologic agents are not only ineffective, but may also cause hemodynamic instability or even death if the wide complex tachycardia turns out to be VT.

- ■ **Wide complex tachycardia from VT:** If the wide complex tachycardia has been shown to be ventricular in origin, the acute treatment is similar to monomorphic VT. The choice of antiarrhythmic agent will depend on the presence or absence of heart failure or left ventricular dysfunction as discussed in Chapter 21, Ventricular Arrhythmias. For stable patients, procainamide and sotalol are preferred agents, although amiodarone is also acceptable and becomes the preferred agent when there is left ventricular dysfunction or heart failure.

- ■ **Diagnosis uncertain:** If the diagnosis of the wide complex tachycardia remains uncertain, calcium channel blockers, beta blockers, or other agents for terminating SVT should not be tried because these agents can cause hemodynamic instability, especially when there is left ventricular dysfunction. In patients who are hemodynamically unstable, electrical cardioversion with appropriate sedation is recommended (Class I). In stable patients, the preferred agents are either procainamide or amiodarone because both agents are effective for VT or SVT. Intravenous procainamide is recommended as initial therapy in stable patients. Intravenous amiodarone is recommended in patients who are hemodynamically unstable, refractory to electrical cardioversion, or if the arrhythmia is recurrent in spite of IV procainamide. Lidocaine is reserved for wide complex tachycardia in patients with poor left ventricular function associated with acute MI or myocardial ischemia. Electrical cardioversion is also an option even if the patient is hemodynamically stable or if the patient does not respond to the chosen antiarrhythmic medication (Table 22.1).

- ■ Electrolyte abnormalities, myocardial ischemia, blood gas, and other metabolic disorders should be identified and corrected. Medications that may be proarrhythmic should be eliminated.

## Prognosis

- ■ Prognosis for VT is worse than SVT. Sustained VT is usually associated with structural cardiac disease such as acute myocardial infarction, cardiomyopathy, or other myocardial diseases resulting in impaired systolic function. The presence of ventricular tachycardia in this setting is associated with a high mortality. These patients are candidates for implantation

### TABLE 22.1

**Acute Management of Wide Complex Tachycardia of Uncertain Diagnosis According to the ACC/AHA/ESC Practice Guidelines in the Management of Patients with Supraventricular Arrhythmias**

| Clinical | Recommendation | Level of Recommendation |
|---|---|---|
| Unstable patients | DC electrical cardioversion | Class I |
| Stable patients | Procainamide | Class I |
| | Sotalol | Class I |
| | Amiodarone | Class I |
| | DC cardioversion | Class I |
| | Lidocaine | Class IIb |
| | Adenosine | Class IIb |
| | Beta blockers | Class III |
| | Verapamil | Class III |
| Patients with | Amiodarone | Class I |
| poor LV function | DC cardioversion | Class I |
| | Lidocaine | |

All pharmacologic agents are given intravenously.
ACC, American College of Cardiology; AHA, American Heart Association; ESC, European Society of Cardiology; LV, left ventricular; DC, direct current.

of automatic implantable defibrillator. Overall prognosis depends on the underlying cardiac disease and severity of left ventricular dysfunction.

■ If the wide complex tachycardia is due to SVT, prognosis is the same as for narrow complex SVT.

## Suggested Readings

2005 American Heart Association guidelines for cardiopulmonary resuscitation and emergency cardiovascular care. Part 7.3: management of symptomatic bradycardia and tachycardia. *Circulation.* 2005;112[Suppl]:IV-67–IV-77.

Akhtar M. Electrophysiologic bases for wide complex tachycardia. *PACE.* 1983;6:81.

Baltazar RF, Javillo JS. Images in cardiology. Ventriculo-atrial Wenckebach during wide complex tachycardia. *Clin Cardiol.* 2006;29:513.

Blomstrom-Lundqvist C, Scheinman MM, Aliot EM, et al. ACC/AHA/ESC Guidelines for the management of patients with supraventricular arrhythmias—executive summary. A report of the American College of Cardiology/American Heart Association Task Force on Practice Guidelines, and the European Society of Cardiology Committee for Practice Guidelines (Writing Committee to Develop Guidelines for the Management of Patients with Supraventricular Arrhythmias) *J Am Coll Cardiol.* 2003;42:1493–1531.

Brugada P, Brugada J, Mont L, et al. A new approach to the differential diagnosis of a regular tachycardia with a wide QRS complex. *Circulation.* 1991;83:1649–1659.

Edhouse J, Morris F. ABC of clinical electrocardiography. Broad complex tachycardia—part I. *BMJ.* 2002;324:719–722.

Edhouse J, Morris F. ABC of clinical electrocardiography. Broad complex tachycardia—part II. *BMJ.* 2002;324:776–779.

Garratt CJ, Griffith MJ, Young G, et al. Value of physical signs in the diagnosis of ventricular tachycardia. *Circulation.* 1994; 90:3103–3107.

Gozensky C, Thorne D. Rabbit ears: an aid in distinguishing ventricular ectopy from aberration. *Heart Lung.* 1975;3:634.

Griffith MJ, Garratt CJ, Mounsey P, et al. Ventricular tachycardia as default diagnosis in broad complex tachycardia. *Lancet.* 1994;343:386–388.

Guidelines 2000 for cardiopulmonary resuscitation and emergency cardiovascular care, an international consensus on science. The American Heart Association in Collaboration with the International Liaison Committee on Resuscitation. 7D: the tachycardia algorithms. *Circulation.* 2000;102[Suppl I]:-I-158–I-165.

Harvey WP, Ronan JA, Jr. Bedside diagnosis of arrhythmias. *Prog Cardiovasc Dis.* 1966;8:419–445.

Stewart RB, Bardy GH, Greene HL. Wide complex tachycardia: misdiagnosis and outcome after emergent therapy. *Ann Intern Med.* 1986;104:766–771.

Surawicz B, Uhley H, Borun R, et al. Task Force I: standardization of terminology and interpretation. *Am J Cardiol.* 1978; 41:130–144.

Tchou P, Young P, Mahmud R, et al. Useful clinical criteria for the diagnosis of ventricular tachycardia. *Am J Med.* 1988;84: 53–56.

Wellens HJ. Electrocardiographic diagnosis of arrhythmias. In: Topol EJ, ed. *Textbook of Cardiovascular Disease.* 2nd ed. Philadelphia: Lippincott William & Wilkins; 2002:1665–1683.

Wellens HJJ, Bar FWHM, Lie KI. The value of the electrocardiogram in the differential diagnosis of a tachycardia with a widened QRS complex. *Am J Med.* 1978;64:27–33.

Wellens HJJ, Conover MB. Wide QRS tachycardia. In: *The ECG in Emergency Decision Making.* Philadelphia: WB Saunders Co; 1992:37–72.

WHO/ISC Task Force. Definition of terms related to cardiac rhythm. *Am Heart J.* 1978;95:796–806.

Zipes DP, Camm AJ, Borggrefe M, et al. ACC/AHA/ESC 2006 guidelines for management of patients with ventricular arrhythmias and the prevention of sudden cardiac death: a report of the American College of Cardiology/American Heart Association Task Force and the European Society of Cardiology Committee for Practice Guidelines (Writing Committee to Develop Guidelines for Management of Patients with Ventricular Arrhythmias and the Prevention of Sudden Cardiac Death). *J Am Coll Cardiol.* 2006,48:e247–e346.

# Acute Coronary Syndrome: ST Elevation Myocardial Infarction

## The Electrocardiogram (ECG) in Acute Coronary Syndrome

- When a patient presents to the emergency department with chest discomfort or symptoms suspicious of acute myocardial infarction (MI), the standard of care requires that a full 12-lead ECG be obtained and interpreted within 10 minutes after the patient enters the medical facility. The ECG can provide the following useful information in patients with acute coronary syndrome:
  - The ECG is the only modality capable of making a diagnosis of ST elevation MI. It is the most important tool in defining the onset of the coronary event and the urgency for immediate revascularization. It serves as the only basis for deciding whether or not the patient is a candidate for thrombolytic therapy or primary angioplasty. It therefore remains central to the decision making process in managing patients with acute coronary syndrome.
  - It provides useful information on whether or not reperfusion therapy has been successful.
  - It can identify the culprit vessel, localize whether the lesion is proximal or distal, and therefore predicts the extent of jeopardized myocardium. Localizing the culprit vessel will also help in predicting potential complications that may inherently occur based on the geographic location of the MI.

- It is the simplest and most useful tool in the diagnosis of right ventricular MI.
- It is the most useful modality in identifying several complications of acute MI, including the various atrioventricular and intraventricular conduction abnormalities as well as the different bradycardias and tachycardias, which are frequent during hospitalization especially after the initial onset of symptoms.

- In this era of modern and expensive technology, the ECG remains the most important and least expensive modality in evaluating and managing patients suspected of having acute symptoms from coronary artery disease. The ECG therefore remains the cornerstone in evaluating and managing patients with acute coronary syndrome and continues to provide very useful information that is not obtainable with other more expensive technologies.

## Acute Coronary Syndrome

- It is well recognized that acute coronary syndrome is caused by rupture of an atheromatous plaque, resulting in partial or total occlusion of the vessel lumen by a thrombus. Depending on how severely the coronary flow is compromised, varying degrees of myocardial ischemia will occur resulting in ST elevation MI, non-ST elevation MI, or unstable angina (Fig. 23.1).

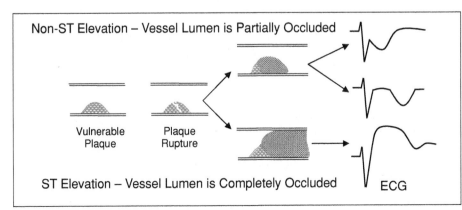

**Figure 23.1: Electrocardiogram Changes of Acute Coronary Syndrome.** Complete occlusion of the vessel lumen by a thrombus causes ST elevation whereas partial occlusion of the vessel lumen will result in ST depression, T-wave inversion, or other less-specific ST and T-wave abnormalities.

**Figure 23.2: Myocardial Ischemia with ST Elevation.** ST elevation from an occlusive thrombus is persistent and generally does not resolve with coronary vasodilators, whereas ST elevation from coronary vasospasm is usually transient and responds to coronary vasodilators.

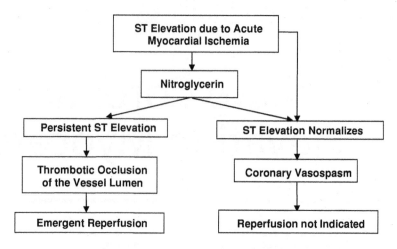

- **ST elevation MI:** Acute ischemia associated with elevation of the ST segment indicates complete occlusion of the vessel lumen by a thrombus with complete cessation of coronary blood flow. When this occurs, myocardial necrosis with elevation of cardiac markers is always expected.
- **Non-ST elevation:** When acute ischemia is associated with ST depression, T wave inversion or other less specific ST and T wave abnormalities, partial or incomplete occlusion of the vessel lumen by a thrombus has occurred. This type of ischemia may or may not be accompanied by cellular necrosis. When there is cellular necrosis, with increased cardiac markers in the circulation, non-ST elevation MI is present. When there is no evidence of myocardial necrosis, the clinical picture is unstable angina. The diagnosis of myocardial necrosis is based on the presence of increased cardiac troponins in the circulation. Regardless of symptoms or ECG findings, the diagnosis of acute MI is not possible unless these cardiac markers are elevated.

## ST Segment Elevation

- Acute coronary syndrome with elevation of the ST segment is almost always from complete occlusion of the vessel lumen by a thrombus resulting in complete cessation of coronary flow. It can also occur when there is coronary vasospasm (Fig. 23.2).
  - **ST elevation from occlusive thrombus:** ST elevation from an occlusive thrombus almost always results in cellular necrosis. Cardiac markers are expected to be always elevated. Unless the occluded vessel is immediately reperfused, pathologic Q waves will occur. ST elevation MI therefore is synonymous with a Q-wave MI.

- **ST elevation from coronary vasospasm:** ST elevation from coronary vasospasm, also called Prinzmetal angina, is usually transient and can be reversed with coronary vasodilators such as nitroglycerin. Myocardial necrosis usually does not occur unless vasospasm becomes prolonged lasting more than 20 minutes.
- The presence of ST segment elevation accompanied by symptoms of myocardial ischemia indicates that the whole thickness of the myocardium is ischemic. This type of ischemia is also called transmural ischemia.
- Example of ST elevation due to coronary vasospasm is shown below (Figs. 23.3 and 23.4). The pattern of ST elevation is identical and cannot be differentiated from the ST elevation associated with an occlusive thrombus.

## ECG Changes in ST Elevation MI

- **ST elevation from an occlusive thrombus:** When a coronary artery is totally occluded by a thrombus, complete cessation of blood flow occurs. Unless adequate collaterals are present, all jeopardized myocardial cells supplied by the coronary artery will undergo

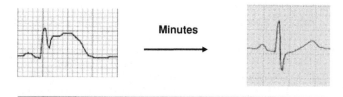

**Figure 23.3: Coronary Vasospasm.** ST elevation from coronary vasospasm is indistinguishable from ST elevation from an occlusive thrombus. ST elevation from coronary vasospasm, however, is usually transient and can be reversed by nitroglycerin, whereas ST elevation from an occlusive thrombus is usually persistent and unresponsive to coronary vasodilators.

**A.**

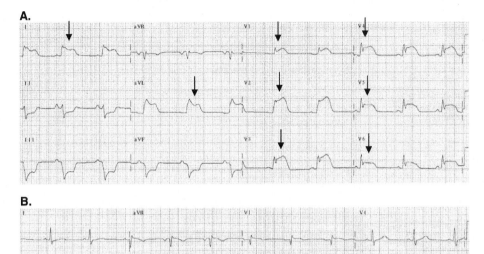

**B.**

**Figure 23.4:  Coronary Vasospasm.** Electrocardiogram **A** and **B** are from the same patient. **(A)** ST elevation in multiple leads (*arrows*), which may be due to an occlusive thrombus or coronary vasospasm. **(B)** After nitroglycerin was given. The ST segment elevation has completely resolved within minutes consistent with coronary vasospasm. Coronary angiography showed smooth walled coronary arteries with no occlusive disease.

irreversible necrosis, usually within 6 hours after the artery is occluded.

■ Necrotic changes in the myocardium are usually not microscopically evident during the first 6 hours after symptom onset. The cardiac troponins may not even be elevated in the circulation in some patients. The ECG, however, will usually show the most dramatic changes at this time. The ECG therefore is the most important modality in triaging patients with chest pain symptoms and is crucial to the diagnosis of ST elevation MI. It also serves as the main criteria in deciding whether or not thrombolytic agent or primary coronary angioplasty is needed.

■ When a coronary artery is completely occluded, the following sequence of ECG changes usually occurs unless the occluded artery is immediately reperfused (Fig. 23.5):

  ■ Peaked or hyperacute T waves (Fig. 23.5A)

  ■ Elevation of the ST segments (Fig. 23.5B,C)

  ■ Changes in the QRS complex with development of pathologic Q waves or decrease in the size or amplitude of the R waves (Fig. 23.5D)

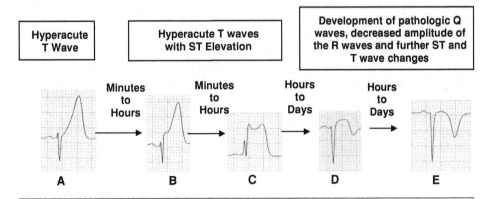

**Figure 23.5:   ST Elevation Myocardial Infarction (MI).** Giant or hyperacute T waves mark the area of ischemia **(A–C)** followed by ST elevation **(B, C)**, diminution of the size of the R wave **(D)** or development of pathologic Q waves **(E)** and inversion of the T waves **(D, E)**. The evolution of ST elevation MI from hyperacute T waves to the development of pathologic Q waves may be completed within 6 hours after symptom onset or may evolve more slowly for several days.

**Figure 23.6:    (A) Hyperacute T Waves.** The initial electrocardiogram (ECG) of a patient presenting with acute onset of chest pain is shown. Tall, hyperacute T waves (*arrows*) are seen in $V_1$ to $V_4$ with elevation of the ST segments in $V_{3-4}$. Note that the hyperacute T waves are confined to the distribution of the occluded vessel and are usually the first to occur before the ST segments become elevated. Subsequent ECGs are shown in **(B–D). (B) ST elevation Myocardial Infarction (MI).** This tracing was recorded 15 minutes after the initial ECG. In addition to the hyperacute T waves, ST elevation has developed in $V_1$ to $V_4$ (*arrows*). (*continued*)

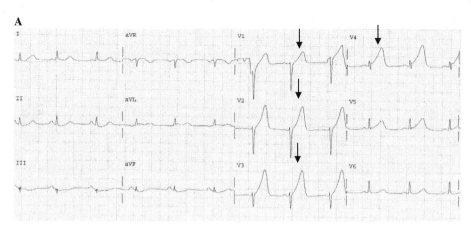

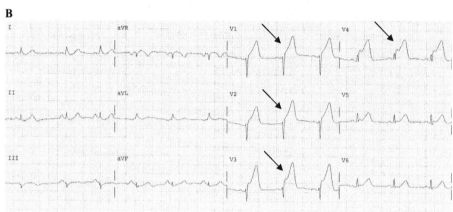

- Further changes in the ST segment and T waves (Fig. 23.5D,E)
- **Peaked or hyperacute T waves:** One of the earliest ECG abnormalities to occur in ST elevation MI is the development of tall and peaked T waves overlying the area of ischemia (Fig. 23.6A). These hyperacute T waves usually precede or accompany the onset of ST segment elevation and are useful in identifying the culprit vessel and timing the onset of acute ischemia.
- **ST segment elevation:** Hyperacute T waves are accompanied or immediately followed by ST segment elevation. ST segment elevation with symptoms of chest discomfort indicates an acute process. The leads with ST elevation are usually adjacent to each other and mark the area of injury and are helpful in identifying the culprit vessel. The extent of ST segment elevation is also helpful in predicting the severity of myocardial involvement.

## Thrombolytic Therapy

- ST elevation from acute coronary syndrome is a medical emergency requiring immediate reperfusion of the occluded artery with a thrombolytic agent or with primary percutaneous coronary intervention (PCI). The extent of myocardial necrosis can be minimized if reperfusion of the occluded artery is timely and successful.
- **Thrombolytic Therapy:** According to American College of Cardiology (ACC)/American Heart Association (AHA) guidelines, thrombolytic therapy is indicated up to 12 hours after onset of symptoms. It may even be extended to 24 hours if the patient's symptoms persist or the chest pain is "stuttering" (waxing and waning) and the ST segments remain elevated at the time of entry. The thrombolytic agent should be infused within 30 minutes after the patient enters the medical facility on his own (door to needle time) or within 30 minutes after contact with emergency service personnel (medical contact to needle time).
  - The best results are obtained if the thrombolytic agent is given within 1 to 2 hours after symptom onset because thrombolytic therapy is time dependent and is more effective when given early.
  - The criteria for initiating a thrombolytic agent in a patient with symptoms of acute ischemia are ST segment elevation or new (or presumably new) onset left bundle branch block (LBBB).
    - **ST segment elevation:**

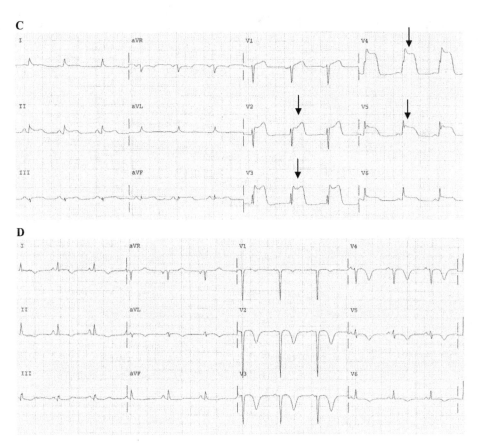

**Figure 23.6:** (*Continued*) **(C) ST Elevation MI.** The above ECG was recorded approximately 1.5 hours from the initial ECG (see **A**). The ST segments continued to evolve even after thrombolytic therapy. ST elevation has become more pronounced in $V_2$ to $V_6$ and slight elevation of the ST segments is noted in II, III, and aVF. Hyperacute T waves are still present in $V_2$ to $V_5$ (*arrows*). **(D) ST Elevation MI.** ECG recorded 13 days later. QS complexes or decreased amplitude of the r waves are seen in $V_1$ to $V_5$. The ST segments are isoelectric and the T waves are inverted from $V_{1–6}$ and leads I, II, and aVL.

- □ ST elevation >1 mm in any two or more adjacent precordial or limb leads.
- □ ST elevation is measured at the J point. The J point is the junction between the terminal portion of the QRS complex and beginning of the ST segment. The preceding T-P segment serves as baseline for measuring the ST elevation. The PR interval is used if the T-P segment is too short or is obscured by a U wave or a P wave of sinus tachycardia.
- □ **New-onset LBBB:** The presence of LBBB will mask the ECG changes of acute MI. If the LBBB is new or presumably new and accompanied by symptoms of acute myocardial ischemia, thrombolytic therapy is indicated.
- Thrombolytic therapy is not indicated (and may be contraindicated) in patients with acute ischemia associated with ST depression or T wave inversion even if the cardiac markers (troponins) are elevated.
- The ECG is the most important modality not only in selecting patients for thrombolytic therapy but also in monitoring successful response to therapy. One of the earliest signs of successful reperfusion during thrombolytic therapy is relief of chest pain and resolution of the initial ST segment elevation by at least 50% within 60 to 90 minutes after initiation of therapy (Fig. 23.7). If ST segment resolution does not occur within 90 minutes after initiating thrombolytic therapy, rescue PCI should be considered.

- Other signs of successful reperfusion include T wave inversion occurring during the first hours of reperfusion therapy and the presence of accelerated idioventricular rhythm.

## Primary Angioplasty

- **Primary PCI:** Primary PCI requires immediate cardiac catheterization and is the preferred method for revascularizing patients with ST elevation MI (Fig. 23.8). The ACC/AHA guidelines recommend that primary PCI should be performed within 90 minutes after first medical contact with emergency personnel (door to balloon or medical contact to balloon) time. Unlike thrombolysis, it is more effective in reestablishing coronary blood flow regardless of the duration of symptoms. It is the preferred method in patients who are unstable, are hemodynamically decompensated, when symptoms exceed 3 hours in duration or the diagnosis of ST elevation MI is in doubt.

**Figure 23.7:   ST Elevation My-
ocardial Infarction.**
Electrocardiogram (ECG) **A** was
recorded before thrombolytic therapy. ST segment elevation is present
in II, III, aVF, and $V_{4-6}$ (*arrows*) with ST
depression in $V_{1-2}$. **(B)** Taken 1 hour
after thrombolytic therapy. ST elevation in the inferolateral leads have
resolved and inverted T waves are
now present in lead III, both are signs
of successful reperfusion.

**A.** Initial ECG

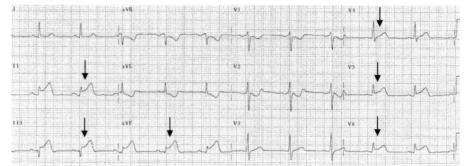

**B.** One hour after initial ECG

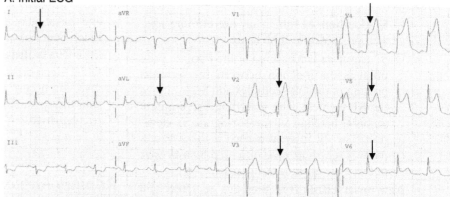

**Figure 23.8:   ST Elevation
Myocardial Infarction.** Electrocardiogram (ECG) **A** shows ST elevation in $V_{2-6}$, I and aVL (*arrows*). Coronary angiography showed
completely occluded proximal left
anterior descending coronary artery.
ECG **B** was recorded 4 hours after
successful percutaneous coronary
intervention. The ST segment elevation has normalized without developing pathologic Q waves, a sign of
successful reperfusion.

A. Initial ECG

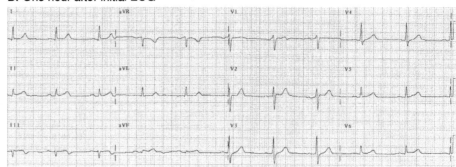

B. After Percutaneous Coronary Intervention

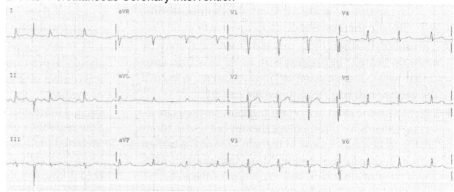

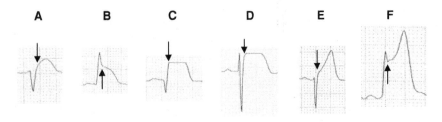

**Figure 23.9:  ST Elevation.** ST elevation MI may show different patterns in different leads and may appear convex or coved (**A, B**), horizontal or plateau (**C, D**), oblique (**E**), or concave (**F**) with a dart and dome configuration. Arrows point to the J points, which are all elevated.

## ST Elevation MI

- ST elevation MI generally indicates the presence of a large infarct. The extent of the infarct is proportional to the number of leads with ST segment elevation. ST elevation MI is associated with a lower ejection fraction, higher incidence of heart failure, and a higher immediate and in-hospital mortality when compared with non-ST elevation MI or unstable angina.

- ST elevation MI may present with several ECG patterns (Fig. 23.9). Although the characteristic example of ST elevation MI is an ST segment that is coved or convex upward (Fig. 23.9A,B), the ST elevation may be horizontal or plateau (Fig. 23.9C,D), or it may be oblique, resembling a ski-slope (Fig. 23.9E) or concave (Fig. 23.9F).

- **Tombstone pattern:** "Tombstoning" is a type of ST elevation MI where the ST segment is about the same level as the height of the R wave and top of the T wave (Figs. 23.4A and 23.6C). The QRS complex, ST segment, and T wave therefore blends together to form a large monophasic complex similar to the shape of a transmembrane action potential (Fig. 23.9C,D). Although this pattern of ST elevation has been shown to indicate a grave prognosis when compared with other patterns of ST segment elevation, it is consistent with the observation that the extent of muscle damage is proportional to the magnitude of ST elevation. Tombstoning is more commonly associated with acute anterior MI. Involvement of the left anterior descending coronary artery is usually proximal and is more severe and extensive than when other patterns of ST elevation are present.

- **Reciprocal ST depression:** One of the features of ST elevation MI that distinguishes it from other causes of ST elevation is the presence of reciprocal ST depression. Reciprocal ST depression is the flip side image recorded directly opposite the lead with ST elevation.

  - For example, if ST elevation occurs in lead III (+120°), a flip side image will be recorded directly opposite lead III at –60° (Fig. 23.10).

- Because there is no standard limb lead representing –60°, aVL (–30°), which is closest to –60° and almost directly opposite lead III, will show reciprocal ST depression (Figs. 23.11 and 23.12).

- Similarly, if ST elevation is present in aVL, reciprocal ST depression will occur in lead III because lead III is the closest lead directly opposite aVL.

- ST segment elevation always points to the area of injury. It is the primary abnormality even if reciprocal ST depression is more pronounced than the ST elevation.

## Localizing the Infarct

- **The coronary arteries:** Although variation in coronary anatomy commonly occurs, three epicardial coronary

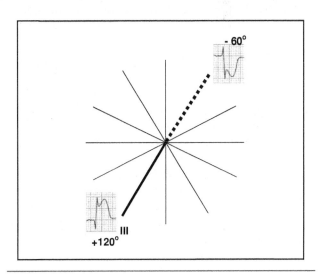

**Figure 23.10:  Reciprocal ST Depression.** When ST elevation from myocardial ischemia is recorded in any lead, a flip side image is recorded directly opposite the lead. In the above example, ST elevation is recorded in lead III (+120°), reciprocal ST depression is also recorded at –60°. Because there is no frontal lead representing –60°, lead aVL, which is adjacent to –60°, will exhibit the most pronounced reciprocal change (see Figs. 23.11 and 23.12).

## ECG Changes in ST Elevation MI

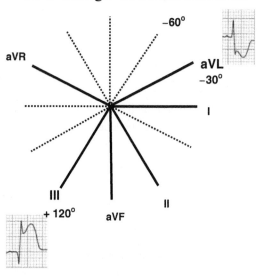

**Figure 23.11:   Reciprocal ST Depression.** ST elevation in lead III is associated with reciprocal ST depression directly opposite lead III. Because lead aVL is the closest lead opposite lead III, aVL will show the most pronounced reciprocal ST depression among the standard electrocardiogram (ECG) leads. The standard limb lead ECG is shown in Figure 23.12.

arteries are generally present. Each artery supplies specific regional areas in the heart. These areas are topographically represented by the following groups of leads:

- **Left anterior descending (LAD) coronary artery:** The LAD supplies the anterior, anteroseptal or anterolateral wall of the left ventricle (LV) (leads $V_1$-$V_6$, I, and aVL).
- **Right coronary artery (RCA):** The RCA supplies the inferior wall (leads II, III, and aVF), often posterolateral wall of the LV (special leads $V_7$, $V_8$, $V_9$). The RCA is the only artery that supplies the right ventricular free wall (special leads $V_{3R}$ to $V_{6R}$).
- **Left circumflex (LCx) coronary artery:** The LCx supplies the anterolateral (leads I, aVL, $V_5$, and $V_6$) and posterolateral (special leads $V_7$, $V_8$, $V_9$) walls of the LV. In 10% to 15% of patients, it supplies the inferior wall of the LV (leads II, III, and aVF).
- The following groups of leads represent certain areas of the heart:
  - $V_{1-2}$: ventricular septum.
  - $V_{2-4}$: anterior wall of the LV. $V_2$ overlaps the septum and anterior wall and is both a septal and anterior lead.
  - $V_1$-$V_3$: anteroseptal wall of the LV.
  - $V_4$-$V_6$, I, and aVL: anterolateral wall of the LV.
  - $V_4$-$V_6$: lateral wall of the LV. $V_4$ overlaps the anterior and lateral walls of the LV and is both an anterior and lateral lead.

- $V_7$-$V_9$: (special leads) posterolateral wall of the LV.
- $V_{3R}$ to $V_{6R}$: (special right-sided precordial leads) right ventricle.
- I and aVL: basal anterolateral or high lateral wall of the LV.
- II, III, and aVF: inferior or diaphragmatic wall of the LV.
- Not all the areas of the heart are represented by the 12-lead ECG. The areas not represented include the right ventricle and posterolateral wall of the LV. Special leads $V_{3R}$ to $V_{6R}$ and $V_7$ to $V_9$ are needed to record these areas, respectively. ST elevation involving the posterolateral wall of the LV is suspected when there is ST depression in leads $V_1$ to $V_3$.
- ST segment elevation points to the area of injury and is helpful in identifying the infarct related artery. Acute MI presenting as ST depression is frequently associated with multivessel coronary disease and is less specific in localizing the culprit vessel.

## Myocardial Distribution of the Three Main Coronary Arteries

- The myocardial distribution of the three coronary arteries is shown in Figure 23.13.

## Left Anterior Descending Coronary Artery

- **Anatomy:** The left main coronary artery divides into two large branches: the LAD and the LCx coronary arteries. The LAD courses toward the apex through the anterior interventricular groove and supplies the anterior wall of the LV. The artery may continue to the inferoapical wall by wrapping around the apex of the LV (Fig. 23.14).
- **First branch:** The first branch of the LAD is the first diagonal artery. This branch runs parallel to the LCx coronary artery and supplies the basal anterolateral wall of the LV. If the first diagonal is a large branch, complete occlusion of this artery causes ST elevation in leads I and aVL with reciprocal ST depression in III and aVF. These ECG changes may be indistinguishable from that due to occlusion of a small LCx coronary artery.
- **Second branch:** The second branch of the LAD is the first septal branch. This artery may be the first instead of the second branch. The artery penetrates the ventricular septum perpendicularly and supplies the basal septum including the proximal conduction system. Involvement of the first septal perforator

will cause ST elevation in $V_1$. It may also involve the conduction system causing new onset right bundle branch block.

- **Anterior MI:** Depending on the location of the coronary lesion and whether the LAD is large or small, complete occlusion of the LAD will cause extensive anterior MI with varying degrees of ST elevation in $V_1$ to $V_6$ as well as leads I and aVL.

  - **Before the first branch:** If the LAD is occluded proximally at the ostium or before the first branch (first diagonal), ST elevation will occur in $V_1$ to $V_4$ (or up to $V_6$) and leads I and aVL from extensive anterior MI. The ST elevation in leads I and AVL represent involvement of the first diagonal branch and is usually accompanied by reciprocal ST depression in III and aVF (Figs. 23.15 and 23.16).

  - **Between the first and second branches:** If the lesion is distal to the first diagonal (but proximal to the first septal branch), ST elevation will include $V_1$ to $V_4$ but not leads I and aVL consistent with acute anteroseptal MI. ST elevation in $V_1$ indicates involvement of the first septal branch (Fig. 23.17).

  - **After the second branch:** If the lesion is distal to the first diagonal and first septal branches, ST elevation will involve $V_2$-$V_4$ but not $V_1$ or I and aVL consistent with anterior often called apical MI.

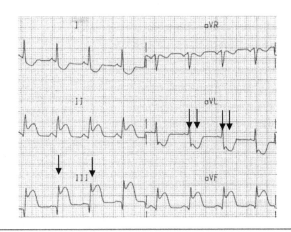

**Figure 23.12: Reciprocal ST Depression.** ST elevation is present in leads II, III, and aVF and is most marked in lead III (*arrows*). Reciprocal ST depression is most pronounced in aVL (*double arrows*) because aVL is almost directly opposite lead III (see Fig. 23.11).

- **Occlusion of the first diagonal branch:** If a large first diagonal branch is the only artery occluded, and the LAD is spared, ST elevation is confined to leads I and aVL consistent with high lateral MI, which involves the base of the LV (Fig. 23.18).

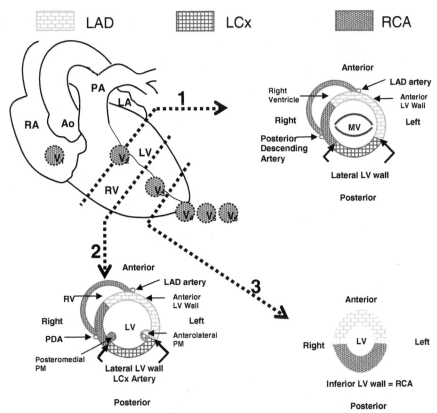

2: Short Axis, LV Papillary Muscle

3: Short Axis, LV Apex

**Figure 23.13: Myocardial Distribution of the Coronary Arteries.** The diagrams summarize the myocardial distribution of the three coronary arteries. The diagram in the upper left represents the frontal view of the heart. The left ventricle is transected by three lines labeled 1, 2, and 3. **Line 1** is at the level of the mitral valve which corresponds to the base of the left ventricle. The short axis view is shown on the upper right diagram. **Line 2** corresponds to the mid-ventricle and the short axis is shown at the lower left. **Line 3** corresponds to the apex of the left ventricle and the short axis is shown at the lower right. Ao, Aorta; LA, left atrium; LV, left ventricle; LAD, left anterior descending; LCx, left circumflex; LV, left ventricle; MV, mitral valve; PA, pulmonary artery; PDA, posterior descending artery; PM, papillary muscle; RA, right atrium; RCA, right coronary artery; $V_1$ to $V_6$, the precordial electrodes superimposed on the heart.

**Figure 23.14: Diagrammatic Representation of the LAD and its Branches.** The left main coronary artery divides into two main branches: the LAD and LCx coronary arteries. The LAD courses through the anterior interventricular groove. It gives diagonal branches laterally and septal branches directly perpendicular to the interventricular septum. LA, left atrium; LAD, left anterior descending artery; LCx, left circumflex; LV, left ventricle; RA, right atrium; RV, right ventricle.

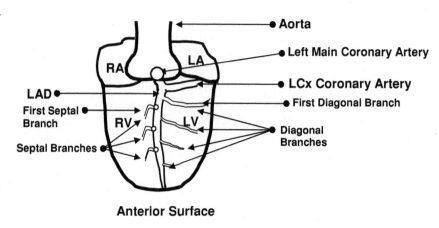

**Anterior Surface**

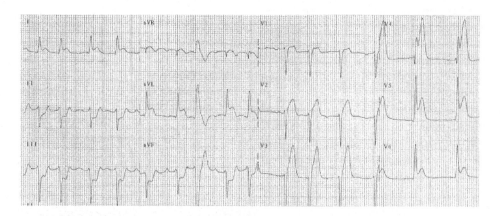

**Figure 23.15: Extensive Anterior Myocardial Infarction (MI).** ST elevation is present in leads $V_{1-6}$, I, and aVL. Cardiac catheterization showed complete occlusion of the proximal left anterior descending (LAD) artery. Note that the ST elevation in I and aVL is due to involvement of the first diagonal branch, which is usually the first branch of the LAD. ST depression in II, III, and aVF is a reciprocal change due to ST elevation in I and aVL.

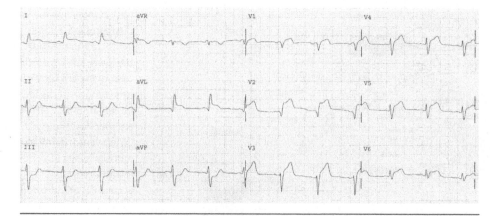

**Figure 23.16: Extensive Anterior Myocardial Infarction.** ST elevation is present in $V_{1-6}$, I, and aVL. Coronary angiography showed complete occlusion of the proximal LAD. This electrocardiogram is similar to that in Figure 23.15.

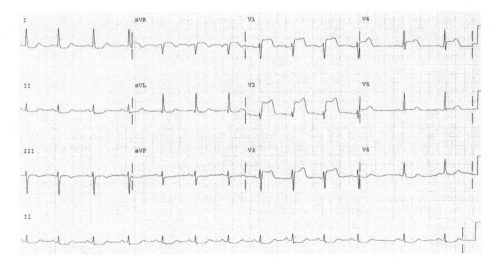

**Figure 23.17:** **Left Anterior Descending (LAD) Artery Occlusion Distal to the First Diagonal Branch.** The electrocardiogram shows acute anteroseptal myocardial infarction with ST segment elevation confined to $V_1$ to $V_4$. This is due to occlusion of the LAD distal to the first diagonal branch (no ST elevation in I and aVL) but proximal to the first septal branch (ST elevation is present in $V_1$).

## LAD Coronary Artery

- Two ECGs showing anterior MI from occlusion of the LAD. The first ECG in Figure 23.16 shows ST elevation in I and aVL from occlusion of the LAD before the first diagonal branch. The second ECG in Figure 23.17 shows anterior MI without ST elevation in I and aVL because of occlusion of the LAD after the first diagonal branch.

- Figure 23.18 shows occlusion confined to the first diagonal branch of the LAD, resulting in high lateral wall MI. ST elevation is present in leads I and aVL only. The ST segment depression in leads III and aVF are reciprocal changes due to the elevated ST segments in I and aVL.

- If the LAD is a long artery, it may wrap around the apex and continues to the inferoapical wall of the LV. Occlusion of a wrap around LAD may cause ST elevation and

eventually Q waves not only in the anterior wall but also inferiorly in II, III, and aVF (Fig. 23.19).

## LCx Artery

- **Anatomy:** The LCx coronary artery circles the left atrioventricular (AV) groove laterally between the left atrium and LV and gives branches that supply the anterolateral and posterolateral walls of the LV (Fig. 23.20). The artery may be small and may terminate very early. In 10% to 15% of cases, the LCx continues posteriorly toward the crux of the heart and down the posterior interventricular groove as the posterior descending coronary artery. When this occurs, the LCx is the dominant artery and supplies not only the inferior

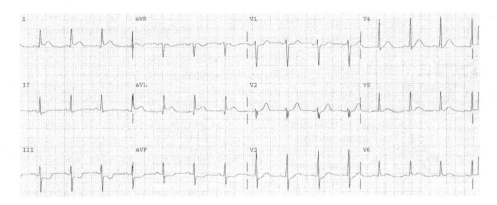

**Figure 23.18:** **Acute High Lateral Myocardial Infarction from Isolated Lesion Involving the First Diagonal Branch of the Left Anterior Descending (LAD) Artery.** ST segment elevation is confined to leads I and aVL. Coronary angiography showed complete occlusion of the first diagonal branch of the LAD. The LAD itself is patent. Occlusion of the first diagonal branch of the LAD causes ST elevation in I and aVL with reciprocal ST depression in III and aVF.

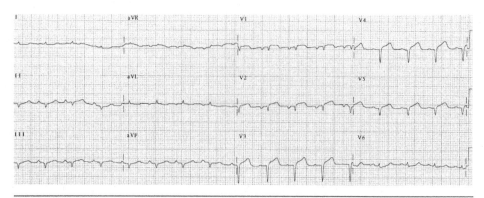

**Figure 23.19: Anterior and Inferior Myocardial Infarction.** QS complexes with ST elevation is noted in $V_1$ to $V_5$ (*anterior wall*) and also in leads II, III, and aVF (*inferior wall*) due to an occluded left anterior descending artery that wraps around the apex of the left ventricle extending to the inferoapical left ventricular wall. The right coronary artery is small but patent.

wall of the LV but also gives rise to the artery to the AV node. Occlusion of the LCx artery will cause:

- **Anterolateral MI:** When the LCx coronary artery is occluded proximally, ST elevation will occur in leads I, aVL, $V_5$, and $V_6$. The MI is confined to the area bounded by the two papillary muscles posterolaterally from the base to the proximal two thirds of the LV (Fig. 23.21). The ST elevation may occur only in leads I and aVL and may be difficult to differentiate from an occluded first diagonal branch of the LAD (Figs. 23.18 and 23.22).

- **Posterolateral MI:** The posterolateral wall of the LV is not directly represented by any standard ECG lead. When posterolateral MI occurs, reciprocal ST depression is noted in $V_1$-$V_3$. $V_5$, and $V_6$ may show ST elevation (Fig. 23.23).

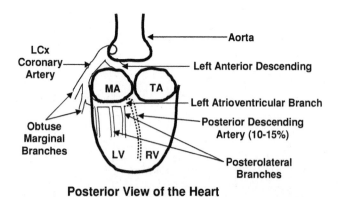

**Figure 23.20: Left Circumflex (LCx) Coronary Artery.** The diagram represents the LCx artery and its main branches. In 10% to 15% of patients, the LCx artery is the dominant artery by continuing as the posterior descending artery (*dotted lines*) and supplying the artery to the AV node. LV, left ventricle; MA, mitral annulus; RV, right ventricle; TA, tricuspid annulus.

- The myocardial distribution of the LCx coronary artery is shown in Fig. 23.21. Acute MI from occlusion of the LCx coronary artery is shown in the ECG in Figure 23.22.

- **Posterolateral MI:** Occlusion of the LCx artery can cause posterior, straight posterior, or posterolateral MI. Because there are no leads representing the posterolateral wall of the LV, a posterolateral MI is suspected in the 12-lead ECG when there is ST depression in $V_1$ to $V_3$. These leads are directly opposite the posterolateral wall and will show reciprocal ST depression when a posterior MI is present. Posterior MI can be confirmed by placing extra electrodes in $V_7$, $V_8$, and $V_9$ ($V_7$ is located at the left posterior axillary line, $V_8$ at the tip of the left scapula, and $V_9$ at the left of the spinal column in the same horizontal plane as $V_{4-6}$). These special leads will show Q waves with ST elevation if a posterolateral MI is present. Prominent R waves may or may not be present in the anterior precordial leads (Fig. 23.23).

- Although ST depression is not an indication for thrombolytic therapy, ST depression in $V_1$ to $V_3$ may be due to posterior MI, which represents a true ST elevation MI. Before thrombolytic therapy is given, leads $V_{7-9}$ should be recorded to verify that the ST depression in $V_{1-3}$ is due to posterior MI and not from subendocardial injury involving the anterior wall of the LV.

- ST elevation confined to leads I and aVL usually indicate lateral MI due to involvement of the LCx coronary artery (Fig. 23.24). ST elevation in leads I, aVL, $V_5$, and $V_6$ is often accompanied by ST elevation in $V_7$ to $V_9$ and reciprocal ST depression in $V_1$ to $V_3$ from posterolateral MI. ST elevation in $V_6$ is usually accompanied by ST elevation in $V_7$ to $V_9$ because these leads are adjacent to $V_6$ (Figs. 23.25 and 23.26).

- Figure 23.26 shows the importance of recording special leads $V_7$ to $V_9$ when a posterolateral MI is suspected.

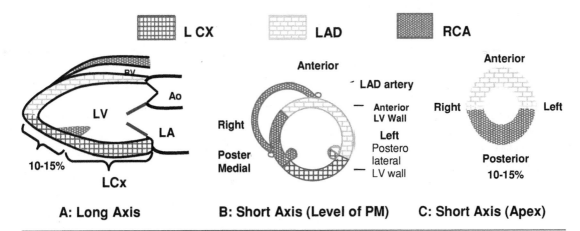

L CX    LAD    RCA

**A: Long Axis**    **B: Short Axis (Level of PM)**    **C: Short Axis (Apex)**

**Figure 23.21:** **Myocardial Distribution of the Left Circumflex (LCx) Coronary Artery.** The LCx coronary artery supplies the territory represented by the purple checkered lines. These include the proximal two thirds (base and midportion) of the lateral wall of the left ventricle. In 10% to 15% of patients, the LCx is the dominant artery and continues inferiorly to the apex of the left ventricle as the posterior descending coronary artery **(A)** long axis view. **(C)** Short axis view of the apex. Ao, aorta; LA, left atrium; LAD; left anterior descending coronary artery; LCx, left circumflex; LV, left ventricle; PM, papillary muscle; RV, right ventricle.

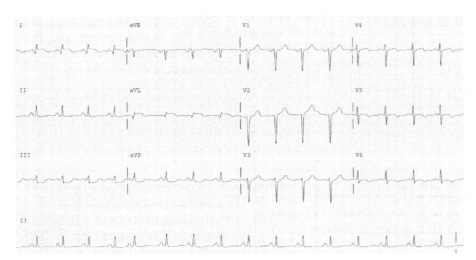

**Figure 23.22:** **High Lateral Myocardial Infarction (MI).** Q waves with elevation of the ST segments are confined to leads I and aVL. The ST depression in III and aVF is reciprocal to the ST elevation in I and aVL. This represents high lateral MI resulting from occlusion of the left circumflex coronary artery. This electrocardiogram finding can also occur when there is occlusion of the first diagonal branch of the left anterior descending coronary artery (see Fig. 23.18).

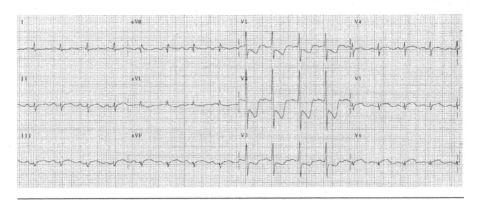

**Figure 23.23:** **Acute Posterolateral Myocardial Infarction (MI).** There is marked depression of the ST segments in $V_1$ to $V_3$ with tall R waves in $V_{1-2}$. The amplitude of the R waves in $V_{5-6}$ is diminished and the ST segments are elevated. This represents an acute posterolateral MI from an occluded left circumflex coronary artery. The ST depression and tall R waves in $V_1$-$V_3$ are reciprocal changes due to the posterior MI. Anterior subendocardial injury and straight posterior MI can be differentiated by recording $V_{7-9}$, which will show ST elevation if posterior MI is present. This distinction is important because ST elevation MI involving the posterior wall of the left ventricle may require thrombolysis, whereas anterior wall subendocardial injury does not.

**Figure 23.24: Acute High Lateral Myocardial Infarction.** ST segment elevation is noted in I and aVL with reciprocal ST depression in III and aVF from occlusion of the left circumflex coronary artery. The ST depression in II, III, and aVF is reciprocal to the ST elevation in I and aVL.

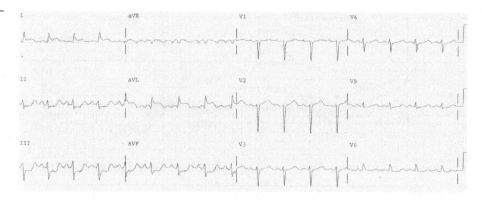

The standard 12-lead ECG shows ST depression in $V_1$ to $V_3$ and ST elevation in $V_5$ and $V_6$. Special leads $V_7$ to $V_9$ recorded posteriorly shows Q waves with ST segment elevation similar to $V_6$. These changes are consistent with a transmural posterolateral MI. The coronary angiogram confirmed the presence of a completely occluded LCx artery.

- **Inferior MI:** Acute inferior MI is due to occlusion of the RCA in 85% to 90% of patients but it can occur in 10% to 15% of patients when the LCx is the dominant artery. In acute inferior MI, the ST segments are elevated in II, III, aVF. If the LCx is the culprit vessel, the ST elevation in lead II is greater than or equal to the ST elevation in lead III (Fig. 23.27).

- If the LCx is small and nondominant, occlusion of the artery may not show any ECG changes (Fig. 23.28). Thus, a normal ECG does not exclude acute MI especially when the LCx is the culprit vessel because most of the area supplied by the LCx is not represented in the standard 12-lead ECG.

## Right Coronary Artery

- **Anatomy:** The RCA courses around the medial AV groove between the right atrium and right ventricle and supplies acute marginal branches to the right ventricle. In 85% to 90% of cases, it is the dominant artery in that it gives rise to the artery to the AV node before continuing posteriorly toward the apex of the LV as the posterior descending artery, which supplies the inferior wall of the LV. The artery often continues posterolaterally beyond the crux to the opposite (lateral or left) AV groove and sends posterolateral branches to the LV (Fig. 23.29).

- Total occlusion of the RCA will cause the following ECG changes:
  - **Inferior MI:** ST elevation in leads II, III, and aVF with reciprocal ST depression in I and aVL (Fig. 23.30).
  - **Inferolateral MI:** ST elevation in leads II, III, aVF, $V_5$, and $V_6$. ST elevation in $V_5$-$V_6$ suggests that the lateral wall of the LV is also involved (Figs. 23.31 and 23.32).

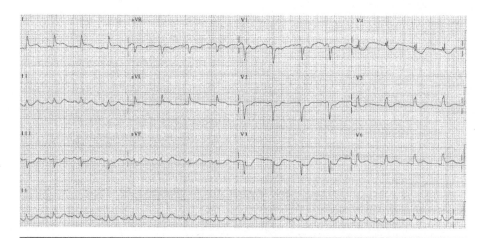

**Figure 23.25: Acute Posterolateral Myocardial Infarction (MI).** ST depression is present in $V_1$-$V_4$. These changes can represent subendocardial injury involving the anterior wall or ST elevation MI involving the posterior wall of the left ventricle. The presence of ST elevation in $V_6$, I, and aVL favors acute posterolateral MI rather than anterior wall injury. This can be confirmed by recording $V_{7-9}$, which will show ST elevation if posterior MI is present.

A: Standard 12 lead ECG

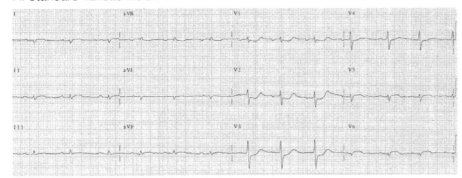

B: Precordial leads V₁ to V₉

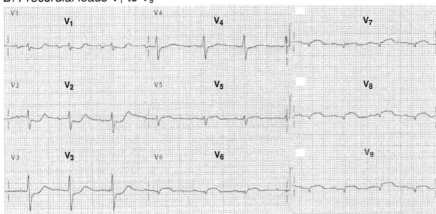

**Figure 23.26: Posterolateral Myocardial Infarction (MI) and Special Leads V₇₋₉.** Electrocardiogram (ECG) **A** is a 12-lead ECG of a 58-year-old male presenting with chest pain. There is ST elevation in leads I, V₅, and V₆, and ST depression in V₁₋₃. **(B)** The same as ECG A and shows only the precordial leads together with V₇ to V₉. ST elevation is present in V₆ as well as V₇, V₈, and V₉ consistent with acute posterolateral MI. These examples show the importance of recording special leads V₇ to V₉ in confirming the diagnosis of posterolateral MI. ECG courtesy of Kittane Vishnupriya, MD.

■ **Inferoposterior MI:** ST elevation in leads II, III, and aVF with ST depression in V₁ to V₃. Reciprocal ST depression in V₁-V₃ indicates the presence of a posterolateral MI (Figs. 23.33 and 23.34). Tall R waves may develop in V₁ or V₂, although this usually occurs much later several hours after the acute episode. Special leads V₇₋₉ will record ST elevation and tall hyperacute T waves during the acute episode.

■ ST depression in V₁-V₃ may be due to ST elevation MI involving the posterolateral wall (Figs. 23.33A and 23.34). It may also be due to subendocardial injury involving the anterior wall of the LV. To differentiate one from the other, leads V₇ to V₉ should be recorded. If posterolateral ST elevation MI is present, V₇ to V₉ will record ST segment elevation. If there is subendocardial injury involving the anterior wall, the ST segments will not be elevated in V₇ to V₉.

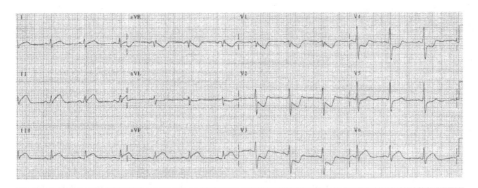

**Figure 23.27: Acute Inferior Myocardial Infarction (MI) from Occlusion of the Left Circumflex Coronary Artery.** Note that the ST elevation in lead II is more prominent than lead III. Additionally, the ST segment is isoelectric in aVL and minimally elevated in lead I. ST depression is present in V₁ to V₃ with ST elevation in V₆ from posterolateral MI.

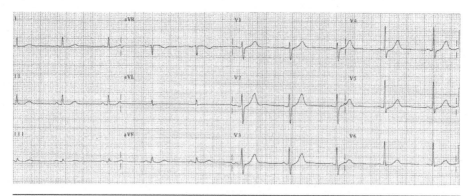

**Figure 23.28: Acute Myocardial Infarction with Normal Electrocardiogram (ECG).** The ECG is from a 56-year-old male who presented with acute persistent chest pains. Serial ECGs were all normal although the cardiac markers were elevated. The coronary angiogram showed completely occluded left circumplex corona artery (LCx). Among the three coronary arteries, LCx coronary disease is the most difficult to diagnose electrocardiographically.

## Acute Inferior MI

- **Inferior MI:** In 85% to 90% of patients with acute inferior MI, the culprit vessel is the RCA and in the remaining 10% to 15%, the LCx coronary artery. Inferior MI can also occur when a long LAD that goes around the apex of the LV is occluded resulting in anterior MI that extends to the inferoapical wall (Fig. 23.19).

- **RCA and inferior MI:** The following ECG findings indicate that the RCA is the culprit vessel when inferior MI is present.

    - **Right ventricular MI (RVMI):** The presence of RVMI always indicates RCA involvement. RVMI is possible only when the proximal RCA is occluded. It is diagnosed by the presence of ST elevation ≥1 mm in any of the right sided precordial leads $V_{3R}$ to $V_{6R}$, with lead $V_{4R}$ the most sensitive (Fig. 23.35). If right-sided precordial leads were not recorded, $V_1$ should be examined for ST segment elevation. Occlusion of the LCx will not result in RVMI because the LCx circles the lateral AV groove and does not supply branches to the right ventricle (diagram in Fig. 23.20).

    - **ST elevation in lead III > II:** When the RCA is totally occluded, the highest ST elevation will be recorded in lead III (Fig. 23.36). This is based on the anatomical location of the RCA, which circles the right AV groove, and is closer to lead III than lead II in the frontal plane. This is in contrast to the LCx coronary artery, which is closer to lead II than lead III because it circles the left or lateral AV groove.

    - **Reciprocal ST depression in aVL > lead I:** Because lead III has the highest ST elevation when the RCA is occluded, the most pronounced ST depression will be recorded opposite lead III at −60°. Because aVL (at −30°) is adjacent to −60°, aVL will record the deepest reciprocal ST depression if the RCA is the culprit vessel.

- **LCx and inferior MI:** If a dominant LCx is the cause of the inferior MI, ST elevation in lead III is not taller than lead II and the ST segments are isoelectric (or may be elevated) in aVL and lead I as shown in Figure 23.27. ST elevation in leads II, III, and aVF with ST depression in $V_2$ and $V_3$ also favors a LCx lesion since the LCx supplies posterolateral branches to the LV, which is diametrically opposite $V_2$ and $V_3$. However, if the LCx is small and the RCA is the dominant artery, the RCA may continue beyond the crux to the left AV groove to supply posterolateral branches to the LV.

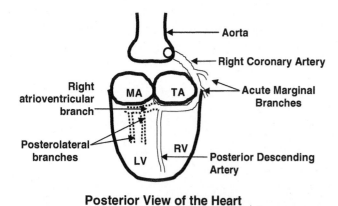

**Posterior View of the Heart**

**Figure 23.29: Diagrammatic Representation of a Dominant Right Coronary Artery (RCA).** The RCA continues posteriorly as the posterior descending artery and often goes beyond the crux to supply posterolateral branches to the left ventricle (*dotted lines*). LV, left ventricle; MA, mitral annulus; RV, right ventricle; TA, tricuspid annulus.

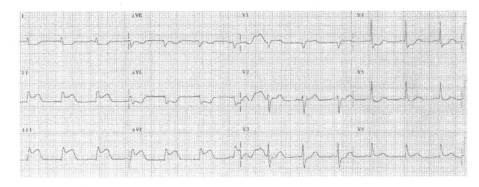

**Figure 23.30:    Acute Inferior Myocardial Infarction (MI).** ST segment elevation is present in II, III, and aVF with reciprocal ST depression in I and aVL consistent with acute inferior MI. This is due to occlusion of the right coronary artery.

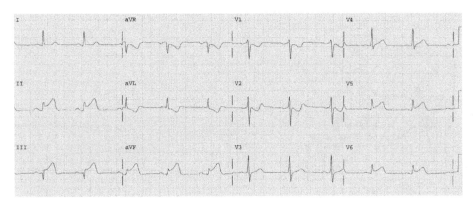

**Figure 23.31:    Acute Inferolateral Myocardial Infarction.** The ST segments are elevated in leads II, III, and aVF with reciprocal ST depression in aVL. ST segments are elevated in $V_5$ and $V_6$ with ST segment depression in $V_1$ and $V_2$. Coronary angiography showed complete occlusion of the proximal right coronary artery.

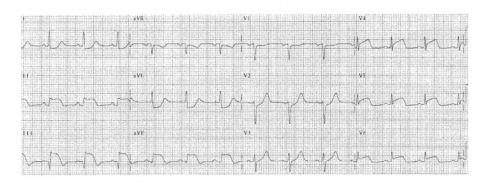

**Figure 23.32:    Acute Inferolateral Myocardial Infarction.** ST elevation is noted in II, III, aVF, and $V_4$ to $V_6$ with reciprocal ST depression in I and aVL. The findings are similar to those in Figure 23.31.

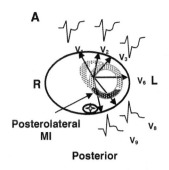

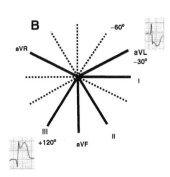

**Figure 23.33:    Posterolateral Myocardial Infarction (MI).** Posterolateral MI is a true ST segment elevation MI. This is suspected when there is ST segment depression in $V_{1-3}$ **(A)**. The ST depression in $V_{1-3}$ is a reciprocal pattern due to ST elevation in the posterolateral wall similar to the reciprocal pattern seen in aVL when there is ST elevation in lead III **(B)**. Posterolateral MI can be verified by recording special leads $V_{7-9}$, which will confirm the presence of ST elevation in this area.

**Figure 23.34: Acute Inferoposterior Myocardial Infarction (MI).** ST segments are elevated in II, III, and aVF with reciprocal ST depression in leads I and aVL consistent with an acute inferior MI. There is also ST depression in $V_1$ to $V_4$ and ST elevation in $V_6$ from posterolateral MI. The P waves (*arrows*) are completely dissociated from the QRS complexes because of AV block.

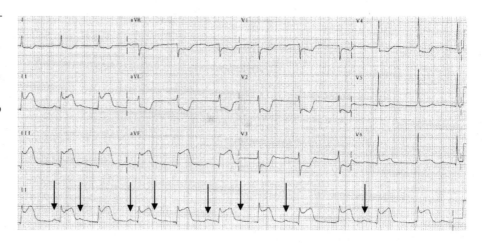

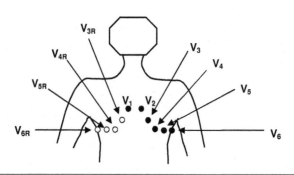

**Figure 23.35: Right-Sided Precordial Leads.** The right-sided precordial leads are labeled $V_{3R}$ to $V_{6R}$ (*open circles*). The leads are obtained by repositioning the standard precordial electrodes $V_{3-6}$ (*dark circles*) to the right side of the chest. Leads $V_1$ and $V_2$ remain in their original location.

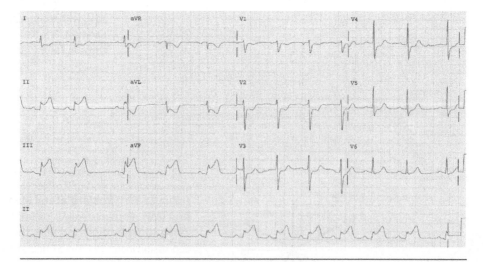

**Figure 23.36: Acute Inferior Myocardial Infarction (MI).** The 12-lead electrocardiogram shows ST segment elevation in II, III, and aVF with reciprocal ST depression in I and aVL from acute inferior MI. There is also reciprocal ST depression in $V_2$ and $V_3$ from involvement of the posterior wall of the left ventricle. Note that the ST elevation in lead III is higher than the ST elevation in lead II and ST depression in aVL is deeper than the ST depression in I, suggesting that the culprit vessel is the right coronary artery. The right-sided precordial leads are shown.

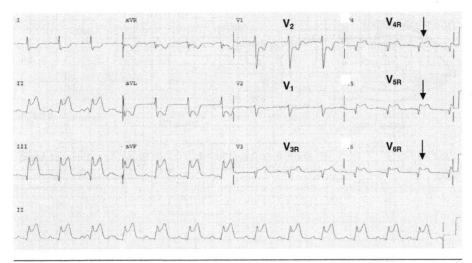

**Figure 23.37:   Acute Inferior MI with Right Ventricular Myocardial Infarction (RVMI).**  The diagnosis of RVMI is based on the presence of ≥1 mm ST elevation in any of the right sided precordial leads $V_{3R}$ to $V_{6R}$ (*arrows*). The electrocardiogram shows at least 1 mm of ST elevation in $V_{4R}$, $V_{5R}$, and $V_{6R}$ consistent with RVMI. It is not necessary to switch $V_1$ and $V_2$, as was done above when recording right-sided precordial leads. The presence of RVMI suggests that the culprit vessel is the proximal right coronary artery.

## Right Ventricular Myocardial Infarction

- **RVMI:** RVMI is a common complication of acute inferior MI. If the initial ECG confirms the diagnosis of acute inferior MI, right-sided precordial leads should be recorded immediately (Fig. 23.37). This is a Class I indication according to the 2004 ACC/AHA guidelines on ST elevation MI. If right-sided precordial leads are not immediately recorded, ST elevation in the right precordial leads may disappear within 10 hours after symptom onset in approximately half of patients with RVMI.

- Right sided precordial leads are recorded by repositioning the precordial leads $V_3$, $V_4$, $V_5$, and $V_6$ to the right side of the chest in the same standard location as that on the left (Fig. 23.35). Right-sided precordial leads are not routinely recorded if there is no evidence of acute inferior MI.

- Any ST elevation ≥1 mm in any of the right sided precordial leads $V_{3R}$ to $V_{6R}$ is consistent with RVMI. These leads, especially $V_{4R}$, are the most sensitive and most specific for the diagnosis of RVMI.

- RVMI is possible only when the proximal RCA is occluded. It does not occur when the distal RCA or LCx coronary artery is involved. This is important prognostically because occlusion of the proximal RCA usually implies the presence of a larger infarct and is associated with a high incidence of AV nodal block when compared to occlusion of a nondominant LCx or distal RCA.

- **RVMI:** Very often, right-sided precordial leads are not recorded at the time of entry. These leads are special leads and are not routine in a regular 12-lead ECG.

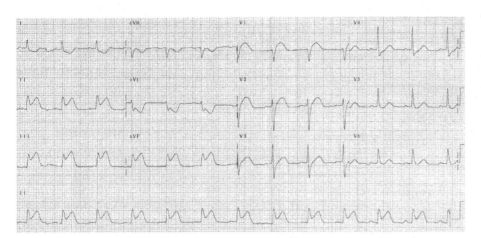

**Figure 23.38:   Right Ventricular Myocardial Infarction (RVMI).** The diagnosis of RVMI should always be suspected in the standard 12-lead electrocardiogram when acute inferior MI is present. ST elevation in lead III greater than lead II and presence of ST elevation in $V_1$ indicate RVMI as shown above. If the ST elevation in $V_1$ extends to $V_2$ or $V_3$, it may resemble acute anterior MI.

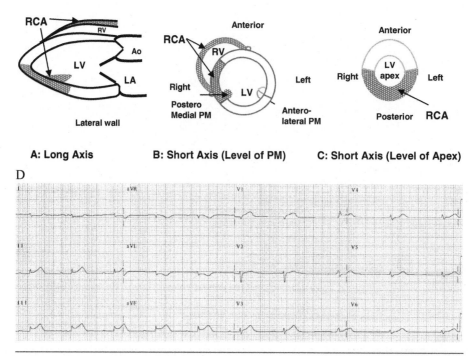

**Figure 23.39:** **(A) Myocardial Distribution of the Right Coronary Artery (RCA).** The red stippled areas represent myocardial distribution of the RCA. These include the right ventricular free wall, lower one-third of the posterolateral wall **(A, B)**, inferior half of the ventricular septum **(B)** and the posterior portion of the LV apex **(C)**. Note that the posteromedial PM **(B)** is supplied only by the RCA, whereas the anterolateral PM is supplied by two arteries, the LAD and LCx. Ao, aorta; LA, left atrium; LAD, left anterior descending; LCx, left circumflex; LV, left ventricle; PM, papillary muscle; RV, right ventricle. **(D) Electrocardiogram (ECG) of RCA Involvement.** Twelve-lead ECG showing a proximally occluded RCA. There is inferior myocardial infarction (MI) with ST elevation in lead III taller than lead II and ST depression in aVL more pronounced than lead I. Even when right sided precordial leads are not recorded, the presence of right ventricular MI can be diagnosed by the ST elevation in $V_1$.

Even if they were recorded, they may be recorded much later and not within the limited time window in which RVMI can be diagnosed. RVMI can be suspected if the initial standard 12-lead ECG will show the following changes:

- **ST elevation in lead III is greater than lead II:** This suggests that the RCA (and not the LCx), is the cause of the inferior MI (Figs. 23.30, 23.38, and 23.39B).

- **ST elevation is present in $V_1$** (Figs. 23.30 and 23.38): Although $V_1$ is not a very sensitive lead for the diagnosis of RVMI when compared with $V_{4R}$, $V_1$ is also a right-sided precordial lead. Thus, ST elevation in $V_1$ during acute inferior MI may be the only indication that an RVMI is present if right-sided precordial leads were not recorded in the ECG. The ST elevation may extend to $V_3$ resembling anterior MI (Fig. 23.38).

- Conversely, RVMI is not possible if the LCx coronary artery is the culprit vessel. If the LCx artery is the culprit vessel, ST elevation in III is not greater than lead II.

ST depression is not present in aVL and ST elevation may be present in lead I (Fig. 23.27).

- The myocardial distribution of the RCA is summarized in Figures 23.39A-C. The RCA is the dominant artery when it is the origin of the posterior descending coronary artery. This occurs in 85% to 90% of all patients. It supplies the whole inferior wall from base to apex and is the only artery that supplies the right ventricular free wall (Fig. 23.39A).

- Figures 23.39D shows the ECG of a patient with occluded proximal RCA. The presence of RVMI can be recognized even when the right-sided precordial leads are not recorded.

## Complications of Acute MI

- The ECG can provide very useful information not only in correctly identifying the culprit coronary artery but also in predicting possible complications based on the

| TABLE 23.1 | | | |
|---|---|---|---|
| **ST Elevation, MI Location, and Possible Complications** | | | |
| Leads with ST Elevation | Location of the MI | Infarct-Related Artery | Possible Complications |
| II, III, aVF | Inferior wall of the left ventricle | RCA in 85% to 90%<br><br><br><br><br>LCx in 10% to 15% | RCA = VT/VF, RVMI, bradyarrhythmias including sinus bradycardia, hypotension and AV block, LV dysfunction, postero-medial papillary muscle dysfunction, or rupture<br>Dominant LCx: VT/VF, LV dysfunction, AV block but no RVMI or papillary muscle dysfunction |
| I and aVL | High lateral | LCx or first diagonal branch of LAD | VT/VF, LV dysfunction |
| $V_1$–$V_4$ | Anteroseptal | LAD | VT-VF, extensive LV dysfunction, RBBB $\pm$ fascicular block, cardiogenic shock |
| $V_5$–$V_6$ + I, aVL | Lateral | LCx | VT/VF, LV dysfunction |
| ST depression in $V_1$–$V_3$ $\pm$ tall R waves | Posterior or straight posterior | LCx , RCA also possible | VT/VF, LV dysfunction |
| II, III, aVF + $V_{3R}$, $V_{4R}$, or $V_{5R}$ | RVMI | Proximal RCA | VT/VF, AV block, bradycardia, hypotension, atrial infarction |

AV, atrioventricular; LAD, left anterior descending; LCx, left circumflex; LV, left ventricular; PM, papillary muscle; RBBB, right bundle branch block; RCA, right coronary artery; RVMI, right ventricular MI; VT/VF, ventricular tachycardia/ventricular fibrillation.

geographic location of the acute MI. Table 23.1 identifies the location of the MI based on the leads with ST elevation, identifies the infarct related artery, and the possible complications associated with the MI.

■ **Ventricular tachycardia (VT) or ventricular fibrillation (VF):** Most deaths from acute MI occur suddenly usually during the first hour after onset of symptoms due to VF (Fig. 23.40). More than half of these deaths occur even before the patient is able to reach a medical facility.

■ **Sustained VT or VF within the first 48 hours:** In-hospital mortality is increased among patients with acute MI who develop VT/VF. Survivors of VT/VF occurring within 48 hours after onset of acute MI have the same long-term prognosis compared with a similar group of patients without VT/VF. In these patients, VT/VF is due to electrical instability associated with acute myocardial injury, which may resolve after the acute injury has subsided.

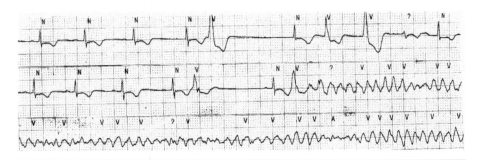

**Figure 23.40:    Ventricular Fibrillation.** This rhythm strip was obtained from a 54-year-old male with ST elevation myocardial infarction. His initial electrocardiogram is shown in Figure 23.18. He developed ventricular fibrillation while he was being monitored in the emergency department. His timely arrival to the hospital allowed him to be resuscitated successfully. The coronary angiogram showed total occlusion of the first diagonal branch of the left anterior descending artery, which was successfully stented. He left the hospital without neurologic sequelae and only minimal myocardial damage.

**Figure 23.41:    Accelerated Idioventricular Rhythm.** The 12-lead electrocardiogram (ECG) in **A** shows normal sinus rhythm and acute inferior MI. **(B)** The same patient a few minutes after ECG **A** was recorded, showing accelerated idioventricular rhythm.

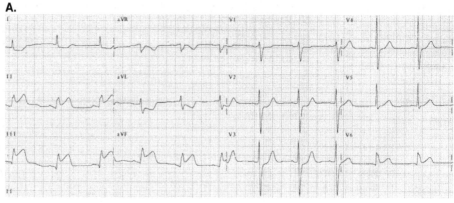

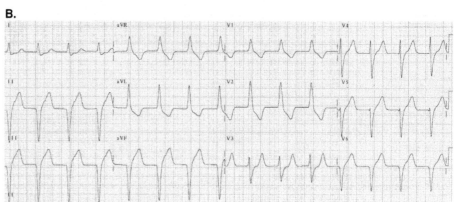

- **Sustained VT or VF after 48 hours:** Survivors of cardiac arrest due to VT/VF occurring after 48 hours of acute MI continue to be at risk for VT/VF. Unless the arrhythmia has been shown to be due to electrolyte abnormalities or due to recurrent acute ischemia, which are reversible, these patients are at high risk for developing recurrence of VT/VF and will benefit from implantation of an automatic defibrillator even without electrophysiologic testing.

- One of the most important factors that determine the prognosis of patients with acute MI is the extent of myocardial damage. The presence of severe myocardial damage and a low left ventricular ejection fraction predisposes to ventricular arrhythmias, which may cause sudden death.

- **Other ventricular arrhythmias:** Some arrhythmias may be related to reperfusion after successful thrombolysis and should be recognized. The most frequent ECG finding associated with successful reperfusion is accelerated idioventricular rhythm (AIVR).

- **AIVR:** AIVR is a ventricular rhythm with a rate of 60 to 110 beats per minute (bpm). AIVR commonly occurs as a reperfusion arrhythmia and is more commonly seen after thrombolysis rather than with primary PCI. It occurs with about equal frequency in patients with acute inferior (Fig. 23.41) and anterior MI (Fig. 23.42).

The arrhythmia is generally benign and does not require any therapy.

- AIVR may be difficult to recognize and may be mistaken for ventricular tachycardia or new onset bundle branch block (Fig. 23.42). In AIVR, the QRS complexes are not preceded by P waves or there is complete AV dissociation. This may result in decreased cardiac output because atrial contraction no longer contributes to left ventricular filling.

- **Acute inferior MI and AV block:** When acute inferior MI causes AV block, the AV block is at the level of the AV node (Figs. 23.43 and 23.44).

## Acute MI and Right Bundle Branch Block (RBBB)

- Among 26,003 patients with acute MI studied in GUSTO-1 (Global Utilization of Streptokinase and tPA for Occluded Coronary Arteries), 289 patients (1.1%) had RBBB. Most of these patients with RBBB had anterior MI. In 133 patients, only RBBB was present. In 145 patients, left anterior fascicular block was also present. Only 11 patients had RBBB with left posterior fascicular block.

A.

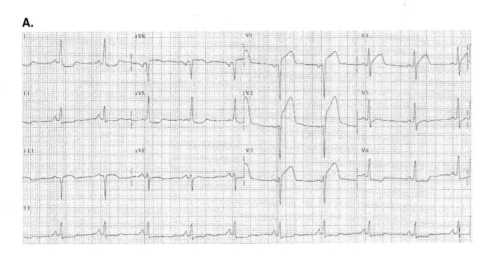

B.

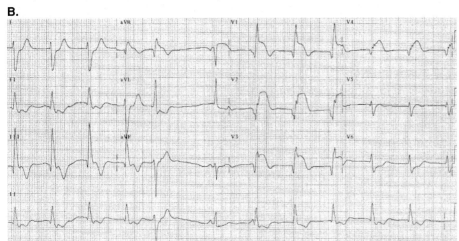

**Figure 23.42:    Accelerated Idioventricular Rhythm.** Electrocardiogram (ECG) **A** shows normal sinus rhythm with acute anteroseptal MI. ECG **B** shows a sudden change in the configuration of the QRS complexes with tall R waves in $V_1$ and a rightward shift in the axis of the QRS complex in the frontal plane due to accelerated idioventricular rhythm. This ECG can be mistaken for new-onset right bundle branch block with left posterior fascicular block.

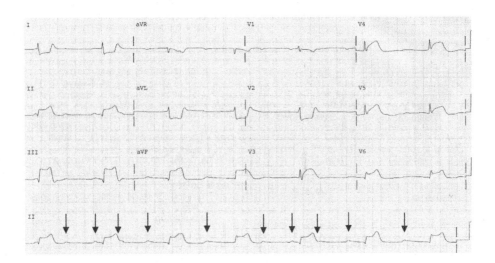

**Figure 23.43:    Acute Inferior Myocardial Infarction (MI) and Complete Atrioventricular (AV) Block.** The P waves (*arrows*) and QRS complexes are completely dissociated consistent with complete AV block. When complete AV block occurs in the setting of an acute inferior MI, the AV block is at the level of the AV node. The AV block is usually reversible and permanent pacing is usually not indicated.

**Figure 23.44:** **Acute Inferolateral Myocardial Infarction with 2:1 Atrioventricular (AV) Block.** The electrocardiogram shows 2:1 AV block. The arrows identify the second P wave that is not conducted.

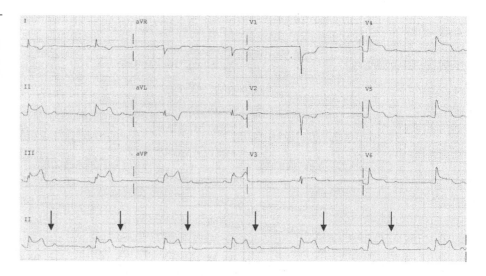

- **Changes in the ST segment and T wave when there is (RBBB):** The diagnosis of acute MI is not difficult when there is RBBB. Changes in the Q waves, ST segment, and T waves continue to be useful.

  - **RBBB without MI:** In RBBB without MI, the ST segments and T waves are normally **discordant** (opposite in direction) in relation to the terminal portion of the QRS complex. Thus, in $V_1$, the T waves are normally inverted and the ST segments are depressed because terminal R' waves are present when there is RBBB. In $V_6$, the T waves are upright and the ST segments are elevated since terminal S waves are present (Figs. 23.45A and 23.46).

  - **RBBB with acute MI:** When ST elevation MI is complicated by RBBB, the ST segments become **concordant** (same direction) in relation to the ter-

minal portion of the QRS complex. Thus, in anterior MI, the ST segments are elevated in $V_1$ and often in $V_2$ because terminal R' waves are normally present in these leads. Similar concordant changes may be noted in leads II, III, and aVF when there is inferior MI (Figs. 23.47 and 23.48B).

- Two examples of RBBB are shown in Figure 23.46, in which the RBBB is uncomplicated without evidence of MI. Note the presence of normally discordant ST segments and T waves. The second patient has inferior MI complicated by RBBB (Fig. 23.47). Note the presence of concordant ST elevation in leads III, aVF, and $V_1$, and concordant ST depression in leads I, aVL, and $V_2$.

- **Q wave changes:** RBBB does not interfere with the diagnosis of acute ST elevation MI. Changes in the

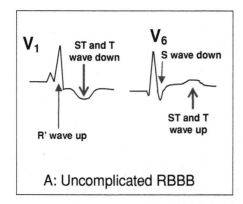

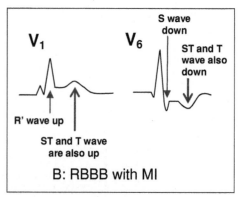

**Figure 23.45:** **ST-T Changes in Right Bundle Branch Block (RBBB).** **(A)** In uncomplicated RBBB, the ST segment and T wave are normally discordant (opposite in direction) to the terminal portion of the QRS complex. **(B)** When ST elevation myocardial infarction occurs, the ST segment (and T wave) becomes concordant (same direction) in relation to the terminal portion of the QRS complex.

A. RBBB without MI

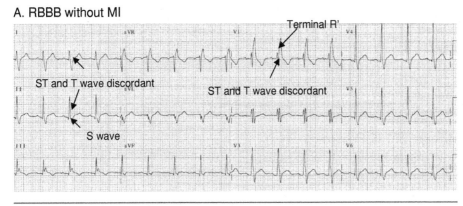

**Figure 23.46:** **Right Bundle Branch Block (RBBB) without Myocardial Infarction.** In uncomplicated RBBB without ST elevation MI, the ST segments and T waves are normally discordant. Thus, the ST segments and T waves are inverted in $V_1$ because the QRS complex ends with a terminal R' wave. In leads I and II, the ST segments are normally elevated and T waves are upright because the QRS complex ends with an S wave. These ST-T abnormalities are secondary to the presence of RBBB.

Q waves or QRS complexes remain useful and can be used for diagnosis. This is unlike LBBB, where the QRS complexes are significantly altered by the conduction abnormality making diagnosis of ST elevation MI by ECG extremely difficult.

## Anterior MI and AV Block

■ Acute anterior MI can result in varying degrees of AV block. The AV block is usually preceded by intraventricular conduction defect, more commonly RBBB with or without fascicular block. The AV block is usually infranodal, at the level of the bundle of His or at the level of the bundle branches or fascicles. These pa-

tients usually have extensive myocardial damage and significantly higher mortality than those without AV block. Implantation of permanent pacemakers in these patients may prevent bradycardia, but may not alter the overall prognosis since there is extensive myocardial damage, which can result in malignant ventricular arrhythmias (Figs. 23.49 and 23.50).

■ Figures 23.49A,B and 23.50A,B are from the same patient. There is acute anterior MI complicated by RBBB. The patient went on to develop complete AV dissociation (Fig. 23.50A) and subsequently sustained VT (Fig. 23.50B). Patients with acute anterior MI complicated by intraventricular conduction defect usually have extensive myocardial damage and are prone to develop VT/VF. The patient received a permanent pacemaker and an automatic defibrillator.

RBBB with Acute Inferior MI

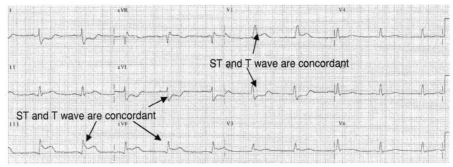

**Figure 23.47:** **Right Bundle Branch Block (RBBB) with ST Elevation Myocardial Infarction (MI).** When RBBB with ST elevation MI is present, the ST segments and T waves become concordant. Thus, the ST segments (and T waves) are elevated in leads III, aVF, and in $V_1$ because the QRS complex ends with an R wave and the ST segments are depressed in leads I, aVL, and $V_2$ because the QRS complex ends with an S wave.

**Figure 23.48:** **(A) Acute Anteroseptal Myocardial Infarction (MI).** ST elevation is present in $V_{1-5}$ consistent with occlusion of the left anterior descending artery proximal to the first septal perforator. The anterior MI was subsequently complicated by RBBB as shown by the electrocardiogram (ECG) in **B. (B) Acute MI with RBBB and Left Anterior Fascicular Block.** This ECG was obtained 14 hours later from the same patient in **(A)**. The QRS complexes are wider and a qR pattern has developed in $V_1$ to $V_4$. There is also left axis deviation. These changes are consistent with acute anterior MI, RBBB, and left anterior fascicular block. Note that the diagnosis of acute ST elevation MI is possible even in the presence of RBBB.

A
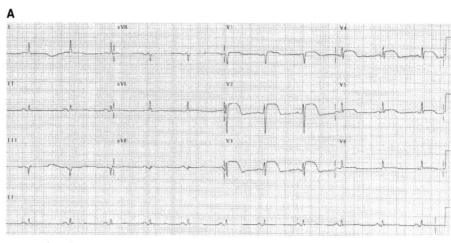

B
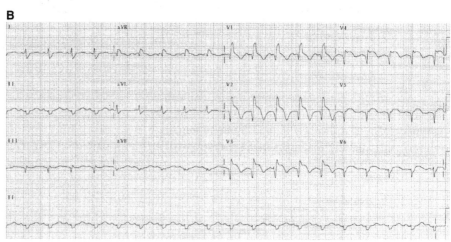

**Figure 23.49:** **Right Bundle Branch Block (RBBB) and Acute Myocardial Infarction (MI).** Electrocardiogram (ECG) **A** and **B** are from the same patient. **(A)** Baseline ECG showing left anterior fascicular block. **(B)** ECG taken a few weeks later showing acute anteroseptal MI complicated by RBBB. The diagnosis of acute MI is based on the presence of pathologic Q waves in $V_1$ to $V_5$ and concordant ST elevation in $V_1$ to $V_3$. There is also first-degree atrioventricular block and left anterior fascicular block, which in the presence of RBBB may suggest trifascicular block.

A: Baseline ECG Prior to MI
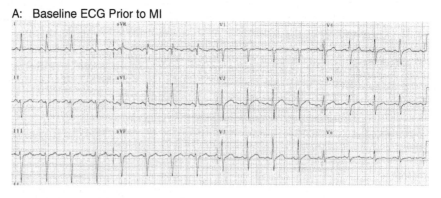

B: Acute MI + RBBB + LAFB + $1^0$ AV Block
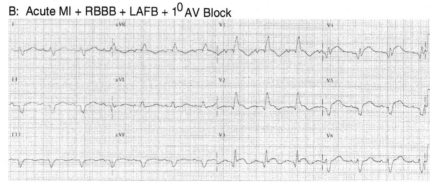

A: Complete AV Dissociation

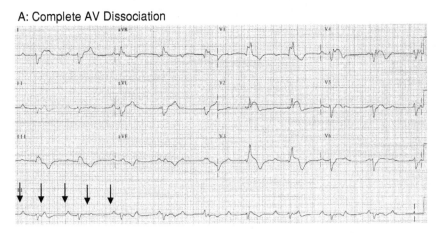

B. Ventricular Tachycardia

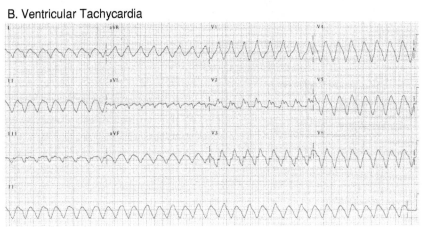

**Figure 23.50:   Acute Myocardial Infarction and Atrioventricular (AV) Block.** Electrocardiograms **A** and **B** are from the same patient as Figure 23.49. **(A)** Complete AV dissociation (the P waves are marked by the arrows). **(B)** Ventricular tachycardia occurring 5 days later. The patient was successfully resuscitated and was discharged with a permanent pacemaker and automatic implantable defibrillator.

## Acute MI and LBBB

- **LBBB:** When LBBB complicates acute MI, the ECG changes of ST elevation MI may not be recognized because it is concealed by the conduction abnormality. This makes diagnosis of acute MI extremely difficult using the ECG. Among 26,003 patients studied in GUSTO-1, 131 patients (0.5%) developed LBBB. Acute

MI in patients with LBBB can be recognized by the following ECG findings (Figs. 23.51–23.55):

- **Concordant ST segment:** In uncomplicated LBBB (LBBB without MI), the ST segments are normally discordant (Fig. 23.51A,B). Thus, the ST segments are depressed in leads with tall R waves and are elevated in leads with deep S waves. When LBBB is complicated by acute MI, the ST segments become concordant (same direction as the QRS complexes)

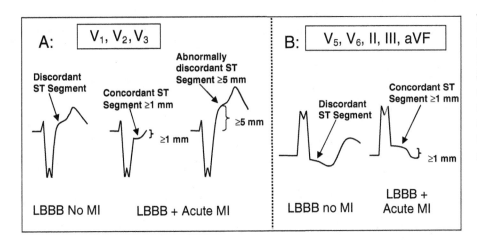

**Figure 23.51:   Acute Myocardial Infarction (MI) and Left Bundle Branch Block (LBBB).** When there is complete LBBB, the presence of concordant ST segment deviation ≥1 mm **(A, B)** and discordant ST elevation ≥5 mm **(A)** are consistent with acute MI when accompanied by symptoms of acute ischemia.

**Figure 23.52: Acute Anteroseptal Myocardial Infarction (MI).** The initial electrocardiogram (ECG) **(A)** shows acute anteroseptal MI. ECG **(B)** taken a few hours later show left bundle branch block with concordant ST elevation ≥1 mm in lead aVL (*arrow*).

A. Initial ECG:

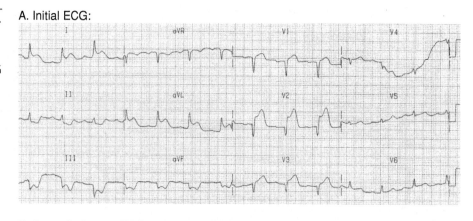

B. Same Patient as ECG A showing LBBB:

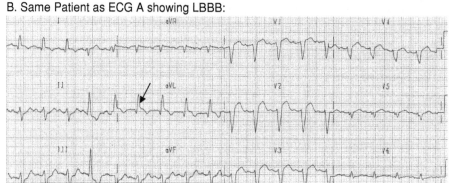

and measure ≥1 mm. Thus, ST segment depression ≥1 mm in leads with deep S waves ($V_1$, $V_2$, or $V_3$; Fig. 23.51A) or ST elevation ≥1 mm in leads with tall R waves ($V_5$, $V_6$, and often in II, III, and aVF; Fig. 23.51B) are consistent with acute ST elevation MI.

- **Discordant ST segment:** Acute MI can also be diagnosed if the ST segments are abnormally discordant (opposite direction to the QRS complexes) and measure ≥5 mm. Thus, ST elevation ≥5 mm in any lead with deep S waves such as $V_1$ to $V_3$ is consistent with acute MI when accompanied by symptoms of acute ischemia (Fig. 23.51A).

- The two ECGs (Figs. 23.54 and 23.55) show discordant ST segments. In Figure 23.54, discordant ST segment elevation of more than 5 mm is present in $V_2$ and $V_3$.

These ECG changes are associated with symptoms of acute ischemia. In Figure 23.55, there is concordant ST segment depression in $V_4$, which is accepted as a criterion for acute MI. In addition, there is also discordant ST segment depression of 5 mm in $V_5$. Presently, discordant ST depression ≥5 mm is not included in the literature as a criterion for acute MI in the presence of LBBB.

## Common Mistakes in ST Elevation MI

- **Other causes of ST elevation:** There are several other causes of ST elevation other than acute MI. These entities

**Figure 23.53: Acute Myocardial Infarction (MI) and Left Bundle Branch Block (LBBB).** LBBB is present with wide QRS complexes measuring >0.12 seconds. Concordant ST segment elevation >1 mm is present in leads with tall R waves including $V_5$, $V_6$, and leads II, III, and aVF (*arrows*) consistent with acute ST elevation MI.

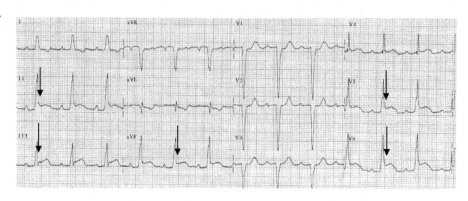

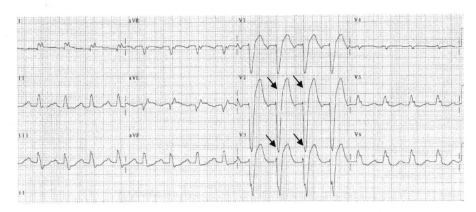

**Figure 23.54: Acute Myocardial Infarction (MI) and Left Bundle Branch Block (LBBB).** LBBB is present with discordant ST segment elevation >5 mm in $V_2$ and in $V_3$ (arrows), which in the presence of symptoms chest pain indicate acute MI.

should be recognized especially when thrombolytic agents are being considered as therapy for the acute MI.

- Normal elevation of the ST segment at the transition zone
- Early repolarization
- LBBB
- Left ventricular hypertrophy (LVH)
- Acute pericarditis
- Left ventricular aneurysm
- Electrolyte abnormalities: hyperkalemia and hypercalcemia
- Wolff-Parkinson-White (WPW) syndrome
- Osborn wave of hypothermia
- Brugada ECG
- Others: Pacemaker rhythm, ectopic ventricular complexes, Takotsubo cardiomyopathy, tumors or trauma involving the ventricles.

■ **ST elevation at the transition zone:** Elevation of the ST segment is common in normal individuals at the precordial transition zones $V_2$, $V_3$, or $V_4$. The transition zone is at the mid-precordial leads, where the R wave becomes equal to the S wave as the precordial electrodes move up from $V_1$ to $V_6$. The ST segments in these transition leads have upsloping configuration and are usually not isoelectric. The elevation of the ST segment is a normal and expected finding and should not be considered a variant of normal (Fig. 23.56).

■ **Early Repolarization:** J point elevation with ST elevation from early repolarization is common in normal individuals. The ST elevation is usually seen in the precordial leads and can be mistaken for transmural myocardial injury. The following are the characteristic features of early repolarization:

- ST elevation is commonly seen in leads $V_2$ to $V_6$ and also in leads II, III, and aVF. The ST elevation is concave upward (Fig. 23.57).
- Early repolarization is not accompanied by reciprocal depression of the ST segment.
- A prominent notch is usually inscribed at the terminal portion of the QRS complex in leads with ST elevation (Fig. 23.57).
- The ST elevation usually becomes isoelectric or less pronounced during tachycardia and becomes more accentuated during bradycardia (Figs. 23.58 and 23.59).
- The T waves in $V_6$ are usually tall when compared with the height of the ST segment. Thus, the ratio between the height of ST segment and that of the T wave is usually ≤25 % in $V_6$. This ratio is helpful when pericarditis is being considered. Elevation of the ST segments in pericarditis is usually prominent. Thus,

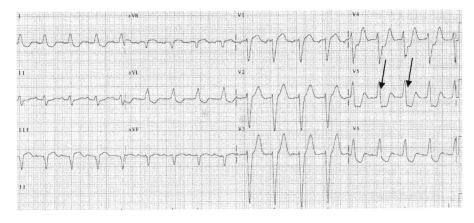

**Figure 23.55: Discordant Pattern.** This patient ruled in for acute myocardial infarction (MI) with markedly elevated troponins. The electrocardiogram shows left bundle branch block (LBBB) with concordant ST segment depression >1 mm in $V_4$. There is also discordant ST segment depression ≥5 mm in $V_5$ (arrows). Discordant ST depression is presently not included as a criterion for acute MI when there is LBBB.

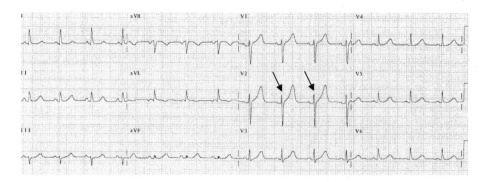

**Figure 23.56:   Normal ST Elevation at the Transition Zone.** Elevation of the ST segment is common in normal individuals at the transition zone which is usually in $V_2$, $V_3$, or $V_4$ (*arrows*). This is a normal finding often described as "high take-off" of the ST segment. Very often, the T waves are also peaked and taller than the R wave at the transition zone. This is also a normal finding.

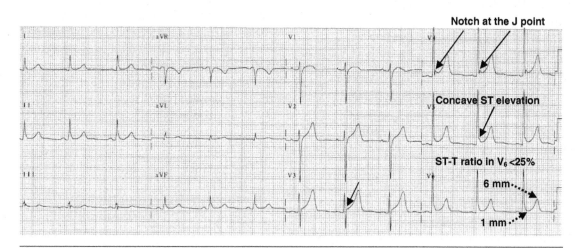

**Figure 23.57:   Early Repolarization.** ST segment elevation is noted in $V_3$ to $V_6$ (*arrows*), which can be mistaken for acute myocardial injury. There is no reciprocal ST depression in any lead and a prominent notch is present at the end of the R wave in $V_4$. Note that the height of the ST segment in $V_6$ measures 1.0 mm and the height of the T wave measures 6 mm (ST elevation/T wave ratio <25%). A ratio ≤25% suggests early repolarization. If pericarditis is being considered, the ratio is >25% because the height of the T waves is generally lower in pericarditis.

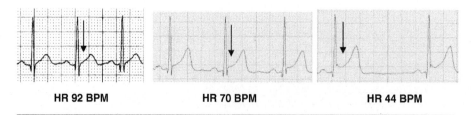

**HR 92 BPM**          **HR 70 BPM**          **HR 44 BPM**

**Figure 23.58:   Early Repolarization during Holter Monitoring.** Three rhythm strips with different heart rates are shown above in the same patient undergoing Holter monitoring. Note that there is more pronounced ST segment elevation because of early repolarization when the heart rate is slower than when the heart rate is faster. Arrows point to the ST segment elevation. HR, heart rate.

**A: Baseline ECG (HR 84 BPM)**    **B: Maximal Exercise (HR 146 BPM)**

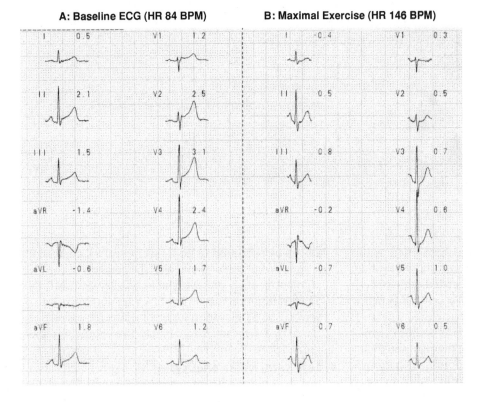

**Figure 23.59: Early Repolarization Before and During Maximal Exercise. (A)** A 12-lead baseline electrocardiogram from a 56-year-old male. The baseline heart rate was 84 beats per minute. ST segments were elevated in II, III, aVF, and $V_2$ to $V_6$. **(B)** The same patient during maximal exercise. Heart rate was 146 beats per minute. The ST segments have become isoelectric.

when the ratio between the height of the ST segment compared with that of the height of the T wave is >25% in $V_6$, pericarditis is the more likely diagnosis.

- In early repolarization, the ST segment elevation is more prominent when the heart rate is slower as shown in Figures 23.58 and 23.59.

- **Hyperkalemia:** Hyperkalemia can cause elevation of the ST segment in the ECG (see Chapter 25, Electrolyte Abnormalities). The ST segment elevation can be mistaken for acute ST elevation MI (Fig. 23.60). When ST segment elevation of this magnitude occur during hyperkalemia, the serum potassium level is usually >8 mEq/L.

- **LBBB:** In LBBB, the ST segments and T waves are normally discordant with the QRS complex. Thus, ST segment elevation and upright T waves are recorded in leads with deep S waves such as $V_1$ to $V_3$ and ST depression with inverted T waves recorded in leads with tall R waves such as $V_5$ or $V_6$ (Fig. 23.61).

- **LVH:** When LVH is present, the ST segment and T wave become discordant. ST depression and T wave inversion are recorded in leads with tall R waves; ST elevation and upright T waves are recorded in leads with deep S waves. Thus, ST elevation is usually present in $V_1$ to $V_3$ because deep S waves are normally expected in these leads when there is LVH (Fig. 23.62).

- **Brugada ECG:** The Brugada ECG is an electrocardiographic abnormality confined to leads $V_1$ and $V_3$. There is RBBB configuration with rSR′ pattern in $V_1$ or $V_2$. The J point and ST segment are elevated measuring ≥1 mm, with a coved or upward convexity terminating into an inverted T wave (Fig. 23.63).

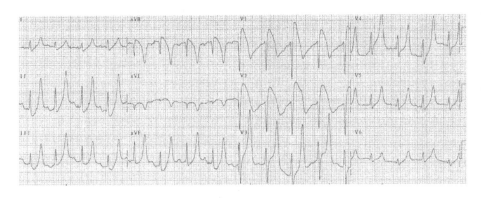

**Figure 23.60: ST Elevation from Hyperkalemia.** The electrocardiogram can be mistaken for acute myocardial infarction (MI) resulting from the marked ST-T changes resembling acute ST elevation MI. Note the presence of peaked T waves in virtually all leads.

**Figure 23.61: ST Elevation from Left Bundle Branch Block (LBBB).** In LBBB, ST elevation (*arrows*) is usually seen in leads with deep S waves such as V₁ to V₃.

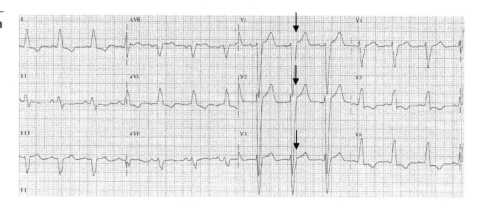

- **Brugada ECG:** The Brugada ECG associated with symptoms of VT/VF is called the Brugada syndrome. The Brugada syndrome is not associated with structural heart disease or prolonged QTc, but is a genetic disease that can cause sudden cardiac death. The abnormality is the result of a defect in the sodium channel of myocytes in the epicardium of the right ventricle and is inherited as an autosomal dominant pattern. The ST elevation in V₁ and in V₂ may be saddle shaped or triangular instead of coved in configuration and the ECG abnormality may wax and wane (Fig. 23.64A,B). The significance as well as prognosis of asymptomatic patients with the Brugada ECG is unknown since not all patients with the Brugada ECG will develop ventricular arrhythmias or syncope (see Chapter 21, Ventricular Arrhythmias).

- **Hypothermia:** Hypothermia is characterized by J point elevation. The J point marks the end of the QRS complex and beginning of the ST segment. A markedly elevated J point is also known as J wave or Osborn wave. The J wave is shaped like a letter "h." The magnitude of the J point elevation follows the severity of the hypothermia (Fig. 23.65A) and disappears when the temperature is restored to normal (Fig. 23.65B).

- **Acute pericarditis:** Acute pericarditis or inflammation of the pericardium is associated with diffuse ST segment elevation (Fig. 23.66A). The ST elevation usu-

ally involves almost all leads. Reciprocal ST depression is confined to leads V₁ and aVR. Depression of the P-R segment is often present. Unlike ST elevation MI, the ST elevation in acute pericarditis does not evolve into q waves. The ST elevation usually persists for a week followed by T wave inversion. It may take another week or more before the inverted T waves revert to normal.

- **Left ventricular aneurysm:** ST segment elevation that does not resolve after acute transmural MI usually suggests the presence of a left ventricular aneurysm. The ST segment elevation is present in leads with Q waves. The T waves are usually inverted. Almost all aneurysms are located at the anteroapical wall of the LV and, much less commonly, the base of the inferior wall. The elevation of the ST segment is usually permanent (Fig. 23.67). In this era of reperfusion therapy, the presence of a left ventricular aneurysm should be suspected in patients with ST elevation MI when pathologic Q waves occur and the ST elevation does not resolved within a few days.

- **Pacemaker-induced ventricular complexes:** ST elevation is also seen in pacemaker captured ventricular complexes (Fig. 23.68) and ectopic ventricular rhythms. The ST elevation is secondary to the abnormal activation of the ventricles.

- **Takotsubo cardiomyopathy:** Takotsubo cardiomyopathy (CMP), also called left ventricular apical

**Figure 23.62: ST Elevation from Left Ventricular Hypertrophy (LVH).** Elevation of the ST segment in LVH is frequently seen in V₂ and V₃, as shown by the arrows.

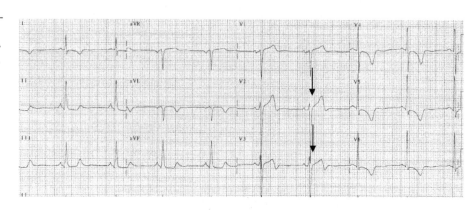

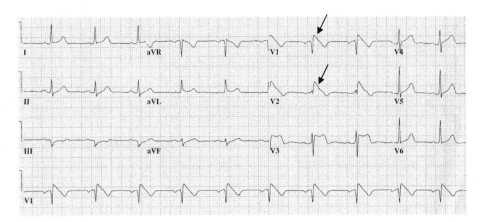

**Figure 23.63: Brugada Electrocardiogram (ECG) with Convex ST Segment.** The Brugada ECG has a right bundle branch block pattern in $V_1$ to $V_3$ with J point elevation, coved ST segment, and inverted T waves (*arrows*). Courtesy of Athol Morgan, MD.

ballooning syndrome, is increasingly becoming more recognized as a clinical entity characterized by substernal chest pain accompanied by ECG changes identical to the ECG of acute coronary syndrome. These includes ST elevation, ST depression, T wave inversion and development of pathologic Q waves. The most common presentation is ST elevation involving the anterior precordial leads. These ECG changes are accompanied by mild troponin elevation. Unlike acute coronary syndrome, which results from thrombotic occlusion of the coronary artery, Takotsubo CMP is associated with normal coronary arteries.

There is ballooning of the anteroapical left ventricular wall and compensatory hyperkinesis of the basal segments. This angiographic appearance resemble an octopus trap (takotsubo) and is usually reversible. Although originally described in Japan it is increasingly recognized in Europe and the United States, mostly in post-menopausal women who have experienced physical or emotional distress. The cause of the CMP is uncertain although it is probably related to excessive sympathetic stimulation, microcirculatory dysfunction, or myocardial stunning resulting from severe multivessel coronary spasm.

**A.**

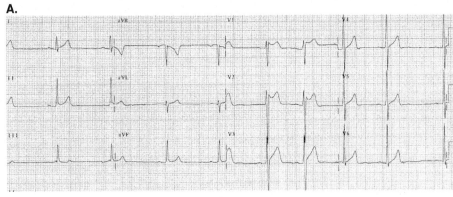

**B.**

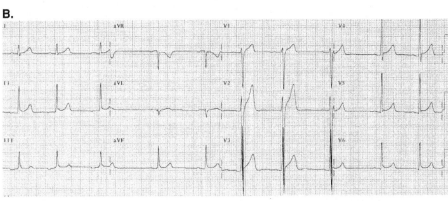

**Figure 23.64: Brugada Electrocardiogram (ECG) with Concave ST Segment.** The ST elevation in $V_1$ and $V_2$ **(A)** is concave (saddle back), which is another type of ST elevation in the Brugada ECG. **(B)** The saddle back pattern has disappeared.

**Figure 23.65: Hypothermia.**
The initial electrocardiogram (ECG) shows Osborn waves (*arrows*) representing elevation of the J point due to hypothermia. There is also sinus bradycardia with a rate of 50 beats per minute. ECG **B** was taken 4 hours after the initial ECG. The Osborn waves have disappeared.

A. a

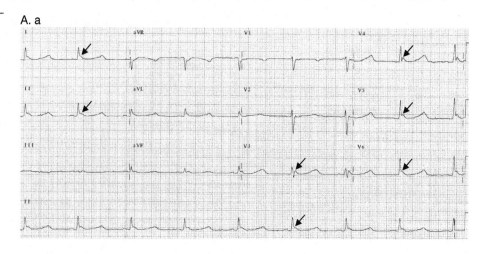

B. 4 hours later

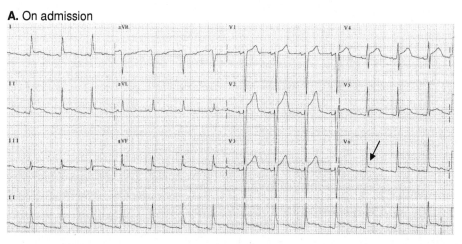

**Figure 23.66: Acute Pericarditis.**
The initial electrocardiogram (ECG) **(A)** on admission shows diffuse ST elevation in almost all leads consistent with acute pericarditis. The ST-T ratio in $V_6$ is >25% (*arrow*). ECG **(B)** was obtained 4 to 5 weeks later showing ST depression, T inversion but no pathologic Q waves.

**A.** On admission

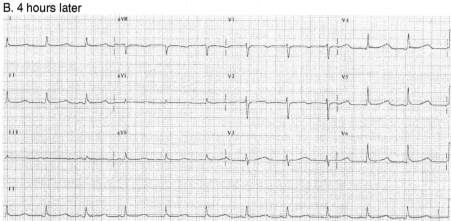

**B.** 5 weeks later

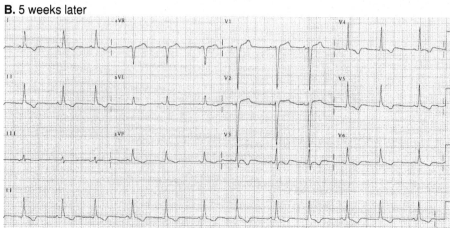

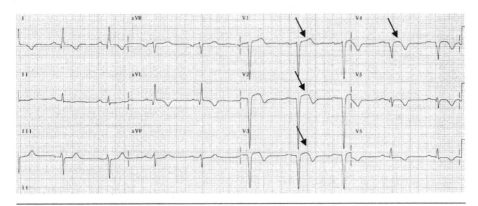

**Figure 23.67:    Left Ventricular Aneurysm.** ST segment elevation persists more than 5 years after acute ST elevation myocardial infarction from left ventricular aneurysm. Note that the ST segment elevation is confined to leads with pathologic Q waves V$_1$ to V$_4$ (*arrows*). The ST segments have an upward convexity and the T waves are inverted. Echocardiogram and nuclear perfusion scans confirmed the presence of an anteroapical left ventricular aneurysm.

## Q Waves

- **Q waves:** Q waves associated with acute ST elevation MI generally indicate transmural myocardial necrosis, which is a more advanced stage of myocardial involvement. Q waves, which mark the area of transmural necrosis, signify permanent myocardial damage. Although Q waves are the usual sequelae of ST elevation MI, not all patients with ST elevation MI will develop Q waves. Additionally, some patients with non-ST elevation MI may develop Q waves. Thus, ST elevation MI is a more concise terminology instead of Q-wave MI.

- The development of Q waves during ST elevation MI may take a few hours to several days, depending on collateral flow. When collaterals are absent or are inadequate, Q waves may develop very early, within a few hours after symptom onset and may be present when the initial ECG is recorded (Fig. 23.69). Similar to ST elevation, pathologic Q wave serves as a useful marker in identifying the infarct related coronary artery, even after the ST-T abnormalities have resolved. Pathologic Q waves may be recorded unexpectedly in a routine ECG and may be the only marker that a previous MI had occurred.

- The presence of Q waves during ST elevation MI is not a contraindication to thrombolytic therapy. Progression of ST elevation MI to a Q wave MI may be prevented if reperfusion is timely and successful.

- **Normal Q waves:** Q waves may be normal or abnormal. Normal Q waves represent activation of the ventricular septum in a left to right direction (see Chapter 6. Depolarization and Repolarization). These Q waves are often called septal Q waves. Septal Q waves are normally recorded in leads located at the left side of the ventricular septum including V$_5$, V$_6$, and leads I and aVL. The size of the normal Q wave is variable and depends on the thickness of the ventricular septum. In normal individuals, the Q waves are usually narrow measuring <0.03 seconds in duration and are <25% of the height of the R wave. Q waves in lead III do not represent septal Q waves. Thus, the Q waves in lead III may be wide and deep but are not necessarily pathologic even when it exceeds 0.03 seconds in duration.

- **Abnormal Q waves:** The differential diagnosis of abnormal Q waves is limited to a few conditions.

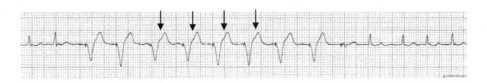

**Figure 23.68:    ST Elevation from Pacemaker-Induced Ventricular Rhythm.** Lead II rhythm strip showing ST elevation during pacemaker captured ventricular complexes (*arrows*) but not in normally conducted complexes. The ST segment elevation is secondary to abnormal activation of the ventricles.

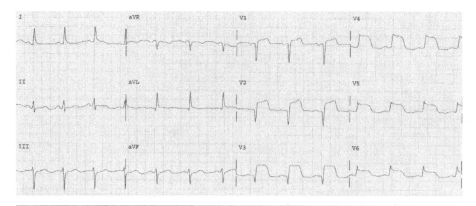

**Figure 23.69:** **Acute Anteroseptal Myocardial Infarction (MI).** Initial electrocardiogram of a patient with chest pain showing deep Q waves in $V_1$ to $V_3$ with marked ST elevation across the precordium consistent with acute extensive anterior MI. Note the early appearance of QS complexes in $V_1$ to $V_3$, suggesting the presence of transmural myocardial necrosis involving the anteroseptal wall. Coronary angiography showed complete occlusion of the left anterior descending coronary artery after the first diagonal branch.

These include transmural MI, idiopathic hypertrophic subaortic cardiomyopathy, LVH, abnormal activation of the ventricles from WPW syndrome, LBBB and fascicular blocks, myocardial scarring from cardiomyopathy, infiltrative disease involving the myocardium, or when the rhythm is ectopic or pacemaker induced.

## Pathologic Q Waves

- **Pathologic Q waves from transmural myocardial necrosis:** Pathologic Q waves from transmural necrosis are easy to identify during the acute episode when they are accompanied by ST elevation and T-wave abnormalities. However, when the MI is remote and the ST-T abnormalities have resolved, Q waves from transmural necrosis may be difficult to differentiate from normal septal Q waves. The following are the features of pathologic Q waves due to transmural myocardial necrosis or clinically established MI according to a joint European Society of Cardiology and American College of Cardiology committee proposal.
  - In leads I, II, aVL, aVF, $V_4$, $V_5$, or $V_6$: a pathologic Q wave should measure $\geq 0.03$ seconds in duration. The abnormal Q wave must be present in any two contiguous leads and should be $\geq 1$ mm deep.
  - In $V_1$, $V_2$, and $V_3$: any Q wave is pathologic regardless of size or duration.
  - QRS confounders such as LBBB, LVH, and WPW syndrome should not be present.

- Similar to ST segment elevation, pathologic Q waves are specific in localizing the area of the transmural MI. Some Q waves, however, are not permanent. Contraction of the scar tissue may occur during the healing process and may cause the Q waves to become narrower and may even disappear.
- **Inferior MI:** The diagnosis of inferior MI is based on the following:
  - Q in II and aVF are $\geq 0.03$ seconds in duration and are $\geq 1$ mm deep.
  - Q in Lead III $\geq 0.04$ seconds in duration or the Q waves have an amplitude of 5 mm or $\geq 25\%$ of the height of the R wave plus a Q wave in aVF that is $\geq 0.03$ seconds in duration and $\geq 1$ mm deep.
  - A QS complex in lead III alone, no matter how deep or wide, is not enough to make a diagnosis of inferior MI.
- **Anterior MI:** The diagnosis of anterior MI is based on the following:
  - **Q waves in $V_1$:** Although the 2000 European Society of Cardiology (ESC)/ACC proposal on the redefinition of MI mentions that any size Q wave is abnormal in $V_1$, $V_2$, or $V_3$, the more recent 2007 ESC/American College of Cardiology Foundation (ACCF)/AHA/World Health Federation (WHF) consensus document on the universal definition of MI considers a QS complex in $V_1$ as a normal finding. Q waves in $V_1$ and in $V_2$ have also been shown to be normal in some patients with chronic pulmonary disease because the diaphragm is displaced downward. It may also be a normal finding when the electrodes are inadvertently misplaced at a higher location at the second instead of the fourth intercostal space.

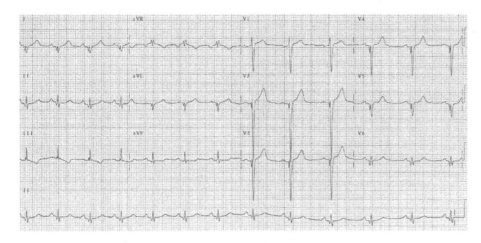

**Figure 23.70: Pathologic Q waves due to Idiopathic Hypertrophic Subaortic Stenosis (IHSS).** Pathologic Q waves are noted in $V_{2-6}$, as well as in leads I and aVL from idiopathic hypertrophic cardiomyopathy. The Q waves in IHSS represent normal activation of an unusually thick septum, which is often two to three times thicker than a normal septum. These Q waves can be mistaken for anterolateral myocardial infarction.

- **Q waves in $V_1$ To $V_3$:** When Q waves are present in $V_1$ to $V_3$, they are pathologic regardless of size or duration since normal septal q waves are not normally recorded in all three leads. Other causes of q waves such as LVH, fascicular block, LBBB, and WPW ECG should be absent.

- **Poor R wave progression:** The size of the R wave does not increase from $V_1$ to $V_4$. This may be due to anterior MI, although this finding is less specific for anterior MI because this may be caused by several other conditions that can cause clockwise rotation (see Chapter 4, The Electrical Axis and Cardiac Rotation).

- **Posterior or inferobasal MI:** Posterior MI will show tall R waves in $V_1$ or $V_2$. The tall R waves are reciprocal changes due to the presence of deep Q waves over the posterior wall. If special leads $V_7$ to $V_9$ are recorded, QS complexes will be present. Other causes of tall R waves in $V_1$ and $V_2$ are further discussed in Chapter 4, The Electrical Axis and Cardiac Rotation.

- **Lateral MI:** Q waves $\geq 0.03$ seconds in I and aVL or in $V_5$ and $V_6$ or in all four leads are pathologic and consistent with lateral MI.

## Other Causes of Pathologic Q Waves

- **Pathologic Q waves resulting from idiopathic hypertrophic subaortic stenosis (IHSS):** When there is excessive thickening of the ventricular septum such as IHSS, the septal Q waves become exaggerated and can be mistaken for Q waves of MI (Fig. 23.70).

- **Pathologic Q waves from preexcitation:** The presence of preexcitation (WPW ECG) can also cause abnormal Q waves that can be mistaken for MI (Fig. 23.71).

- **Pathologic Q waves from LBBB:** Activation of the LV is abnormal when there is LBBB. In LBBB, deep QS complexes in $V_{1,2,3}$ and often in leads II, III, and aVF are not necessarily pathologic (Fig. 23.72). However, any size Q wave in $V_5$ and $V_6$ is pathologic when there is LBBB because the ventricular septum is activated from right to left and Q waves should not be present in these leads. In LBBB, Q waves in $V_{5,6}$ indicate a septal infarct (Fig. 23.73).

- **Pathologic Q waves resulting from ectopic ventricular rhythms:** Accelerated idioventricular rhythm, ventricular tachycardia, or ventricular pacemaker rhythm may cause Q waves from abnormal activation of the ventricles.

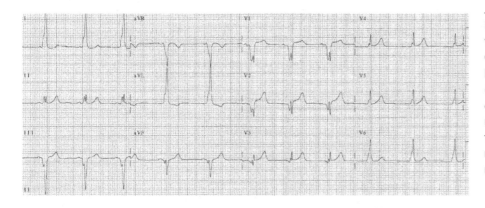

**Figure 23.71: Pathologic Q waves from Preexcitation.** Deep Q waves are seen in $V_1$, $V_2$, $V_3$, and leads III and aVF from preexcitation (Wolff-Parkinson-White electrocardiogram). These Q waves represent delta waves directed posteriorly and inferiorly can be mistaken for anteroseptal or inferior myocardial infarction.

**Figure 23.72: Q Waves in Left Bundle Branch Block (LBBB).** QS complexes are present in leads III, aVF, and V₁ to V₃ (*arrows*), which can be mistaken for myocardial infarction. These QS complexes are not pathologic and do not indicate a Q wave infarct when LBBB is present.

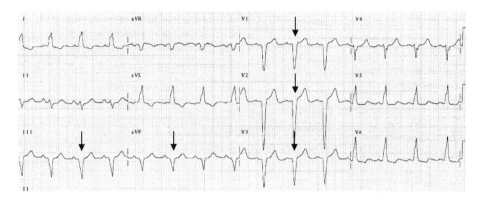

## Acute Coronary Syndrome

### ECG Findings ECG Findings of ST Elevation Myocardial Infarciton

- The ECG of acute coronary syndrome can be divided into two types:
  - ST segment elevation
  - Non-ST segment elevation
    - □ ST segment depression
    - □ T-wave inversion
    - □ Other less specific ST and T wave abnormalities
- ECG changes of ST elevation myocardial infarction:
  - ST segment elevation of ≥1 mm in two or more adjacent leads
  - New or presumed new-onset LBBB
  - Development of pathologic Q waves

### ST Elevation versus Non-ST Elevation

- Acute coronary syndrome is usually the result of rupture of an atherosclerotic plaque resulting in obstruction of the vessel lumen by a thrombus. Depending on the severity of coronary obstruction, thrombotic occlusion of the vessel lumen may cause varying degrees of myocardial ischemia, which can

be divided into those with and those without ST elevation. These two ECG abnormalities have distinctive pathologies and have different prognostic and therapeutic significance.

- **ST segment elevation:** Acute coronary syndrome with ST elevation in the ECG indicates that one of the three epicardial coronary arteries is totally occluded with TIMI 0 flow (Thrombolysis in Myocardial Infarction grade flow indicating no antegrade flow beyond the point of occlusion). Thrombotic occlusion of the vessel lumen with ST segment elevation almost always results in cellular necrosis with elevation of the cardiac troponins in the circulation. If myocardial perfusion is not restored in a timely manner, changes in the QRS complex with development of Q waves or decreased amplitude of the R waves will occur. Acute coronary syndrome from coronary vasospasm can also cause ST elevation although coronary vasospasm is usually transient and responds to coronary vasodilators such as nitroglycerin.

- **Non-ST segment elevation:** When the vessel lumen is partially occluded by a thrombus, myocardial ischemia may or may not occur depending on the severity of coronary artery obstruction, presence of collateral flow and myocardial demand for oxygen. Even if the vessel lumen is partially occluded if myocardial oxygen demand does not exceed its blood supply, myocardial ischemia may not develop. If myocardial ischemia occurs, it may or may not result in myocardial necrosis.

**Figure 23.73: Left Bundle Branch Block (LBBB) and Septal Q Waves.** When there is LBBB, septal Q waves should not be present in V₅ or V₆ or in leads I or aVL. When Q waves are present in these leads (*arrows*), no matter how small or microscopic, these Q waves are pathologic and indicate a septal myocardial infarction.

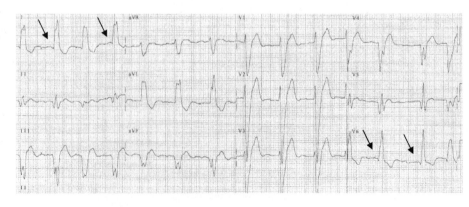

- ☐ **Non-ST elevation MI:** Partial occlusion of the vessel lumen accompanied by cellular necrosis indicates non-ST elevation MI. The most important marker of cellular necrosis is increased cardiac troponins in the circulation. The diagnosis of non-ST elevation MI is not established unless these cardiac markers are elevated. The ECG will show ST segment depression, T wave inversion, or less-specific ST and T wave abnormalities. Occasionally, the ECG may not show any significant abnormalities.

- ☐ **Unstable angina:** In unstable angina, the ECG changes are identical to that of non-ST elevation MI, although the cardiac troponins are not elevated in the circulation.

- ■ **Acute MI:** With the advent of troponins as a marker of myocardial necrosis, acute MI was redefined in 2000 by a consensus document of the ESC/ACC and again in 2007 by the ESC/ACCF/AHA/WHF, as *myocardial necrosis in a clinical setting consistent with myocardial ischemia.*

  - ■ **Myocardial necrosis:** Myocardial necrosis is based on the rise and/or fall of cardiac troponins.

  - ■ **Myocardial ischemia:** Evidence of myocardial ischemia is based on any of the following:
    - ☐ Clinical symptoms of ischemia
    - ☐ ECG changes indicative of new ischemia, which includes any of the following:
      - ☐ New ST-T changes
      - ☐ New LBBB
      - ☐ Development of pathologic Q waves
    - ☐ Imaging abnormalities
    - ☐ New loss of viable myocardium
    - ☐ New regional wall motion abnormality

- ■ Thus, increased in cardiac troponins in the circulation is the most important marker of myocardial necrosis. The diagnosis of acute MI is not possible unless the troponins are elevated. If sudden cardiac death occur before blood samples for troponins could be obtained or before troponins become elevated, acute MI is diagnosed by the associated symptoms and ECG changes of myocardial ischemia.

## Clinical Implications

- ■ ST segment elevation from acute coronary syndrome indicates complete obstruction of the vessel lumen. Therapy requires that coronary blood flow be restored immediately. T-wave inversion and ST segment depression indicate less severe form of myocardial ischemia from a combination of diminished coronary blood flow and increased myocardial oxygen demand. Immediate therapy for T-wave inversion and ST segment depression is directed toward stabilizing the thrombus and lowering myocardial demand for oxygen.

- ■ **ST segment elevation:** Thrombotic occlusion of the vessel lumen with persistent elevation of the ST segment is always associated with troponin elevation. Unless adequate collaterals are present or unless the occluded coronary artery is immediately reperfused, virtually all myocardial cells supplied by the totally occluded artery become irreversibly damaged within 6 hours after symptom onset. No significant pathologic abnormalities in the myocardium may be detected microscopically, if the patient dies suddenly within this period. The ECG, however, is very useful in identifying the presence of acute transmural ischemia and in timing the various stages of the infarct.

  - ■ **Hyperacute T waves:** Hyperacute T waves are usually the earliest ECG abnormality to occur in ST elevation MI. The presence of peaked and tall T waves overlying the area of ischemia often occur very early during the initial onset of symptoms and is often helpful in timing the onset of an acute ischemic process. The hyperacute T waves may be due to local hyperkalemia or presence of an electrical gradient between normal and injured myocardial cells during electrical systole.

  - ■ **ST Elevation:** When ST elevation is present, it is usually the most striking abnormality in the ECG during the acute phase of myocardial ischemia. The magnitude of ST elevation is measured at the J point. ST elevation is usually confined to leads geographically representing the territory supplied by the occluded artery. Thus, the presence of ST elevation is helpful in identifying the infarct related artery. The greater the number of leads with ST elevation and the more pronounced the ST elevation, the more severe the myocardial ischemia and the more extensive the myocardial damage. Myocardial ischemia, which is reversible, may be severe and relentless and transition to necrosis, which is irreversible, may be completed within 6 to 24 hours after onset of symptoms. This transition is highly variable and often unpredictable because of collateral flow and remodeling within the thrombus. For example, if the thrombus undergoes spontaneous lysis and rethrombosis, the symptoms and ECG findings may wax and wane and the above sequence of evolution may take several days or even weeks before the infarct is finally completed.

  - ■ **Q waves:** ST elevation MI generally results in the development of pathologic Q waves or diminution in the size of the R waves. Q waves are pathologic when they measure $\geq 0.03$ seconds in duration and are at least $\geq 1$ mm deep in leads I, II, AVF, aVL, and $V_4$ to $V_6$. Any size Q wave is pathologic when present in $V_2$ and also in $V_3$. The presence of pathologic q waves indicates transmural necrosis, which is usually permanent. Although ST elevation MI is synonymous with Q wave MI, Q waves may not always occur especially if the occluded coronary artery is revascularized in a timely fashion. Additionally, approximately 25% of patients with non-ST elevation MI may develop Q waves; thus, non-ST elevation MI rather than Q wave MI is the preferred terminology.

## Identifying the Infarct-Related Artery

- ■ ST segment elevation or pathologic Q waves in the ECG is useful in identifying the location of the infarct-related artery.

- When ST elevation or Q waves are localized in the anterior precordial leads $V_1$ to $V_4$ (or to $V_6$), acute anterior MI is present. This identifies the LAD artery as the culprit vessel. The ESC/ACC task force on the redefinition of acute MI requires that ST elevation in $V_1$ to $V_3$ should be present in at least two leads and should measure $\geq 2$ mm in contrast to other leads which requires only 1 mm of ST elevation.

- When ST elevation or pathologic Q waves occur in leads II, III, and aVF, acute inferior MI from occlusion of the posterior descending coronary artery is present. The RCA is the culprit vessel in 85% to 90% of patients with acute inferior MI and the LCx coronary artery in the remaining 10% to 15%. Inferior MI may also occur when there is anterior MI because the LAD may circle the apex of the LV and extend inferoapically. This is not a true inferior MI because the posterior descending coronary artery is not involved. This is merely an extension of the anterior MI.

- When ST elevation or pathologic Q waves are confined to leads I and aVL or leads $V_5$ and $V_6$, acute lateral MI is present and identifies the LCx coronary artery as the culprit vessel. This is often associated with ST depression in $V_2$ and in $V_3$.

- The posterolateral wall of the LV is not represented in the standard 12-lead ECG. Acute posterolateral MI with ST segment elevation in $V_7$, $V_8$, and $V_9$ may not be recognized because these leads are not routinely recorded. It is usually suspected when there is ST elevation in $V_6$ and ST depression in $V_2$ and $V_3$. Tall R waves may also be present in $V_1$ and $V_2$, which are reciprocal changes due to the presence of deep Q waves posterolaterally. This usually identifies the LCx as the culprit lesion, although, occasionally, it may be due to a dominant RCA.

## LAD Coronary Artery

- **Area supplied:** The LAD is a large artery that supplies the whole anterior wall of the LV. It is the main blood supply to the intraventricular conduction system including the bundle of His, bundle branches, and distal fascicular system.

- **Anatomy:** The LAD courses through the anterior interventricular groove and supplies the ventricular septum and anterior wall of the LV.

  - The length of the LAD can be short (terminates before the apex), medium (terminates at the apex), or large (wraps around the apex and continues to the inferior wall of the LV).

  - The first branch of the LAD is the first diagonal ($D_1$), which courses laterally between the LAD and left circumflex coronary artery. Usually one to three diagonal branches are given off by the LAD. $D_1$ is often the largest diagonal branch and supplies the base of the anterolateral wall of the LV.

  - The second branch is the first septal branch ($S_1$). $S_1$ may be the first instead of the second branch. About three to five septal branches arise at right angles from the LAD

and directly insert perpendicularly into the myocardium and supply the anterior two thirds of the ventricular septum. $S_1$ supplies the basal anteroseptal region of the LV and is the main blood supply of the distal His bundle and proximal left and right bundle branches.

- **Occlusion of the proximal LAD:** The following is a summary of the ECG findings when complete occlusion involves the proximal LAD:

  - **Occlusion of the LAD before the first branch ($D_1$ or $S_1$):**

    □ ST elevation in $V_1$ to $V_4$ (anteroseptal) and leads I and aVL (basal lateral or high lateral wall). Because the first septal branch or $S_1$ supplies the base of the ventricular septum, ST elevation will occur in $V_1$.

    □ ST elevation in aVL. Because the first diagonal branch or $D_1$ supplies the base of the lateral wall, ST elevation will occur in aVL.

    □ Reciprocal ST depression is present in III and aVF (from ST elevation in aVL, which is diametrically opposite lead III)

    □ If ST elevation is confined to $V_1$ to $V_3$, reciprocal ST depression may be present in $V_5$ or $V_6$.

    □ Complete RBBB may occur.

    □ If the LAD is large and extends to the left ventricular apex and contiguous inferior wall, ST elevation may occur in leads II, III, and aVF (acute inferior MI), in addition to the ST elevation in the precordial leads.

    □ ST elevation may be present in aVR.

  - **Occlusion of the LAD distal to the first diagonal and first septal branches:**

    □ Occlusion of the LAD distal to $D_1$ and $S_1$ results in a less extensive infarct compared with a more proximal lesion and will cause ST elevation only in $V_2$ to $V_4$.

    □ ST elevation will not occur in $V_1$ nor lead aVL or lead I because the first septal and first diagonal branches are spared. Because ST elevation is not present in lead aVL, reciprocal ST depression will not occur in lead III.

- **Common Complications Associated with Acute Anterior MI:**

  - **Tachyarrhythmias:** Ventricular fibrillation is the most common cause of death usually within the first few hours after symptom onset. Although ventricular tachycardia and fibrillation can occur in any patient with acute MI, acute anterior myocardial infarction is more commonly associated with tachyarrhythmias including sinus tachycardia, ventricular tachycardia, and ventricular fibrillation in contrast to inferior MI, which is usually associated with bradyarrhythmias such as sinus bradycardia and varying degrees of AV block.

  - **Intraventricular conduction defects:** Occlusion of the LAD proximal to the first septal branch can jeopardize the conduction system and can cause transient or permanent conduction abnormalities.

☐ **RBBB with or without fascicular block:** This is usually from the involvement of the first septal branch of the LAD. Diagnosis of acute MI in the presence or RBBB is not difficult because activation of the LV is not altered.

☐ **LBBB:** LBBB is less frequently seen as a complication of MI compared with RBBB. Although LAD disease is commonly expected to cause LBBB, LBBB complicating acute MI are usually non-anterior in location with the lesion more commonly associated with the right rather than left coronary artery as shown in the subset analysis of patients with acute MI in the GUSTO-1 databases. The diagnosis of acute MI in the presence of LBBB is difficult because the LV is activated abnormally from the right bundle branch. This was previously discussed in Chapter 10, Intraventricular Conduction Defect: Bundle Branch Block.

■ **Complete AV block:** When complete AV block occurs in the setting of acute anterior MI, the AV block is infranodal because the LAD supplies most of the distal intraventricular conduction system. The AV block is often preceded by RBBB with or without fascicular block. Prognosis remains poor even with temporary or permanent pacing because occlusion of the LAD complicated by RBBB is usually an extensive MI. Atropine does not reverse the AV block because the conduction abnormality is infranodal, at the His-Purkinje level. The indication for the implantation of permanent pacemakers in patients with intraventricular conduction defect and AV block associated with acute MI is discussed under treatment.

■ **LV dysfunction and pump failure:** Acute anterior MI is associated with a higher incidence of heart failure and cardiogenic shock. Cardiogenic shock usually occurs when at least 40% of the left ventricular myocardium is involved. Heart failure and cardiogenic shock are more common with acute anterior MI because acute anterior MI is generally a large infarct.

■ **Late ventricular arrhythmias and sudden death:** Patients with extensive myocardial damage and severe left ventricular dysfunction who survive their MI are at high risk for ventricular arrhythmias and sudden death. These complications are more frequently seen in patients with anterior MI.

## LCx Artery

■ **Anatomy and area supplied:** The LCx coronary artery circles around the left or lateral AV groove and sends three or more obtuse marginal branches to the lateral wall of the LV. It continues posteriorly as the posterior AV artery sending three or more posterolateral branches to the LV. In 10% to 15% of patients, the LCx artery continues as the posterior descending coronary artery, which supplies the inferior wall of the LV. When this occurs, the pattern of coronary distribution is described as left dominant.

■ **Occlusion of the LCx:** The following is a summary of the ECG changes when the LCx coronary artery is occluded:

■ Acute lateral MI with ST elevation (or pathologic Q waves) in I and aVL or $V_5$ and $V_6$ with or without ST depression in $V_1$ to $V_3$.

■ Acute inferior MI with ST elevation or pathologic Q waves in II, III, and aVF if the LCx artery is the dominant artery.

■ No significant ECG changes. When acute MI is diagnosed clinically without significant ECG changes, the culprit vessel is usually the LCx coronary artery.

■ Unless there is unusual variation in coronary anatomy, occlusion of the LCx coronary artery does not result in right ventricular infarction.

■ Straight posterior MI or acute posterolateral MI with prominent q waves and ST elevation in special leads $V_7$, $V_8$, and $V_9$. Tall R waves may be present in $V_1$ and $V_2$ with reciprocal ST depression from $V_1$ to $V_3$.

☐ If the MI involves the basal posterior wall of the LV or is directly posterior or posterolateral, the ECG will show reciprocal ST depression in $V_1$ to $V_3$ because these leads are diametrically opposite the posterior or posterolateral wall. Unfortunately, ST depression in $V_1$ to $V_3$ can be mistaken for ischemia involving the anterior wall of the LV rather than a transmural posterior MI. This dilemma can be resolved by recording extra leads $V_7$, $V_8$, and $V_9$, which overlie the posterolateral wall of the LV. Leads $V_7$ to $V_9$ will show ST elevation if an acute transmural posterolateral MI is present but not when there is anterior wall ischemia and injury. ST elevation of 0.5 mm is significant because of the wider distance between these leads in relation to the heart. ST elevation in $V_7$ to $V_9$ makes the patient a candidate for thrombolytic therapy.

☐ Tall R waves in $V_1$ to $V_2$ may also occur although these changes usually develop several hours later.

■ **Common Complications Associated with Acute Lateral or Posterolateral MI:**

■ **Tachyarrhythmias:** Ventricular tachycardia and ventricular fibrillation can occur similar to any acute MI during the first few hours after onset of symptoms.

■ **Left ventricular dysfunction:** This can occur as a complication if the artery is large and supplies a significant portion of the myocardium.

■ **AV block:** AV can occur at the level of the AV node only if the LCx coronary artery is dominant and there is associated inferior MI.

## Right Coronary Artery

■ **Anatomy and area supplied:** The right coronary artery (RCA) courses around the right or medial AV groove and gives acute marginal branches to the right ventricle. The RCA is the dominant artery in 85% to 90% of cases by continuing posteriorly to the crux of the heart and giving rise to a branch that supplies the AV node and the posterior descending artery, which supplies the inferior wall of the LV. The

RCA often continues beyond the crux toward the left AV groove as the right posterior AV artery, which gives posterolateral branches to the LV.

- **Occlusion of the RCA:**
  - Occlusion of the RCA will cause acute inferior MI with ST elevation in II, III, and aVF.
  - ST elevation in $V_5$ and $V_6$ may occur because of posterolateral involvement of the LV.
  - Reciprocal ST depression in $V_1$ to $V_3$ with inferior MI suggests the presence of a posterolateral MI. This can be verified by recording extra precordial leads $V_7$, $V_8$, and $V_9$ which will show ST elevation consistent with a transmural posterolateral MI (see LCx Coronary Artery Occlusion).
- Acute inferior MI is usually due to occlusion of the RCA, except in some patients where the LCx is the dominant artery. Occlusion of the proximal RCA can cause right ventricular infarction, which does not occur if the LCx coronary artery is the culprit vessel. Inferior MI complicated by right ventricular infarction is a large infarct with a high mortality of 25% to 30% compared with inferior MI without RV infarction, which has a mortality of approximately 6%.
- Acute inferior MI from occlusion of the RCA can be differentiated from acute inferior MI due to occlusion of the LCx coronary artery by the following ECG findings:
  - If ST elevation in lead III > lead II, the RCA is the culprit vessel. This is based on the anatomical location of the RCA, which circles the right AV groove and is closer to lead III than lead II whereas the LCx circles the left AV groove and is closer to lead II than lead III. Thus, if ST elevation in lead III > lead II, the proximal or mid RCA is the culprit vessel, whereas if ST elevation in lead II > lead III or ST elevation in III is not greater than II, the LCx artery is the culprit vessel.
  - ST depression in lead aVL > lead I, RCA is the culprit lesion. This is corollary to the observation mentioned previously, that lead III has a higher ST elevation when the RCA is the culprit vessel. Because lead III is diametrically opposite aVL, reciprocal ST depression will be more pronounced in aVL than in lead I.
  - RV infarction can occur only if the proximal or mid RCA is occluded (but not the LCx or distal RCA). The presence of RV infarct is best diagnosed by recording right sided precordial leads.
- **Complications of Acute Inferior MI:**
  - **VT and VF:** This is similar to the complications of any acute MI.
  - **Bradyarrhythmias and AV block:** Sinus bradycardia and other sinus disturbances are very common findings in acute inferior MI and are more common when the RCA is involved. The RCA carries vagal afferent fibers, which can cause sinus bradycardia due to reflex stimulation rather than due to direct suppression of sinus node function. Varying degrees of AV block (first, second, and third degree) can occur with acute inferior MI. The AV

block is at the level of the AV node because the RCA supplies the AV node in 85% to 90% of patients and by the LCx in the remaining 10% to 15%. AV block at the level of the AV node has a better prognosis than AV block occurring in the distal conduction system. AV block occurring during the first few hours of a myocardial infarct is usually due to a vagal mechanism and has a better prognosis compared to AV block occurring late post-MI.

- **Intraventricular conduction defect:** Intraventricular conduction defect (IVCD), either RBBB or LBBB, may occur as a complication of acute MI. IVCD complicating acute MI is usually associated with an extensive MI and mortality is much higher when compared with patients who do not develop IVCD. These patients have higher incidence of asystole, AV block, VF, both primary and late, as well as cardiogenic shock. The IVCD may be transient or persistent. When the IVCD is transient, the prognosis seems to be similar to patients who never developed the conduction abnormality. Acute (new-onset) LBBB or a previously existent (old) LBBB may conceal the ECG changes of acute MI, whereas the ECG diagnosis of acute MI can be recognized even when RBBB is present.
- **Atrial ischemia or infarction:** Atrial branches to the right atrium are usually supplied by the RCA which can result in atrial ischemia or infarction when there is occlusion of the proximal RCA. The acute onset of atrial fibrillation may be the only clue that atrial infarction had occurred. Atrial infarction can also be diagnosed when depression of the P-Q segment is present in the setting of acute inferior MI.
- **Papillary muscle rupture:** Most papillary muscle rupture involves the posteromedial papillary muscle because it has a single blood supply originating from the RCA. The anterolateral papillary muscle is less prone to rupture because it has dual blood supply from the LAD and LCx coronary arteries. Papillary muscle rupture is rare but is incompatible with life because of acute severe mitral regurgitation.
- **RVMI:** RVMI can occur only with acute inferior infarction due to occlusion of the proximal or probably mid-RCA. It does not occur when the lesion involves the distal RCA or LCx coronary artery.
  - ☐ When acute inferior MI is diagnosed, RVMI should always be routinely excluded by recording right-sided precordial leads. The right-sided precordial leads should be recorded immediately, because the ECG changes in half of patients with RVMI may resolve within 10 hours after the onset of symptoms. Right-sided precordial leads are the most sensitive, most specific, and the least expensive procedure in the diagnosis of RVMI. ST elevation of $\geq 1$ mm in any of the right-sided precordial leads is diagnostic of RVMI with lead $V_{4R}$ the most sensitive. Changes in the QRS complex is not a criteria for the diagnosis of RVMI because the right ventricle does not contribute significantly in the generation of the QRS complex.

☐ If right-sided precordial leads were not recorded or were recorded late during the course of the MI, the diagnosis of RVMI may be missed. Using the standard 12-lead ECG, RVMI is suspected when ST elevation in lead III is greater than lead II (suggesting proximal RCA occlusion) and ST elevation is present in $V_1$.

☐ RVMI often presents with a special hemodynamic subset of patients with acute MI who can develop the clinical triad of hypotension, jugular neck vein distension, and clear lungs. This subset of patients can be mistaken for cardiogenic shock. The presence of Kussmaul sign characterized by distension of the neck veins during inspiration is diagnostic of RVMI when acute inferior MI is present. Approximately one third to one half of patients with acute inferior MI have RVMI but only 10% to 15% of patients with RVMI will manifest the hemodynamic abnormality. The hemodynamic picture of RVMI usually disappears after a few weeks, suggesting that the RVMI is due to myocardial stunning rather than necrosis. The thin-walled right ventricle has a lower oxygen demand and may partially receive its blood supply from the blood within the right ventricular cavity, thus limiting the extent of myocardial necrosis.

## Treatment

■ The ECG remains the most useful test in planning the initial strategies in the therapy of a patient with acute coronary syndrome. If a patient presents to a medical facility with symptoms of acute ischemia, the ACC/AHA guidelines recommend that the ECG should be obtained and interpreted within 10 minutes after patient entry. If ST elevation is present in the initial ECG and patient is having symptoms due to myocardial ischemia, 0.4 mg of sublingual nitroglycerin should be given immediately, if not previously given, and repeated every 5 minutes for three doses. This is a Class I indication according to the ACC/AHA guidelines on ST elevation MI. Nitroglycerin is helpful in excluding vasospasm as the cause of the ST segment elevation. If the ST elevation persists after three successive doses, immediate reperfusion of the occluded artery with a thrombolytic agent or with primary PCI should be considered without waiting for the results of cardiac troponins. Although acute coronary syndrome with ST segment elevation is almost always associated with increased troponins in the circulation, the troponins may not be elevated in some patients presenting to the hospital within 6 hours after symptom onset.

■ **Thrombolytic therapy:** Thrombolytic therapy or primary PCI should be considered if the chest pain is at least 20 minutes in duration.

  ■ The following are the ECG criteria for immediate thrombolytic therapy or PCI:

    ☐ ST elevation >1 mm is present in any two adjacent leads.

    ☐ New or presumably new-onset LBBB associated with symptoms of ischemia.

    ☐ ST segment depression even in the presence of cellular necrosis (elevated cardiac troponins) is not an indication for thrombolytic therapy. The only exception is ST segment depression in $V_1$ to $V_3$, which may represent a straight posterior or posterolateral infarct. A posterior infarct is a transmural infarct and can be verified by the presence of ST elevation in leads $V_7$ to $V_9$.

■ Virtually all myocardial cells supplied by the infarct related artery become necrotic within 6 hours after symptom onset, unless collateral flow is adequate. Thus, if thrombolytic therapy is elected, it should be given within 30 minutes after patient entry to the emergency department (door to needle time) or first contact with emergency personnel (medical contact to needle time). Thrombolytic therapy is most effective when given within 2 hours after symptom onset. With further delay, the benefits of any type of reperfusion therapy decline.

■ The therapeutic window for thrombolytic therapy is up to 12 hours after symptom onset. This may be extended to 24 hours for some patients who continue to have stuttering symptoms of chest pain with persistent ST elevation.

■ Absolute contraindications to thrombolytic therapy according to the 2004 ACC/AHA guidelines include: any prior intracranial hemorrhage, known structural cerebrovascular lesion such as arteriovenous malformation, known malignant intracranial neoplasm either primary or metastatic, ischemic stroke within 3 months, suspected aortic dissection, active bleeding or bleeding diathesis other than menses, and significant closed head or facial trauma within 3 months.

■ Relative contraindications include history of chronic severe, poorly controlled hypertension, severe uncontrolled hypertension on presentation (systolic blood pressure >180 mm Hg or diastolic blood pressure >110 mm Hg), history of prior ischemic stroke >3 months, dementia or known intracranial pathology that is not included under absolute contraindications, traumatic or prolonged cardiac resuscitation >10 minutes, major surgery <3 weeks, recent (within 2 to 4 weeks) internal bleeding, noncompressible vascular punctures, pregnancy, active peptic ulcer, current use of anticoagulants (the higher the International Normalized Ratio, the higher the risk of bleeding), and prior exposure (>5 days) to streptokinase/anistreplase or prior allergic reaction to these agents.

■ Intracerebral hemorrhage is a major complication and is expected to occur in approximately 1% of patients receiving thrombolytic therapy. It is fatal in up to two thirds of patients with this complication. Patients older than 65 years, a low body weight of <70 kg, and alteplase (as opposed to streptokinase) as the thrombolytic agent, are associated with higher incidence of intracerebral hemorrhage.

■ There are five thrombolytic agents approved for intravenous use: (1) tissue plasminogen activator or tPa (alteplase),

(2) recombinant tissue plasminogen activator or rtPa (reteplase), (3) tenecteplase, (4) streptokinase, and (5) anistreplase. Alteplase, reteplase, and tenecteplase are plasminogen activators. These are selective agents that specifically convert plasminogen to plasmin and are given concomitantly with intravenous heparin infusion. Streptokinase and anistreplase do not require heparin infusion because these nonselective thrombolytic agents can cause depletion of the coagulation factors and produce massive amounts of fibrin degradation products, which have anticoagulant properties. If patient is a high risk for systemic emboli such as the presence of a large infarct, atrial fibrillation, left ventricular thrombus, or previous embolus, Activated partial thromboplastin time should be checked 4 hours after these nonselective thrombolytic agents have been given and heparin started when activated partial thromboplastin time is <2 times control (or <70 seconds).

- Additional medical therapy for ST elevation MI include:

  - **Aspirin:** The initial dose of aspirin is 162 to 325 mg orally. This should be given immediately even before the patient arrives to a medical facility. Plain aspirin (not enteric coated), should be chewed. Maintenance dose of 75 to 162 mg daily is continued indefinitely thereafter.

    - If the patient is allergic to aspirin, clopidogrel should be given as a substitute.

    - In patients undergoing coronary bypass surgery, aspirin should be started within 48 hours after surgery to reduce closure of the saphenous vein grafts.

    - Patients who have PCI with stents placed should initially receive the higher dose of aspirin at 162 to 325 mg daily for one month for bare metal stent, 3 months for sirolimus and 6 months for paclitaxel eluting stent and continued at a dose of 75 to 162 mg daily indefinitely.

  - **Clopidogrel:** Similar to aspirin, clopidogrel is considered standard therapy and is a Class I recommendation in patients with acute coronary syndrome including patients with ST elevation MI with or without reperfusion therapy according to the 2007 focused update of the ACC/AHA 2004 guidelines for ST elevation MI. The maintenance dose is 75 mg orally daily for a minimum of 14 days and reasonably up to a year. The loading dose is 300 mg orally, although in elderly patients >75 years especially those given fibrinolytics, the loading dose needs further study.

    - In patients undergoing coronary bypass surgery, clopidogrel should be discontinued at least 5 days and preferably for 7 days unless the need for surgery outweighs the risk of bleeding.

  - **Unfractionated heparin:** When unfractionated heparin is given concomitantly with a selective thrombolytic agent such as tPA, rtPA, or tenecteplase, the recommended dose is 60 U/kg given as an IV bolus. The initial dose should not exceed 4,000 U. This is followed by a maintenance dose of 12 U/kg/hour not to exceed 1,000 U/hour for patients weighing more than 70 kg. Activated partial thromboplastin time should be maintained to 50 to 70 seconds or 1.5 to 2 times baseline. Heparin is usually given for 48 hours, but may be given longer if there is atrial fibrillation, left ventricular thrombi, pulmonary embolism, or congestive heart failure. Platelets should be monitored daily. When given to patients not on thrombolytic therapy, the dose is 60 to 70 U/kg bolus followed by maintenance infusion of 12 to 15 U/kg/hour. According to the ACC/AHA 2007 revised guidelines on unstable angina and non-ST elevation MI, patients who did not receive thrombolytic therapy may receive other types of heparin other than unfractionated heparin for the whole duration of hospitalization or for a total of 8 days. This includes low-molecular-weight heparin (enoxaparin) and fondaparinux.

    - **Enoxaparin:** An initial 30 mg IV bolus is followed by a subcutaneous injection of 1 mg/kg every 12 hours. For patients older than 75 years of age, the initial bolus is omitted and the subcutaneous dose is 0.75 mg/kg every 12 hours. The dose should be adjusted if the serum creatinine is ≥2.5 mg/dL in men and ≥2.0 mg/dL in women.

    - **Fondaparinux:** The initial dose is 2.5 mg IV followed by subcutaneous doses of 2.5 mg once daily up to the duration of hospitalization or a maximum of 8 days provided that the creatinine is <3.0 mg/dL.

  - **Nitroglycerin:** Nitroglycerin is initially given sublingually unless the patient is hypotensive with a blood pressure <90 mm Hg or heart rate is <50 bpm or there is suspected RVMI. Intravenous nitroglycerin is given when there are symptoms of ongoing ischemia or congestive heart failure or for uncontrolled hypertension.

  - **Oxygen:** Oxygen supplementation is given to improve arterial saturation.

  - **Morphine sulfate:** Morphine sulfate is the analgesic of choice with a Class I recommendation for pain relief for ST elevation MI but only a Class IIa recommendation for non-ST elevation MI. The dose is 2 to 4 mg IV and repeated in increments of 2 to 8 mg at 5- to 15-minute intervals.

  - **Beta blockers:** Beta blockers should be given orally in the first 24 hours unless the patient has contraindications to beta blocker therapy such as PR interval >0.24 seconds, second-degree AV block or higher, signs of heart failure, or low cardiac output and bronchospastic pulmonary disease. This is given a Class I recommendation in the ACC/AHA guidelines. Beta blockers have been shown to decrease the incidence of ventricular arrhythmias after acute MI. Beta blockers may be administered IV if hypertension is present. This carries a Class IIa recommendation.

  - **Antagonists of the renin-angiotensin system:** The use of angiotensin-converting enzyme inhibitors is a Class I recommendation in patients with ST elevation MI. It should be given orally (not IV) and continued indefinitely in patients with ST elevation MI with left ventricular ejection fraction ≤40% and patients with hypertension, diabetes, or chronic renal disease in the absence of contraindications to angiotensin-converting enzyme inhibitor therapy. Angiotensin receptor blockers, specifically valsartan or candesartan, may be given if the patient cannot tolerate angiotensin-converting enzyme inhibitors. The routine use of angiotensin-converting enzyme inhibitors or angiotensin receptor blockers is reasonable in patients with acute ST elevation MI without any of the above indications. This carries a Class IIa recommendation.

- **Aldosterone antagonist:** Aldosterone antagonists (eplerenone in post-MI patients and spironolactone in patients with chronic heart failure), have been shown to reduce mortality. The 2007 focused update of the ACC/AHA 2004 guidelines on ST elevation MI gives a Class I recommendation for the use of aldosterone blockers to patients with ejection fraction of $\leq 40\%$ and have either diabetes or heart failure unless there is renal dysfunction (serum creatinine $\geq 2.5$ mg/dL in men and $\geq 2.0$ mg/dL in women and potassium $\geq 5.0$ mEq/L).

- **Cholesterol-lowering agents:** Statins or if contraindicated, other lipid-lowering agents, should be given to lower low-density lipoprotein cholesterol to $<100$ mg/dL in all patients and further lowering to $<70$ mg/dL is reasonable in some patients.

- **IIB/IIIA inhibitors:** Other antiplatelet agents such as IIB/IIIA inhibitors (abciximab, eptifibatide, and tirofiban) are not indicated in the treatment of ST elevation MI unless the patient is being readied for primary PCI. The use of standard dose IIB/IIIA inhibitor (abciximab) in combination with half-dose thrombolytic agent (reteplase) has not been shown to improve mortality in the short term (30 days) or long term (1 year) compared with the use of the thrombolytic agent alone.

- **Primary PCI:** Primary PCI is the most effective reperfusion method and has now become the standard therapy for reperfusing ST elevation MI in centers that are capable of doing the procedure in a timely fashion. The success rate of being able to reperfuse the occluded artery with primary PCI is $>90\%$, whereas the 90-minute patency rate with thrombolytic therapy is approximately 65% to 75%. Unfortunately, PCI can be performed only in centers with interventional cardiac catheterization laboratories, and in some states, only when backup cardiac surgery is available. The most recent 2007 focused update of the ACC/AHA guidelines on ST elevation MI reemphasizes the previous recommendation that reperfusion of the occluded artery should be started as early as possible since the greatest benefit of any type of reperfusion therapy depends on the shortest time in which complete reperfusion is achieved. Therefore, the delay in performing PCI should be considered when deciding whether thrombolytic therapy or primary PCI is the best modality of reperfusion. Thus, if the patient is admitted to a hospital that is capable of doing PCI, the procedure should be performed within 90 minutes after first medical contact. If the patient is admitted to a facility that is not capable of doing PCI and it is not possible to perform PCI within 90 minutes with interhospital transfer, thrombolytic therapy should be given unless contraindicated, within 30 minutes of hospital presentation.

Transfer to another hospital with PCI capabilities should be considered when:

- Thrombolytic therapy is contraindicated.
- PCI can be performed within 90 minutes (door to balloon time) of first medical contact.
- Thrombolytic therapy had been tried but failed to reperfuse the occluded artery (rescue PCI).
- PCI is also the therapy of choice when the patient is hemodynamically unstable especially when there is cardiogenic shock or pump failure, onset of symptoms is more than 3 hours or the diagnosis of ST elevation MI is in doubt.

- **Facilitated PCI:** This involves the administration of heparin in high doses, IIb/IIIa antagonists, fibrinolytic agents in less than full doses or a combination of the agents discussed previously before PCI is attempted. Full dose thrombolytic therapy followed by immediate PCI may be harmful and is not recommended (Class III recommendation according to the 2007 focused update ACC/AHA 2004 guidelines for the management of patients with ST elevation MI). These antithrombotic agents are given to improve patency of the occluded coronary artery. Facilitated PCI is performed if primary PCI is not available within 90 minutes after first medical contact. This is usually performed when the patient is initially admitted to a hospital without PCI capabilities and interhospital transfer is being planned to a facility that is capable of doing PCI.

- **Cardiac pacemakers and acute MI:**

  - In patients with acute MI complicated by AV block, implantation of permanent pacemakers depends on the location of the AV block (which should be infranodal), rather than the presence or absence of symptoms. Most patients with infranodal block have wide QRS complexes. However, when AV block is persistent and is associated with symptoms, the AV block may or may not be infranodal before a permanent pacemaker is implanted.

  - Whenever a patient who has survived an acute MI becomes a candidate for permanent pacemaker, two other conditions should be answered. These include the need for biventricular pacing because most of these patients will have an intraventricular conduction defect and the need for implantable cardioverter defibrillator (ICD) because most of these patients have left ventricular dysfunction.

  - **Indications of implantation of permanent pacemaker after acute MI:** The following are indications for insertion of a permanent pacemaker following acute ST elevation MI according to the ACC/AHA/Heart Rhythm Society (HRS) 2008 guidelines for device-based therapy of cardiac rhythm abnormalities and the ACC/AHA 2004 guidelines for the management of ST elevation MI.

    - Class I recommendation:
      - Persistent second-degree AV block in the His-Purkinje system with bilateral bundle-branch block or third-degree AV block within or below the His-Purkinje system.

- Transient advanced second- or third-degree AV block at the infranodal level and associated bundle branch block. An electrophysiologic study may be necessary if the site of the block is uncertain.
  - Persistent and symptomatic second- or third-degree AV block.
  - Class IIb recommendation:
    - Persistent second- or third-degree AV block at the level of the AV node.
  - Class III recommendation: permanent pacing is not recommended in the following conditions:
    - Transient AV block without intraventricular conduction defect.
    - Transient AV block in the presence of isolated left anterior fascicular block.
    - Acquired left anterior fascicular block in the absence of AV block.
    - Persistent first-degree AV block in the presence of bundle branch block, old or indeterminate.

- **Ventricular and supraventricular tachycardia:** The treatment of ventricular and supraventricular tachycardia following acute MI is similar to the general management of these arrhythmias in patients without ischemic heart disease.

- **Implantation of ICD after acute MI:** In patients with acute MI, the following are indications for implantation of ICD according to the ACC/AHA 2004 guidelines for the management of ST elevation MI:
  - Class I recommendation:
    - Patients with VF or hemodynamically significant VT more than 2 days after acute MI not from reversible ischemia or from reinfarction.
    - Left ventricular ejection fraction of 31% to 40% at least 1 month after acute MI even in the absence of spontaneous VT/VF or have inducible VT/VF on electrophysiological testing.
  - Class IIa recommendation:
    - Left ventricular dysfunction (ejection fraction ≤30%) at least 1 month after acute MI and 3 months after coronary artery revascularization.
  - Class IIb recommendation:
    - Left ventricular dysfunction (ejection fraction 31% to 40%) at least 1 month after acute ST elevation MI without additional evidence of electrical instability such as nonsustained VT.
    - Left ventricular dysfunction (ejection fraction 31% to 40%) at least 1 month after acute ST elevation MI and additional evidence of electrical instability such as nonsustained VT but do not have inducible VF or sustained VT on electrophysiologi testing.
  - Class III recommendation: ICD is not indicated when ejection fraction is >40% at least 1 month after acute ST elevation MI.

- **RVMI:** Left ventricular preload may be diminished from right ventricular failure and volume is needed to optimize diastolic filling and cardiac output. Treatment of RVMI therefore usually requires adequate hydration with IV fluids.
  - The use of nitroglycerin may further reduce preload and potentiate the hemodynamic abnormalities associated with RVMI and should be used cautiously when acute inferior MI is present. It is contraindicated if systolic blood pressure is <90 mm Hg or heart rate is <50 bpm.
  - Acute inferior MI complicated by RVMI involves not only the right ventricle but may be associated with significant left ventricular dysfunction. If left ventricular output is low and LV filling pressure is high (high pulmonary wedge pressure), inotropic support with dopamine or dobutamine should be considered.
  - Complete AV block may occur as a complication of RVMI because the artery to the AV node is usually compromised when there is occlusion of the proximal or mid-RCA. If the AV block is associated with a low ventricular rate of <50 bpm or patient is hemodynamically unstable with low output, atropine is the drug of choice. The dose is 0.5 to 1.0 mg IV repeated every 3 to 5 minutes until a total dose of 3 mg (0.04 mg/kg) is given within a period of 3 hours. This dose can result in complete vagal blockade and need not be exceeded. Doses of <0.5 mg should be discouraged because it may slow instead of increase heart rate by stimulation of the vagal nuclei centrally resulting in parasympathomimetic response. If AV block does not respond to atropine, temporary dual chamber pacing to preserve AV synchrony may be needed to optimize left ventricular output because ventricular performance is dependent on atrial contribution to left ventricular filling.

## Prognosis

- Acute MI continues to be the leading cause of death and disability in spite of the advances in the diagnosis and therapy of coronary disease. About half of all deaths from acute MI will occur during the initial hours after the onset of symptoms with most deaths from ventricular fibrillation. Most deaths occur before the patients are able to reach a medical facility. Of those who survive and are able to seek medical care, prognosis is dependent on the extent and severity of myocardial damage.

- ST elevation MI is more extensive than non-ST elevation MI resulting in a lower ejection fraction, higher incidence of heart failure, ventricular arrhythmias, and higher immediate and in-hospital mortality of up to 10% compared with non-ST elevation MI, which has a lower incidence of the above complications and a lower in-hospital mortality of 1% to 3%.

## Suggested Readings

Anderson JL, Adams CD, Antman EM, et al. ACC/AHA 2007 guidelines for the management of patients with unstable angina/non-ST-elevation myocardial infarction. *J Am Coll Cardiol.* 2007;50:e1–157.

Antman EM, Anbe DT, Armstrong PW, et al. ACC/AHA guidelines for the management of patients with ST elevation myocardial infarction: executive summary: a report of the ACC/AHA Task Force on Practice Guidelines (Committee to Revise the 1999 Guidelines on the Management of Patients with Acute Myocardial Infarction). *J Am Coll Cardiol.* 2004;44:671–719.

Antman EM, Hand M, Armstrong PW, et al. 2007 Focused update of the ACC/AHA 2004 guidelines for the management of patients with ST elevation myocardial infarction. *J Am Coll Cardiol.* 2008;51:210–247.

Assali AR, Sclarovsky S, Hertz I, et al. Comparison of patients with inferior wall acute myocardial infarction with versus without ST-segment elevation in leads $V_5$ and $V_6$. *Am J Cardiol.* 1998;81:81–83.

Balci B, Yesildag O. Correlation between clinical findings and the "tombstoning" electrocardiographic pattern in patients with anterior wall acute myocardial infarction. *J Am Coll Cardiol.* 2003;92:1316–1318.

Birnbaum Y, Sclarovsky S, Solodky A, et al. Prediction of the level of left anterior descending coronary artery obstruction during anterior wall acute myocardial infarction by the admission electrocardiogram. *Am J Cardiol.* 1993;72:823–826.

Birnbaum Y, Solodky A, Hertz I, et al. Implications of inferior ST-segment depression in anterior acute myocardial infarction: electrocardiographic and angiographic correlation. *Am Heart J.* 1994;127:1467–1473.

Braunwald E, Antman EM, Beasley JW, et al. ACC/AHA guidelines for the management of patients with unstable angina and non-ST segment elevation myocardial infarction: a report of the ACC/AHA Task Force on Practice Guidelines (Committee on the Management of Patients with Unstable Angina). *J Am Coll Cardiol.* 2000;36:970–1062.

Braunwald E, Antman EM, Beasley JW, et al. ACC/AHA 2002 guideline update for the management of patients with unstable angina and non-ST segment elevation myocardial infarction: Summary article: a report of the ACC/AHA Task Force on Practice Guidelines (Committee on the Management of Patients with Unstable Angina. *Circulation.* 2002;106:1893–1900.

Brugada R, Brugada J, Antzelevitch C, et al. Sodium channel blockers identify risk for sudden death in patients with ST segment elevation and right bundle branch block but structurally normal hearts. *Circulation.* 2000;101:510–515.

Dunn MI, Lipman BS. Myocardial Infarction, injury and ischemia. In: *Clinical Electrocardiography.* 8th ed. Chicago: Year Book Medical Publishers, Inc; 1989:160–209.

Edhouse J, Brady WJ, Morris F. ABC of clinical electrocardiography. Acute myocardial infarction—part II. *BMJ.* 2002;324:963–966.

Engelen DJ, Gorgels AP, Cheriex EC, et al. Value of the electrocardiogram in localizing the occlusion site in the left anterior descending coronary artery in acute anterior myocardial infarction. *J Am Coll Cardiol.* 1999;34:389–395.

Epstein AE, DiMarco JP, Ellenbogen KA, et al. ACC/AHA/HRS 2008 guidelines for device-based therapy of cardiac rhythm abnormalities: a report of the American College of Cardiology/American Heart Association Task Force on Practice Guidelines (Writing Committee to Revise the ACC/AHA/NASPE 2002 Guideline Update for Implantation of Cardiac Pacemakers and Antiarrhythmia Devices). *Circulation,* 2008; 117:e350–e408.

Ginzton LE, Laks MM. The differential diagnosis of acute pericarditis from normal variant: new electrocardiographic criteria. *Circulation.* 1982;65:1004–1009.

Goldberger AL. Electrocardiogram in the diagnosis of myocardial ischemia and infarction. 2007 UpToDate.

Goldberger AL. Pathogenesis and diagnosis of Q waves in the electrocardiogram. 2007 UpToDate.

Goldberger A, Goldberger E. Myocardial ischemia and infarction I and II. In: *Clinical Electrocardiography.* 5th ed. Mosby-Year Book, Inc; 1994:87–122.

Gregoratos G, Abrams J, Epstein AE, et al. ACC/AHA/NASPE 2002 guideline update for implantation of cardiac pacemakers and antiarrhythmia devices: summary article. *Circulation.* 2002;106:2145–2161.

Guo XH, Yap YG, Chen LJ, et al. Correlation of coronary angiography with "tombstoning" electrocardiographic pattern in patients after acute myocardial infarction. *Clin Cardiol.* 2000;23:347–352.

Hertz, I, Assali AR, Adler Y, et al. New electrocardiographic criteria for predicting either the right or left circumflex artery as the culprit coronary artery in inferior wall acute myocardial infarction. *Am J Cardiol.* 1997;80:1343–1345.

The Joint European Society of Cardiology/American College of Cardiology Committee. Myocardial infarction redefined—a consensus document of the joint European Society of Cardiology/American College of Cardiology Committee for the Redefinition of Myocardial Infarction. *J Am Coll Cardiol.* 2000;36:959–969.

Kontos MC, Desai PV, Jesse RL, et al. Usefulness of the admission electrocardiogram for identifying the infarct-related-artery in inferior wall acute myocardial infarction. *Am J Cardiol.* 1997;79:182–184.

Kosuge M, Kimura K, Ishikawa T, et al. Electrocardiographic criteria for predicting total occlusion of the proximal left anterior descending coronary artery in anterior wall acute myocardial infarction. *Clin Cardiol.* 2001;24:33–38.

Kosuge M, Kimura K, Ishikawa T, et al. New electrocardiographic criteria for predicting the site of coronary artery occlusion in inferior wall acute myocardial infarction. *Am J Cardiol.* 1998;82:1318–1322.

Kulkarni AU, Brown R, Ayoubi M, et al. Clinical use of posterior electrocardiographic leads: A prospective electrocardiographic analysis during coronary occlusion. *Am Heart J.* 1996;131:736–741.

Kyuhyun W, Asinger RW, Marriott HJL. ST-segment elevation in conditions other than acute myocardial infarction. *N Engl J Med.* 2003;349:2128–2135.

Kurisu S, Sato H, Kawagoe T, et al. Tako-tsubo-like left ventricular dysfunction with ST-segment elevation: a novel cardiac syndrome mimicking acute myocardial infarction. *Am Heart J.* 2002;143:448–455.

Matetsky S, Freimark D, Chouraqui P, et al. Significance of ST segment elevations in posterior chest leads (V$_7$ to V$_9$) in patients with acute inferior myocardial infarction: application for thrombolytic therapy. *J Am Coll Cardiol.* 1998;31:506–511.

Matsuo K, Akahoshi M, Nakashima E, et al. The prevalence, incidence and prognostic value of the Brugada-type electrocardiogram. A population based study of four decades. *J Am Coll Cardiol.* 2001;38:765–770.

Mirvis DM, Goldberger AL. Electrocardiography. In: Zipes DP, Libby P, Bonow RO, Braunwald E, eds. *Braunwald's Heart Disease: A Textbook of Cardiovascular Medicine.* 7th ed. Philadelphia: Elsevier Saunders; 2005:107–148.

Morris F, Brady WJ. ABC of clinical electrocardiography. Acute myocardial infarction—part I. *BMJ.* 2002;324:831–834.

Pitt B, Remme W, Zannad F, et al., for the Eplerenone Post-Acute Myocardial Infarction Heart Failure Efficacy and Survival Study investigators. Eplerenone, a selective aldosterone blocker, in patients with left ventricular dysfunction after myocardial infarction. *N Engl J Med.* 2003;348:1309–1321.

Reeder GS, Kennedy HL. Diagnosis of an acute myocardial infarction. 2007 UpToDate.

Ryan TJ, Antman EM, Brooks NH, et al. 1999 update: ACC/AHA guidelines for the management of patients with acute myocardial infarction: executive summary and recommendations: a report of the American College of Cardiology/American Heart Association Task Force on Practice Guidelines (Committee on Management of Acute Myocardial Infarction). *Circulation.* 1999;100:1016–1030.

Ryan TJ, Anderson JL, Antman EM, et al. American College of Cardiology/American Heart Association guidelines for the management of patients with acute myocardial infarction: a report of the American College of Cardiology/American Heart Association Task Force on Practice Guidelines (Committee on Management of Acute Myocardial Infarction). *J Am Coll Cardiol.* 1996;28:1328–1428.

Sabatine MS, Cannon CP, Gibson M, et al. Addition of clopidogrel to aspirin and fibrinolytic therapy for myocardial infarction with ST-segment elevation. *N Engl J Med.* 2005; 352;1179–1189.

Sgarbossa EB, Pinski SL, Topol EJ, et al. Acute myocardial infarction and complete bundle branch block at hospital admission: clinical characteristics and outcome in the thrombolytic era. *J Am Coll Cardiol.* 1998;31:105–110.

Sgarbossa EB, Pinski SL, Barbagelata A, et al. Electrocardiographic diagnosis of evolving acute myocardial infarction in the presence of left bundle-branch block. *N Engl J Med.* 1996;334:481–487.

Sgarbossa EB, Wagner GS. Electrocardiography. In: Topol EJ, ed. *Textbook of Cardiovascular Medicine.* 2nd ed. Philadelphia: Lippincott Williams & Wilkins; 2002:1329–1363.

Smith SC, Allen J, Blair SN, et al. AHA/ACC guidelines for secondary prevention for patients with coronary and other atherosclerotic vascular disease: 2006 update. *Circulation.* 2006;113:2363–2372.

Surawicz B, Parikh SR. Prevalence of male and female patterns of early ventricular repolarization in the normal ECG of males and females from childhood to old age. *J Am Coll Cardiol.* 2002;40:1870–1876.

Thygesen K, Alpert JS, White HD, et al. ESC/ACCF/AHA/WHF expert consensus document. Universal definition of myocardial infarction. *J Am Coll Cardiol.* 2007;50:2173–2195.

Virmani R, Burke AP. Pathology of myocardial ischemia, infarction, reperfusion and sudden death. In: Zipes DP, Libby P, Bonow RO, Braunwald E, eds. *Braunwald's Heart Disease: A Textbook of Cardiovascular Medicine.* 7th ed. Philadelphia: Elsevier Saunders; 2005:107–148.

Wimalaratna HSK. "Tombstoning" of ST segment in acute myocardial infarction. *Lancet.* 1993;342:496 [letter].

Wang K, Asinger RW, Marriott HJL. ST-segment elevation in conditions other than acute myocardial infarction. *N Engl J Med.* 2003;349:2128–2135.

Zimetbaum PJ, Josephson ME. Use of the electrocardiogram in acute myocardial infarction. *N Engl J Med.* 2003;348: 933–940.

Zimetbaum PJ, Krishnan S, Gold A, et al. Usefulness of ST-segment elevation in lead III exceeding that of lead II for identifying the location of the totally occluded coronary artery in inferior wall myocardial infarction. *Am J Cardiol.* 1998;82:918–919.

Zipes DP, Camm AJ, Borggrefe M, et al. ACC/AHA/ESC 2006 guidelines for management of patients with ventricular arrhythmias and the prevention of sudden cardiac death: executive summary: a report of the American College of Cardiology/American Heart Association Task Force and the European Society of Cardiology Committee for Practice Guidelines (Writing Committee to Develop Guidelines for Management of Patients with Ventricular Arrhythmias and the Prevention of Sudden Cardiac Death). *Circulation.* 2006;114:1088–1132.

# Acute Coronary Syndrome: Non-ST Elevation Myocardial Infarction and Unstable Angina

- **Acute coronary syndrome:** Acute coronary syndrome is usually from plaque rupture, resulting in varying degrees of myocardial ischemia. The electrocardiogram (ECG) provides useful information that cannot be obtained with other diagnostic procedures and is the most important modality in the initial management of patients with this disorder.

- **ECG findings:** Patients with acute coronary syndrome can be classified according to their ECG presentation and include those with ST segment elevation and those without ST elevation.

  - **ST elevation:** Almost all patients with acute coronary syndrome with ST segment elevation will develop myocardial necrosis with increased cardiac troponins in the circulation. These patients have an occluded coronary artery with completely obstructed flow and are candidates for immediate reperfusion with a thrombolytic agent or with primary percutaneous coronary intervention (PCI). This was discussed in Chapter 23, Acute Coronary Syndrome: ST Elevation Myocardial Infarction.

  - **Non-ST elevation:** Patients with acute coronary syndrome without ST segment elevation usually have ST depression, T-wave inversion, or less-specific ST and T wave abnormalities. Some patients may not show any changes in the ECG. These patients will either have unstable angina with no evidence of myocardial necrosis or non-ST elevation myocardial infarction (MI) when evidence of myocardial necrosis is present. The presence or absence of myocardial necrosis is based on whether or not cardiac troponins are elevated in the circulation. Unstable angina and non-ST elevation MI have the same pathophysiology, similar ECG findings, similar clinical presentation, and similar management and are discussed together.

- The ECG is also helpful in providing prognostic information in acute coronary syndrome based on the initial presentation.

- Patients with acute coronary syndrome accompanied by ST segment elevation carries the highest risk of death during the acute phase.

- Patients presenting with ST segment depression have the highest overall mortality over a period of 6 months.

- Patients with isolated T wave inversion or those with no significant ECG abnormalities incur the lowest risk.

## The Normal T Wave

- **The normal T wave:** The T wave normally follows the direction of the QRS complex. Thus, in leads where the R waves are tall, the T waves are also tall. In leads where the S waves are deep and the R waves are small, as in leads III or aVL, the T waves may be flat or inverted. Determining the direction or axis of any wave in the ECG such as the QRS complex was previously discussed in Chapter 4, The Electrical Axis and Cardiac Rotation.

  - **Frontal plane:** In the frontal plane, the axis of the normal T wave is within 45° of the axis of the QRS complex (Figs. 24.1 and 24.2). This is also called the QRS/T angle, which is the angle formed between the axis of the QRS complex and that of the T wave. When this angle is increased, myocardial ischemia should be considered, although this is usually not a specific finding. The tallest T wave in the limb leads is approximately 5 mm but could reach up to 8 mm.

  - **Horizontal plane:** In the horizontal plane, the axis of the normal T wave is within 60° of the axis of the QRS complex. Calculation of the T-wave axis in the horizontal plane is usually not necessary, because the T waves are expected to be upright in most precordial leads other than $V_1$ or $V_2$. If the T waves are inverted in $V_1$, $V_2$, and also in $V_3$, this is abnormal (Fig. 24.3), except in children and young adults.

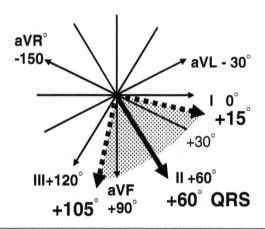

**Figure 24.1: Axis of the T Wave in the Frontal Plane.** If the axis of the QRS is 60°, the T wave should be within 45° (*shaded*) to the left or right of the axis of the QRS complex as shown.

Because the precordial leads are closer to the heart than the limb leads, the T waves are taller in the precordial leads, especially $V_2$–$V_4$, and usually measure up to 10 mm but can reach up to 12 mm.

- **The normal T wave:**
  - In Figure 24.2, the axis of the T wave and QRS complex is almost 0°. Although the T wave is inverted in lead III (arrows), this is not abnormal because the axis of the T wave is within 45° of the axis of the QRS complex. In the horizontal plane, the T wave is inverted in $V_1$ and upright in $V_2$ to $V_6$. This is also a normal finding.
  - In Figure 24.3, the T waves are inverted in $V_1$, $V_2$ and $V_3$ (arrows). This is abnormal in adults. However, inversion of the T wave from $V_1$ to $V_3$ is entirely normal in children. This T-wave inversion may normally persist through adulthood in some patients and is called persistent juvenile pattern.

## Abnormal T Waves

- **T waves:** Figure 24.4 shows different examples of T waves, both normal and abnormal.

- **Normal T wave:** A normal T wave is upright and asymmetric. The initial upstroke is inscribed slowly and the terminal downstroke is inscribed more rapidly (Fig. 24.4A).
- **Ischemic T waves:** Figure 24.4B–D show typical ischemic T waves. Ischemic T waves are symmetrical. They are symmetrically tall when the ischemia is subendocardial and are deeply symmetrically inverted, measuring at least 2 mm when the ischemia is subepicardial or transmural. These T-wave abnormalities when accompanied by symptoms of myocardial ischemia may or may not be associated with troponin elevation.
- **Nonspecific T waves:** The other T-wave abnormalities shown in Figure 24.4E–G are nonspecific. These include T waves that are inverted but are <2 mm in amplitude. They may nevertheless occur as the only ECG abnormality associated with acute myocardial ischemia and may or may not be associated with troponin elevation. It is also possible that the ECG may not show any definite abnormalities when there is myocardial ischemia.

- Interpretation of any T-wave abnormality should always include all available clinical information because the T-wave abnormalities are not always from ischemia, even if they look typical for myocardial ischemia.
- **Abnormal T-wave changes from myocardial ischemia:** When coronary blood flow is diminished or when myocardial oxygen demand exceeds blood supply, changes in the T waves are the earliest to occur. Electrocardiographically, changes confined to the T waves indicate myocardial ischemia, which may be subendocardial or transmural.
  - **Subendocardial ischemia:** Myocardial ischemia is subendocardial when it is localized to the subendocardial area. It is usually manifested in the ECG as peaking of the T waves over the area of ischemia.
  - **Transmural ischemia:** The ischemia is transmural or subepicardial when it involves the whole thickness of the myocardium. This is usually manifested in the ECG as deeply and symmetrically inverted T waves over the area of ischemia.

**Figure 24.2: T Wave Axis in the Frontal Plane.** Although the T waves are inverted in lead III (*arrows*), the axis of the T wave is within 45° of the axis of the QRS complex (QRS axis 0°, T wave axis –5°), thus the T wave inversion in lead III is expected. This is not an abnormal finding.

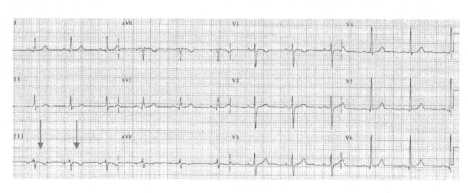

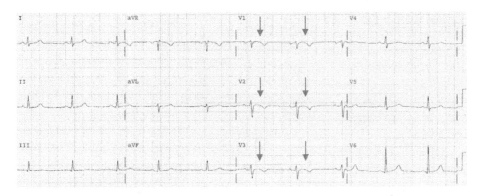

**Figure 24.3:    Persistent Juvenile Pattern.** The electrocardiogram is from a 25-year-old asymptomatic female showing inversion of the T wave in $V_1$ to $V_3$ (*arrows*). This is a normal finding in children, which may normally persist to adulthood and is called persistent juvenile pattern.

■ **Subendocardial ischemia:** The typical pattern of subendocardial ischemia is the presence of tall and symmetrically peaked T waves (Fig. 24.5). The configuration of the T wave is similar to that of hyperkalemia except that in subendocardial ischemia, the base is usually broad and the QT interval is slightly prolonged. Peaking of the T waves is confined to the area of ischemia unlike hyperkalemia where peaking is generalized (Fig. 24.6). Peaking of the T waves may also occur in fluoride intoxication and left ventricular hypertrophy from volume overload such as aortic regurgitation. It can also occur as a normal finding (Fig. 24.7) or when there is a metabolic abnormality (Fig. 24.8) especially over the precordial transition zone $V_2$ to $V_4$. Thus, peaking of the T wave is not specific for myocardial ischemia.

■ **Transmural ischemia:** T waves that are symmetrically and deeply inverted may indicate transmural ischemia, which involves the whole thickness of the myocardium. In transmural or subepicardial ischemia, the T wave is pointed downward, often resembling an arrowhead. If the T wave is divided equally into two halves by drawing a perpendicular line at the middle of the T wave, the left half of the inverted T wave resembles the other

half. The ST segment may or may not be depressed. The QTc may be slightly prolonged (Fig. 24.9). When acute symptoms of ischemia are also present, these T waves may or may not be associated with troponin elevation. When troponins are elevated in the circulation, non-ST elevation MI or more specifically a T-wave infarct is present; otherwise, the T wave changes are due to unstable angina.

■ **Other causes of deep T-wave inversion:** There are several other causes of deep and symmetrical T-wave inversion other than myocardial ischemia. These include hypertrophic cardiomyopathy especially the apical type, pericarditis, pulmonary embolism, mitral valve prolapse, metabolic conditions, electrolyte disorders, and effect of drugs such as tricyclic antidepressants and antiarrhythmic agents. It can also be due to noncardiac conditions such as cerebrovascular accidents or other craniocerebral abnormalities, peptic ulcer perforation, acute cholecystitis, and acute pancreatitis. It may even be a variant of normal especially in young African American males. Deep symmetrical inversion of the T wave, therefore, is not specific and does not necessarily imply that the T-wave abnormality is due to transmural myocardial ischemia.

■ Figure 24.10 is the initial ECG of a patient who presented with chest discomfort. There was deep and symmetrical T-wave inversion across the precordium. The cardiac troponins were elevated consistent with non-ST elevation MI or, more specifically, a T-wave infarct.

■ Figure 24.11 is the 12-lead ECG of a 37-year-old woman, without history of cardiac disease and is 6 months postpartum when she developed cerebral hemorrhage. Deep T-wave inversion is noted in the limb and precordial leads resembling transmural ischemia.

■ **Secondary ST and T wave abnormalities:** The abnormality in the T wave as well as the ST segment is secondary if it is caused by abnormal depolarization of the ventricles, as would occur when there is bundle branch block, ventricular hypertrophy, preexcitation of the ventricles, or when the rhythm is ectopic or induced by a ventricular pacemaker. These secondary ST

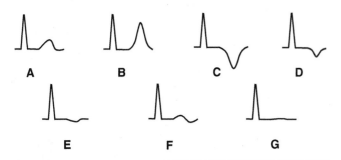

**Figure 24.4:    T Waves. (A)** Normal T wave. **(B)** Peaked T waves from subendocardial ischemia. **(C)** Classical deep T-wave inversion due to transmural ischemia. **(D)** Symmetrically but less deeply inverted T wave also due to transmural ischemia. **(E)** Shallow T-wave inversion **(F)** Biphasic T wave. **(G)** Low, flat, or isoelectric T wave. Although the T-wave configuration of **B, C,** and **D** suggests myocardial ischemia, these T-wave abnormalities may also be due to other causes.

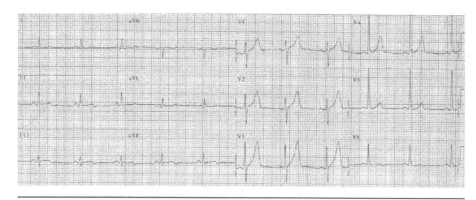

**Figure 24.5:    Subendocardial Ischemia.**  Peaking of the T waves is confined to $V_1$ to $V_4$ consistent with subendocardial ischemia involving the anterior wall. Note also that the T waves are taller in $V_1$ than in $V_6$ and are biphasic in leads II, III, and aVF. Peaking of the T waves mark the area of ischemia and can occur as the initial manifestation of acute coronary syndrome before the onset of ST segment elevation.

**Figure 24.6:    Hyperkalemia.**
Peaking of the T waves from hyper-kalemia (serum potassium = 6.6 mEq/L). In subendocardial ischemia, the abnormally peaked T waves are localized to the ischemic area. In hy-perkalemia, peaking of the T waves is generalized (*arrows*).

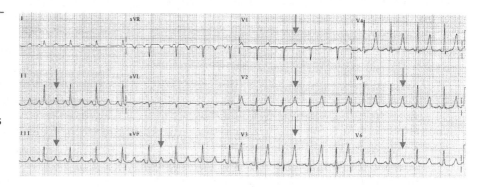

**Figure 24.7:    Peaked T Waves.**
Routine electrocardiogram obtained from an asymptomatic middle-age male. Peaked T waves are present representing a normal variant. Peaked T waves are often associated with early repolarization. Potassium level was 3.8 mEq/L.

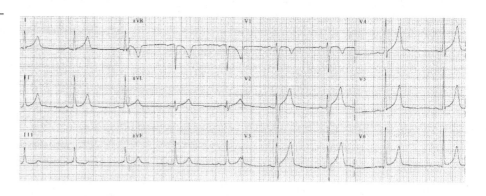

**Figure 24.8:    Giant T Waves.**
Twelve-lead electrocardiogram (ECG) of a 33-year-old alcoholic man show-ing giant T waves with prolonged QTc. The T waves are tall and peaked with a broad base. The cause of the ECG abnormality was thought to be due to alcohol or associated metabolic abnormality.

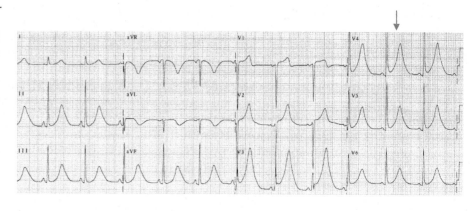

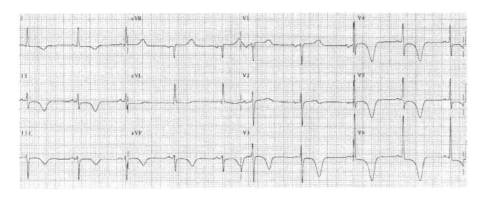

**Figure 24.9: Transmural Myocardial Ischemia.** The T-wave changes shown are typical of transmural ischemia. Ischemic T waves are deeply inverted, usually measuring >2 mm and resemble the tip of an arrowhead as shown in $V_3$ to $V_6$.

and T-wave abnormalities are therefore associated with abnormal QRS complexes, unlike myocardial ischemia, which is a primary repolarization disorder. Figures 24.12 and 24.13 are examples of secondary ST and T-wave abnormalities. In Figure 24.12, the T waves are inverted because of left ventricular hypertrophy; in Figure 24.13, from preexcitation of the ventricles.

## Mechanism of Normal and Abnormal T Waves

- **Normal myocardium:** Because the Purkinje fibers are located subendocardially, depolarization of the myocardium is endocardial to epicardial in direction. A surface electrode overlying the myocardium will record a tall QRS complex. Although the epicardium is the last to be depolarized, it is the earliest to recover because it has the shortest action potential duration when compared to other cells in the myocardium. Because the direction of repolarization is epicardial to endocardial, this causes the T wave to be normally upright (Fig. 24.14A).
- **Myocardial ischemia:** Myocardial ischemia may alter the direction of repolarization depending on the severity of the ischemic process. This will cause changes that are confined to the T waves.

- **Subendocardial ischemia:** When myocardial ischemia is confined to the subendocardium, the direction of depolarization and repolarization is not altered and is similar to that of normal myocardium. The repolarization wave however is delayed over the area of ischemia causing the T wave to become taller and more symmetrical (Fig. 24.14B). These changes are confined to the ischemic area.
- **Transmural ischemia:** When the whole thickness of the myocardium is ischemic, the direction of the repolarization wave is not only reversed that of normal but also travels slowly causing the T wave to be deeply and symmetrically inverted (Fig. 24.14C).

## The ST Segment

- The normal ST segment is isoelectric and is at the same level as the TP and PR segments. The ST segment is abnormal when it is elevated or depressed by ≥1 mm from baseline or the configuration changes into a different pattern. Electrocardiographically, alteration involving the ST segment indicates a more advance stage of myocardial ischemia and is called myocardial injury.
- **ST elevation:** Acute coronary syndrome with ST elevation indicates that one of the three epicardial coronary arteries is totally occluded with TIMI 0 flow

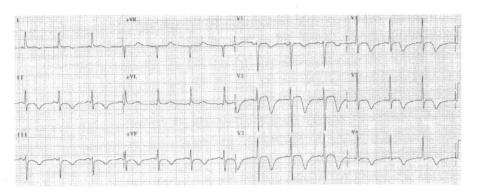

**Figure 24.10: T-Wave Inversion from non-ST Elevation MI.** The T waves are symmetrically and deeply inverted in most leads. These electrocardiogram changes are associated with elevation of the cardiac troponins consistent with non-ST elevation myocardial infarction or, more specifically, a T-wave infarct.

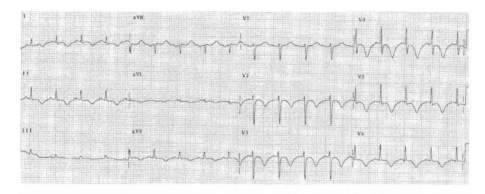

**Figure 24.11:  T-Wave Inversion from Cerebrovascular Accident Hemorrhage.** The electrocardiogram (ECG) is from a 37-year-old woman 6 months postpartum who developed a left occipital hemorrhage. Note that the T-wave inversion is deep and symmetrical in $V_2$ to $V_6$ and also in leads I, II, and aVF resembling transmural myocardial ischemia. Note the similarity of this ECG from that in Figure 24.10.

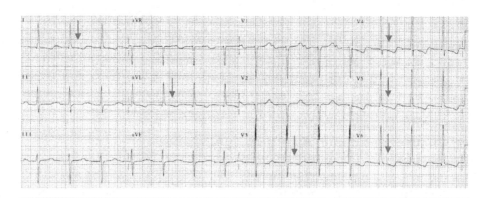

**Figure 24.12:  Secondary ST and T-Wave Abnormality.** The electrocardiogram shows left ventricular hypertrophy. Tall R waves are present with downsloping ST depression and T wave-inversion (*arrows*). These ST-T changes are secondary to abnormal activation of the ventricles.

**Figure 24.13:  Secondary T-Wave Abnormality.** Twelve-lead electrocardiogram showing preexcitation. The ST-T abnormalities (*arrows*) are secondary to abnormal activation of the ventricles.

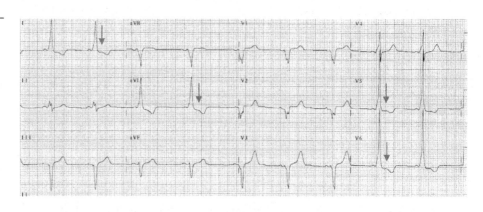

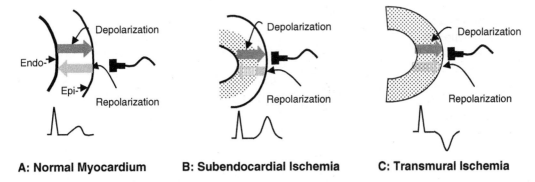

**A: Normal Myocardium    B: Subendocardial Ischemia    C: Transmural Ischemia**

**Figure 24.14:** **(A) The T Wave** Normal myocardium. Depolarization starts from endocardium to epicardium since the Purkinje fibers are located subendocardially. Repolarization is reversed and is epicardial to endocardial, thus the T wave and QRS complex are both upright. **(B) Subendocardial Ischemia.** The shaded portion represents the area of ischemia. The direction of depolarization and repolarization is similar to normal myocardium. After the repolarization wave reaches the ischemic area, the repolarization wave is delayed causing the T wave to be tall and symmetrical. **(C) Transmural Ischemia.** The direction of repolarization is reversed that of normal and is endocardial to epicardial resulting in deeply and symmetrically inverted T waves.

indicating no perfusion or antegrade flow beyond the point of occlusion. Thrombotic occlusion of the vessel lumen with ST segment elevation almost always results in cellular necrosis with elevation of the cardiac troponins in the circulation. ST elevation electrocardiographically indicates transmural or subepicardial injury, which involves the whole thickness of the myocardium.

- **ST depression:** ST depression from acute coronary syndrome electrocardiographically indicates subendocardial myocardial injury. Unlike ST elevation, which is almost always accompanied by cellular necrosis, ST depression may or may not be associated with troponin elevation. ST depression may be horizontal (Fig. 24.15A,B), downsloping (C,D), scooping (E), slow upsloping (F), or fast upsloping (G). Typical ST depression from subendocardial injury is usually

horizontal (A,B), downsloping (C), or slow upsloping (F) accompanied by depression of the J point. These types of ST segment depression, however, may be caused by other conditions that may be cardiac or noncardiac and similar to T-wave inversion, are not specific for myocardial injury.

- The typical ST depression associated with acute coronary syndrome has a horizontal or downsloping configuration with depression of the J point of at least 1 mm as shown in Figures 24.15A–C, 24.16, and 24.17. Other types of ST segment depression are less specific.

- Unlike ST elevation, ST depression from acute myocardial injury, even when accompanied by troponin elevation, is not an indication for thrombolytic therapy. It usually indicates multivessel coronary disease, including significant stenosis of the left main coronary artery.

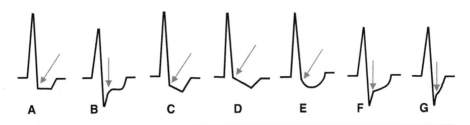

**A    B    C    D    E    F    G**

**Figure 24.15:    ST Segment Depression.** **(A, B)** Horizontal ST depression. **(C, D)** Downsloping ST segment depression. **(E)** Scooping ST segment depression frequently from digitalis effect. **(F)** Slow upsloping ST segment depression. **(G)** Fast upsloping ST segment depression frequently a normal finding. **(A, B, C, F)** Typical ischemic ST depression. **(D)** Left ventricular strain frequently associated with left ventricular hypertrophy. Arrows indicate the J point.

**Figure 24.16: ST Segment Depression.** Horizontal ST depression is seen in leads I and II and horizontal to downsloping ST depression in $V_3$ to $V_6$ consistent with subendocardial injury. Serial troponins were not elevated and the patient's symptoms were consistent with unstable angina.

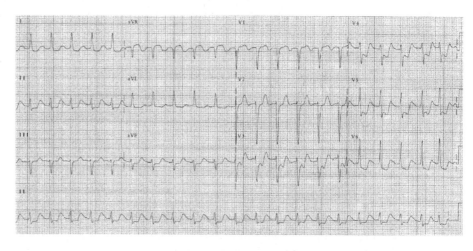

## ST Segment Depression

- **ST depression in $V_1$ to $V_3$:** Acute coronary syndrome with ST segment depression in the ECG is a contraindication to thrombolytic therapy. One exception is ST segment depression in $V_1$ to $V_3$, which may represent a true posterolateral ST elevation MI from total occlusion of the left circumflex coronary artery (Fig. 24.17). When ST segment depression is present in $V_1$ to $V_3$, special leads $V_7$ to $V_9$ should be recorded to exclude a true posterolateral MI, which represents a true ST elevation MI. This has been previously discussed in Chapter 23, Acute Coronary Syndrome: ST Elevation Myocardial Infarction (see Fig. 23.26A,B). Because leads $V_7$ to $V_9$ are not routinely recorded, ST depression confined to $V_1$ to $V_3$ can be mistaken for non-ST elevation MI or unstable angina.

- **Occlusion of the left main coronary artery:** Total occlusion of the left main coronary artery is usually fatal and most patients do not survive to reach a medical facility. Total or subtotal occlusion of the left main coronary artery will show diffuse ST segment depression in multiple leads especially $V_4$ to $V_6$ and in leads I, II, and aVL. Leads aVR and $V_1$ show elevation of the ST segments with ST elevation in aVR > ST elevation in $V_1$ (Fig. 24.18, arrows). Because these leads are not adjacent to each other, thrombolytic therapy is not indi-

cated. This type of ST segment depression may also occur when there is severe triple vessel disease. These ECG changes indicate extensive myocardial injury that will require aggressive therapy including early coronary revascularization.

- **Digitalis effect:** The scooping type of ST depression, as shown in Figure 24.19, is usually from digitalis effect.

- **Secondary ST segment depression:** Secondary ST depression from left ventricular hypertrophy with strain pattern is shown in Figure 24.20.

## Mechanism of ST Elevation and ST Depression

- Deviation of the ST segment as a result of myocardial ischemia has been ascribed to two different mechanisms namely systolic current of injury or diastolic current of injury.

## Systolic Current of Injury

- **ST elevation and ST depression from systolic current of injury:** When the myocardial cells are

**Figure 24.17: ST Segment Depression in the Anterior Precordial Leads.** The ST depression in the anterior precordial leads may represent anterior subendocardial injury, although this may also represent a true ST elevation myocardial infarction involving the left ventricle posterolaterally.

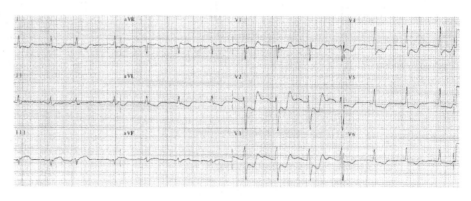

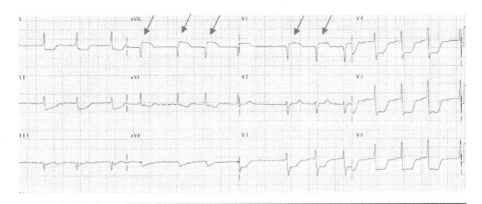

**Figure 24.18:    ST Depression from Subtotal Occlusion of the Left Main Coronary Artery.**  Twelve-lead electrocardiogram (ECG) shows atrial fibrillation and marked ST depression in multiple leads including $V_3$ to $V_6$ and leads I, II, aVL, and aVF. There is also elevation of the ST segment in leads $V_1$ and aVR. The ST elevation in aVR is higher than the ST elevation in $V_1$ (*arrows*). This type of ECG is frequently associated with subtotal occlusion of the left main coronary artery or its equivalent.

A

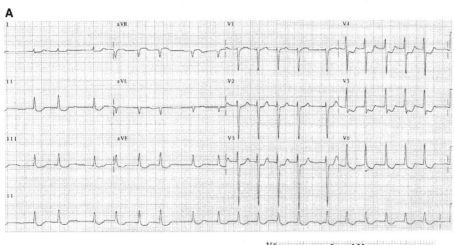

**Figure 24.19:    ST Segment Depression from Digitalis. (A)** The ST depression in leads II and $V_6$ (*arrows*) has a scooping or slow downsloping pattern. This type of ST depression is due to digitalis. **(B)** Leads II and $V_6$ are magnified to show the ST depression.

B    Lead II            Lead $V_6$

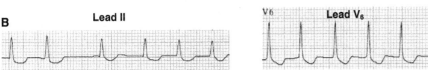

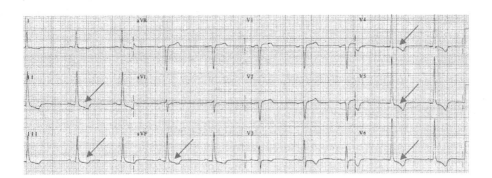

**Figure 24.20:    Left Ventricular Hypertrophy:**  Twelve-lead electrocardiogram showing left ventricular hypertrophy (LVH) with downsloping ST depression from left ventricular strain. The J point is not depressed and the ST segments have a downsloping configuration with upward convexity (*arrows*). This type of LVH is usually seen in patients with hypertension and is often described as pressure or systolic overload.

ST elevation due to systolic current of injury

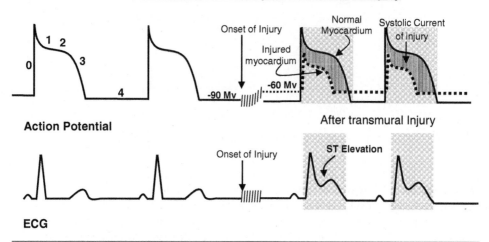

**Figure 24.21: Systolic Current of Injury.** The upper row represents transmembrane action potentials before and after myocardial injury and the lower row the corresponding electrocardiogram (ECG). A change in resting potential from –90 to approximately –60 mV will occur when cells are injured. A less negative resting potential causes the amplitude and duration of the action potential to diminish when compared to normal cells. This difference in potential creates a current of injury during electrical systole (corresponding to phases 1–3 of the action potential equivalent to the ST segment and T wave in the ECG) between normal and injured myocardium. This current flows from normal myocardium toward the injured myocardium. Thus, if the injury is subepicardial or transmural, the current of injury is directed toward the overlying electrode resulting in ST elevation. (0 to 4 represent the different phases of the action potential.)

ST elevation due to diastolic current of injury

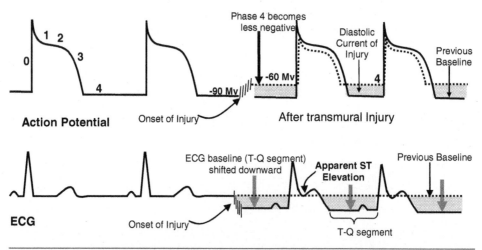

**Figure 24.22: Diastolic Current of Injury.** The yellow shaded areas in the upper and lower diagrams represent electrical diastole showing a change in resting potential from –90 to –60 mV after myocardial injury. Because the resting potential of injured cells is less negative, the cells are relatively in a state of partial depolarization. Thus, the extracellular membrane of the injured cells is more negative (less positive) compared with that of normal myocardium causing a diastolic current of injury directed away from the injured myocardium. This diastolic current of injury causes the TQ segment to be displaced downward away from the overlying electrode. When all cells are discharged during systole, the potential gradient between injured and normal cells is diminished, shifting the electrocardiogram baseline to its original position, resulting in apparent ST elevation.

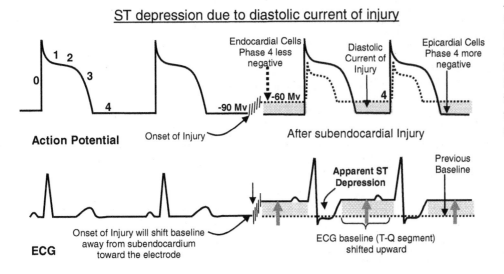

**Figure 24.23:  ST Segment Depression.** When there is subendocardial injury, the ST segment is depressed because the baseline is shifted upward away from the injured subendocardium toward the direction of the recording electrode. See text.

injured, the resting potential of injured cells is less negative compared with normal cells. A less negative resting potential will diminish the height, amplitude, and duration of the action potential (Fig. 24.21). This difference in the action potential between normal cells and injured cells creates a current of injury during electrical systole (phases 1–3 or ST segment and T wave in the ECG) that is directed *toward the injured myocardium*. Thus, if the injury is transmural or subepicardial, the injury current is directed subepicardially resulting in elevation of the ST segment in the recording ECG electrodes that overlie the area of injury (Fig. 24.21). If the injury is confined to the subendocardium, the current of injury is directed subendocardially, away from the recording electrodes, resulting in depression of the ST segment.

## Diastolic Current of Injury

- **Apparent ST segment elevation from diastolic current of injury:** The resting potential of injured myocardial cells is less negative compared with normal

cells. This difference in potential occurs during phase 4, which corresponds to the TQ segment in the ECG. Because the injured cells have a less negative resting potential, they will have a more negative (less positive) extracellular charge relative to normal myocardium. This difference in potential between normal and injured myocardium will create an electrical gradient during diastole that is directed *away from the injured cells*, toward the more positive normal myocardium. This causes the ECG baseline (TQ segment) to shift downward, away from the surface electrode overlying the area of injury (Fig. 24.22). During systole, all myocardial cells are discharged, erasing the potential difference between injured cells and normal cells. This will cause the ECG to compensate and return the ST segment to its previous baseline before the injury, resulting in apparent ST elevation. The opposite will occur if the injury is subendocardial.

- **Apparent ST segment depression from diastolic current of injury:** The mechanism of ST segment depression from subendocardial injury is shown in Figure 24.23. When there is subendocardial injury, phase 4 or resting potential of the injured subendocardial

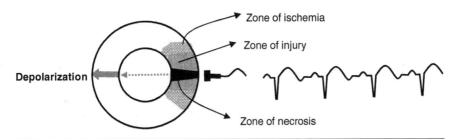

**Figure 24.24:  Q Waves.** Diagrammatic representation of a transmural infarct. The necrotic area (*black*) involves the whole thickness of the myocardium and consists of cells that cannot be depolarized. Thus, an electrode overlying the necrotic area will normally record the electrical activity on the opposite side of the myocardium (*red arrow*), resulting in q waves.

myocardial cells is less negative when compared with normal myocardial cells. This difference in potential between normal and injured myocardium will create an electrical gradient during diastole. Because the injured cells are in a state of partial depolarization, a diastolic current of injury is directed *away from the injured subendocardium* toward the normal subepicardium causing the TQ segment to shift upward toward the surface electrode overlying the ischemic area. During systole, all myocardial cells are discharged simultaneously, erasing the diastolic gradient between injured cells and normal cells. This will cause the ECG to compensate and return the ST segment to its previous baseline before the injury, resulting in apparent ST segment depression (Fig. 24.23).

- In summary, the direction of *systolic* current of injury is always *toward* the injured myocardium, whereas *diastolic* current of injury, equivalent to the TQ segment, is always directed *away* from the injured myocardium.

## Q Waves

- **Pathologic Q waves:** Pathologic Q waves can be prevented if the ischemic process is relieved within a timely fashion. However, if myocardial injury progresses, myocardial necrosis will occur resulting in pathologic Q waves. Electrocardiographically, Q waves indicate transmural myocardial necrosis, which signify permanent myocardial damage and are usually not reversible. However, some Q waves may reverse because of contraction of the scar tissue during the healing process. Additionally, the injured myocardium may be temporarily stunned during the acute episode and may be unable to conduct an electrical impulse locally, which may be transient and reversible. Pathologic Q waves is the usual sequelae of ST elevation MI, although it may also occur in approximately 25% of patients with non-ST elevation MI. Abnormal Q waves have been previously discussed in Chapter 23, Acute Coronary Syndrome: ST Elevation Myocardial Infarction.
- **Summary of the evolution of the ECG in acute coronary syndrome:**
  - **T-wave abnormalities:** Alterations confined to the T waves indicate *myocardial ischemia*. These T-wave abnormalities are reversible. However, if the ischemic process continues unabated, alterations in the ST segment will follow.
  - **ST segment abnormalities:** Changes involving the ST segment suggest a more advance stage of myocardial ischemia and indicate *myocardial injury*. Alterations involving the ST segment and T wave may be reversible. However, if the ischemic process continues unrelieved, changes in the QRS complex will follow.

- **Q waves:** Q waves indicate the presence of *myocardial necrosis* and are usually not reversible.

## Non-ST Elevation MI and Unstable Angina

### ECG of Non-ST Elevation MI and Unstable Angina

1. J point and ST segment depression of ≥1 mm below baseline.
2. Symmetrically inverted T waves measuring ≥2 mm.
3. The ST and T wave abnormalities may be less specific.

### Mechanism

- **Normal ventricular myocardium:** Unlike the single muscle cell where depolarization and repolarization occur in the same direction, depolarization and repolarization of the normal ventricular myocardium occur in opposite directions. Thus, depolarization of the myocardium is endocardial to epicardial because the impulse originates from the Purkinje fibers, which are located subendocardially. An electrode overlying the myocardium will record a tall QRS complex. Although the epicardium is the last to be depolarized, it is the earliest to recover because it has shorter action potential duration compared to other cells in the myocardium. Thus, the repolarization wave travels from epicardium to endocardium, away from the recording electrode resulting in upright T wave in the ECG. In addition to the shorter action potential duration of epicardial cells, there are other reasons why the epicardium recovers earlier than the endocardium, even if the epicardium is the last to be depolarized.
  - The subendocardium has a higher rate of metabolism, thus requiring more oxygen when compared with the epicardium.
  - The subendocardium is the deepest portion of the myocardium and is farthest from the coronary circulation.
  - The subendocardium is immediately adjacent to the ventricular cavities. Because the ventricles generate the highest pressure in the cardiovascular system, the subendocardium is subject to a higher tension than the epicardium.
  - Repolarization (the ST segment and T wave) occurs during systole when the myocardium is mechanically contracting. There is no significant myocardial perfusion during systole especially in the subendocardium at the time of repolarization.
- **Myocardial ischemia:** Myocardial ischemia is a pathologic condition resulting from an imbalance between oxygen supply and demand. Depending on the severity of myocardial ischemia, the ECG changes may involve the T wave, the ST segment, or the QRS complex. Changes confined to the T waves are traditionally called myocardial ischemia. Alterations in the ST segment are described as myocardial injury and when

the QRS complex is altered with development of pathologic Q waves or decreased amplitude of the R wave, the abnormality is myocardial necrosis.

- **Changes involving the T waves:** Changes affecting only the T waves indicate myocardial ischemia, which may be subendocardial resulting in tall T waves or transmural resulting in deeply inverted T waves. An abnormal T wave associated with troponin elevation is consistent with non-ST elevation MI or more specifically, a T-wave infarct.

  - **Subendocardial ischemia:** The endocardial cells immediately adjacent to the ventricular cavities are able to extract nutrients directly from blood within the ventricles. Thus, it is the deeper subendocardial cells and not the endocardium itself that are at risk for myocardial ischemia. When there is subendocardial ischemia, the repolarization wave is not significantly altered and normally starts from epicardium to endocardium resulting in upright T waves. The repolarization wave, however, is delayed after it reaches the ischemic area, causing the T wave to be symmetrical and taller than normal in leads overlying the area of ischemia.

  - **Transmural or subepicardial ischemia:** If the ischemia is transmural involving the whole thickness of the myocardium, the direction of the repolarization wave is reversed, starting from endocardium to epicardium, causing the T wave to become deeply inverted instead of upright. Because the duration of the action potential of ischemic cells becomes longer than normal, the repolarization wave travels slowly causing the T wave to be symmetrical with slightly prolonged QT.

- **Changes involving the ST segment:** Changes in the ST segment indicate myocardial injury, which is a more advanced form of myocardial ischemia. Myocardial injury may be transmural resulting in ST segment elevation or it may be subendocardial, resulting in ST segment depression.

  - **Transmural or subepicardial injury:** Transmural or subepicardial injury causes the ST segment to become elevated. ST elevation is a more severe form of myocardial injury, which is almost always associated with troponin elevation consistent with ST elevation MI. Elevation of the ST segment may be due to systolic or diastolic current of injury.

    - **Systolic current of injury:** Systolic current of injury occurs during phases 1 through 3 of the action potential corresponding to the ST segment and T wave in the ECG. *Systolic current of injury always points to the direction of the injured myocardium.* This causes the ST segment to become elevated in leads overlying the area of injury.

    - **Diastolic current of injury:** Diastolic current of injury occurs during phase 4 of the action potential corresponding to the T-Q segment in the ECG. *Diastolic current of injury is always directed away from the area of injury.* Thus, the baseline or T-Q segment of the ECG is shifted downward, away

from the recording surface electrode overlying the area of injury. During electrical systole corresponding to the QT interval in the ECG, all cells are depolarized, eliminating all the electrical charges of both injured cells and normal cells. This will cause the ECG to compensate and return the ST segment back to its previous baseline before the injury, resulting in apparent ST elevation. In pericarditis, only the epicardial cells are injured. The endocardial cells remain preserved. A diastolic current of injury will flow from epicardium to endocardium, away from the injured area and away from the recording surface electrodes. This will similarly cause the baseline T-Q segment to shift downward. During electrical systole, apparent ST segment elevation will occur as the ECG returns to its previous baseline.

  - **Subendocardial injury:** Subendocardial injury depresses the ST segment and represents a less severe form of myocardial injury involving the subendocardium. ST depression with troponin elevation is non-ST elevation MI. More specifically, it is an ST depression MI. Depression of the ST segment may be due to systolic or diastolic current of injury.

    - **Systolic current of injury:** *Systolic current of injury always flows toward the area of injury.* Thus, a current of injury flows from normal myocardium (subepicardium) toward the subendocardium, *away* from the recording surface electrode, resulting in depression of the ST segment.

    - **Diastolic current of injury:** *Diastolic current of injury flows in the opposite direction, which is away from the injured myocardium.* Thus, during electrical diastole, the current of injury will flow away from subendocardium toward normal myocardium (subepicardium) in the direction of the recording electrode, shifting the T-Q segment upward. During electrical systole, all cells are discharged, eliminating the potential difference between injured cells and normal cells. This will cause the ECG to compensate and return the ST segment downward to its previous baseline before the injury, resulting in apparent ST depression.

- **Changes involving the QRS complex:** If myocardial ischemia is not relieved and collateral flow is not adequate, myocardial injury will progress irreversibly to myocardial necrosis resulting in alteration of the QRS complex. Thus, changes in the QRS complex resulting in pathologic Q waves or diminished amplitude of the R wave represent transmural myocardial necrosis. These changes are usually permanent. Cells that are necrotic or infarcted do not depolarize or conduct electrical activity. If an electrode is positioned over a necrotic myocardium, Q waves or QS complexes will be recorded, which represent activation of normal myocardium away and opposite the infarcted area, causing a negative deflection in the ECG.

## Clinical Implications

- Myocardial ischemia with elevation of the ST segment is due to complete occlusion of the vessel lumen. When blood supply is completely interrupted for a duration of more than 20 minutes, myocardial necrosis always occurs and troponin elevation is always expected.

- Myocardial ischemia with depression of the ST segment or inversion of the T wave may be due to either diminished coronary flow or increased myocardial oxygen demand or a combination of both. It may also be due to a completely occluded artery, but has collateral flow. These ST and T wave abnormalities may or may not be associated with troponin elevation, depending on the severity of myocardial ischemia. When cardiac troponins are elevated in the circulation, non-ST elevation MI is present. If the troponins are not elevated, the clinical picture is one of unstable angina. These patients with non-ST elevation MI or unstable angina may not show any abnormalities in the ECG.

- Unlike ST segment elevation and pathologic Q waves, T-wave inversion is not specific for myocardial ischemia. Although deep and symmetrical T-wave inversions measuring ≥2 mm are typical for myocardial ischemia, ischemic-looking T waves may be seen in patients without ischemic heart disease.

- ST depression from myocardial injury usually measures ≥1 mm. The ST depression may be horizontal, downsloping, or slow upsloping in configuration. The J point (junction between the QRS complex and ST segment) should be depressed by ≥1 mm if the ST depression is from myocardial ischemia. ST depression is less specific if the J point is not depressed or if the J point is depressed by <0.5 mm. ST depression is not only the result of myocardial ischemia, but could also be due to the effect of drugs such as digitalis, antiarrhythmic agents, Ritalin, and tricyclic antidepressants. ST depression can also occur in patients with cardiac diseases not due to ischemia such as left ventricular hypertrophy, electrolyte abnormalities, mitral valve prolapse, and other noncardiac abnormalities, including anemia.

- The severity of ST depression and T wave inversion provide important diagnostic and prognostic information. For example, patients with ST depression ≥0.5 mm have higher morbidity and mortality compared to patients with T wave inversion or those without ECG findings.

- Although ST elevation MI is synonymous with a Q wave MI, not all patients with ST elevation will develop Q waves. Additionally, approximately 25% of patients with non-ST elevation MI will also develop Q waves. The rest (75%) will have a non-Q wave MI. Thus, ST elevation MI and non-ST elevation MI are preferred over Q wave and non-Q wave MI. Similarly, Hurst emphasizes that non-ST elevation MI, which is the terminology used in the American College of Cardiology/American Heart Association (ACC/AHA) guidelines, does not specify the abnormality present in the ECG. Thus, when a non-ST elevation MI occurs, he prefers to identify the infarct either as a T-wave MI or ST depression MI rather than a non-ST elevation MI.

- The infarct related artery can be predicted using the 12-lead ECG when there is ST elevation MI, T-wave MI, or Q-wave MI. Identifying the culprit vessel is more difficult when the MI is associated with ST segment depression. Very often, myocardial ischemia with ST segment depression is due to multivessel coronary disease, including the possibility of a significant left main coronary artery lesion.

## Treatment

- Unlike ST elevation MI, which indicates that the coronary artery is completely occluded and there is urgency in immediately establishing coronary flow with a thrombolytic agent or primary PCI, non-ST elevation MI and unstable angina indicate that the coronary artery is partially occluded, resulting in imbalance between oxygen supply and demand. Thus, the patient can be initially risk stratified so that patients who are high risk for reinfarction or death should undergo an early invasive strategy, whereas patients who are not identified as being high risk can undergo an early conservative approach.

  - **Early conservative:** The early conservative approach includes mainly medical therapy. Cardiac catheterization is reserved only when there is evidence of continuing ischemia either spontaneously occurring or exercise induced in spite of intensive medical therapy.

  - **Early invasive:** The early aggressive approach includes medical therapy and an early invasive strategy with cardiac catheterization and revascularization of the occluded vessel performed within 4 to 24 hours after the patient is hospitalized regardless of the presence or absence of continuing ischemia.

- **High-risk patients:** According to the ACC/AHA 2007 guidelines for the management of patients with unstable angina and non-ST elevation MI, high-risk patients include any of the following findings:

  - Recurrent angina or ischemia at rest or with low-level activities despite intensive medical therapy

  - Elevated cardiac biomarkers

  - New or presumably new ST depression

  - Signs or symptoms of heart failure or new or worsening mitral regurgitation

  - High-risk findings from noninvasive testing

  - Hemodynamically unstable patient

  - Sustained ventricular tachycardia

  - Left ventricular dysfunction with ejection fraction of <40%

  - Previous PCI within 6 months

  - Prior coronary artery bypass surgery

  - High risk score using risk stratification models

- **Antiplatelet and anticoagulant therapy:** Antithrombotic agents are the mainstay in the therapy of patients with non-ST

**TABLE 24.1**

**Summary of the Initial and Maintenance Doses of Aspirin and Clopidogrel according to the American College of Cardiology/American Hospital Association 2007 Guidelines on Non-ST Elevation Myocardial Infarction and Unstable Angina**

| | Medically Treated (No Stent) | Percutaneous Coronary Intervention | | |
|---|---|---|---|---|
| | | Bare Metal Stent | Sirolimus Stent | Paclitaxel Stent |
| Aspirin (initial dose) | 162–325 mg | 162–325 mg | 162–325 mg | 162–325 mg |
| Minimum duration | | 162–325 mg for ≥1 month | 162–325 mg for ≥3 months | 162–325 mg for ≥6 months |
| Maintenance dose | 75–162 mg daily indefinitely | 75–162 mg daily indefinitely | 75–162 mg daily indefinitely | 75–162 mg daily indefinitely |
| Clopidogrel (initial dose) | 300–600 mg loading dose | 300–600 mg loading dose | 300–600 mg loading dose | 300–600 mg loading dose |
| Minimum duration | 75 mg daily for ≥1 month | 75 mg daily for ≥1 month | 75 mg daily for ≥12 months | 75 mg daily for ≥12 months |
| Maintenance dose | Ideally up to 12 months | Ideally up to 12 months | Ideally up to 12 months | Ideally up to 12 months |

elevation MI and unstable angina, whether or not an early conservative or a more aggressive strategy is used.

- **Aspirin:** Aspirin should be given as soon as possible, often in the prehospital setting when diagnosis of acute coronary syndrome is suspected. The initial dose of aspirin is 162 to 325 mg of plain (nonenteric coated) aspirin given orally.

  □ **Medically treated patients:** Among patients who are treated medically and are not stented, aspirin is continued at a dose of 75 to 162 mg daily indefinitely.

  □ **Stented patients:** In patients undergoing PCI with stent placement, the dose of enteric-coated aspirin depends on the type of stent used.

  □ **Bare metal stent:** Aspirin is given at a dose of 162 to 325 mg daily given for at least 1 month if a bare metal stent was deployed. This is followed by 75 to 162 mg daily indefinitely.

  □ **Drug-eluting stent:** The dose of aspirin is 162 to 325 mg daily for at least 3 months if a sirolimus-coated stent was deployed and for at least 6 months for paclitaxel-coated stent. This is followed by a maintenance dose of 75 to 162 mg daily indefinitely.

- **Clopidogrel:** The loading dose of clopidogrel is usually 300 mg given orally. A higher loading dose of 600 to 900 mg inhibits platelets more rapidly, although its safety and clinical efficacy needs to be established.

  □ **Medically treated patients:** Among medically treated patients who are not stented, 75 mg of clopidogrel is given daily for at least 1 month and ideally up to 1 year. Clopidogrel should not be given or should be discontinued for 5 to 7 days in patients undergoing coronary bypass surgery.

  □ **Bare metal stent:** Clopidogrel is given at a maintenance dose of 75 mg/day for at least 1 month and ideally up to 1 year for patients who have bare metal stents.

  □ **Drug-eluting stent:** The maintenance dose is 75 mg daily for at least 1 year.

- Table 24.1 summarizes the initial dose, minimum duration, and maintenance dose of aspirin and clopidogrel according to the ACC/AHA 2007 guidelines on non-ST elevation MI and unstable angina.

- **Unfractionated heparin or low-molecular-weight heparin**

  □ **Patients undergoing PCI:** Intravenous unfractionated heparin or subcutaneous low-molecular-weight heparin in addition to aspirin and clopidogrel is a Class I recommendation in patients undergoing PCI. Enoxaparin, a low-molecular-weight heparin, is preferred to unfractionated heparin except when there is renal failure or when bypass surgery is planned within 24 hours. The use of bivalirudin or fondaparinux also receives a Class I recommendation.

  □ **Patients not undergoing PCI:** The use of unfractionated heparin, enoxaparin, and fondaparinux among patients who are treated conservatively also receives a Class I recommendation. Fondaparinux is the preferred agent when there is increased risk of bleeding. Enoxaparin and fondaparinux is preferred over unfractionated heparin unless bypass surgery is being planned within 24 hours.

- **IIb/IIIa antagonists:**

  □ **Patients undergoing PCI:** The use of IIb/IIIa platelet antagonists such as abciximab (ReoPro), eptifibatide

(Integrilin), or tirofiban (Aggrastat) is a Class I indication for patients with acute coronary syndrome undergoing PCI.

☐ **Patients not undergoing PCI:** For patients not undergoing PCI, IIb/IIIa antagonists can also be given as medical therapy to high-risk patients in addition to aspirin and clopidogrel. Patients appear to benefit with tirofiban or eptifibatide (Class IIb recommendation), but not with abciximab. The use of abciximab, therefore, as medical treatment of acute coronary syndrome in patients who are not undergoing PCI is not recommended (Class III).

■ **Thrombolytic agents:** Thrombolytic agents such as alteplase, streptokinase, reteplase, or tenecteplase are contraindicated in non-ST elevation MI and unstable angina.

■ In addition to the use of antiplatelet agents, the general medical therapy of non-ST elevation MI and unstable angina is similar to that of ST elevation MI because both entities have the same pathophysiologic substrate: plaque rupture with thrombotic occlusion of the vessel lumen. General medical therapy for patients with non-ST elevation MI and unstable angina are similar and include:

■ **Oxygen:** Oxygen is initially given to patients with hypoxemia or arterial oxygen saturation of <90% or those of questionable respiratory status.

■ **Nitroglycerin:** Nitroglycerin 0.4 mg sublingual tablets or spray 5 minutes apart for 3 doses followed IV if there are symptoms of ischemia. The IV infusion is started at 10 mcg/minute and increased by 10 mcg/minute every 3 to 5 minutes until symptoms are improved or systolic blood pressure drops. No definite maximum dose is recommended although the top dose is usually 200 mcg/minute.

■ **Morphine:** Morphine sulfate 1 to 5 mg IV may be given if chest pain is not relieved after three sublingual nitroglycerin tablets or chest pain recurs in spite of anti-ischemic therapy. This may be repeated every 5 to 30 minutes if necessary. Although morphine sulfate continues to be a Class I indication for patients with ST elevation MI, the more recent ACC/AHA 2007 guidelines on non-ST elevation MI has downgraded the use of morphine for ischemic pain associated with non-ST elevation MI and unstable angina from Class I to Class IIa.

■ **Beta blockers:** The latest 2007 AHA/ACC guidelines recommend that beta blockers should be given orally within the first 24 hours when there are no contraindications. Contraindications to beta blocker therapy include PR interval >0.24 seconds, second degree atrioventricular block or higher, severe left ventricular dysfunction, or history of asthma. The agent should be gradually titrated in patients with moderate left ventricular dysfunction. Intravenous beta blockers should be used cautiously and avoided when there is heart failure, hypotension, or hemodynamic instability.

■ **Renin-angiotensin antagonists:** Angiotensin-converting enzyme inhibitors or angiotensin receptor blockers and aldosterone antagonists should be given when there is associated left ventricular dysfunction in the absence of contraindications.

■ **Statins:** Statins to lower the low-density lipoprotein to a target goal of <70 mg/dL.

■ Patients who continue to have ischemia, the following agents or procedures can be given:

■ A combination of nitrates and beta blockers are the drugs of choice for myocardial ischemia.

■ Calcium blockers are second- or third-line agents:

☐ Calcium channel blockers may be given if ischemia is not relieved by nitrates and beta blockers.

☐ Nondihydropyridine calcium antagonists such as verapamil and diltiazem are given when beta blockers are contraindicated.

☐ Calcium channel blockers should not be given when there is evidence of left ventricular dysfunction.

☐ Intra-aortic balloon pump may be used for severe ischemia not responsive to medical therapy.

☐ Oxygen and morphine sulfate is usually given as part of general medical therapy

## Prognosis

■ Non-ST elevation MI and unstable angina have a lower in-hospital mortality of approximately 1% to 3% when compared with ST elevation MI. Myocardial involvement is less extensive and left ventricular systolic function is usually preserved.

■ Non-ST elevation MI is associated with a higher recurrence of cardiovascular events after hospital discharge compared with ST elevation MI and exacts a higher post-hospital mortality. Although ST elevation MI has a higher initial mortality, overall mortality of ST and non-ST elevation MI will be similar after a 2- to 3-year follow-up. Patients with non-ST elevation MI and unstable angina who are high risk for cardiovascular events should be identified so that they can be revascularized.

## Suggested Readings

Anderson JL, Adams CD, Antman EM, et al. ACC/AHA 2007 guidelines for the management of patients with unstable angina/non-ST elevation myocardial infarction: a report of the American College of Cardiology/American Heart Association Task Force on Practice Guidelines (Writing Committee to Revise the 2002 Guidelines for the Management of Patients with Unstable Angina/Non-ST Elevation Myocardial Infarction). *J Am Coll Cardiol.* 2007;50:e1–e157.

Birnbaum Y, Solodky A, Hertz I, et al. Implications of inferior ST-segment depression in anterior acute myocardial infarction: electrocardiographic and angiographic correlation. *Am Heart J.* 1994;127:1467–1473.

Braunwald E, Antman EM, Beasley JW, et al. ACC/AHA guidelines for the management of patients with unstable angina and non-ST segment elevation myocardial infarction: a report of the ACC/AHA Task Force on Practice Guidelines (Committee on the Management of Patients with Unstable Angina). *J Am Coll Cardiol*. 2000;36:970–1062.

Braunwald E, Antman EM, Beasley JW, et al. ACC/AHA 2002 guideline update for the management of patients with unstable angina and non-ST segment elevation myocardial infarction: Summary article: a report of the ACC/AHA Task Force on Practice Guidelines (Committee on the Management of Patients with Unstable Angina. *Circulation*. 2002;106:1893–1900.

Channer K, Morris F. ABC of clinical electrocardiography. Myocardial ischaemia. *BMJ*. 2002;324:1023–1026.

Dunn MI, Lipman BS. Myocardial Infarction, injury and ischemia. In: *Clinical Electrocardiography*. 8th ed. Chicago: Year Book Medical Publishers, Inc; 1989:160–209.

Edhouse J, Brady WJ, Morris F. ABC of clinical electrocardiography. Acute myocardial infarction-Part II. *BMJ*. 2002;324:963–966.

Goldberger A, Goldberger E. Myocardial ischemia and infarction I and II. *Clinical Electrocardiography*. 5th ed. St. Louis: Mosby-Year Book, Inc. 1994:87–122.

Grines CL, Bonow RO, Casey DE, et al. Prevention of premature discontinuation of dual antiplatelet therapy in patients with coronary artery stents: a science advisory from the American Heart Association, American College of Cardiology, Society for Cardiovascular Angiography and Interventions, American College of Surgeons, and American Dental Association, with representation from the American College of Physicians. *J Am Coll Cardiol*. 2007;49:734–739.

Hurst JW. Abnormalities of the S-T segment—part I. *Clin Cardiol*. 1997;20:511–520.

Hurst JW. Abnormalities of the S-T segment—part II. *Clin Cardiol*. 1997;20:595–600.

Hurst JW. Thoughts about the ventricular gradient and its current clinical use (part I of II). *Clin Cardiol*. 2005;28:175–180.

Hurst JW. Thoughts about the ventricular gradient and its current clinical use (part II of II). *Clin Cardiol*. 2005;28:219–224.

Hurst JW. Thoughts about the abnormalities in the electrocardiogram of patients with acute myocardial infarction with emphasis on a more accurate method of interpreting ST segment displacement: part I. *Clin Cardiol*. 2007;30:381–390.

Hurst JW. Thoughts about the abnormalities in the electrocardiogram of patients with acute myocardial infarction with emphasis on a more accurate method of interpreting ST segment displacement: part II. *Clin Cardiol*. 2007;30:443–449.

The Joint European Society of Cardiology/American College of Cardiology Committee. Myocardial infarction redefined—a consensus document of the joint European Society of Cardiology/American College of Cardiology Committee for the redefinition of myocardial infarction. *J Am Coll Cardiol* 2000;36:959–969.

Mirvis DM, Goldberger AL. Electrocardiography. In: Zipes DP, Libby P, Bonow RO, et al, eds. *Braunwald's Heart Disease, A Textbook of Cardiovascular Medicine*. 7th ed. Philadelphia: Elsevier/Saunders; 2005:107–148.

Morris F, Brady WJ. ABC of clinical electrocardiography. Acute myocardial infarction—part I. *BMJ*. 2002;324:831–834.

Nomenclature and criteria for diagnosis of ischemic heart disease. Report of the Joint International Society and Federation of Cardiology/World Health Organization task force on standardization of clinical nomenclature. *Circulation*. 1979;59:607–609.

Sgarbossa EB, Wagner GS. Electrocardiography. In: Topol EJ, ed. *Textbook of Cardiovascular Medicine*. 2nd ed. Philadelphia: Lippincott Williams & Wilkins; 2002:1329–1363.

Wagner GS. Ischemia and injury due to insufficient blood supply. In: *Marriott's Practical Electrocardiography*. 10th ed. Philadelphia: Lippincott Williams & Wilkins; 2001:163–178.

Yan G-X, Antzelevitch C. Cellular basis for the normal T wave and the electrocardiographic manifestations of the long-QT syndrome. *Circulation*. 1998;98:1928–1936.

Yan G-X, Lankipalli RS, Burke JF, et al. Ventricular repolarization components on the electrocardiogram. Cellular basis and clinical significance. *J Am Coll Cardiol*. 2003;42:401–409.

# Electrolyte Abnormalities

## Hyperkalemia

- Among the various electrolyte abnormalities, hyperkalemia, hypokalemia, hypercalcemia, and hypocalcemia are the only disorders that can cause reliable diagnostic changes in the electrocardiogram (ECG). These ECG changes can be recognized well before the results of the laboratory tests become available. The severity of these electrolyte abnormalities usually parallels the changes in the ECG.

- A simple rule to remember regarding the effect of these electrolyte abnormalities on the ECG is that when increased levels are present (hyperkalemia or hypercalcemia), the QT interval is shortened. Inversely, when decreased levels of these electrolytes are present (hypokalemia or hypocalcemia), the QT interval is prolonged. Figure 25.1 shows the ECG abnormalities associated with each of these electrolyte disorders.

- The normal level of serum potassium varies from 3.3 to 5.3 millimoles per liter (mmol/L), also expressed as milliequivalents per liter (mEq/L). Hyperkalemia implies the presence of higher than normal levels of serum potassium.

- Among the electrolyte disorders, hyperkalemia is the most fatal. It also exhibits the most remarkable changes in the ECG. The ECG abnormalities generally reflect the increasing severity of the hyperkalemia, thus the ECG is useful not only in the diagnosis of this electrolyte disorder, but is also helpful in determining the intensity in which hyperkalemia should be treated.

- Figure 25.2 is a diagrammatic representation of the ECG changes associated with increasing levels of potassium in the serum.

  - **Mild hyperkalemia (<6.0 mmol/L):** Peaking of the T waves occurs and may be the earliest and only abnormality that can be recognized. The QT interval is normal or shortened (Fig. 25.2B).

  - **Moderate hyperkalemia (6.0 to 7.0 mmol/L):** More pronounced peaking of the T waves occur, QRS complexes widen, P waves become broader with diminished amplitude, and PR interval lengthens resulting in atrioventricular (AV) block (Fig. 25.2C).

**Figure 25.1: Electrolyte Abnormalities.** Only disorders of potassium and calcium can be reliably diagnosed in the electrocardiogram. When the serum level of these electrolytes is increased (hyperkalemia and hypercalcemia), the QT interval is shortened, whereas when the serum level is low (hypokalemia and hypocalcemia), the QT interval is prolonged.

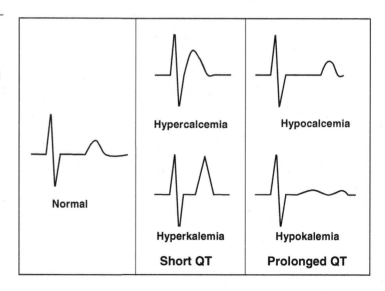

Normal

Hypercalcemia

Hypocalcemia

Hyperkalemia

Hypokalemia

Short QT

Prolonged QT

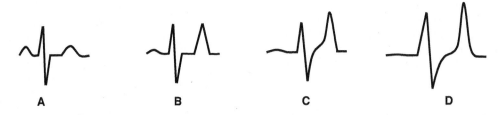

**Figure 25.2:** **The Electrocardiogram of Hyperkalemia.** Diagram depicts the electrocardiogram changes as the level of hyperkalemia increases. **(A)** Normal, **(B)** mild to moderate hyperkalemia, **(C)** moderate, and **(D)** severe hyperkalemia.

- **Severe hyperkalemia (>7.0 mmol/L):** P waves become unrecognizable, further widening of the QRS complex occurs, S and T waves merge with a very short ST segment resulting in a sinusoidal wave, ST segment may be elevated in $V_{1-2}$ and mistaken for acute ischemic injury, and, finally, slowing of the heart rate, asystole, or ventricular flutter can occur (Fig. 25.2D).

- **Mild hyperkalemia (<6.0 mmol/L):** Peaking of the T waves is the earliest to occur and is the most characteristic ECG pattern of hyperkalemia. Hyperkalemic T waves are often described as "tented" because they closely resemble the shape of a tent. The T waves are tall and symmetrical with a pointed tip and a narrow base (Fig. 25.3–25.5). The QT interval is generally short, unless coexisting abnormalities such as hypocalcemia or myocardial disease are present.

- **Moderate hyperkalemia (6.0 to 7.0 mmol/L):** As the level of serum potassium increases, the amplitude of the T wave also increases and often the height of the T wave becomes taller than the R wave. The T waves are tallest in precordial leads $V_{2-4}$, because of the proximity of these leads to the myocardium (Figs. 25.5–25.7).

- The onset of the P wave and QRS abnormalities is more difficult to predict than the T wave changes. In general, the P waves and QRS complexes start to widen when moderate hyperkalemia is present, as conduction through the atria and ventricles becomes delayed (Fig. 25.7).

- **Severe hyperkalemia (>7.0 mmol/L):** When the potassium level increases to >7.0 mmol/L, the amplitude of the P wave decreases until the P waves are no longer detectable. The absence of P waves in spite of normal sinus rhythm is due to marked slowing of the sinus impulse across the atria or the sinus impulse traveling through specialized internodal pathways. Sinoventricular rhythm is the term used to describe sinus rhythm without any discernible P waves. Sinoventricular rhythm is impossible to distinguish from junctional rhythm when the QRS complexes are narrow or from accelerated ventricular rhythm when the QRS complexes are wide.

- Other ECG changes associated with severe hyperkalemia are shown in Figs. 25.7 through 25.15:
  - Further widening of the QRS complex, shortening of the ST segment and fusion of the S wave with the T wave resembling a sine wave (Figs. 25.7, 25.12, and 25.13).
  - P waves completely disappear in spite of the rhythm being normal sinus, resulting in sinoventricular rhythm (Figs. 25.8, 25.10–25.15).
  - ST segment elevation mimicking acute ischemic injury can occur, especially in the right sided precordial leads $V_{1-2}$ (Fig. 25.9).
  - Severe bradycardia (Figs. 25.10–25.15) or ventricular flutter/fibrillation may occur.

- Figures 25.11 through 25.13 are from the same patient showing increasing levels of potassium.

- Figures 25.14 and 25.15 show very high potassium levels, which can lead to cardiac arrest.

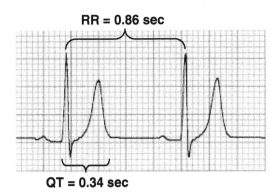

**RR = 0.86 sec**

**QT = 0.34 sec**

**Figure 25.3:** **"Tented" T waves.** The most distinctive abnormality in hyperkalemia is the presence of tented T waves characterized by tall, peaked, and symmetrical T waves with a narrow base and short QT interval. In the above example, the QT interval measures 0.34 seconds.

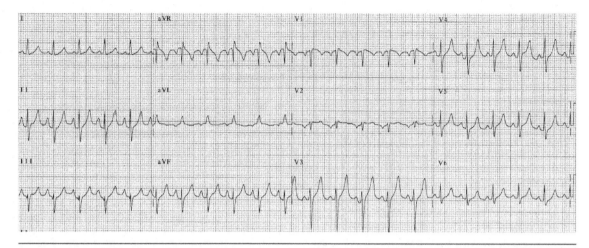

**Figure 25.4:  Mild Hyperkalemia.** The most significant electrocardiogram finding of mild hyperkalemia is the presence of peaked T waves in virtually all leads with upright T waves as shown.

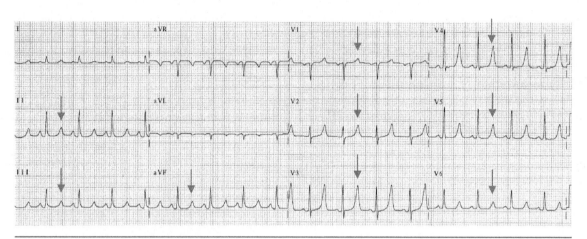

**Figure 25.5:  Moderate Hyperkalemia.** Potassium level is 6.6 mmol/L. Peaking of the T waves (*arrows*) is noted diffusely. The T waves are tented with a pointed tip and a narrow base. The T waves measure 10 mm in $V_3$ and are taller than the QRS complexes.

**A.** Before therapy ($V_1$-$V_6$)    **B.** After therapy ($V_1$-$V_6$)

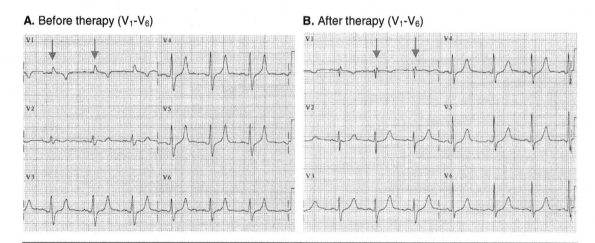

**Figure 25.6:  Wide QRS Complex.** **(A)** Before therapy, the potassium level is 6.6 mmol/L. The QRS complexes in the precordial leads are wide measuring 124 milliseconds. The R waves are upright in $V_1$ (*arrows*). **(B)** Posttherapy, potassium level is 4.6 mmol/L. The QRS complexes are narrower and the tall R waves in $V_1$ are no longer present (*arrows*). ms, milliseconds.

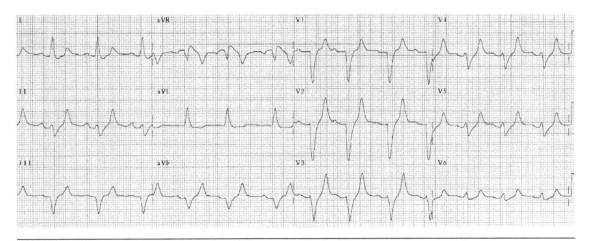

**Figure 25.7:    Severe Hyperkalemia with Widening of the QRS Complexes.** Potassium level is 7.6 mmol/L. The PR interval is slightly prolonged. The QRS complexes are wide with marked peaking of the T waves. The S wave continues directly into the T wave in leads II, aVF, and $V_2$ to $V_5$, resembling a sine wave.

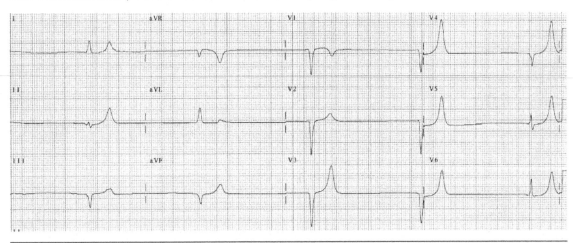

**Figure 25.8:    Marked Bradycardia in a Patient with Severe Hyperkalemia.** Potassium level is 8.3 mmol/L. The QRS complexes are widened and are not preceded by P waves. There is marked peaking of the T waves, which is the hallmark of hyperkalemia. The rhythm is often called junctional, but is impossible to differentiate from sinoventricular rhythm, which is sinus rhythm without discernible P waves.

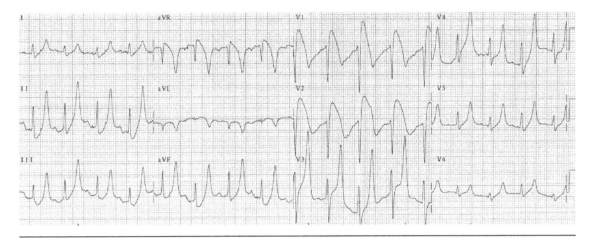

**Figure 25.9:    Severe Hyperkalemia with ST Elevation in $V_1V_2$ Resembling Acute ST Elevation Myocardial Infarction.** Potassium level is 8.6 mmol/L. The T waves are markedly peaked in all leads especially $V_1$ to $V_5$, II, III, and aVF. The T wave in $V_3$ measures almost 25 mm and most T waves are taller than the QRS complexes. ST segment elevation in $V_{1-2}$ can be mistaken for acute myocardial infarction or the ST elevation associated with the Brugada electrocardiogram.

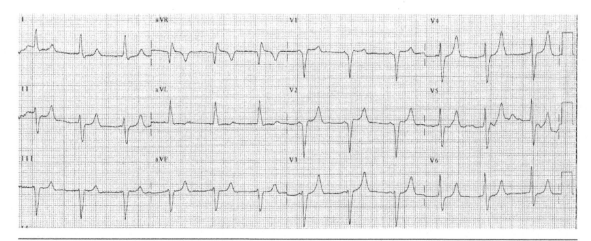

**Figure 25.10:    Absent P waves and Wide QRS Complexes in Severe Hyperkalemia.** Potassium level is 9.0 mmol/L. P waves are absent and the QRS complexes are wide with a left bundle branch block configuration. The rhythm is often called sinoventricular, although this is difficult to differentiate from accelerated idioventricular rhythm.

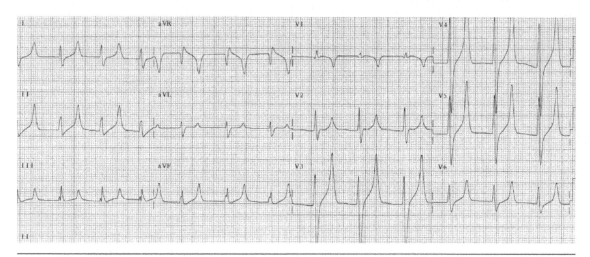

**Figure 25.11:    Generalized Peaking of the T Waves is the Hallmark of Hyperkalemia.** Potassium level is 8.7 mmol/L. In hyperkalemia, peaking of the T waves is generalized, occurring in almost all T waves that are upright. Note that some of the T waves are taller than the QRS complexes.

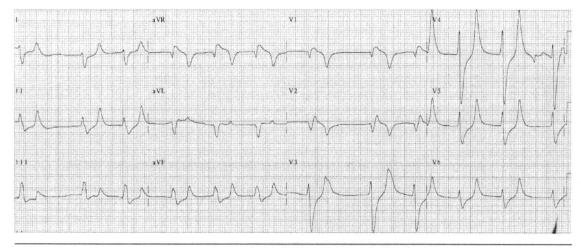

**Figure 25.12:    The Presence of Sine Waves Indicate that the Hyperkalemia is Severe.** Potassium level is 8.9 mmol/L. Note that the sine waves are formed by the short ST segment causing the S waves to continue into the T waves. These are seen in both limb and precordial leads.

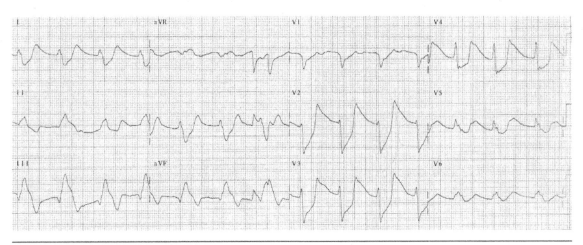

**Figure 25.13:   Marked Widening of the QRS Complexes Indicates More Advanced Hyperkalemia.** Potassium level is >10.0 mmol/L.

## ECG Findings of Hyperkalemia

1. Increased amplitude and peaking of the T waves. This is the earliest, most consistent, and most characteristic ECG abnormality associated with hyperkalemia. T-wave peaking persists and worsens with increasing levels of hyperkalemia.

2. The QT interval is short or normal.

3. As hyperkalemia worsens, the QRS complexes widen.

4. The P wave becomes broader and the amplitude becomes lower.

5. AV conduction becomes prolonged.

6. The P waves eventually disappear resulting in sinoventricular rhythm.

7. The S wave continues into the T wave resulting in a sine wave configuration.

8. Cardiac arrest from marked bradycardia, asystole, or ventricular flutter/fibrillation.

## Mechanism

- The normal serum potassium varies from 3.3 to 5.3 mmol/L. Hyperkalemia occurs when serum potassium exceeds 5.3 mmol/L. When extracellular potassium is increased, the ratio between intracellular and extracellular potassium is decreased and the resting membrane potential becomes less negative ($<-90$ mV). This will affect the height and velocity of phase

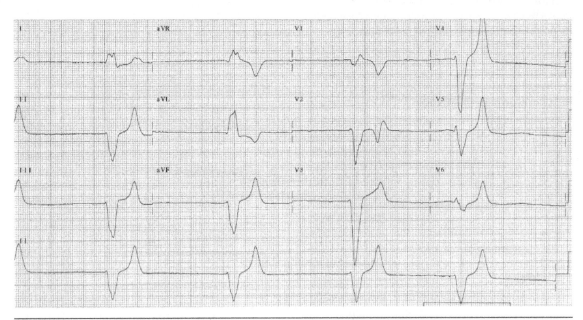

**Figure 25.14:   Slow Ventricular Rhythm and Unusually Wide QRS Complexes.** Potassium level is >10 mmol/L. The rhythm is unusually slow at <30 beats per minute with unusually wide QRS complexes with a left bundle branch block pattern, peaked T waves, and no P waves. This rhythm usually precedes asystole or ventricular fibrillation.

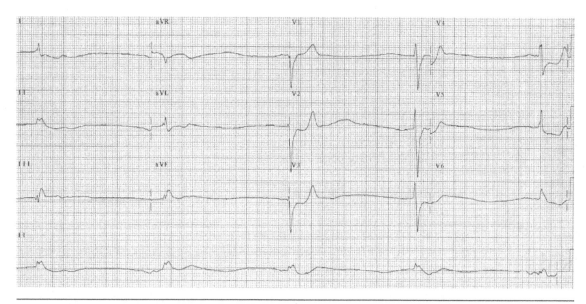

**Figure 25.15:   Marked Bradycardia with Wide Complexes, a Late Manifestation of Severe Hyperkalemia.** The initial potassium level is unknown. After the patient was resuscitated, the potassium level was checked and found to be 8.8 mmol/L. The QRS complexes are wide with a very slow ventricular rate of 26 beats per minute. No P waves can be identified. Peaking of the T waves persists in $V_2$ and $V_3$.

0 of the action potential. Slowing in conduction velocity in the atria and ventricles will cause widening of the P wave and QRS complex. As the severity of the hyperkalemia further increases, the resting potential becomes less and less negative resulting in further widening of the QRS complex and P wave. Hyperkalemia also shortens phase 2, which is equivalent to the plateau phase of the action potential. This will shorten the ST segment in the ECG resulting in a shorter QT interval. It also causes a more rapid phase 3 or steeper downslope of the action potential resulting in peaking of the T waves.

■ Although the ECG findings may not consistently correlate with the level of serum potassium, the following are the ECG findings associated with increasing severity of hyperkalemia:

■ **Mild hyperkalemia: <6.0 mmol/L**

☐ Increased amplitude with peaking of the T waves is the first abnormality to be detected when the potassium level rises between 5 and 6 mmol/L. Hyperkalemic T waves are typical and diagnostic in that the T waves are tall and pointed with a narrow base and a normal or short QT. The T waves become taller and more peaked as the level of hyperkalemia progresses. The diagnosis of hyperkalemia is untenable unless the above T-wave abnormalities are present. The T waves are often taller than the R waves in precordial leads $V_2$ to $V_4$.

☐ The QT or corrected QT interval (QTc) is normal or shortened. It is prolonged only when hyperkalemia is associated with other electrolyte abnormalities such as hypocalcemia or when there is associated myocardial disease. This combination of hyperkalemia and hypocalcemia is commonly seen in patients with chronic renal disease.

■ **Moderate hyperkalemia: 6.0 to 7.0 mmol/L**

☐ Widening of the P wave and QRS complex starts to occur when the potassium level exceeds 6.0 mmol/L. Widening of the QRS complex may be mistaken for bundle branch block. Widening of the QRS complex associated with hyperkalemia is reversible after the electrolyte abnormality is corrected unlike preexistent bundle branch block, which is persistent.

☐ Broadening of the P waves occurs when there is slowing of conduction of the impulse across the atria. When the P wave starts to widen, slight prolongation of the PR interval and varying degrees of AV block may occur.

■ **Severe Hyperkalemia: >7.0 mmol/L**

☐ With increasing levels of serum potassium, further widening of the QRS complex occurs accompanied by shortening of the ST segment. The wide QRS complex will eventually merge into the tall and peaked T wave resembling a sine wave. The ST segments are often elevated in $V_{1-2}$ and may be mistaken for acute ST elevation myocardial infarction.

☐ Even when the rhythm remains normal sinus, the P wave may not be evident in the ECG. The absence of P waves in hyperkalemia even when the rhythm remains normal sinus is called sinoventricular rhythm. The absence of P waves may be due to slow conduction of the sinus impulse across the atria or the sinus impulse being conducted through special internodal tracts between the sinus node and AV node. Because the QRS complexes are no longer preceded by P waves, the rhythm is impossible to differentiate from AV junctional rhythm (when the QRS complexes are narrow) or accelerated idioventricular rhythm (when the QRS complexes are wide). Cardiac arrest may occur when the potassium level exceeds 8.5 mmol/L. This is preceded by marked slowing of the heart rate, further widening of the QRS complexes, asystole, or ventricular flutter/fibrillation.

## Clinical Implications

- Potassium is the major intracellular ion in the body. Approximately 98% of the total amount of potassium is intracellular and the remaining 2% extracellular. This difference in concentration between intracellular and extracellular potassium is due to the presence of sodium potassium adenosine triphosphatase pump where 3 units of sodium is pumped out of the cell in exchange for 2 units of potassium. The ratio between intracellular and extracellular potassium makes the resting membrane potential negative at approximately –90 mV.

- Increased extracellular potassium may be due to increased potassium load, worsening renal function, or acute shift of intracellular potassium extracellularly. Increased potassium in the diet by itself rarely causes hyperkalemia. Some drugs can also cause hyperkalemia when there is renal dysfunction. These include potassium supplements, potassium sparing diuretics (triamterene and amiloride), aldosterone antagonists (spironolactone and eplerenone), angiotensin-converting enzyme inhibitors, angiotensin receptor blockers, and nonsteroidal anti-inflammatory agents including the selective cyclo-oxygenase 2 inhibitors. More commonly, hyperkalemia is due to renal failure. It may also be the result of acute shift of intracellular potassium to the extracellular space as when cells are damaged from hemolysis or rhabdomyolysis. Acidosis can also cause a shift of $H^+$ ions into the cell in exchange for potassium that moves out of the cell. For every 0.1 unit decrease in blood pH, the level of potassium in the serum increases by approximately 0.5 mmol/L.

- Among the electrolyte abnormalities, hyperkalemia causes the most remarkable ECG abnormalities. The ECG changes frequently parallel the severity of the electrolyte disorder. The expected ECG findings, however, may not correlate well with the potassium level because the effect of hyperkalemia on the ECG depends on several factors and not just the serum potassium level. These include the baseline level of potassium, the rate of rise of potassium in the blood, coexisting electrolyte abnormalities, coexisting metabolic abnormalities, and the presence or absence of myocardial disease.

- Mild or moderate hyperkalemia is usually asymptomatic. When significant hyperkalemia occurs usually >7.0 mmol/L, symptoms include generalized weakness, paralysis, respiratory failure from respiratory muscle weakness, and cardiac arrest.

- Among all the electrolyte abnormalities, hyperkalemia is the most fatal. Because severe hyperkalemia can be diagnosed in the ECG, this will allow emergency treatment of the electrolyte abnormality even before the results of the laboratory become available.

- Similarly, the ECG is useful in the diagnosis of pseudohyperkalemia. The laboratory may mistakenly report a high potassium level not the result of actual hyperkalemia but from hemolysis after the blood is collected. If there are no associated ECG changes, the diagnosis of hyperkalemia is unlikely. This will obviate the need for unnecessary therapy.

## Therapy

- Treatment should be tailored according to the severity of the hyperkalemia. The ECG abnormalities together with the serum potassium level serve as useful guide in dictating the intensity of management.

- The American Heart Association (AHA) guidelines of cardiopulmonary resuscitation and emergency cardiovascular care recommend the following for the treatment of hyperkalemia.

- **Mild hyperkalemia, potassium level <6.0 mmol/L:** Potassium level <6.0 mmol/L is seldom of great concern. The only therapy that may be needed is to identify the cause of the hyperkalemia so that further increases in serum potassium can be prevented. In addition, therapy may include removal of potassium from the body.

  - **Loop diuretics:** Furosemide 40 to 80 mg IV or bumetanide 1 mg IV to enhance excretion of potassium.

  - **Cation-exchange resin:** Sodium polystyrene sulfonate (Kayexalate) is given orally or by retention enema. The oral dose can vary from 15 to 60 g daily. Fifteen grams is given orally one to four times per day. Sorbitol 20%, 10 to 20 mL is given every 2 hours or as needed to prevent constipation. Lower doses of Kayexalate of 5 to 10 g may be given up to three times per day without laxative therapy. If the patient is unable to take the resin orally, it can be given as retention enema, 30 to 50 g every 6 hours in a warm emulsion such as 50 mL 70% sorbitol mixed with 100 to 150 mL tap water and retained for at least 30 to 60 minutes. Each gram of Kayexalate removes approximately 1 mmol of potassium and takes at least 30 minutes to 2 hours to take effect. The resin binder carries a high sodium load and should be given cautiously to patients in congestive heart failure. The resin can also bind other cations such as magnesium and calcium. These electrolytes should be monitored together with the level of serum potassium. Patients on digitalis should be monitored closely since hypokalemia can aggravate digitalis toxicity.

- **Moderate hyperkalemia, potassium level 6.0 to 7.0 mmol/L:** When moderate hyperkalemia is present, therapy should be more emergent. In addition to eliminating the cause of the hyperkalemia and removal of excess potassium from the blood with loop diuretics and cation exchange resins, the level of serum potassium can be lowered more rapidly by shifting extracellular potassium intracellularly.

  - **Glucose plus insulin:** Twenty-five grams of glucose (50 mL 50% dextrose) is mixed with 10 units of regular insulin. The solution is injected IV for over 15 to 30 minutes. Ten units of regular insulin can also be mixed with 500 mL 10% glucose. The solution is given IV for 60 minutes. The effect may last for 4 to 6 hours.

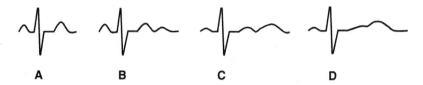

**Figure 25.16:** **The Electrocardiogram of Hypokalemia.** **(A–D)** Varying levels of serum potassium. **(A)** Normal level of serum potassium. **(B)** Mild hypokalemia. A prominent U wave is present. **(C)** Moderate hypokalemia. The U wave becomes more prominent than the T wave. **(D)** Severe hypokalemia. There is fusion of the T and U waves.

- **Sodium bicarbonate:** 50 mEq is given IV over 5 minutes. Sodium bicarbonate lowers extracellular potassium by shifting potassium into the cells. This agent is more effective when hyperkalemia is associated with metabolic acidosis. The effect may last for 2 hours and may be repeated as necessary.
- **Nebulized albuterol:** 10 to 20 mg nebulized over 15 minutes. B₂ agonists shifts extracellular potassium intracellularly and the effect may last for ≥2 hours. If insulin is being given concomitantly, albuterol can attenuate its hypoglycemic effect.
- **Severe hyperkalemia and critical hyperkalemia, potassium level >7.0 mmol/L:** When serum potassium level exceeds 7.0 mmol/L or when the ECG abnormalities include absent P waves and changes in the QRS, ST segment and T waves, AV block or slowing of the heart rate, treatment of hyperkalemia should be very aggressive because severe hyperkalemia may cause lethal arrhythmias and cardiac arrest. The following agents are given in order of priority according to the AHA guidelines.
  - **Calcium chloride:** 10% 5 to 10 mL (500 to 1,000 mg) given IV over 2 to 5 minutes. Calcium does not lower the level of serum potassium but will stabilize myocardial membrane against the toxic effects of potassium, thereby lowering the risk of fatal arrhythmias including ventricular fibrillation. The effect of calcium is immediate but lasts only for 20 to 40 minutes and repeated dosing may be needed.
  - **Sodium bicarbonate:** 50 mEq given IV over 5 minutes. This should be injected using a separate tubing or IV line from that used for calcium chloride.
  - **Glucose plus insulin:** Mix 10 units of regular insulin with 50 mL 50% dextrose. The solution is given IV over 15 to 30 minutes.
  - **Nebulized albuterol:** 10 to 20 mg nebulized over 15 minutes.
  - **Loop diuretics:** as above.
  - **Kayexalate enema:** 15 to 60 g plus sorbitol given orally or rectally as above.
  - **Dialysis:** If above therapy is unsuccessful, emergent dialysis should be considered especially in patients with renal failure even if not previously on dialysis.

## Prognosis

- Severe hyperkalemia is the most fatal among all electrolyte abnormalities and is a medical emergency. Overall prognosis of hyperkalemia depends on the potassium level, efficacy of therapy, and comorbidities associated with the hyperkalemia. The presence of diabetic ketoacidosis and renal failure as the cause of the hyperkalemia often confer a poor prognosis.

## Hypokalemia

- Hypokalemia is defined as the presence of serum potassium that is lower than normal. The normal value for serum potassium is 3.3 to 5.3 mmol/L.
- The most important ECG finding in hypokalemia is the presence of prominent U waves. As the hypokalemia becomes more profound, the amplitude of the T wave becomes lower as the size of the U wave becomes larger until both T and U waves bond together and become indistinguishable (Figs. 25.16 and 25.17).
- **Normal U wave:** The U wave follows the T wave and is the last component of ventricular repolarization. The normal U wave is small measuring less than a quarter of the size of the T wave. The exact origin of the normal U wave is uncertain but is most probably from the repolarization of the Purkinje fibers.
- **Hypokalemic U wave:** The U wave in hypokalemia is large and pathologic. It is much larger than the T wave and its origin is not the same as that of the normal U wave. It has been shown that in hypokalemia, the normal T wave becomes interrupted, splitting into two components. The T wave represents the first component and the U wave the second component. Thus, the Q-U interval truly represents the actual QT interval and is prolonged. The QT interval represents only the first component of the split T wave, and is equal to or even shorter than the normal QT interval (Figs. 25.18–25.21).

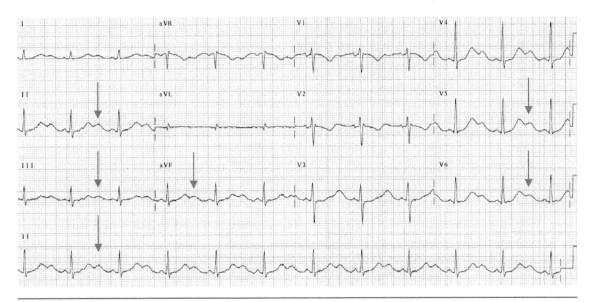

**Figure 25.17: Prominent U Waves in Hypokalemia.** Potassium level is 2.7 mm/L. The 12-lead electrocardiogram shows the classical finding of hypokalemia characterized by prominent U waves (*arrows*). Fusion of the T and U waves is seen in V₃; thus, the T and U waves become indistinguishable.

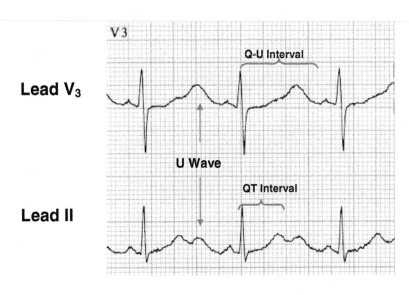

**Figure 25.18: The QT and the Q-U Interval in Hypokalemia.** Lead V₃ and lead II were simultaneously recorded. In lead II, the U waves are separately inscribed from the T waves and the two humps resemble the back of a camel. If the QT interval is measured in lead II, the QT interval is short since it represents only the first component of a split T wave. It does not represent the real QT interval. In V₃, the U waves are very prominent and can not be separated from the T wave. This QU interval represents the actual QT interval and is prolonged. The 12-lead electrocardiogram is shown in Figure 25.17.

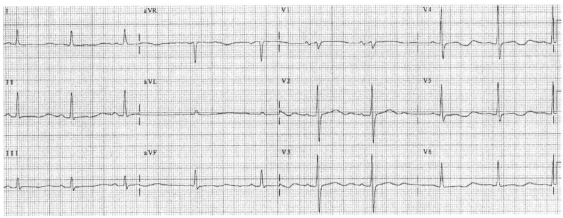

**Figure 25.19: Prolonged QU Interval in Hypokalemia.** Potassium level is 3.1 mmol/L. The U waves are prominent in V₂₋₆ with prolonged QU interval.

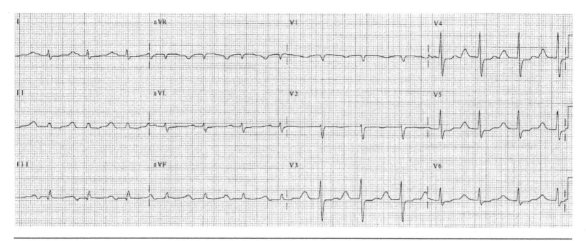

**Figure 25.20: Prominent U Waves and Prolonged QU Interval in Hypokalemia.** Potassium level is 2.8 mmol/L. The U waves are more prominent than the T waves and are most prominent in $V_3$ to $V_5$. The QU interval is prolonged.

## ECG Findings of Hypokalemia

1. Prominent U waves
2. Nonspecific ST depression and T-wave flattening as the U wave becomes more prominent
3. Prolongation of the QU interval
4. Fusion of the T and U waves
5. Ventricular arrhythmias, especially torsade de pointes

## Mechanism

■ The ratio between intracellular and extracellular potassium determines the resting potential of a cell, which is normally –90 mV. When there is hypokalemia, extracellular potassium is decreased and the ratio between intracellular and extracellular potassium becomes higher. Thus, the cells become more negative than –90 mV and the resting potential is hyperpolarized. This will cause lengthening of the duration of the action potential resulting in a longer QT interval in the surface ECG. This will increase the frequency of ventricular arrhythmias especially torsade de pointes.

■ The ECG hallmark of hypokalemia is the presence of prominent U waves and prolongation of the QU interval. As hypokalemia worsens, the T wave flattens, a U wave emerges, and a seesaw effect between the amplitude of the T and U wave occurs. As the U wave grows larger, the T wave becomes smaller. Merging of the T and U waves eventually occur; thus, the T and U waves become indistinguishable from one another.

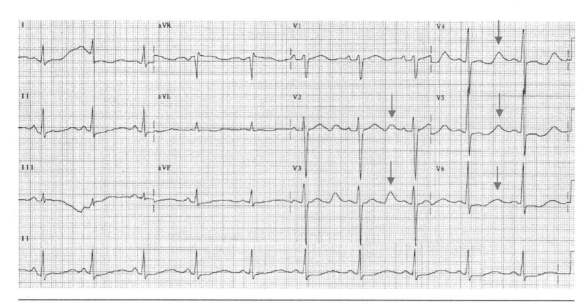

**Figure 25.21: Hypokalemia with "Roller Coaster" ST-T Configuration.** Potassium level is 1.7 mmol/L. The T waves have merged with the U waves in $V_{4-6}$. The QU interval is prolonged with a "roller coaster" configuration in $V_{2-6}$.

- In hypokalemia, phase 3 of the transmembrane action potential is less steep causing a small or attenuated intramyocardial voltage gradient, resulting in low T waves. This is opposite to that of hyperkalemia, where phase 3 has a steeper slope, which translates into a higher intramyocardial voltage gradient, resulting in T waves that are taller and more peaked.

- According to Yan et al., the mechanism of a pathologic U wave resulting from hypokalemia is different from the mechanism of a normal U wave. When hypokalemia is present, the abnormal T-U complex has been shown to be due to splitting of the ascending limb of the normal T wave into two components. The first component of the split T wave is the original T wave and the other component becomes a separate U wave, which is actually the other half of the split T wave. If only the QT interval is measured, which represents only the first component of the bifid T wave, the QT interval is equal to or even shorter than the normal QT interval. Thus, in hypokalemia, measurement of the true QT interval should include the U wave and is measured as the QU interval.

## Clinical Implications

- The normal level of potassium in the blood is 3.3 to 5.3 mmol/L. Hypokalemia refers to the presence of lower than normal potassium in the blood, which is <3.3 mmol/L.

- The normal daily intake of potassium varies from 80 to 120 mEq/day. Almost 90% of dietary potassium is excreted by the kidneys and the rest by the gastrointestinal (GI) tract.

- Hypokalemia usually occurs from potassium loss in the kidneys, frequently brought about by chronic diuretic therapy or potassium loss in the GI tract as a result of frequent vomiting, continuous gastric suction, or diarrhea.

- Hypokalemia also occurs when there is acute shift of extracellular potassium intracellularly from metabolic alkalosis or drugs such as insulin and beta agonists. Alkalosis causes extracellular potassium to move into the cell in exchange for $H^+$, resulting in a lower level of serum potassium. Metabolic alkalosis decreases serum potassium by 0.8 mmol/L for every 0.1 unit increase in pH above normal. Acidosis causes a reverse effect with intracellular potassium moving out of the cell in exchange for $H^+$. Thus, an acidotic patient with a normal potassium level is expected to develop hypokalemia once the acidosis is corrected.

- Symptoms of hypokalemia usually occur when significant electrolyte depletion has occurred. This is usually manifested as generalized weakness, fatigue, and paralysis. In patients who are being weaned off a respirator, it is important that potassium level should be checked because hypokalemia can cause muscle weakness that can result in respiratory failure. If hypokalemia is present, the electrolyte abnormality should be corrected. Hypokalemia can affect the muscles of the GI tract, resulting in ileus or constipation. It can also affect the muscles of the lower extremities, resulting in leg cramps and paresthesias.

- Arrhythmias including torsade de pointes and pulseless electrical activity may occur when the QT (or QU) interval is prolonged.

## Therapy

- Because potassium is predominantly an intracellular ion, hypokalemia may occur even when total body potassium is normal or higher than normal. Generally however, when hypokalemia is present and is from chronic loss of potassium, a decrease in serum potassium of 1 mmol/L is equivalent to a deficit of approximately 150 to 400 mmol of body potassium.

- Therapy of hypokalemia includes identification and correction of the underlying abnormality.

- Aggressive intravenous replacement of potassium may be associated with hyperkalemia and cardiac arrhythmias. Thus, intravenous administration of potassium is preferred when arrhythmias are present or when hypokalemia is severe (<2.5 mEq/L). Oral replacement is given if the patient is clinically stable without arrhythmias and the potassium level is ≥2.5 mmol/L because administration of potassium orally is much safer and can be given in higher doses.

- Replacement therapy of approximately 200 to 300 mmol potassium is needed to increase the serum potassium level by 1 mmol/L. However, it may take several days to correct the electrolyte abnormality because the administered potassium is also excreted in the urine. Since intravenous replacement of potassium can potentially cause cardiac arrhythmias, the AHA guidelines recommend the following:

  - The maximum infusion of potassium should not exceed 10 to 20 mmol/hour and should be infused under continuous cardiac monitoring.

  - Potassium when given >20 mmol/hour should be infused with a central line. This concentration of potassium may be painful when given IV because it may cause sclerosis of the veins. The tip of the central catheter should not extend to the right atrium or ventricle because this may cause local hyperkalemia.

  - If severe life-threatening arrhythmias are present and a more rapid infusion is necessary, an initial infusion of 10 mmol IV is given over 5 minutes and repeated once if necessary.

- Potassium is preferably mixed with non-glucose solutions to prevent insulin secretion, which can shift potassium intracellularly.

- Hypokalemia is usually associated with other electrolyte abnormalities, especially hypomagnesemia. When there is hypomagnesemia, it might be difficult to correct the potassium deficiency because magnesium is necessary for the movement of electrolytes in and out of the cell including potassium; therefore, correcting both electrolyte abnormality should be done simultaneously.

- The use of potassium sparing diuretics should be considered in hypokalemic patients requiring long term diuretic therapy.

## Prognosis

- Hypokalemia can cause ventricular arrhythmias and may be fatal if left uncorrected. It is usually from aggressive use of diuretics or gastrointestinal losses. Unlike patients with

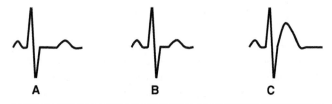

**Figure 25.22:** **The Electrocardiogram of Hypercalcemia.** Diagrammatic representation of the electrocardiogram changes associated with hypercalcemia. **(A)** Normal. **(B)** Hypercalcemia: the ST segment is shortened because of shortening of phase 2 of the action potential. **(C)** Hypercalcemia with ST segment elevation. Fusion of the QRS complex and T wave occur due to further shortening of the ST segment.

hyperkalemia, the renal function in hypokalemic patients is usually preserved. After the hypokalemia is corrected, prognosis will depend on the underlying cause of the hypokalemia.

## Hypercalcemia

- Hypercalcemia refers to the presence of elevated calcium level above normal. The normal level of total serum calcium varies from 8.5 to 10.5 mg/dL or for ionized calcium 4.2 to 4.8 mg/dL.

- When extracellular calcium is increased, the duration of the action potential is shortened. Shortening of the action potential duration results in shortening of the QT interval.

- The ECG findings of hypercalcemia include (Figs. 25.22 and 25.23):
  - Shortening of the QT interval. This is due to shortening of phase 2 of the action potential corresponding to the ST segment in the ECG.
  - Elevation of the ST segment especially in the precordial leads. This may be mistaken for acute ischemic injury.

## ECG Findings of Hypercalcemia

1. Short QT interval from shortening of the ST segment
2. Flattened and widened T wave with ST elevation
3. Prolonged P-R interval
4. Widened QRS complex
5. Increased QRS voltage
6. Notching of the terminal portion of the QRS complex from a prominent J wave
7. AV block progressing to complete heart block and cardiac arrest when serum calcium >15 to 20 mg/dL.

## Mechanism

- Increasing levels of serum calcium may cause changes in the ECG. Unlike hyperkalemia, in which the ECG changes are more dramatic, the ECG abnormalities associated with hypercalcemia are less specific and should not be used as the basis for making the diagnosis of hypercalcemia.
  - Hypercalcemia shortens the duration of the action potential of the myocyte, resulting in a shortened QT interval. This usually occurs when the serum calcium is >13 mg/dL. Because the duration of ventricular systole is shortened, ventricular refractoriness is shortened, rendering the

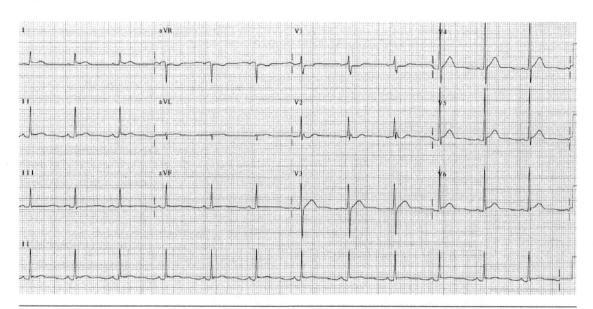

**Figure 25.23:** **The ST and T Wave Configuration in Hypercalcemia.** Total calcium level is 16.0 mg/dL. Note the short ST segment and ST elevation in $V_3$ to $V_6$. Prominent J wave or Osborn wave may also occur when there is hypercalcemia.

patient more prone to arrhythmias. It also renders patients more susceptible to the toxic effects of digitalis.

- Hypercalcemia initially increases inotropicity and chronotropy by causing increased calcium influx and decreases calcium egress in the myocyte. However, as serum calcium further increases to levels >15 to –20 mg/dL, myocardial contractility becomes depressed.
- Very high levels of calcium, >15 to 20 mg/dL, may result in arrhythmias most commonly bradycardia and complete heart block.

## Clinical Significance

- Calcium is the most common mineral in the body; 99% of the total amount of calcium is stored in bones. The remaining 1% is distributed in the sera, 50% of which is bound to albumin and the rest available as ionized calcium. Total serum calcium is affected by the level of serum albumin. When serum albumin is low, total calcium is low. Inversely, when serum albumin is high, the total calcium level is high. The level of ionized calcium, however, is not affected by the level of serum albumin and is more important in causing signs and symptoms of calcium excess or deficiency.
- Pseudohypercalcemia can occur when there is profound dehydration, causing increased binding of calcium by albumin. This will result in increased total serum calcium but the level of ionized calcium remains normal. This can also occur in some patients with multiple myeloma.
- The normal level of total serum calcium is 8.5 to 10.5 mg/dL and of ionized calcium 4.2 to 4.8 mg/dL. Hypercalcemia indicates the presence of high levels of serum calcium above the normal range. When real hypercalcemia is suspected, the level of ionized calcium should be checked. Ionized calcium is collected anaerobically, adjusted to a normal pH of 7.4, and is often reported as normalized calcium.
- The level of ionized calcium is actively regulated by the endocrine system. When there is hypocalcemia, enhanced secretion of parathyroid hormone (PTH) increases osteoclastic activity and bone resorption, thus increasing the level of calcium in the blood. PTH also promotes absorption of calcium in the GI tract by activating Vitamin D and decreases excretion of calcium in the kidneys by promoting tubular reabsorption. Inversely, when there is increased level of calcium, PTH secretion is inhibited and calcitonin is released, which will lower serum calcium by reducing osteoclastic activity and increasing the deposition of calcium in the bones and at the same time increase excretion of calcium by the kidneys.
- Ionized calcium is affected by pH, whereas total calcium is not. When there is metabolic or respiratory alkalosis, $H^+$ is shifted from plasma proteins to serum to buffer the increased bicarbonates. More ionized calcium will become protein-bound to neutralize the more negatively charged plasma protein, thus decreasing the level of ionized calcium. The reverse happens when there is acidosis: ionized calcium increases in the serum.

- The two most common causes of hypercalcemia accounting for more than 90% of cases are hyperparathyroidism and malignancy.
  - Hyperparathyroidism may be primary from an autonomously hyperfunctioning parathyroid gland (primary hyperparathyroidism) or secondary from chronic renal disease (secondary hyperparathyroidism).
  - Hypercalcemia of malignancy is due to increased osteoclastic activity, resulting in increased bone resorption. This may be due to increased hormonelike substances in the blood or direct invasion of tumor cells into the bone.
    - ☐ Humoral hypercalcemia: from increase in PTH-like substances in the blood, resulting in increase osteoclastic activity and bone resorption. This type of hypercalcemia is seen in squamous cell cancer of the lungs, head and neck, and often renal and ovarian cancer.
    - ☐ Bone metastasis: direct bone metastasis may also result in increased bone resorption most commonly the result of breast cancer or multiple myeloma.
  - Other causes of hypercalcemia include use of drugs such as thiazide diuretics, lithium, and vitamins A and D or sarcoidosis and other granulomatous diseases.
- There are usually no physical findings associated with the hypercalcemia itself. Symptoms of hypercalcemia usually do not occur until the serum calcium reaches 12 mg/dL or higher. Hypertension is common in patients with hypercalcemia and is a common manifestation in patients with primary hyperparathyroidism. At serum levels of 12 to 15 mg/dL, weakness, apathy, fatigue, depression, and confusion may occur. GI symptoms of constipation and dysphagia are common. A higher incidence of dyspepsia and peptic ulcer disease may occur because of a calcium-mediated increase in gastrin secretion. As hypercalcemia becomes more severe, dehydration may occur because hypercalcemia decreases renal concentrating capacity, resulting in polyuria and polydipsia. Finally, neurologic symptoms characterized by hallucinations, disorientation, and coma may develop. Although symptoms of hypercalcemia are usually neuromuscular, cardiac manifestations may occur, including AV block and cardiac arrest.

## Therapy

- Treatment is directed toward the underlying cause of the hypercalcemia. Therapy for hypercalcemia is essential when the calcium level is >12 mg/dL, especially when the patient is symptomatic. Therapy is mandatory at levels >15 mg/dL, regardless of symptoms.
- Excessive increase of calcium in the blood causes polyuria and GI symptoms, especially in patients with malignancy, resulting in dehydration. This enhances reabsorption of calcium in the kidneys, thus further worsening hypercalcemia. Patients with hypercalcemia are therefore volume-contracted; proper hydration with restoration of extracellular volume promotes calcium excretion.

■ **Saline diuresis:** In symptomatic patients with severe hypercalcemia >15 mg/dL who have reasonably preserved cardiovascular and renal function and are dehydrated, the 2005 AHA guidelines for cardiopulmonary resuscitation and emergency cardiovascular care recommends intravenous infusion of 300 to 500 mL/hour of 0.9% saline until any fluid deficit is corrected or until patient starts to diurese adequately. After the patient is properly hydrated, IV hydration is continued at 100 to 200 mL/hour to maintain adequate diuresis and promote calcium excretion. At least 3 to 4 L is usually needed in the first 24 hours. Other electrolytes, especially potassium and magnesium, should be monitored carefully.

■ **Loop diuretics:** Loop diuretics (e.g., furosemide [20–40 mg 2 to 4 times daily] or bumetanide [1 to 2 mg twice daily]), may be used in patients with heart failure, although their use in the treatment of the hypercalcemia itself is controversial and should be used only after appropriate volume repletion with normal saline. Thiazide diuretics should not be substituted for loop diuretics because they prevent calcium excretion.

■ **Calcitonin:** Calcitonin lowers serum calcium by inhibiting bone resorption and promoting urinary calcium excretion.

■ **Bisphosphonates:** Biphosphonic acid lowers serum calcium by inhibiting osteoclastic bone resorption. The following bisphosphonates are commonly used in the treatment of hypercalcemia associated with malignancy.

■ **Pamidronate:** Pamidronate is given as an intravenous infusion. It can be combined with calcitonin to provide a longer effect. There is risk of renal toxicity if given rapidly or in high doses.

■ **Zoledronic acid:** Zoledronic acid is preferred as it is more potent than pamidronate. It can be infused over a shorter period. The drug can also cause renal damage if the infusion is given rapidly or in high doses. Renal function should be reassessed if a second infusion is necessary. Patients receiving the infusion should be properly hydrated.

■ **Steroids:** Glucocorticoids reduce calcium level by several mechanisms. They inhibit intestinal absorption, increase urinary excretion of calcium, and have cytolytic effect to some tumor cells, especially multiple myeloma and other malignancies. They also inhibit calcitriol production by mononuclear cells in lungs and lymph nodes; thus, they are effective in hypercalcemia associated with granulomatous diseases and occasionally with lymphoma.

■ **Phosphates:** Phosphates are given orally to prevent calcium absorption. It combines with calcium to form complexes that limits its absorption. It also increases calcium deposition in bones.

■ **Hemodialysis:** Hemodialysis should be considered when there is need to promptly decrease the level of serum calcium in patients with heart failure or renal failure who cannot tolerate saline infusion. The dialysis fluid should be altered because the conventional dialysis solution may have a composition that may not be ideally suited for rapid correction of the electrolyte abnormality.

## Prognosis

■ Prognosis depends on the underlying condition. Hypercalcemia is commonly associated with malignancy; thus, the intensity of therapy should be individualized and should consider the overall clinical picture.

## Hypocalcemia

■ Hypocalcemia is defined as a calcium level below the normal range. The normal serum calcium level varies from 8.5 to 10.5 mg/dL and the normal level of ionized calcium is 4.2 to 4.8 mg/dL.

■ When the level of extracellular calcium is decreased, the following ECG changes occur:

■ The QT interval is prolonged. Prolongation of the QT interval is due to prolongation of phase 2 of the action potential, which corresponds to the ST segment in the ECG. Thus, prolongation of the QT interval is mainly due to prolongation of the ST segment. The T wave is not significantly affected. Terminal inversion of the T waves may occur (Figs. 25.24–25.27).

■ Heart block may occur when the hypocalcemia is more severe.

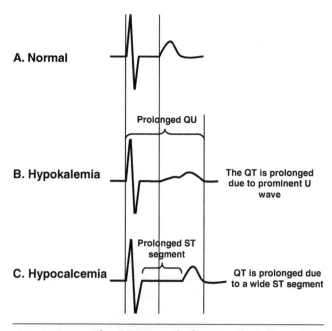

**Figure 25.24:    The QT Interval of Hypocalcemia and Hypokalemia.** In hypokalemia, the prolongation of the QT or QU interval is due to the presence of prominent U waves **(B)**. In hypocalcemia, prolongation of the QT interval is primarily due to lengthening of the ST segment **(C)**.

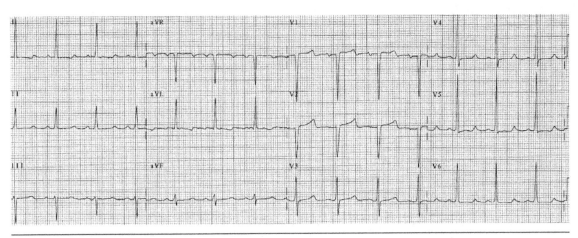

**Figure 25.25: Prolonged ST Segment in Hypocalcemia.** Total serum calcium is 7.6 mg/dL. The QT interval is prolonged from lengthening of the ST segment. The T waves are narrow as shown in V₄ to V₆.

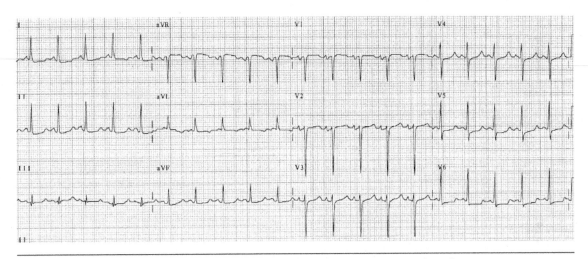

**Figure 25.26:   ST Segment and T Wave Changes Associated with Hypocalcemia.** Serum calcium is 7.2 mg/dL. The QT interval is prolonged with ST depression and narrow T waves.

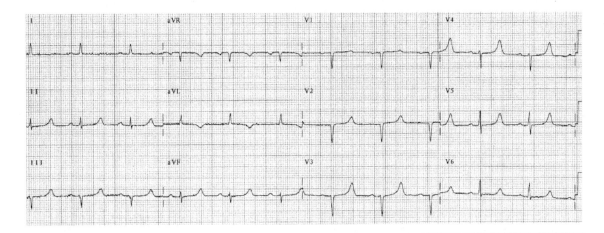

**Figure 25.27:   Hypocalcemia and Hyperkalemia.** Potassium level is 5.6 mmol/L and total calcium is 6.8 mg/dL. This electrolyte abnormality is commonly seen in renal failure. The T waves are peaked due to hyperkalemia and QTc is prolonged measuring 491 milliseconds from hypocalcemia.

## ECG Abnormalities of Hypocalcemia

1. Prolonged QT interval due to lengthening of the ST segment.
2. Flat ST segment and terminal T-wave inversion.
3. Heart block and ventricular fibrillation when hypocalcemia is severe.

## Mechanism

- ECG findings include:
  - Prolongation of the QT interval. Prolongation of the QT interval is due to lengthening of phase 2 of the action potential. Because phase 2 of the action potential corresponds to the ST segment, prolongation of the QT interval is mainly from lengthening of the JT interval, which represents the interval between the end of the QRS complex and the end of the T wave. Although the ST segment lengthens, the size of the T wave is not altered. This is the most diagnostic ECG abnormality associated with hypocalcemia. This is in contrast to hypokalemia where a prominent U wave is present resulting in prolongation of the QT (QU) interval. Other ECG findings include flat ST segment, widening of the QRS complex, and AV block. Ventricular fibrillation may occur when hypocalcemia is severe.

## Clinical Implications

- Hypocalcemia refers to a low level of serum calcium below the normal range of 8.5 to 10.5 mg/dL (or 2.1 to 2.6 mmol/L). It is also defined as below the normal level of ionized calcium, which is 4.2 to 4.8 mg/dL (or <1.0 mmol/L).
- The recommended daily calcium is 1,200 mg. Hypocalcemia can occur when there is:
  - Decreased intake or diminished absorption of calcium: Vitamin D is necessary for absorption of calcium in the GI tract. Vitamin D deficiency can occur in patients who are not exposed to sunlight or do not have adequate vitamin D in the diet. In chronic renal failure, there is defective hydroxylation of vitamin D to active vitamin D. Secondary increase in PTH may occur in an effort to maintain serum calcium levels.
  - Parathyroid hormone deficiency: This is usually the result of inadvertent removal of the parathyroid glands during thyroid surgery. The parathyroid glands are also affected by tumor or by infiltrative disorders, such as hemochromatosis or sarcoidosis.
  - Alkalosis: Metabolic or respiratory alkalosis decreases the level of ionized calcium.
  - Chelation of calcium with citrate and other substances: Hypocalcemia may occur following transfusion of >6 units of citrated blood. Increased phosphates from acute renal failure and exogenous bicarbonates and free fatty acids during acute pancreatitis can also result in chelation of calcium.
- Signs and symptoms of hypocalcemia are dependent not only on the level of free or ionized calcium, but also on the rapidity in which calcium declines. In renal patients, hypocalcemia may not be clinically manifest because of coexistent acidosis, which increases the level of ionized calcium and may abruptly manifest only when the acidosis is corrected.

- Symptoms of hypocalcemia usually do not occur until the level of ionized calcium falls below 0.7 mmol/L. This includes generalized irritability, hyperreflexia, muscle cramps, tetany, carpopedal spasm, seizures, and neuromuscular excitability characterized by a positive Chvostek and Trousseau signs.
  - Chvostek sign is elicited by tapping the facial nerve on the face anterior to the ear resulting in twitching of the facial muscles on the same side.
  - Trousseau sign involves inflating a blood pressure cuff above the systolic pressure for 3 minutes, resulting in muscular contraction with flexion of the wrist, thumbs, and metacarpophalangeal joints and hyperextension of the fingers.
- Although symptoms of hypocalcemia are predominantly neuromuscular and include weakness, tetany, confusion and seizures, hypocalcemia can also cause arrhythmias, decrease in myocardial contractility, heart failure, and hypotension.
- Hypocalcemia usually develops in association with other electrolyte abnormalities such as hyperkalemia and hypomagnesemia. The combination of hypocalcemia and hyperkalemia is commonly seen in patients with renal failure.

## Therapy

- Treatment of hypocalcemia includes measurement of the ionized level of serum. When symptoms are present, calcium should be given intravenously even before the result of ionized calcium is available. Between 100 and 300 mg of elemental calcium is given intravenously, which will increase serum calcium for 1 to 2 hours; thus, repeated doses may be necessary. Calcium is given as calcium chloride or calcium gluconate. Calcium chloride has a higher amount of elemental calcium compared to calcium gluconate:
  - Calcium chloride 10% 10 mL contains 360 mg of elemental calcium, whereas calcium gluconate 10% 10 mL contains 93 mg of elemental calcium.
  - Calcium is given IV over 10 minutes (90 to 180 mg elemental calcium) followed by an IV drip of 540 to 720 mg in 500 to 1,000 mL $D_5W$. The serum calcium level should be monitored every 4 to 6 hours and maintained at the low normal range of 7 to 9 mg/dL.
  - Calcium should be injected cautiously to patients receiving digitalis because it may cause digitalis toxicity.
- If symptoms are not present, oral calcium supplements 1 to 4 g daily in divided doses may suffice.
- Therapy includes correction of other electrolyte abnormalities because calcium entry into the cells is dependent on the presence of normal levels of magnesium and potassium.

## Prognosis

- Prognosis of patients with hypocalcemia will depend on the underlying medical condition.

## Suggested Readings

2005 American Heart Association guidelines for cardiopulmonary resuscitation and emergency cardiovascular care. Part 10.1: life-threatening electrolyte abnormalities. *Circulation.* 2005;112:IV-121–I-125.

Agus ZS. Etiology of hypercalcemia. 2008 UpToDate. www.utdol.com.

Agus ZS, Berenson JR. Treatment of hypercalcemia. 2008 UpToDate. www.utdol.com.

Dagogo-Jack S. Mineral and metabolic bone disease. In: Carey CF, Lee HH, Woeltje KF, eds. *The Washington Manual of Medical Therapeutics.* 29th ed. Philadelphia: Lippincott Williams & Wilkins; 1998:441–455.

Gibbs MA, Wolfson AB, Tayal WS. Electrolyte disturbances. In: Marx JA, ed. *Rosen's Emergency Medicine, Concepts and Clinical Practice.* 5th ed. St. Louis: Mosby; 2002:1724–1744.

Inzucchi SE. Understanding hypercalcemia. *Postgrad Med.* 2004; 115:69–76.

Palmer BF. Managing hyperkalemia caused by inhibitors or the renin-angiotensin-aldosterone system. *N Engl J Med.* 2004; 351:585–592.

Rose BD. Clinical manifestations and treatment of hyperkalemia. 2008 UpToDate. www.utdol.com.

Rose BD. Clinical manifestations and treatment of hypokalemia. 2008 UpToDate. www.utdol.com.

Rutecki GW, Whittier FC. Recognizing hypercalcemia: the "3-hormone, 3-organ rule." *J Crit Illness.* 1998;13:59–66.

Singer GG. Fluid and electrolyte management. In: Carey CF, Lee HH, Woeltje KF, eds. *The Washington Manual of Medical Therapeutics.* 29th ed. Philadelphia: Lippincott Williams & Wilkins; 1998:39–60.

Urbano FL. Signs of hypocalcemia: Chvostek's and Trousseau's signs. *Hosp Physician.* 2000;36:43–45.

Yan GX, Shimizu W, Antzelevitch C. Cellular basis for the normal T-wave and the electrocardiographic manifestations of the long-QT syndrome. *Circulation.* 1998;98:1921–1927.

Yan GX, Lankipalli RS, Burke JF, et al. Ventricular repolarization components of the electrocardiogram, cellular basis and clinical significance. *J Am Coll Cardiol.* 2003;42: 401–409.

Zaloga GP, RR Kirby, WC Bernards, et al. Fluids and electrolytes. In: Civetta JM, Taylor RW Kirby RR, eds. *Critical Care.* 3rd ed. Philadelphia: Lippincott-Raven Publishers; 1997:413–429.

# The ECG of Cardiac Pacemakers

## Types of Pacemakers

- Most physicians or paramedical personnel who are not familiar with artificial pacemakers will find any discussion on cardiac pacemakers difficult and complicated. This chapter will provide a simplified and basic discussion of the electrocardiogram (ECG) of cardiac pacemakers.

- Artificial cardiac pacemakers are electronic devices that were clinically introduced for the treatment of symptomatic bradyarrhythmias. The device consists of a generator and one or more electrodes. The generator includes the circuitry and power supply, which are encased in a sealed container made of stainless steel or titanium. It is usually the size of a cigarette lighter and is implanted subcutaneously in the pectoral or subclavicular region. The generator is connected to the heart by electrodes, which are inserted transvenously into the right atrium, right ventricle, or to both chambers.

- **Initial classification:** Permanent cardiac pacemakers were initially classified as atrial, ventricular, or dual chamber pacemakers (Fig. 26.1).

  - **Atrial:** An atrial pacemaker is a single chamber device consisting of a generator with an electrode inserted into the right atrium.

  - **Ventricular:** A ventricular pacemaker is a single chamber device consisting of a generator with an electrode inserted into the right ventricle.

- **Dual chamber:** A dual chamber pacemaker is a device with two separate electrodes: one in the right atrium and the other in the right ventricle.

## Ventricular Pacemakers

- **Single chamber ventricular pacemaker:** A basic knowledge of the function of a single chamber pacemaker is essential. This will serve as a foundation in understanding the ECG of the more complicated devices. Single chamber ventricular pacemakers were the earliest pacemakers that were put into clinical use for the treatment of complete atrioventricular (AV) block. These electronic devices can initiate a ventricular rhythm by emitting an electrical impulse directly to the ventricles.

- The electrical impulse is represented in the ECG as a vertical artifact. The presence of a pacemaker artifact is a signal that the pacemaker has discharged and the wide QRS complex that immediately follows indicates that it has captured the ventricles (Figs. 26.2 and 26.3).

## Atrial Pacemaker

- **Single chamber atrial pacemaker:** An atrial pacemaker can be identified in the ECG by the presence of

---

**Figure 26.1: Diagrammatic Representation of the Different Types of Pacemakers.**
**(A)** atrial pacemaker. **(B)** ventricular pacemaker.
**(C)** Dual chamber pacemaker.

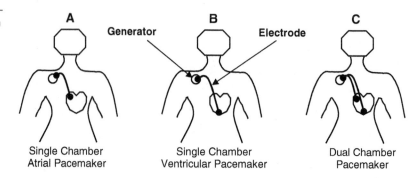

A     Generator     B     Electrode     C

Single Chamber
Atrial Pacemaker

Single Chamber
Ventricular Pacemaker

Dual Chamber
Pacemaker

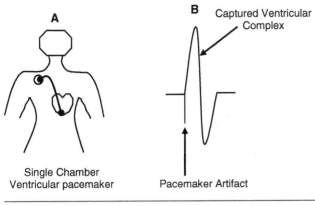

**Figure 26.2:** **Single Chamber Ventricular Pacemaker.** **(A)** Diagrammatic representation of a single chamber ventricular pacemaker. The electrocardiogram generated by a ventricular pacemaker is shown in **(B)**. Arrow points to the pacemaker artifact, which generates a wide QRS complex representing a captured ventricular impulse.

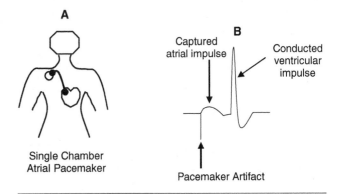

**Figure 26.4:** **Single Chamber Atrial Pacemaker.** **(A)** A diagrammatic representation of an atrial pacemaker. **(B)** The electrocardiogram generated by an atrial pacemaker. The pacemaker stimulus is followed by a P wave, which represents a pacemaker captured atrial complex. If atrioventricular conduction is intact, the P wave is followed by a normally conducted QRS complex.

a pacemaker artifact similar to that of a ventricular pacemaker. The pacemaker signal however is immediately followed by a P wave (instead of a QRS complex), which indicates that the pacemaker has captured the atrium (Figs. 26.4 and 26.5).

- Single chamber atrial pacemakers were clinically introduced for the treatment of symptomatic bradyarrhythmias resulting from sick sinus syndrome. When the atrium is stimulated, the impulse can propagate to the ventricles and AV synchrony is preserved. Atrial pacing is, therefore, more physiologic than ventricular pacing.
- Single chamber atrial pacemakers are indicated only when AV conduction is intact. They are not indicated for the treatment of complete AV block.

## Sensing and Pacing Functions

- **Fixed rate pacemakers:** The earliest implantable pacemakers were capable only of stimulating the heart by delivering electrical impulses to the ventricle or atrium. They were not capable of recognizing or sensing the patient's spontaneous rhythm. The device therefore did not have any sensing capabilities and dis-

charged constantly regardless of the patient's rhythm. These pacemakers were called fixed rate or asynchronous pacemakers (Fig. 26.6).

- **Demand pacemakers:** To avoid competition between the pacemaker and the patient's own rhythm, the second-generation pacemakers were equipped with a sensing circuit capable of detecting (or sensing) the patient's intrinsic ventricular or atrial impulses. When a spontaneous ventricular or atrial complex is detected, the pacemaker was inhibited from delivering a stimulus (Fig. 26.7). These devices were called demand or synchronous pacemakers.

## Pacemaker Identification System

- As pacemaker function became increasingly more advanced, a coding system was developed to identify the different modes or functions that a pacemaker is capable of. The first universally accepted pacemaker coding system was developed by the Intersociety Commission on Heart Disease Resources. The initial coding system consisted only of three letters, which identified the type and basic function of the pacemaker.

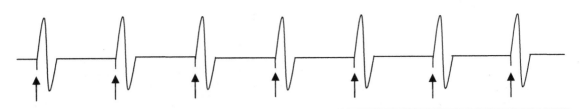

**Figure 26.3:** **Ventricular Pacemaker.** Rhythm strip showing a ventricular pacemaker. Each pacemaker stimulus (*arrow*) is followed by a wide QRS complex representing a pacemaker captured ventricular complex.

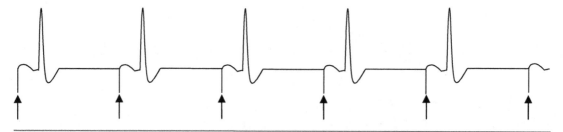

**Figure 26.5:   Atrial Pacemaker.** Rhythm strip showing an atrial pacemaker. Each pacemaker stimulus (*arrows*) is followed by a P wave representing a pacemaker-captured atrial complex.

- The first letter identifies the chamber paced. This could be the A, atrium; V, ventricle; or D, dual (both atrium and ventricle).
- The second letter indicates the chamber sensed. This could be the A, atrium; V, ventricle; D, dual (both chambers); or the number 0, none.
- The third letter describes the pacemaker response to a sensed event that could be I, inhibited; T, triggered; D, dual (atrial inhibited followed by ventricular triggered); or the number 0, none.

- Thus, a fixed-rate, single-chamber ventricular pacemaker, which is a pacemaker without sensing capabilities, is designated as V00 and a demand ventricular pacemaker, which has sensing capabilities, is a VVI or VVT. The same modes can be applied to atrial pacemakers; thus, a fixed rate, single chamber atrial pacemaker is designated as A00 and a demand atrial pacemaker, which has sensing capabilities, is AAI or AAT.
- The various modes or different types of pacemakers are coded below (Table 26.1):
- As pacemaker technology became more complex, the North American Society of Pacing and Electrophysiology and the British Pacing and Electrophysiology Group expanded the pacemaker code from three to five letters (Table 26.2).
  - The fourth letter identifies programmable features of the pacemaker (P, programmability is simple. M,

multiprogrammable when three or more programmable features are present. C, communicating: the pacemaker communicates by transmitting stored information to a programmer as opposed to a programmer sending commands to the pacemaker. R, rate modulating, the pacemaker has features capable of increasing its rate automatically during stress or exercise. 0, none.
  - The fifth letter identifies whether the pacemaker is capable of terminating tachyarrhythmias (P, pacing is used to terminate tachyarrhythmias; S, shock is used to terminate tachyarrhythmias; D or dual, both pacing and shock can terminate an arrhythmia).
- Thus, a VVI pacemaker that has the capacity to vary its rate is a VVIR and the same pacemaker that uses burst pacing to terminate a tachyarrhythmia is a VVIRP.

## Ventricular Pacemakers

- There are three possible single chamber ventricular pacemaker modes: V00, VVI, and VVT.
- **V00 mode:** This is the code for a fixed rate ventricular pacemaker.
  - The first letter, V, stands for ventricle, which is the chamber paced. The second letter, 0, indicates that the device has no sensing capabilities. The

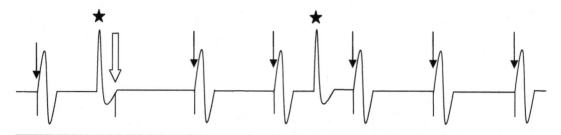

**Figure 26.6:   Fixed Rate Ventricular Pacemaker.** Fixed rate ventricular pacemakers do not have sensing capabilities and stimulate the ventricles constantly (*arrows*), regardless of the patient's underlying rhythm. Rhythm strip shows a fixed rate ventricular pacemaker. Note that the pacemaker is firing constantly causing a pacemaker stimulus to be delivered after a spontaneous ventricular complex (*first star*). The pacemaker impulse was not captured (*block arrow*) because the ventricles are still refractory from the ventricular impulse.

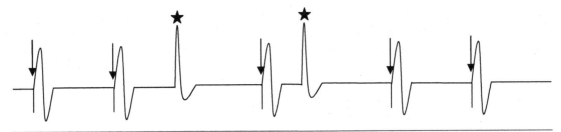

**Figure 26.7:   Demand Ventricular Pacemaker.** Demand ventricular pacemakers are capable of recognizing the patient's intrinsic rhythm. When a spontaneous ventricular complex is detected (*stars*), the pacemaker is inhibited from delivering a stimulus to the ventricle; thus, competition between the pacemaker and the patient's own spontaneous rhythm is prevented.

third letter characterizes the mode of response to a sensed event. Because the pacemaker has no sensing capabilities, the third letter is automatically 0.

- V00, or fixed rate ventricular pacemaker, is the first permanent pacemaker introduced for the treatment of symptomatic AV block. It stimulates the ventricles at a constant rate regardless of the underlying rhythm (Fig. 26.8). Because the pacemaker does not have any sensing capabilities, competition always occurs between the patient's own intrinsic rhythm and that of the constantly delivered pacemaker stimuli. As a result, some pacemaker impulses are delivered to the ventricle even when the ventricles are completely refractory. Other impulses may occur at the end of the T wave of a spontaneous ventricular complex, which corresponds to the vulnerable period of the cardiac cycle (Fig. 26.9). This can potentially precipitate a cardiac arrhythmia.

- **VVI mode:** This is the code for a demand ventricular pacemaker.

- The first letter, V, indicates that the ventricle is the chamber paced. The second letter, V, means that the device is capable of sensing intrinsic impulses from the ventricles. The third letter, I, indicates that the pacemaker is inhibited (meaning that it will not deliver a ventricular stimulus) when it senses a ventricular event.

- VVI pacing is an upgraded version of a V00 pacemaker. It is capable not only of stimulating the ventricles, but is also able to sense impulses originating from the ventricles. When the pacemaker senses a native QRS complex, the pacemaker is inhibited from delivering a pacemaker stimulus. Thus, competition between the patient's rhythm and that of the pacemaker is prevented (Fig. 26.10).

- VVI pacing is the most commonly utilized among the three ventricular pacemaker modes. Even in the era of modern dual chamber pacing, VVI pacing is the pacemaker mode of choice when there is complete AV block and permanent atrial fibrillation (Fig. 26.11).

- **Hysteresis:** In VVI pacing, the interval between two consecutive pacemaker stimuli is constant and is the same as the interval between a sensed ventricular complex and the next pacemaker stimulus (Fig. 26.12). VVI pacemakers, however, can be programmed to have a much longer escape interval. This longer escape interval is called hysteresis and is shown in Figure 26.13.

- Hysteresis was intended to give the patient a chance to manifest his own rhythm, which is often more effective than an artificially paced rhythm. A long hysteresis should not be mistaken for pacemaker malfunction.

- **Oversensing:** In VVI pacing, the pacemaker is inhibited when it senses a native QRS complex. The pacemaker may also be inhibited by extraneous artifacts such as muscle tremors (myopotentials) or electromagnetic interference, especially those generated by large motors. This type of pacemaker inhibition other than

| TABLE 26.1 | | | |
|---|---|---|---|
| **Pacemaker Coding System** | | | |
| Atrial Pacemaker | Ventricular Pacemaker | Dual Chamber Pacemaker | |
| A00 | V00 | DDD | D00 |
| AAI | VVI | DVI | VDD |
| AAT | VVT | DVT | VAT |
| | | DAT | VDT |

The first letter represents the chamber paced, the second letter the chamber sensed, and the third letter the pacemaker response to a sensed event.
A, atrial; V, ventricle; D, dual; 0, none; I, inhibited; T, triggered.

**TABLE 26.2**

**NASPE/BPEG Generic Pacemaker Code**

| Position | I | II | III | IV | V |
|---|---|---|---|---|---|
| Category | Chamber(s) Paced | Chamber(s) Sensed | Response to Sensing | Programmability, Rate Modulation | Antitachyarrhythmia Function(s) |
| | 0 | 0 | 0 | 0 | 0 |
| | A | A | T | P | P* |
| | V | V | I | M | S* |
| | D | D | D# | C | D* |
| | | | | R | |
| Manufacturers' designation only | S, single (A or V) | S, single (A or V) | | | |

NASPE, North American Society of Pacing and Electrophysiology; BPEG, British Pacing and Electrophysiology Group; 0, none; A, atrium; V, ventricle; D, dual (atrium + ventricle); T, triggered; I, inhibited; D#, dual (triggered + inhibited); P, simple programmable; M, multiprogrammable; C, communicating; R, rate modulation; P*, pacing (antitachyarrhythmia); S*, shock; D*, dual (pacing and shock).

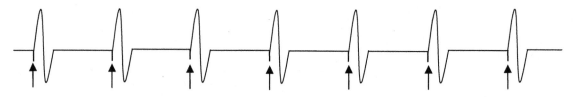

**Figure 26.8: V00 or Fixed Rate Single Chamber Ventricular Pacemaker.** V00 pacemakers operate very satisfactorily when there is no competing rhythm as shown. Note that all pacemaker artifacts (*arrows*) are captured by the ventricles resulting in wide QRS complexes.

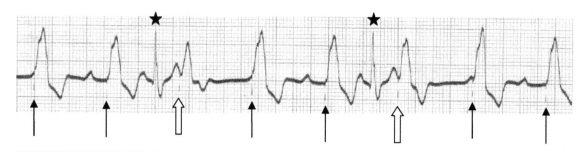

**Figure 26.9: V00 or Fixed Rate Ventricular Pacemaker.** When fixed rate pacing is used, pacemaker artifacts are delivered constantly regardless of the patient's rhythm (*arrows*). If the patient has an intrinsic rhythm (*stars*), some pacemaker artifacts may be delivered at end of the T wave of the preceding intrinsic QRS complex (*block arrows*) corresponding to the vulnerable period of the cardiac cycle.

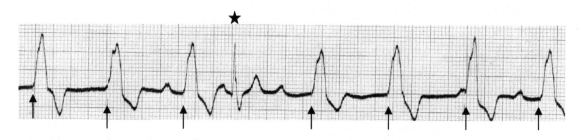

**Figure 26.10: VVI Pacing.** In VVI pacing, the pacemaker is capable of stimulating the ventricles and sensing spontaneous ventricular impulses. The fourth complex is a spontaneous QRS complex (*star*), which was sensed by the pacemaker and was inhibited from delivering a ventricular impulse.

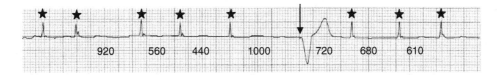

**Figure 26.11: VVI Pacing and Atrial Fibrillation.** The rhythm is atrial fibrillation. The pacemaker was programmed to discharge at a rate of 60 beats per minute and was appropriately inhibited by the first five ventricular complexes. After the fifth complex, a long pause followed, which was appropriately terminated by a pacemaker stimulus resulting in a captured ventricular complex (*arrow*). The long pause measured 1,000 milliseconds, equivalent to a heart rate of 60 beats per minute. The numbers indicate the intervals in milliseconds between the ventricular complexes.

those due to the patient's intrinsic rhythm is called oversensing. Extraneous artifacts, especially those resulting from electromagnetic interference, may inhibit the pacemaker output because the pacemaker erroneously senses these extraneous artifacts as the patient's intrinsic rhythm. Because these electrical artifacts have a faster rate than the programmed rate of the pacemaker, the pacemaker is inhibited and is prevented from delivering a pacemaker output. If the patient is pacemaker-dependent, prolonged inhibition of the pacemaker may result in syncope.

■ Oversensing has been minimized and is no longer a problem with modern-day pacemakers with the use of bipolar instead of unipolar electrodes and insulating the pacemaker generator with a metallic shield to prevent oversensing of myopotentials. Use of electrocautery close to the generator during surgery, however, still poses a potential problem, which can inhibit a pacemaker in VVI mode. This can be prevented by programming the pacemaker to fixed rate mode before the surgery. Applying a magnet over the generator whenever electrocautery is activated can also temporarily convert the pacemaker from VVI mode to a fixed rate or V00 mode (Fig. 26.14).

■ **VVT mode:** This is the code for a ventricular triggered pacemaker.

■ The first letter, V, indicates that the ventricle is the chamber paced. The second letter, V, means that the device is capable of sensing intrinsic impulses from the ventricles. The third letter, T, indicates that the pacemaker is triggered when it senses a ventricular event (meaning that when a ventricular impulse is sensed, the pacemaker will respond by delivering a stimulus).

■ When the pacemaker senses a native ventricular complex, a pacemaker artifact is emitted, which is buried within the sensed QRS complex (Fig. 26.15). A triggered response is the pacemaker's way of acknowledging that the ventricular impulse was sensed. A triggered response within the QRS complex is harmless; however, the frequency of pacemaker output is increased and is not energy efficient. Its main advantage is that when there is oversensing of myopotentials or extraneous artifacts, VVT pacing may prevent asystole in patients who are

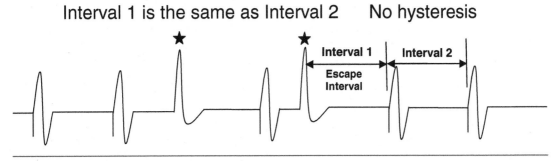

**Figure 26.12: VVI or Ventricular Demand Pacemaker.** VVI pacemakers are capable of sensing spontaneous ventricular impulses (*stars*). When a ventricular impulse is sensed, the escape interval between a spontaneous ventricular complex and the next pacemaker spike (interval 1) is the same as the interval between two consecutive pacemaker spikes (interval 2).

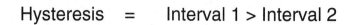

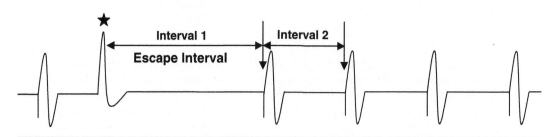

**Figure 26.13: Hysteresis.** Hysteresis is present when the escape interval after a sensed impulse (interval 1) is longer than the interval between two consecutive pacemaker stimuli (interval 2). The presence of hysteresis should not be mistaken for pacemaker malfunction.

pacemaker-dependent by delivering a ventricular output as opposed to a pacemaker in VVI mode, which is inhibited by these extraneous artifacts.

- Triggered responses are no longer used in single chamber pacemakers, but are commonly used in dual chamber pacing. For example, when one chamber such as the atria senses a native atrial complex, the dual chamber pacemaker is triggered to deliver an output to the ventricles after a programmed interval to preserve AV synchrony (see Dual Chamber Pacemakers).

## Atrial Pacemakers

- Atrial pacemakers are similar to ventricular pacemakers except that the pacemaker generator is connected to the atrium instead of the ventricle.
  - **A00 mode:** A00 or fixed rate atrial pacemaker continuously stimulates the atrium regardless of the atrial rhythm (Fig. 26.16).
  - **AAI mode:** In atrial demand pacemaker, the pacemaker is inhibited from delivering a stimulus

when a spontaneous atrial impulse is sensed (Fig. 26.17).

- **AAT mode:** When the pacemaker is atrial triggered, the pacemaker is required to deliver a stimulus coinciding with the sensed P wave when a spontaneous atrial complex is sensed (Fig. 26.18).

## Pacemaker Electrodes

- **Pacemaker electrodes:** Most pacemaker electrodes are endocardial electrodes and are inserted transvenously into the right atrium or right ventricle. The right atrial electrode is usually anchored to the right atrial appendage and the ventricular electrode at the apex of the right ventricle. In rare cases in which transvenous insertion is not possible, a myocardial or epicardial lead is sutured into the atrial or ventricular myocardium using a transthoracic or subcostal approach.
- There are two types of pacemaker electrodes: bipolar and unipolar.
  - **Bipolar:** A bipolar electrode has the stimulating electrode (or cathode) at the tip of the catheter and the negative electrode (or anode) just below the

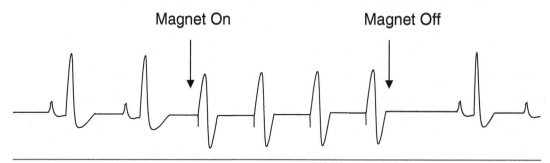

**Figure 26.14: Application of a Magnet.** Application of a magnet to the pacemaker generator will convert the device to a fixed rate mode. Thus, a VVI pacemaker is converted to a V00 pacemaker with application of a magnet as shown above. After the magnet is taken off the pacemaker, the pacemaker reverts to a VVI mode.

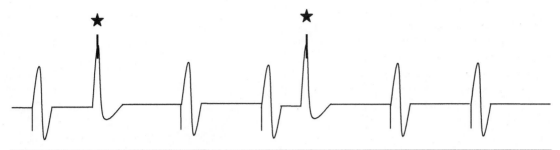

**Figure 26.15:    VVT or Ventricular Triggered Pacemaker.**  A pacemaker in VVT mode paces the ventricles. It can also sense spontaneous impulses from the ventricles. When a ventricular impulse is sensed, the pacemaker is immediately triggered to deliver a pacemaker stimulus as shown by the second and fifth complexes (*stars*). The triggered output is seen as an artifact buried within the patient's own QRS complex.

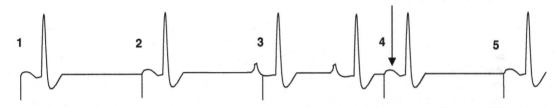

**Figure 26.16:    Atrial Pacemaker in A00 Mode.**  A pacemaker in A00 mode constantly delivers an atrial output regardless of the atrial rhythm. It is not capable of sensing any atrial impulse. The third pacemaker artifact occurred after an intrinsic P wave and was not captured. The fourth pacemaker artifact was able to capture the atrium and the pacemaker induced P wave (*arrow*) was conducted to the ventricles resulting in a normally conducted QRS complex.

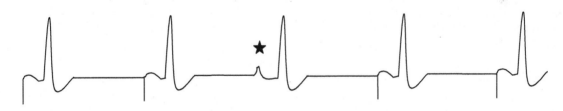

**Figure 26.17:    AAI or Atrial Demand Pacemaker.**  In AAI mode, the atrium is paced. When an atrial P wave is sensed (*star*), the pacemaker is inhibited from delivering an atrial stimulus.

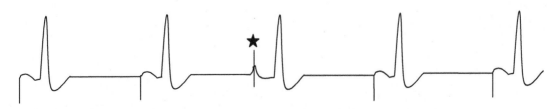

**Figure 26.18:    AAT or Atrial Triggered Pacemaker.**  A pacemaker in AAT mode is similar to a pacemaker in AAI mode except that the pacemaker is triggered to deliver a pacemaker stimulus (*star*) when it senses an atrial event.

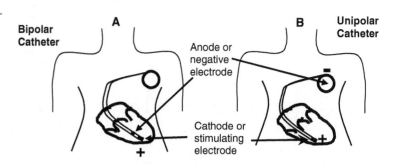

**Figure 26.19: Bipolar and Unipolar Electrodes. (A)** A bipolar electrode. Both positive and negative electrodes are a short distance from each other within the area of the right ventricle. **(B)** A unipolar electrode. The stimulating electrode or cathode is located at the tip of the catheter and the negative electrode is in the metal housing of the pacemaker generator.

cathode at a distance of about 10 mm (Fig. 26.19A). The short distance between the two terminals causes a smaller pacemaker artifact in the ECG and a smaller antenna effect; thus, the pacemaker is less affected by electronic artifacts. Virtually all pacemakers today have bipolar electrodes.

- **Unipolar:** A unipolar electrode has the stimulating electrode (or cathode) at the tip of the catheter and the negative electrode (or anode) in the metal housing of the pacemaker generator (Fig. 26.19B). Because the flow of current extends from the apex of the right ventricle (where the cathode is located), to the pacemaker generator (where the anode is located), the pacemaker artifact is unusually large. The wide distance between the two electrodes also causes a large antenna effect, rendering the pacemaker vulnerable to interference by electromagnetic forces.
- The location of the pacemaker electrode determines the morphology of the QRS complex. Stimulation of the right ventricle will result in a left bundle branch block configuration of the QRS complexes (Fig. 26.20). Stimulation of the left ventricle will generate a QRS

complex with a right bundle branch block configuration (Fig. 26.21). Not all pacemaker-induced right bundle branch block patterns are due to left ventricular pacing, however.

## Pacemaker Syndrome

- **Pacemaker syndrome:** Symptoms of low output, hypotension, and even syncope or near syncope can occur in patients with cardiac pacemakers, especially in VVI mode. This constellation of symptoms during ventricular pacing is called the pacemaker syndrome. Pacemaker syndrome can occur if there is retrograde conduction of the ventricular impulse to the atria (Fig. 26.22), causing both atria and ventricles to contract simultaneously. When the atria contracts against a closed mitral and tricuspid valves, pulmonary venous hypertension, low cardiac output, and reflex hypotension can occur. This can be minimized with insertion of a dual chamber cardiac pacemaker.

**Figure 26.20: Right Ventricular Pacing.** When the stimulating electrode is in the right ventricle, the QRS complexes have a left bundle branch block configuration with deep S waves in $V_1$–$V_2$.

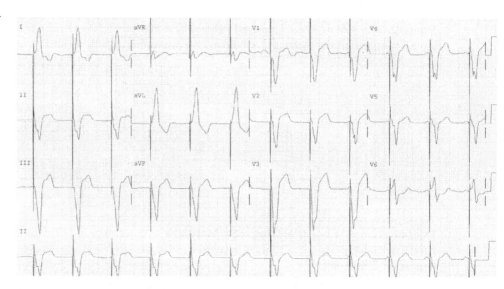

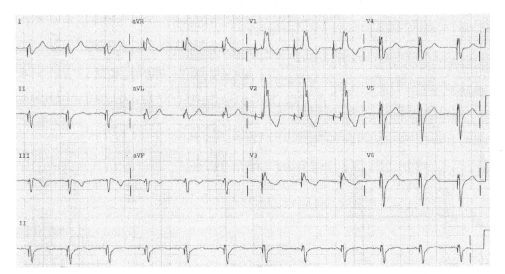

**Figure 26.21:    Left Ventricular Pacing.** A transvenous catheter was inserted into the left ventricle after inadvertently crossing a patent foramen ovale. Note that the QRS complexes in $V_1$ have right bundle branch block configuration indicative of left ventricular pacing.

## Dual Chamber Pacemakers

- **Dual chamber pacemakers:** Dual chamber pacing was introduced to preserve AV synchrony. It has separate electrodes, one in the ventricle and the other in the atrium. Dual chamber pacing is easy to recognize in the ECG when there are two separate pacemaker stimuli, one capturing the atria and the other the ventricles. Its function is more complicated than a single chamber device because it combines atrial and ventricular sensing with atrial and ventricular pacing.

- The different ECG patterns associated with a dual chamber pacemaker are shown in Figure 26.23.
  - Atrial pacing in combination with ventricular pacing
  - Atrial pacing in combination with ventricular sensing
  - Atrial sensing in combination with ventricular pacing
  - Atrial sensing in combination with ventricular sensing

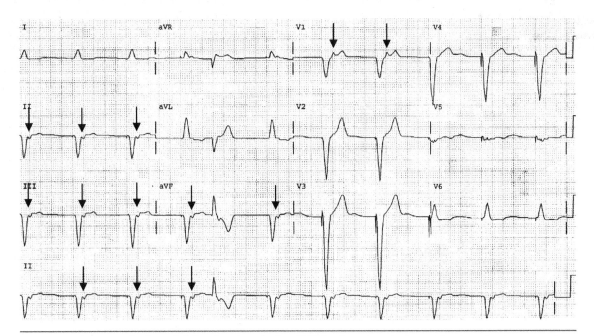

**Figure 26.22:    Ventriculoatrial Conduction during VVI Pacing.** Ventriculoatrial (V-A) conduction or conduction of the ventricular impulse to the atria can occur during ventricular pacing resulting in retrograde P waves. The P waves are seen after the QRS complexes (*arrows*) and are due to retrograde conduction of the ventricular impulse to the atria across the AV conduction system. Pacemaker syndrome is due to simultaneous contraction of both atria and ventricles when there is V-A conduction. V-A conduction is possible even in patients with complete AV block.

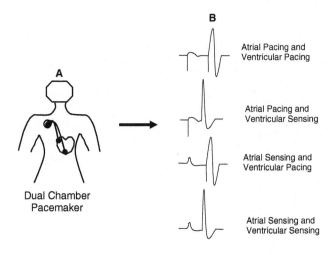

**Possible ECG of Dual Chamber Pacemaker**

**Figure 26.23: Dual Chamber Pacemaker. (A)** A diagrammatic representation of a dual chamber pacemaker. **(B)** The different electrocardiogram patterns associated with a dual chamber pacemaker.

## DDD Pacing

- **DDD Pacing:** Among several dual chamber pacemaker modes, DDD pacing is the most commonly used. It is called universal pacemaker because it is the only pacemaker that can pace and sense both chambers separately. Figures 26.24 through 26.28 show the possible ECG findings associated with DDD pacing.
  - In DDD pacing, the pacemaker is capable of sensing impulses from both atrium and ventricle. When the pacemaker senses an atrial impulse, the atrial channel is inhibited from delivering an atrial stimulus. Inhibition of the atrial channel triggers the ventricular channel to deliver a stimulus to the ventricle after a programmed interval. However, if a spontaneous ventricular impulse is sensed, the pacemaker

will be inhibited from discharging a pacemaker stimulus.
  - DDD pacing is the most physiologic among all available pacemakers and was introduced to preserved AV synchrony.
- Other ECG presentations of DDD pacing are shown in Figs. 26.26–26.28.
- **Indication:** DDD pacing is the pacemaker mode of choice when there is complete AV block with intact sinus function. The pacemaker can track the atrial rate and triggers a ventricular output for every atrial impulse that is sensed. The pacemaker therefore is rate-responsive because spontaneous increase in atrial rate is always followed by a pacemaker-induced ventricular response. Thus, when the patient develops sinus tachycardia during stress or exercise, the ventricular rate increases commensurately, because the pacemaker is committed to deliver a ventricular output after every sensed atrial event (Fig. 26.29).
- **Contraindication:** DDD pacing, however, is not appropriate for all clinical situations. Although DDD pacing is the pacemaker mode of choice among patients with complete AV block with intact sinus function, it is contraindicated when there is permanent atrial fibrillation. DDD pacing is not appropriate when there is atrial flutter or fibrillation because every sensed atrial event will trigger a ventricular output (Figs. 26.30 and 26.31). Furthermore, it is not possible to pace the atrium when there is atrial flutter or atrial fibrillation. In this setting, a VVI pacemaker is the pacemaker mode of choice.
- **Mode switching:** When atrial flutter or fibrillation is paroxysmal or recurrent, some DDD pacemakers are capable of mode switching when the supraventricular arrhythmia is detected. For example, in patients with DDD pacemakers, the pacemaker mode switches automatically from DDD to VVI mode when atrial fibrillation is detected and back to DDD when the arrhythmia spontaneously converts to normal sinus rhythm. If a DDD pacemaker is not capable of automatic mode switching, it should be programmed to a VVI mode.

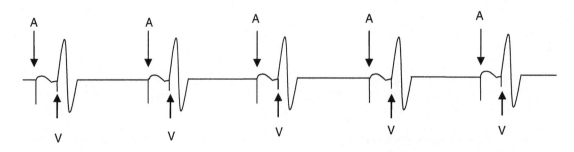

**Figure 26.24: Dual Chamber Pacemaker without any Competing Rhythm.** The presence of separate atrial (A) and ventricular (V) stimuli suggest that the pacemaker is dual chamber. Atrial pacing followed by ventricular pacing is one of the possible electrocardiogram patterns of a DDD pacemaker.

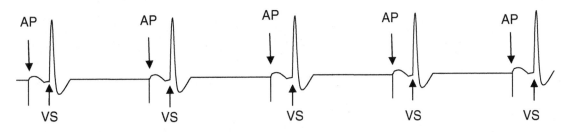

**Figure 26.25:  DDD Pacing: Atrial Pacing Followed by a Spontaneous Ventricular Rhythm.** Another electrocardiogram pattern of DDD pacing is the presence of pacemaker induced atrial complexes, which may conduct normally to the ventricles. The pacemaker senses the normally conducted ventricular complexes (VS) resulting in inhibition of the ventricular output hence no ventricular pacemaker artifact is present. AP, atrial pacing; VS, ventricular sensing.

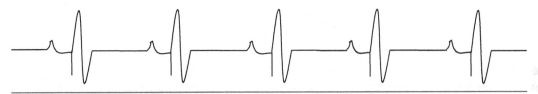

**Figure 26.26:  DDD Pacing: Normal Sinus Rhythm followed by Paced Ventricular Rhythm.** DDD pacing can also present with sinus P waves followed by pacemaker-induced QRS complexes. When sinus rhythm is present, the sensed P waves inhibit the atrial output and at the same time triggers the pacemaker to deliver a ventricular output after a programmed atrioventricular interval. Thus, when sinus tachycardia occurs, every P wave will be followed by a QRS complex.

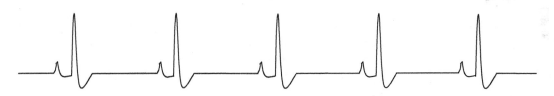

**Figure 26.27:  DDD Pacing: Normal Sinus Rhythm with Normal Atrioventricular Conduction.** In DDD pacing, the presence of spontaneous atrial and ventricular complexes may inhibit the pacemaker output completely. This will allow the patient to manifest his or her own rhythm without evidence of pacemaker activity.

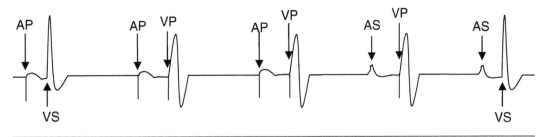

**Figure 26.28:  DDD Pacing.** This rhythm strip summarizes all the possible combinations for DDD pacing. AP, atrial pacing; AS, atrial sensing; VP, ventricular pacing; VS, ventricular sensing.

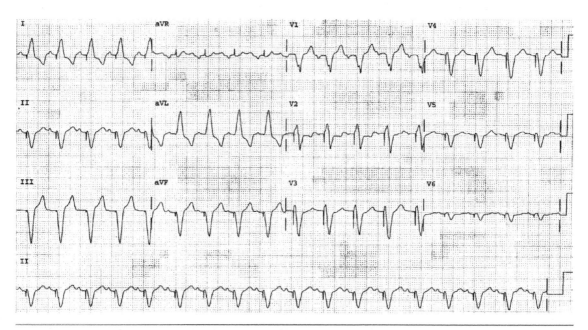

**Figure 26.29: Pacemaker in DDD Mode Tracking Sinus Tachycardia.** Sinus tachycardia is present with upright P waves in leads I, II, and aVF. DDD pacing can track the atrial rate committing the pacemaker to deliver a ventricular output for every sensed atrial event. DDD pacing is the pacemaker of choice when complete atrioventricular block is present with intact sinus node function.

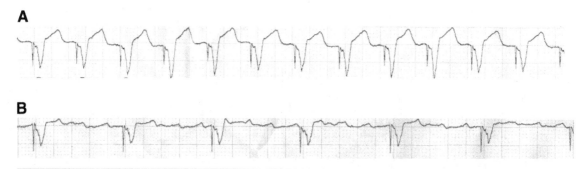

**Figure 26.30: DDD Pacing During Atrial Fibrillation.** During atrial fibrillation, a pacemaker in DDD mode can track the atrial rate and delivers a ventricular output after every sensed atrial event resulting in a fast ventricular rate as shown above. DDD pacing therefore is not appropriate during atrial fibrillation. The pacemaker should be programmed to a VVI mode. See also Figure 26.11.

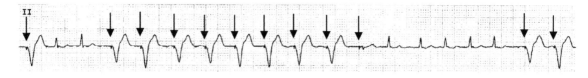

**Figure 26.31: DDD Pacing and Atrial Flutter.** Rhythm strip **A** shows a dual chamber pacemaker in DDD mode in a patient with atrial flutter. Note that the pacemaker rate is relatively fast at approximately 115 per minute. Rhythm strip **B** was taken after the pacemaker was programmed to VVI mode. The rhythm is atrial flutter and the ventricular rate is slower at 60 per minute.

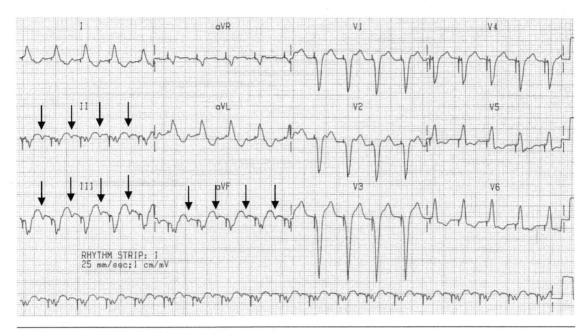

**Figure 26.32: Pacemaker-Mediated Tachycardia.** Twelve-lead electrocardiogram of a patient with pacemaker mediated tachycardia (PMT). PMT is possible only when there is ventriculoatrial (V-A) conduction (*arrows*), which are seen as retrograde P waves in II, III, and aVF. The P waves are sensed by the atrial channel triggering the pacemaker to deliver a ventricular output. Once the ventricles are stimulated, V-A conduction again occurs resulting in PMT.

## Pacemaker-Mediated Tachycardia

■ **Pacemaker-mediated tachycardia:** One of the complications of DDD pacing is pacemaker-mediated tachycardia (PMT) (Fig. 20.32). This tachycardia is possible only when there is ventriculoatrial (V-A) conduction. V-A conduction refers to the conduction of an impulse retrogradely from ventricles to atria through the AV conduction system. V-A conduction has been shown to occur even in the presence of complete AV block.

■ When the ventricle is paced, the ventricular impulse can conduct retrogradely to the atria. The retrograde P wave is sensed by the atrial channel of the pacemaker and commits the pacemaker to deliver a ventricular output, which will again result in retrograde conduction. PMT can also occur in any dual chamber pacemaker in which a sensed atrial event can trigger a ventricular output such as VDD, VAT, and DDT modes.

■ PMT can be terminated by placing a magnet over the pacemaker generator, temporarily converting the pacemaker to a fixed rate or D00 mode or by reprogramming the pacemaker.

■ PMT can also be terminated by programming the pacemaker to DVI or VVI mode. Any programming that renders the atrial channel incapable of sensing retrograde P waves will terminate the tachycardia.

■ If the pacemaker has to remain in DDD mode, the pacemaker can be reprogrammed not to recognize the retrograde P wave. This is done by lengthening the atrial refractory period (ARP). During the ARP, the atrial channel is not able to sense any impulse (Fig. 26.33). The atrial refractory period starts with a paced or sensed atrial activity and continues until ventricular pacing or sensing. The ARP also extends beyond the QRS complex and is called postventricular atrial refractory period (PVARP). The duration of the PVARP is programmable. The PVARP is built into the pacemaker to prevent the atrium from sensing the ventricular output and QRS complex as an atrial event. Lengthening the PVARP will prevent the pacemaker from sensing retrograde P waves because the retrograde P wave will now fall within the atrial refractory period.

■ An endless loop PMT should not be confused with sinus tachycardia during DDD pacing. When sinus tachycardia is present, the P waves are upright in II, III, and aVF (Fig. 26.34A). On the other hand, when PMT is present, the P waves are retrogradely conducted (ventriculoatrial conduction) and will be inverted in leads II, III, and aVF (Fig. 26.34B).

■ Very often, a pacemaker tachycardia can also occur when there is atrial flutter or atrial fibrillation (Figs. 26.30, 26.31, and 26.35).

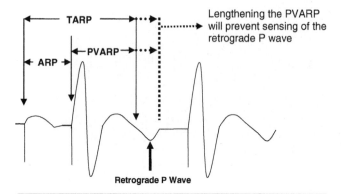

**Figure 26.33: Atrial Refractory Period in DDD Pacing.** The atrial refractory period (ARP) starts with atrial pacing and continues until ventricular pacing or ventricular sensing. This corresponds to the whole atrioventricular or PR interval and indicates the time that the atrial channel is unable to sense any impulse. The ARP also continues beyond ventricular pacing (or sensing). This portion of the atrial refractory period is called the postventricular atrial refractory period (PVARP). The length of the PVARP is programmable. The total atrial refractory period (TARP) includes the ARP and the PVARP. During the TARP, the atrial channel is deft to any impulse. If there is PMT, the PVARP can be programmed to a longer interval (*dotted line*) so that it will not sense the retrograde P wave.

## ECG Pattern of Other Dual Chamber Pacemakers

- The ECG of other, less commonly encountered dual chamber pacemakers are shown.
- **VAT mode:** The pacemaker is an atrial synchronous pacemaker and was one of the earliest dual chamber pacemakers introduced clinically that can preserve AV synchrony (Fig. 26.36).

- When an atrial impulse is sensed, the pacemaker is triggered to deliver a pacemaker stimulus to the ventricles. Thus, the ventricles are stimulated only when a spontaneous atrial impulse is sensed. When there is no spontaneous atrial rhythm, the pacemaker acts like a V00 pacemaker because the pacemaker does not sense ventricular impulses.
- The main drawback of VAT pacing is that sensing occurs only in the atrium. Thus, spontaneous ventricular complexes are not sensed and the pacemaker can deliver electrical stimuli to the ventricles even when there are spontaneous QRS complexes.
- **DVI Pacing:** Also called A-V sequential pacing. It was intended for patients with complete AV block (Fig. 26.37).

- When the pacemaker senses a spontaneous ventricular complex, the pacemaker is inhibited from delivering a stimulus to the ventricles. Thus, the initial pacemaker stimulus is delivered to the atrium after a programmed escape interval. This interval is measured from the last spontaneous or pacemaker induced ventricular complex. After the atrium is paced, the ventricle is sequentially paced; however, if a spontaneous ventricular impulse is sensed, the pacemaker stimulus will be inhibited.
- Unlike VAT pacing in which the ventricles are stimulated even when a spontaneous ventricular complex is present, pacing in DVI mode prevents the pacemaker from delivering a stimulus to the ventricle if the pacemaker senses a spontaneous ventricular impulse. Because DVI pacing is not capable of sensing atrial impulses, AV synchrony is not preserved.
- **VDD mode.** In VDD mode, only the ventricle is paced. Sensing occurs in both chambers. The pacemaker is not capable of pacing the atrium; however, when an atrial impulse is sensed, the pacemaker is triggered to deliver a ventricular output. If the

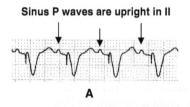

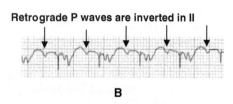

A

B

**Figure 26.34: DDD Pacing During Sinus Tachycardia (A) and Endless Loop Tachycardia (B). (A)** Sinus tachycardia with P waves upright in lead II (*arrows*). The full 12-lead electrocardiogram (ECG) of sinus tachycardia followed by pacemaker induced ventricular response is shown in Figure 26.29. **(B)** Endless loop pacemaker mediated tachycardia. The P waves are inverted in lead II (*arrows*). The full 12-lead ECG of a pacemaker mediated tachycardia is shown in Figure 26.32.

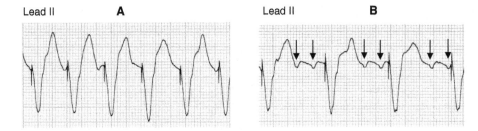

**Figure 26.35:** **DDD Pacing with Mode Switching.** **(A)** A dual chamber pacemaker in DDD mode. Ventricular pacing is seen with a rate of approximately 110 beats per minute, which is the maximum rate that is programmed for the pacemaker. The underlying rhythm is not obvious in the rhythm strip. Because the pacemaker is capable of mode switching, it automatically programs itself into a VVI mode **(B)** with a rate of approximately 70 beats per minute. The underlying rhythm is atrial flutter with atrioventricular block. The flutter waves are marked by the arrows.

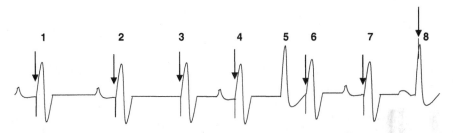

**Figure 26.36:** **VAT mode.** VAT pacing is the first atrial sensing dual chamber pacemaker put into clinical use that is capable of preserving atrioventricular (AV) synchrony. In VAT pacing, the ventricle is the only chamber paced and the atrium is the only chamber sensed. When a spontaneous atrial impulse is sensed, the ventricle is triggered after a programmed AV interval (first, second, fourth, and seventh complexes), thus the pacemaker can track the atrial rate and is rate responsive. Because a sensed P wave always triggers a ventricular output, AV synchrony is preserved. The drawback is that competition can occur when spontaneous ventricular rhythm is present because the pacemaker is not capable of sensing ventricular impulses (fifth and eighth complexes). When there is no atrial activity (third complex), the pacemaker will function in VOO mode. Arrows point to the pacemaker artifacts.

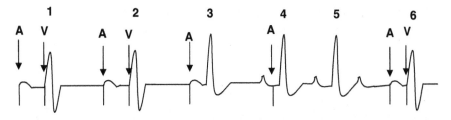

**Figure 26.37:** **DVI Mode.** In DVI pacing, both atria and ventricles are paced. The ventricle is the only chamber sensed. In the absence of a competing rhythm, the atrium and ventricle are sequentially paced and the resulting electrocardiogram is shown in complexes 1 and 2. When a native ventricular impulse is sensed, the ventricular output is inhibited (third, fourth, and fifth complexes). When the ventricular rate drops below a preset rate (distance between third and fourth complexes), the pacemaker is committed to deliver an atrial output regardless of the atrial rhythm. Note that the atrial artifact in four was not followed by a ventricular output because the pacemaker was able to sense the native ventricular complex. It was not able to recognize the P wave in front of the QRS complex because DVI pacing is not capable of sensing atrial impulses (fourth complex). The pacemaker is not rate responsive since the pacemaker is not capable of sensing atrial impulses; thus, atrioventricular synchrony is not preserved. The arrows identify the pacemaker artifacts. (**A** represents atrial pacemaker artifacts and **V** represent ventricular pacemaker artifacts).

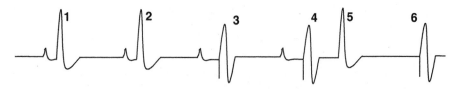

**Figure 26.38:  VDD Mode.** In VDD mode only the ventricle is paced. The pacemaker is capable of sensing impulses from both atrium and ventricle (first two complexes). When an atrial impulse is sensed, the pacemaker is triggered to deliver a ventricular output after a programmed atrioventricular (AV) interval (third and fourth complexes). When a ventricular complex is sensed, the pacemaker is inhibited from delivering a ventricular output (fifth complex). When the atrial rate is fast, the pacemaker can track the atrial rate and is therefore rate responsive similar to a DDD pacemaker. However, when the atrial rate is unusually slow or when there is no atrial activity (pause after the fifth complex), the pacemaker functions in the VVI mode (sixth complex) because the pacemaker is not capable of pacing the atrium and loses its advantage as a dual chamber pacemaker in preserving AV synchrony.

pacemaker senses a spontaneous ventricular complex, it is inhibited from delivering a pacemaker stimulus to the ventricles. The pacemaker will function as a VVI pacer if it does not sense any spontaneous atrial complex (Fig. 26.38).

■ **DDI pacing:** In DDI pacing, the atrial or ventricular outputs are inhibited when atrial or ventricular impulses are sensed. Although atrial sensing occurs, the pacemaker is not triggered to deliver a ventricular stimulus, thus the pacemaker is not rate responsive (Fig. 26.39).

## Pacemaker with Antitachycardia Properties

■ Pacemakers are also capable of terminating ventricular tachycardia. The rhythm strips in Figures 26.40 and 26.41 show a VVIRP pacemaker, which is capable of

terminating ventricular tachycardia with burst pacing. This is usually accomplished by delivering a series of ventricular pacemaker stimuli in an attempt to capture the ventricles during the tachycardia. Figure 26.40 shows ventricular tachycardia terminated successfully by burst pacing.

■ In Figure 26.41, burst pacing was delivered inappropriately during a sinus tachycardia, which was mistaken for ventricular tachycardia. After burst pacing was completed, the rhythm had deteriorated from sinus tachycardia to ventricular tachycardia.

## Biventricular Pacemakers and Cardioverter Defibrillators

■ **Biventricular pacemakers:** Patients with wide QRS complexes resulting from left or right bundle branch

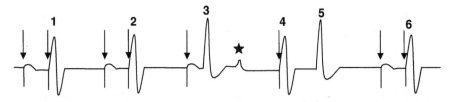

**Figure 26.39:  DDI mode.** Both atrium and ventricle are paced (first two complexes). The pacemaker is capable of sensing impulses from both atrium and ventricle. When an atrial impulse is sensed (*star*), the pacemaker is inhibited from delivering an atrial output. When a ventricular impulse is sensed (third and fifth complexes), the pacemaker is inhibited from delivering a ventricular output. When the atrial rhythm is unusually slow or when there is no atrial activity (pause after the fifth complex), atrial pacing is initiated when the lower rate limit of the pacemaker is reached (sixth complex). This is followed by a ventricular output unless a spontaneous ventricular complex occurs. Although the pacemaker is capable of sensing atrial impulses, the ventricular output is not triggered when an atrial impulse is sensed (*star*). The pacemaker therefore is not rate responsive since it is not capable of increasing the ventricular rate when the atrial rate increases during stress or exercise.

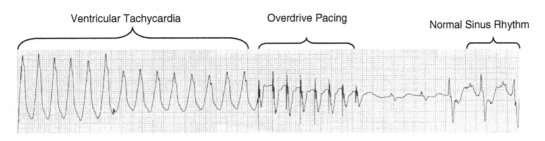

**Figure 26.40:   Overdrive Pacing Terminating Ventricular Tachycardia.** The left side of the tracing shows ventricular tachycardia with a rate of 180 beats per minute. The pacemaker recognizes the ventricular tachycardia and delivers a burst of ventricular pacemaker stimuli, which is faster than the rate of the ventricular tachycardia. The pacemaker successfully captures the ventricles during pacing. When pacing is terminated, the rhythm is successfully converted to a slower ventricular rhythm followed by normal sinus rhythm.

block, severe left ventricular systolic dysfunction (ejection fraction ≤35%), and symptoms of heart failure in spite of optimal medical therapy are candidates for implantation of biventricular pacemakers. Biventricular pacing is performed by pacing both ventricles simultaneously, even in the absence of bradyarrhythmias from AV block or sinus node dysfunction. Biventricular pacing synchronizes ventricular contraction in patients with bundle branch block and has been shown to improve cardiac output in patients with wide QRS complexes who also have severe left ventricular dysfunction. The left ventricle is paced with an electrode inserted through the coronary sinus. The right atrium and right ventricle are paced conventionally. Patients with severe left ventricular dysfunction are also at risk for malignant ventricular arrhythmias. Thus, patients with heart failure requiring biventricular pacemakers are also candidates for implantation of devices with defibrillating properties.

■ **Automatic implantable devices:** Patients who are survivors of cardiac arrest or patients who are high risk for ventricular tachycardia or fibrillation are candidates for implantation of automatic cardioverter defibrillators. These devices are commonly integrated with biventricular pacemakers in patients undergoing car-

diac resynchronization therapy. Thus, automatic implantable defibrillators are commonly integrated with pacemakers and permanent pacemakers are integrated with defibrillating properties, making them capable of treating both bradycardia and tachycardia. An example of a patient with an implantable cardioverter/defibrillator (ICD) whose ventricular tachycardia is terminated by delivery of an electrical shock is shown in Figure 26.42. Although the defibrillator also has pacemaking properties, pacemaker activity was not necessary after successful cardioversion.

## Artificial Cardiac Pacemakers: Clinical Implications

■ Permanent pacemakers were clinically introduced for the treatment of symptomatic bradyarrhythmias from complete AV block and sinus node dysfunction. Single chamber ventricular pacemakers were the first generation of implantable devices used for this purpose. Single chamber ventricular pacemakers, however, do not preserve AV synchrony. Furthermore, ventricular pacing can result in pacemaker syndrome.

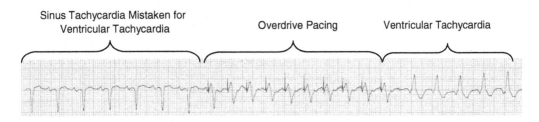

**Figure 26.41:   VVIRP.** Rhythm strip shows a rate responsive VVI pacemaker with features capable of terminating a tachyarrhythmia using burst pacing (VVIRP). In the rhythm strip, the pacemaker mistook the sinus tachycardia for ventricular tachycardia and inappropriately delivered a burst of 10 ventricular pacemaker stimuli, which is successful in capturing the ventricles. When pacing was terminated, the rhythm had changed to ventricular tachycardia as noted at the end of the rhythm strip.

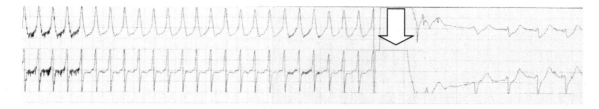

**Figure 26.42:   Automatic Implantable Cardioverter Defibrillator (AICD).** Rhythm strip showing a wide complex tachycardia on the left half of the rhythm strip. The AICD was able to recognize the ventricular tachycardia and automatically delivered an electrical shock (*arrow*) that successfully converted the rhythm to normal sinus (*right side of the tracing*).

■ Pacemaker syndrome is a hemodynamic consequence of ventricular pacing. This is mainly from retrograde or ventriculoatrial conduction of the paced ventricular impulse to the atria. This is characterized by cannon A waves in the neck from contraction of the atria when the mitral and tricuspid valves are closed. Increase in atrial and pulmonary venous pressures can occur when the atria are contracting against a closed AV valve, resulting in shortness of breath as well as reflex drop in blood pressure. This overall symptom complex of hypotension, shortness of breath, and low cardiac output is called the pacemaker syndrome.

■ Single chamber ventricular pacemakers have been replaced by dual chamber pacemakers, which are more physiologic, because AV synchrony is preserved. Although single channel AAI pacemakers can also preserve AV synchrony, they are limited to patients with intact AV conduction and are not indicated in the presence of complete AV block. VVI pacemakers remain the most commonly implanted pacemaker worldwide. In the United States, most pacemakers that are implanted are dual chamber devices in DDD mode.

■ VVI pacing continues to be the pacemaker mode of choice when complete AV block occurs in the setting of permanent atrial fibrillation. DDD pacing is contraindicated because it is not possible to pace the atrium when there is atrial flutter or fibrillation. Furthermore, the presence of atrial flutter or fibrillation will commit the pacemaker to deliver a ventricular output for every sensed atrial event resulting in unnecessary tachycardia.

■ Although single chamber atrial pacemaker is the most appropriate device for patients with sick sinus syndrome, dual chamber pacing in DDD mode is more often used. Sick sinus syndrome is most commonly the result of degenerative disease that affects not only the sinus node but may eventually involve the AV node and distal conduction system.

■ Pacemakers are sometimes inappropriately inhibited by extraneous impulses such as muscle tremors, electrocautery, microwaves, magnetic fields, and other artifacts. Oversensing of these artifacts has been minimized with the use of bipolar electrodes where the anode or negative electrode is mounted just a short distance from the tip of the catheter thus shortening the distance between the two electrodes and the size of the antenna. If electrocautery is performed during a surgical procedure, it should not involve the area of the pacemaker generator. If this cannot be avoided, the pacemaker can be programmed to a fixed rate mode or a magnet can be placed over the generator to temporarily convert the pacemaker to a fixed rate mode. Pacemakers with sensing capabilities (VVI, DDD pacemakers) are temporarily converted to a fixed rate (V00, D00) mode when a magnet is placed over a pacemaker generator.

■ Endless loop or pacemaker-mediated tachycardia can occur with DDD pacing as well as with other modes of pacing such as VDD, VAT, and DDT. The tachycardia can be terminated by reprogramming the pacemaker to other modes such as VVI or DVI or a magnet can be applied to the pacemaker generator, temporarily converting the pacemaker to a fixed rate or D00 mode. If the pacemaker needs to remain in DDD mode, the pacemaker can be programmed not to recognize the retrograde P wave by lengthening the refractory period of the atrial channel.

■ **Permanent pacemakers:** The indications for insertion of permanent pacemakers in patients with acquired AV block are discussed in Chapter 8, Atrioventricular Block; for patients with intraventricular conduction defect, in Chapter 11, Intraventricular Conduction Defect: Trifascicular Block; and for patients with sick sinus syndrome, in Chapter 12, Sinus Node Dysfunction.

■ Whenever there is a need for a permanent pacemaker, two other conditions should always be considered before the permanent pacemaker is implanted: the need for biventricular pacemaker in patients with bundle branch block and the need for ICD in patients with left ventricular dysfunction.

   ■ **Biventricular pacemakers:** Implantation of biventricular pacemaker (also called cardiac resynchronization therapy), is indicated in patients with a QRS duration of >0.12 seconds, who have systolic left ventricular dysfunction (ejection fraction ≤35%) and continue to have symptoms of heart failure (Class III or Class IV) in spite of optimal medical therapy for heart failure. Cardiac resynchronization is performed by pacing both ventricles simultaneously. Simultaneous pacing of both ventricles will significantly decrease the delay in the spread of electrical impulse to both ventricles when there is bundle branch block. Biventricular pacing has been shown to improve cardiac output in patients with wide QRS complexes. The patient should be in normal sinus rhythm so that timing of atrial and ventricular contraction can be synchronized. Although most patients who have received biventricular pacemakers have left bundle branch block, currently, the width of the QRS complex rather than the type of bundle branch block is the main indication for biventricular pacing.

- **Implantable cardioverter defibrillators:** Patients with severe left ventricular dysfunction are at risk for sudden cardiac death due to ventricular tachycardia or ventricular fibrillation. These patients therefore are also candidates for implantation of ICD.

  □ **Secondary prevention:** ICD may be implanted for secondary prevention of sudden cardiac death implying that these patients have experienced and survived a previous episode of cardiac arrest or sustained ventricular tachycardia.

  □ **Primary prevention:** These patients have not experienced any previous arrhythmias or cardiac arrest but are high risk for ventricular tachycardia or ventricular fibrillation. For primary prevention of sudden cardiac death, the following are Class I indications for implantation of ICD according to the American College of Cardiology/American Heart Association/Heart Rhythm Society 2008 guidelines for device-based therapy of cardiac rhythm abnormalities.

    □ Left ventricular ejection fraction <35% due to prior myocardial infarction (MI) who are at least 40 days post-MI and are in New York Heart Association (NYHA) functional Class II or III.

    □ Nonischemic dialated cardiomyopathy with ejection fraction ≤35% and who are in NYHA functional Class II or III.

    □ The following are Class IIa recommendations for primary prevention of sudden cardiac death.

    □ Left ventricular dysfunction due to prior MI who are at least 40 days post-MI, have an ejection fraction <30% and are in NYHA functional Class I.

    □ Selected patients with idiopathic hypertrophic subaortic stenosis who have 1 or more major risk factors for sudden cardiac death. This includes strong family history of sudden cardiac death, abnormal blood pressure response during exercise testing, unusually thick ventricular septum ≥3.0 cm, and spontaneous nonsustained VT or unexplained syncope.

    □ Patients with arrhythmogenic right ventricular dysplasia or cardiomyopathy who have 1 or more risk factors for sudden cardiac death. This includes male gender, severe right ventricular (RV) dilatation and extensive RV involvement, LV involvement, young age (<5 years) and nonsustained ventricular tachycardia during monitoring or induction of ventricular tachycardia during electrophysiologic testing.

- Similar to pacemakers, ICDs may be affected by electromagnetic interferences including those emitted by electronic article surveillance system, which are deployed as antitheft devices in shopping centers. This may cause the ICD to discharge inappropriately if the patient is exposed long enough to the effects of the antitheft device.

## Suggested Readings

Bernstein AD, Camm AJ, Fletcher RD, et al. NASPE/BPEG generic pacemaker code for antibradyarrhythmia and adaptive-rate pacing and antitachyarrhythmia devices. *Pacing Clin Electrophysiol.* 1987;10:794–799.

Epstein AE, DiMarco JP, Ellenbogen KA, et al. ACC/AHA/HRS 2008 guidelines for device-based therapy of cardiac rhythm abnormalities: a report of the American College of Cardiology/American Heart Association Task Force on Practice Guidelines (Writing Committee to Revise the ACC/AHA/NASPE 2002 Guideline Update for Implantation of Cardiac Pacemakers and Antiarrhythmia Devices). *Circulation.* 2008;117:e350–e408.

Gimbel JR, Cox Jr, JW. Electronic article surveillance systems and interactions with implantable cardiac devices: risk of adverse interactions in public and commercial spaces. *Mayo Clin Proc.* 2007;82:318–322.

Hayes DL. Pacemakers. In: Topol EJ, ed. *Textbook of Cardiovascular Medicine.* 2nd ed. Philadelphia: Lippincott Williams & Wilkins; 2002:1571–1596.

Mower MM, Aranaga CE, Tabatznik B. Unusual patterns of conduction produced by pacemaker stimuli. *Am Heart J.* 1967;74:24–30.

Parsonnet V, Furman S, Smyth PD. A revised code for pacemaker identification. Pacemaker Study Group. *Circulation.* 1981;64:60A–62A.

Surawicz B, Uhley H, Borun R, et al. Task Force I: standardization of terminology and interpretation. *Am J Cardiol.* 1978;41:130–144.

# Commonly Used Injectable Pharmacologic Agents

## Adenosine (Adenocard): Pregnancy Category C

- **Indication:** Drug of choice for the conversion of paroxysmal supraventricular tachycardia (PSVT) to normal sinus rhythm.
- **Mechanism of action:** Adenosine is an atrioventricular (AV) nodal blocker and can interrupt supraventricular arrhythmias that are AV node–dependent. It also inhibits the sinus node resulting in depression of sinus node function.
- **Intravenous dose:**
  - Rapid bolus of 6 mg given intravenously as quickly as possible (within 1 to 2 seconds) preferably to a proximal vein. The injection should be followed by a flush of 10 to 20 mL normal saline using a separate syringe. To enhance delivery of the pharmacologic agent to the heart, the arm should be elevated immediately after the injection especially if a distal vein is used.
  - If the supraventricular tachycardia (SVT) is not converted after 1 to 2 minutes, a higher dose of 12 mg is given.
  - If the SVT has not converted, a third and final dose of 12 mg is given.
  - A rhythm strip should always be recorded during injection, which may be useful in the diagnosis of other tachycardias other than paroxysmal SVT (PSVT).
- **Contraindications:**
  - Adenosine can cause bronchoconstriction in patients with asthma or in patients with history of bronchospastic pulmonary disease.
  - Patients with sick sinus syndrome may develop pronounced bradycardia after the PSVT is terminated.
- **Other things you should know about adenosine:**
  - Intravenous doses of more than 12 mg are not recommended.
  - Injection into a central IV line may result in a more pronounced effect. Consider giving a smaller initial dose of 3 mg if adenosine is injected into a central line.

- Carbamazepine and dipyridamole potentiate the effects of adenosine. If the patient is on any of these agents, the initial dose of adenosine should also be reduced to 3 mg.
- Methylxanthines such as caffeine and theophylline is the antidote of adenosine. The usual dose of adenosine may not be effective in patients who are on theophylline. Larger doses are necessary, but should not be given if the patient is taking theophylline for bronchospastic pulmonary disease.
- Sixty percent of patients with PSVT will convert to normal sinus rhythm within 1 minute after an initial bolus of 6 mg and up to 92% after a 12-mg bolus.
- The elimination half-life of adenosine is <10 seconds. Transient periods of asystole, AV block, or bradycardia frequently occur before conversion to normal sinus rhythm. The antidote for adenosine is aminophylline given intravenously. The antidote is rarely needed because the half-life of adenosine is very short.
- When given to patients with wide complex tachycardia, adenosine can depress left ventricular function, but because of its short half-life, its effect is transient and is usually tolerable even in patients with poor left ventricular dysfunction. It receives a Class IIb recommendation by the American College of Cardiology/American Heart Association/European Society of Cardiology guidelines on supraventricular arrhythmias when given to patients with wide complex tachycardia of unknown origin.
- Adenosine should be used cautiously in patients with severe coronary artery disease because adenosine is a potent coronary vasodilator and can cause ischemia by redistributing coronary flow to normal vessels.
- Prolonged asystole, ventricular tachycardia, and ventricular fibrillation may occur.
- Atrial fibrillation can occur in up to 10% of patients and may be catastrophic in a patient with Wolff-Parkinson-White (WPW) syndrome.
- Adenosine does not convert atrial flutter or atrial fibrillation to normal sinus rhythm but can slow

ventricular rate transiently, which may be useful if the diagnosis of the narrow complex tachycardia is uncertain.

# Amiodarone (Cordarone): Pregnancy Category D

- **Indication:** Amiodarone is indicated only for the treatment of ventricular arrhythmias. The use of amiodarone in the treatment of supraventricular arrhythmias and control of ventricular rate in atrial flutter or fibrillation is not recommended by the Food and Drug Administration (FDA) and its use is based solely on published information.
  - **Ventricular arrhythmias:**
    - Amiodarone IV is indicated for the treatment of ventricular tachycardia (VT) in patients with normal left ventricular systolic function and in patients with systolic dysfunction.
    - It is also indicated for the treatment of ventricular fibrillation (VF) and pulseless VT.
    - Indicated for the treatment of wide complex tachycardia of uncertain etiology.
  - **Supraventricular arrhythmias:**
    - Accepted as a second- or third-line agent for the termination of atrial tachycardia from enhanced automaticity including focal atrial tachycardia, multifocal atrial tachycardia, and other types of atrial tachycardia resulting from reentry that are refractory to medical therapy.
    - Although amiodarone is extensively used and is effective in controlling the ventricular rate in atrial fibrillation and converting patients with atrial fibrillation to normal sinus rhythm, it has not been approved by the FDA for these indications.
- **Mechanism of action:** Amiodarone is generally a Class III antiarrhythmic agent, but exhibits all Class I to IV properties of the Vaughan Williams classification. Thus, similar to Class I agents, it is a sodium channel blocker; similar to beta blockers (Class II), it has antisympathetic properties; and similar to Class III agents, it blocks the potassium channel and therefore prolongs the duration of the action potential, slows conduction and prolongs the refractory period. It also has Class IV negative chronotropic effects on AV nodal tissues similar to calcium blockers thereby slowing AV conduction.
- **Intravenous dose:**
  - **Sustained VT or wide complex tachycardia of unknown origin:**
    - Initial bolus: 150 mg given IV rapidly for 10 minutes (150 mg or 3 mL of amiodarone is diluted with 100 mL $D_5W$ and infused over 10 minutes equivalent to 15 mg/minute).
    - This infusion may be repeated every 10 minutes as needed.
  - **Cardiac arrest from pulseless VT or VF:**
    - Initial bolus: Amiodarone is given at a bigger dose of 300 mg diluted to 20 to 30 mL of saline or $D_5W$ given IV push.
    - This may be followed by supplementary boluses of 150 mg IV given by IV push every 3 to 5 minutes.
  - **Next 6 hours:** Follow initial bolus with an IV drip of 1 mg/minute × 6 hours (total = 360 mg). The solution is prepared by adding 900 mg of 18 mL of amiodarone to 500 mL $D_5W$ (or 450 mg in 250 mL $D_5W$).
    - If the arrhythmia keeps recurring, an alternative is to give the solution as 150 mg IV boluses for 10 minutes every 10 to 15 minutes as needed, instead of giving the solution by IV drip.
  - **Next 18 hours:** Continue the IV drip to a lower dose of 0.5 mg/minute × 18 hours (total = 540 mg). The maximum total cumulative dose including dose used in resuscitation should not exceed 2.2 g in the first 24 hours.
  - **After 24 hours:** The intravenous dose is maintained after 24 hours:
    - The infusion is continued at 0.5 mg/minute × 24 hours. Maintenance infusion of 0.5 mg/minute can be continued for several days and if necessary up to 2 to 3 weeks.
    - If patient develops recurrence of the ventricular arrhythmia at any time during infusion, a supplemental bolus of 150 mg diluted with 100 mL $D_5W$ may be given IV over 10 minutes.
    - The maximum daily dose should not exceed 2,100 mg. Intravenous dosing should be switched to oral medication when the arrhythmia has been suppressed.
    - Doses >2,200 mg/24 hours are associated with significant hypotension.
- **Other things you should know about amiodarone:**
  - Amiodarone is the preferred drug for ventricular arrhythmias and some atrial arrhythmias when there is left ventricular systolic dysfunction (ejection fraction ≤40% or when congestive heart failure is present). Amiodarone is indicated only for the treatment of VT/VF but is also effective in the following conditions:
    - It is effective in persistent VT or VF after defibrillation.
    - It is effective in stable monomorphic VT.
    - It is indicated for wide complex tachycardia that has not been diagnosed to be either VT or wide complex SVT.
    - It is effective in regular polymorphic VT (no QT prolongation).

- ☐ It can be used as second- to third-line therapy for conversion of SVT to normal sinus rhythm when other drugs are not effective.
- ☐ It is effective in conversion of atrial fibrillation to normal sinus rhythm.
- ☐ It is also effective in controlling ventricular rate in atrial fibrillation especially in patients with WPW syndrome.
- ▪ Amiodarone prolongs the QTc and is proarrhythmic. Its proarrhythmic effect however is much less than the other antiarrhythmic agents. It should not be administered with other agents that prolong the QTc.
- ▪ The half-life of intravenous boluses varies from 4.8 to 68 hours and becomes longer as tissues become saturated. After steady state is reached, amiodarone has a long and variable half-life from 40 days to 3 to 5 months.
- ▪ It can cause multiple organ toxicity including hepatocellular damage, hyper- or hypothyroidism, optic neuritis, and pulmonary disorders including acute respiratory distress syndrome.
- ▪ Acute hepatocellular injury may occur with doses that are larger than recommended.
- ▪ Its hypotensive and bradycardic effects are frequently related to the rapidity of infusion rather than the dose.
- ▪ It is metabolized through the cytochrome P450 (CYP 450) 3A4 and 2C9 pathways and therefore has the potential for several drug-drug interactions.
  - ☐ Statins (lovastatin, atorvastatin, and simvastatin but not pravastatin or rosuvastatin) are metabolized through the CYP 450 3A4 pathway. Serum concentration of these statins can increase resulting in higher incidence of myopathy or rhabdomyolysis.
  - ☐ Calcium channel blockers such as verapamil and diltiazem are also metabolized through the CYP 450 3A4 pathway. The effects of these agents can be potentiated by amiodarone resulting in significant bradycardia.
  - ☐ CYP 450 3A4 inhibitors such as grapefruit juice, protease inhibitors, and cimetidine may increase the serum levels of amiodarone and can potentially cause amiodarone toxicity.
  - ☐ Agents that accelerate the CYP 450 3A4 metabolic pathway such as rifampin, barbiturates, and St. John's wort may decrease the blood levels of amiodarone making it subtherapeutic.
  - ☐ Amiodarone is also metabolized through the CYP 450 2C9 pathway and therefore competes with the metabolism of warfarin resulting in prolongation of the prothrombin time. The maintenance dose of warfarin should be reduced when amiodarone is started. Patients on warfarin should have prothrombin tests monitored carefully.
  - ☐ Beta blockers in combination with amiodarone can cause profound bradycardia.
  - ☐ Amiodarone can also potentiate the effect of digitalis; hence, the maintenance dose of digoxin should be reduced by half when amiodarone is given.
  - ☐ Effective plasma concentration of amiodarone is between 1 to 2 mcg/mL. The plasma concentration of amiodarone may be helpful in monitoring the efficacy but not toxicity. The effective therapeutic levels of amiodarone overlap with toxic levels and should not exceed 3 to 4 mcg/L.

## Atenolol (Tenormin): Pregnancy Category D

- ▪ **Indication:** Atenolol is indicated in the management of patients with angina pectoris, acute myocardial infarction, and control of hypertension. Although atenolol does not carry indication for termination of SVT or for controlling the ventricular rate in atrial flutter or fibrillation, it is frequently used for this purpose based on published information.
- ▪ **Mechanism of action:** Atenolol is a synthetic selective $\beta_1$ adrenergic blocking agent. When given in high doses, $\beta_1$ receptor blocking agents including atenolol are not specific $\beta_1$ blockers but also blocks $\beta_2$ receptors, which are present in bronchial and vascular smooth muscles.
- ▪ **Dose:** The IV dose of atenolol for patients with acute myocardial infarction (or for the management of supraventricular arrhythmias), is 5 mg IV given slowly over 5 minutes. Injection rate should not exceed 1 mg/minute. A second dose of 5 mg is given IV after 10 minutes if the first dose was well tolerated. The blood pressure, heart rate, and electrocardiogram should be monitored during the intravenous infusion. If the intravenous dose is well tolerated, an oral dose of 50 mg is given 10 minutes after the last IV dose followed by another 50 mg 12 hours later. The maintenance dose is 50 mg twice daily or 100 mg once daily.
- ▪ **Other things you should know about atenolol:**
  - ▪ Unlike metoprolol or propranolol, atenolol is primarily excreted by the kidneys (85%) and is not metabolized or is only minimally metabolized by the liver. Thus, atenolol given orally does not undergo first pass degradation by the liver. When there is renal failure, the dose should be adjusted.
  - ▪ When atenolol is given orally, only approximately 50% is absorbed. The other half is excreted unchanged in the gastrointestinal tract. This is unlike metoprolol where absorption is rapid and complete

when given orally. Metoprolol is primarily metabolized in the liver and 50% of the oral dose is eliminated during first pass.

■ The elimination half-life of atenolol is approximately 7 hours, but is much longer when there is renal dysfunction.

■ Abrupt discontinuation or cessation of any beta blocker, including atenolol, in patients with known coronary disease and symptoms of angina may result in exacerbation of anginal symptoms or occurrence of acute coronary syndrome.

■ The latest 2007 focused update of the American College of Cardiology/American Heart Association 2004 guidelines raises doubt about the safety of intravenous beta blockers in acute ST elevation myocardial infarction and should not be given to patients at increased risk for cardiogenic shock (see Metoprolol).

■ Atenolol is the only beta blocker that receives a category D pregnancy risk classification by the FDA. All other beta blockers receive a category C classification. Sotalol, which also has beta blocking properties, carry a category B classification.

## Atropine Sulfate: Pregnancy Category C

■ **Indication:** According to the 2005 American Heart Association guidelines for cardiopulmonary resuscitation and emergency cardiovascular care, atropine remains the first-line drug for the treatment of acute symptomatic bradycardia. It is indicated for the treatment of acute symptomatic bradyarrhythmia due to sinus node dysfunction, AV nodal block, and increased vagal activity. It is the second drug of choice after epinephrine or vasopressin, in patients with ventricular asystole and pulseless electrical activity.

■ **Mechanism of action:** Atropine is an anticholinergic agent and increases ventricular rate by reversing vagally mediated mechanisms of bradycardia and hypotension.

■ **Dosing:**

   ■ **Asystole:** For asystole or slow pulseless electrical activity, a dose of 1.0 mg is given IV. If not effective, the dose is repeated every 3 to 5 minutes until a maximum dose of 3.0 mg is given. Complete vagal blockade occurs at a total dose of 0.04 mg/kg, which is 2.0 mg for a 50-kg and almost 3.0 mg for a 70-kg patient.

   ■ **Bradycardia from AV block or sinus dysfunction:** The initial dose is 0.5 to 1.0 mg IV every 3 to 5 minutes as needed until the maximum dose is given.

■ **Other things you should know about atropine:**

   ■ For the treatment of bradycardia, doses of <0.5 mg should not be given because small doses of atropine can cause paradoxical slowing of the heart rate.

Small doses of atropine are parasympathomimetic. It stimulates the vagal nuclei, resulting in paradoxical slowing. This paradoxical effect can also occur if injected subcutaneously or intramuscularly. Atropine should always be given IV. If an IV route is not available during cardiac resuscitation, it can be given intratracheally at a dose of 2 to 3 mg diluted with 10 mL normal saline.

■ It is not effective and should not be given to patients with infranodal blocks (AV block below the level of the AV node) such as those due to Mobitz II second-degree AV block and complete AV block below the level of the AV node with wide QRS escape complexes (Class IIb recommendation).

■ Should be avoided in patients with bradycardia from hypothermia.

■ The use of atropine should not delay the insertion of transcutaneous or transvenous pacing in patients with symptomatic bradycardia with low cardiac output.

## Beta Blockers: Beta Blockers are Class II Agents According to the Vaughan Williams Classification of Anti-Arrhythmic Agents

■ Beta blockers that are available intravenously include atenolol, esmolol, metoprolol, and propranolol. These different beta blockers are discussed individually in alphabetical listing.

## Digoxin (Lanoxin): Pregnancy Category C

■ **Indication:** Control of ventricular rate in atrial fibrillation. It is also used for control of ventricular rate in atrial flutter and conversion of PSVT to normal sinus rhythm although these two indications have not been approved by the FDA.

■ **Mechanism of action:**

   ■ Digoxin inhibits sodium-potassium ATPase, which is an enzyme that regulates the exchange of sodium and potassium inside the cells. When ATPase is inhibited, sodium builds up within the cells. Sodium buildup activates the sodium-calcium exchange mechanism. Increase in calcium inside the cell activates the intracellular cytosol system to release more calcium. The increased calcium inside the cell enhances myocardial inotropicity with increased myocardial systolic contraction.

■ Digoxin also affects the cardiovascular system indirectly by its effect on the autonomic nervous system.

  □ It has parasympathetic effects, which inhibits the sinus node, thus slowing the heart rate and slowing conduction at the AV node.

  □ It reduces activity of the sympathetic nervous system and renin-angiotensin-aldosterone-system, thus reducing the activation of the neurohormonal system. This is mediated through baroreceptors sensitization, which causes increased afferent inhibitory activities.

### ■ Intravenous dose:

■ Before giving a full loading dose, first ascertain that the patient is not already on digoxin.

■ The ideal serum therapeutic level of digoxin is 0.7 to 1.1 ng/mL. The dose of digoxin that is needed to achieve this level in a 70-kg man is 0.6 to 1.0 mg (10 to 15 mcg/kg). The total dose depends on the lean body mass (and not total body weight) and renal function. Fifty percent of the total dose is given initially. Subsequent additional doses are given at 6- to 8-hour intervals.

■ Thus, if the patient weighs 70 kg, the total digitalizing dose is approximately 1.0 mg. Half the total dose or 0.5 mg, is given IV followed by another 0.25 mg IV in 6 hours and 0.25 mg IV after another 6 hours. The patient will have received the full digitalizing dose of 1.0 mg in 12 hours.

■ Digoxin is excreted primarily in the kidneys. Renal excretion is dependent on glomerular filtration. In patients with renal dysfunction, the creatinine clearance should be calculated using the Cockroft and Gault formula: Creatinine clearance for men = {(140 − age) + (weight in kg)} divided by 72 × serum creatinine (in mg/mL). The calculated renal clearance for men is multiplied by 0.85 for women.

  □ If the creatinine clearance is ≥90, the normal dosage is unchanged.

  □ If the creatinine clearance is 60 to 89, maintenance dose is 0.125 mg daily.

  □ If the creatinine clearance is 30 to 59, 0.125 mg is given every other day.

  □ If the creatinine clearance is <29, use digoxin very cautiously.

### ■ Other things you should know about digoxin:

■ Intramuscular injection of digoxin is very painful. Parenteral injections therefore should be limited intravenously.

■ Rapid injection or infusion can cause systemic and coronary constriction. Injection of digoxin therefore should be given slowly over 5 minutes or longer and not given as a bolus injection.

■ Serum concentrations of digoxin are not altered significantly by increase in body fat, thus lean body weight and not total body weight correlates best with the distribution space of digoxin.

■ The half-life of digoxin in patients with normal kidney function is 1.5 to 2 days. In anuric patients, it is prolonged to 3.5 to 5 days. Maintenance dosing can be given once per day.

■ Elderly patients, especially those with renal dysfunction, may be difficult to digitalize because maintenance dosing may be difficult; hence, serum digoxin level should be monitored.

■ When assessing for serum digoxin level, blood should be drawn after steady state is reached to allow proper equilibration between serum and tissue levels. Therefore, the level should be assayed just before the next daily dose. If not possible, at least 6 to 8 hours after the last dose should have elapsed regardless whether oral or IV preparation is being given. The serum level will be 10% to 25% lower after 24 hours as compared with 8 hours with once-daily dosing, but minor differences in serum level with twice-daily dosing at 8 or 12 hours after last dose.

■ The initial high levels of digoxin do not reflect the actual concentration at the site of action until a steady state of distribution occurs during chronic use. Serum level reflects pharmacologic effect when serum concentrations are in equilibrium with tissue concentrations.

■ The serum level of digoxin should not exceed 1.3 ng/mL. Higher levels may be necessary to control the ventricular rate in atrial fibrillation as compared with digoxin being given for inotropic support in heart failure; nevertheless, higher serum digoxin levels were associated with a higher mortality in the Digitalis Investigation Group study.

■ Digoxin competes with amiodarone and quinidine. These two drugs are the most significant in increasing the digoxin levels. Therefore, the dose of digoxin should generally be halved when giving digoxin in combination with these drugs. Digoxin level should be monitored.

■ Digitalis has a tendency to increase automaticity and at the same time cause AV block; thus, automatic atrial tachycardia with 2:1 AV block is usually a manifestation of digitalis toxicity. Other arrhythmias associated with digitalis include ventricular ectopy, bidirectional ventricular tachycardia, sinus dysfunction, and all degrees of AV block.

■ Digoxin is not removed by dialysis; therefore, dialysis or exchange transfusion is not effective in treating digitalis toxicity. Most of the drug is bound to tissue and does not circulate freely.

■ Digibind is the antidote for digitalis toxicity. This is given intravenously and the dose is calculated according to the serum digoxin level. Digibind should be given only for life-threatening arrhythmias such as paroxysmal atrial tachycardia with block or significant bradyarrhythmias from AV block or sinus dysfunction.

- Digibind is excreted by the kidneys as a digoxin-Digibind complex. When there is renal failure, the Digibind-digoxin complex may not be excreted or excretion may be significantly delayed. Thus, digitalis toxicity may recur after 72 hours because the effect of Digibind in binding be effective after that time.

- The serum level of digoxin does not reflect the digoxin level after Digibind is given. Thus it is not possible to reassess digoxin toxicity after the antidote is given.

- Slowing of the ventricular rate in patients with heart failure is more pronounce when digoxin is combined with a beta blocker (such as carvedilol) compared with the use of either drug alone.

- Avoid electrical cardioversion if patient is on digoxin. If cardioversion is necessary, use lower current during cardioversion.

## Diltiazem (Cardizem Injectable or Lyo-Jet Syringe): Pregnancy Category C

- **Indication:** Conversion of paroxysmal supraventricular tachycardia to normal sinus rhythm, control of ventricular rate in atrial flutter, or fibrillation or in patients with multifocal atrial tachycardia.

- **Mechanism of action:** Diltiazem, like verapamil, is a nondihydropyridine calcium channel blocker. It increases refractoriness of the AV node and can slow down the rate of the sinus node. It is a negative inotropic agent and can decrease myocardial contractility. It relaxes vascular smooth muscle resulting in peripheral vasodilatation.

- **Intravenous dose:**
  - Initial bolus of 0.25 mg/kg (approximately 15 to 20 mg for a 70-kg patient) given slowly IV over 2 minutes. If not effective, a second dose of 0.35 mg/kg (approximately 20 to 25 mg for a 70-kg patient) may be given after 15 minutes, slowly, IV. The heart rate and blood pressure should be monitored during IV infusion.
  - To prolong the half-life of diltiazem and maintain control of ventricular rate in atrial fibrillation, an intravenous drip of 5 to 15 mg/hour should be started after giving the intravenous bolus.
  - Additional small boluses of $\geq 5$ mg may be given intermittently during infusion if ventricular rate is not optimally controlled with maintenance IV infusion.

- **Other things you should know about diltiazem:**
  - Diltiazem is just as effective as verapamil in converting PSVT to normal sinus rhythm, but is less negatively inotropic and may be used cautiously in patients with left ventricular dysfunction who are not hemodynamically decompensated.
  - The elimination half life of IV diltiazem is approximately 3 to 5 hours and is shorter than verapamil. Because of the relatively short half-life, a maintenance infusion is necessary when controlling the heart rate in atrial fibrillation. The maintenance infusion dose is 5 to 15 mg/hour. While on maintenance infusion, an oral dose should be started within 3 hours after the initial IV dose so that the infusion can be discontinued within 24 hours unless the patient can not take oral medications.
  - Although IV diltiazem may be tolerable in patients with atrial arrhythmias with mild heart failure, they should not be given to patients with acutely decompensated heart failure. Oral nondihydropyridine calcium channel blockers, including oral diltiazem, should not be given when there is left ventricular dysfunction. It should not be given for wide complex tachycardia of unknown origin, sick sinus syndrome, or atrial fibrillation associated with WPW syndrome.
  - Severe bradycardia and hypotension may occur when diltiazem is combined with beta blockers.

## Dobutamine (Dobutrex): Pregnancy Category B

- **Indication:** Dobutamine is indicated for the treatment of heart failure. It is also used off-label for the treatment of bradyarrhythmias and heart block not responsive to atropine, especially in treatment of infranodal AV block.

- **Mechanism of action:** Dobutamine is a synthetic catecholamine with predominantly $\beta_1$ and slight $\beta_2$ adrenergic properties and mild to moderate $\alpha$ properties.

- **Dosing:** Given as IV infusion with an initial dose of 1 mcg/kg/minute and increased to 2.5 to 5.0 mcg/kg/minute. This can be titrated gradually every 3 minutes according to heart rate to a maximum dose of 20 mcg/kg/minute. Higher doses up to 40 mcg/kg/minute can be given but are usually associated with atrial and ventricular arrhythmias. The use of dobutamine for AV block and bradyarrhythmias should only be temporary, before a temporary pacemaker can be inserted. The drug very often comes in premix infusion of 500 mg in 250 mL $D_5W$.

- **Other things you should know about dobutamine:**
    - Dobutamine has a short elimination half-life of 2 minutes and should be given as a continuous intravenous infusion.
    - It is indicated for the treatment of patients with low cardiac output or heart failure. It is also used off-label as temporary measure for treatment of symptomatic bradyarrhythmia before a pacemaker can be inserted. It is the preferred agent in infranodal AV block with wide escape complexes, because atropine is not effective when AV block is infranodal. It can also be tried in patients with symptomatic bradyarrhythmias not responsive to atropine before a pacemaker can be inserted.
    - The chronotropic effect of dobutamine is not as potent as dopamine or isoproterenol and is more often used as an inotropic agent in acute heart failure rather than for its chronotropic effect in patients with bradyarrhythmias or AV block. If dobutamine is not effective in increasing the heart rate, isoproterenol should be given instead.

# Epinephrine: Pregnancy Category C

- **Indication:** Epinephrine is indicated for cardiac arrest due to VF or pulseless VT. It is also indicated for the treatment of anaphylaxis and syncope from complete heart block or hypersensitive carotid sinus and for the treatment of asthma.
- **Mechanism of action:** The drug is a sympathomimetic catecholamine with $\alpha$-, $\beta_1$-, and $\beta_2$-adrenergic activity. It has the most potent $\alpha$-adrenergic effect resulting in intense vasoconstriction, which can result in coronary and cerebral perfusion pressure during cardiopulmonary resuscitation. It is this intense $\alpha$-adrenergic effect that is useful in cardiac arrest.
- **Dose:** According to the 2005 American Heart Association guidelines for cardiopulmonary resuscitation, the dose of epinephrine in cardiac resuscitation is 1 mg given by intravenous or if not possible by intraosseous administration every 3 to 5 minutes. Higher doses may be given to overcome beta blocker or calcium channel overdose. If intravenous or intraosseous administration is not possible during resuscitation, it may be given intratracheally at a dose of 2 to 2.5 mg. Higher doses of epinephrine has not been shown to be more effective than standard doses during cardiopulmonary resuscitation.
    - For anaphylaxis, the drug is given intramuscularly 0.3 mg, which may be repeated if needed. It may also be given subcutaneously at a dose of 0.2 to 1.0 mg.
    - For asthma, the drug is given subcutaneously 0.2 to 0.5 mg. If needed for severe attacks, a second and third dose may be given every 20 minutes for a maximum of three doses.

# Esmolol (Brevibloc): Pregnancy Category C

- **Indication:** Esmolol is indicated for the conversion of SVT to normal sinus rhythm and control of ventricular rate in patients with atrial fibrillation or atrial flutter. Also indicated for the treatment of inappropriate, noncompensatory sinus tachycardia and hypertension that occur during induction and tracheal intubation, during surgery or emergence from anesthesia and postoperative period.
- **Mechanism of action:** Esmolol is a selective $\beta_1$ blocker.
- **Dose:** The dose of esmolol is quite complicated because the drug is very short acting and may need frequent retitration:
    - The initial IV loading dose is 0.5 mg/kg over 1 minute followed by an infusion of 50 mcg/kg/minute for 4 minutes. If effective, the infusion rate is continued. The dose can be titrated depending on the desired ventricular rate during atrial flutter or fibrillation. Thus, the maintenance infusion rate can be increased from 50 to 100 mcg/kg/minute, and after 4 or more minutes to 150 mcg/kg/minute and subsequently up to a maximum of 200 mcg/kg/minute.
    - If the first bolus is not effective, another option is to give a second bolus of 0.5 mg/kg over 1 minute and increase infusion rate by 50 mcg for an infusion rate of 100 mcg/kg/minute for 4 minutes. If effective, continue the infusion rate.
    - If not effective, give a third and final bolus of 0.5 mg/kg over 1 minute and increase infusion rate by 50 mcg for an infusion rate of 150 mcg/kg/minute for 4 minutes. The infusion rate can be increased by 50 mcg/kg/minute to a maximum of 200 mcg/kg/minute.
    - The usual maintenance infusion rate is 50 to 200 mcg/kg/minute. Maintenance infusion can be given for 24 hours if necessary; however, the patient should be monitored for hypotension and bradycardia.
    - A higher maximum maintenance infusion dose of 50 to 300 mcg/kg/minute may be given for the treatment of hypertension.
- **Other things you should know about esmolol:**
    - Esmolol has a very short half-life of only 2 to 9 minutes. The drug is too short-acting, making routine use for control of ventricular rate in atrial flutter and fibrillation difficult to maintain in the medical intensive care unit, more especially when long-term control is necessary. The short half-life, however,

may be advantageous to patients who develop arrhythmia during the perioperative and immediate postoperative period where immediate and short-term control is all that is needed.

■ Esmolol is also indicated for hypertension occurring during the perioperative and immediate postoperative period. For control of hypertension, a higher maintenance infusion dose of up to 250 to 300 mcg/kg/minute may be necessary (see dosing). It can also be given as treatment for noncompensatory sinus tachycardia, which, according to the judgment of the physician, may be inappropriate and needs to be controlled.

■ Dosing is not affected by hepatic or renal disease.

■ Can cause slowing of the sinus node, thus the agent should be given cautiously when there is history of sick sinus syndrome or previous bradycardia.

■ The maximum infusion dose should not exceed 200 mcg/kg/minute and the agent may be continued as an infusion up to 24 hours.

## Ibutilide (Corvert): Pregnancy Category C

■ **Indication:** Rapid conversion of atrial flutter or atrial fibrillation to normal sinus rhythm

■ **Mechanism of Action:** Ibutilide is a Class III antiarrhythmic agent. Class III agents block the potassium channel and therefore prolong the duration of the action potential. Conduction is slowed and atrial and ventricular refractoriness are prolonged. The effect of ibutilide is different when compared to other Class III agents because it prolongs the action potential duration by slowing the inward flow of sodium during repolarization in contrast to most type III agents, which slow the outward flow of potassium.

■ **Dosing:**

■ Before converting atrial flutter or atrial fibrillation to normal sinus rhythm with ibutilide, any patient known to have the arrhythmia for more than 48 hours should first be adequately anticoagulated for at least 3 weeks before attempting conversion to normal sinus rhythm. However, if a more immediate cardioversion seems necessary, a transesophageal echocardiogram should be performed to exclude thrombi in the atria or left atrial appendage. Cardioversion may then be carried out under adequate anticoagulation if no thrombi are demonstrated.

■ For patients weighing ≥60 kg, the dose of ibutilide is 1 mg given intravenously for 10 minutes. For patients weighing <60 kg, the dose is 0.01 mg/kg or a maximum of 0.6 mg. One mg of ibutilide is available as a 10-mL preparation and is injected at a rate of 1 mL/minute. The 10-mL preparation (1 mg) can be injected directly IV (10 minutes) without dilution. It could also be diluted to a larger volume of 50 mL and infused intravenously for 10 minutes.

■ If the arrhythmia has not converted 10 minutes after injection, the same dose can be repeated with the same rate of administration. There is a 50% to 70% chance for atrial flutter and 30% to 50% chance for atrial fibrillation to convert to normal sinus rhythm almost immediately after the drug is administered. If the arrhythmia has not converted after the second dose, no further injections should be given.

■ For postcardiac surgery patients weighing <60 kg, 0.5 mg (0.005 mg/kg per dose) given as a single or double dose, was effective for atrial fibrillation and flutter.

■ **Other things you should know about ibutilide:**

■ Sustained polymorphic ventricular tachycardia (PVT) requiring cardioversion can occur in approximately 1.7% of patients receiving intravenous ibutilide. This arrhythmia can be fatal if not immediately recognized. PVT may or may not be associated with baseline QTc prolongation; the tachycardia is called torsades de pointes.

■ The initial episode of PVT can occur up to 40 minutes after initial infusion, although recurrence of PVT can occur up to 3 hours after initial infusion.

■ Sustained PVT is more common in patients with low ejection fraction or patients with history of congestive heart failure, especially where there is baseline QT prolongation. The drug, therefore, should not be given to patients who are hemodynamically unstable or in heart failure, in patients with recent myocardial infarction or angina, patients with electrolyte and blood gas abnormalities including patients with baseline QT prolongation, or those who are metabolically deranged.

■ Nonsustained PVT occurred in an additional 2.7% of patients and nonsustained monomorphic VT in 4.9%.

■ Cardiac monitoring should be continued for at least 4 hours after infusion or until QTc is back to baseline. Longer monitoring is required for patients with hepatic dysfunction. Prolongation of the QT interval is related to the dose and infusion rate. Patients developing PVT should be monitored for a longer period.

■ The hemodynamic effect of the drug is similar in patients with systolic dysfunction and those without. No significant effect in cardiac output or pulmonary wedge pressure has been noted. The drug has not been shown to increase the duration of the QRS complex.

■ When giving ibutilide, the QTc interval should preferably be <440 milliseconds and the serum potassium at least 4.0 mEq/L. Patients with QTc >440 milliseconds and potassium <4.0 mEq/L were not allowed to participate when clinical trials with ibutilide were conducted.

- Although torsade is the most common arrhythmia associated with the drug, sinus arrest and complete asystole can occur during conversion from atrial flutter or atrial fibrillation to normal sinus rhythm especially in patients with sick sinus syndrome.

- The drug is more effective in atrial flutter than in atrial fibrillation. Approximately 53% of patients with atrial flutter will convert with the first 1 mg dose and 70% after the second dose. In atrial fibrillation, approximately 22% will convert with the first dose and 43% after the second dose. Conversion occurred within 30 minutes after the start of infusion. This is in contrast to intravenous sotalol (1.5 mg/kg), where only 18% of patients with atrial flutter and 10% with atrial fibrillation converted during clinical trials with the drug.

- If atrial flutter or atrial fibrillation has not converted after 90 minutes after the infusion is completed, the patient can be electrically cardioverted if appropriate. Other antiarrhythmic agents can also be started 4 hours after the infusion is completed.

- Patients with more recent onset atrial flutter or atrial fibrillation (within 30 days) have a higher chance of conversion to normal sinus rhythm compared with patients whose arrhythmias were of longer duration. The efficacy of ibutilide has not been tested in patients with atrial flutter or atrial fibrillation longer than 90 days in duration.

## Isoproterenol (Isuprel): Pregnancy Category C

- **Indication:** As a temporizing measure for the treatment of heart block or symptomatic bradyarrhythmias when atropine or dobutamine has failed. It is also given as a temporizing measure for the treatment of torsades de pointes before a pacemaker can be inserted.

- **Mechanism of Action:** Isoproterenol is a β-adrenergic agonist with very potent $\beta_1$ and $\beta_2$ properties. Similar to other β-adrenergic agents, it increases cyclic AMP by stimulating adenyl cyclase, eventually increasing intracellular calcium. It has very potent chronotropic and inotropic properties and prevents bronchospasm.

- **Dose:** Given as an intravenous infusion at 2 to 10 mcg/minute titrated according to the heart rate, It is usually prepared by diluting 1 mg of isoproterenol to 500 mL $D_5W$, resulting in a concentration of 2 mcg/mL.

- **Other things you should know about isoproterenol:**
  - Isoproterenol is the drug of choice for the temporary treatment of infranodal AV block. It shortens the refractory period of the AV node and enhances AV conduction. It also increases automaticity allowing latent pacemakers to become manifest. Because of its serious side effects, it is potentially dangerous to use routinely and should be used cautiously only as a temporizing measure for the treatment of heart block and bradyarrhythmias before a temporary pacemaker can be inserted or after atropine or dobutamine has failed.

  - Isoproterenol is a very potent $\beta_1$- and $\beta_2$-adrenergic agent. It increases automaticity not only of the sinus node but all cells with pacemaking potential, resulting in ectopic rhythms that may dominate over that of the sinus node. It can cause ectopic atrial tachycardia, atrial flutter, atrial fibrillation, and ventricular tachycardia or fibrillation even in patients with structurally normal hearts.

  - Isoproterenol increases inotropicity and cardiac output and markedly increases oxygen consumption. It can provoke ischemia in patients with coronary disease and can provoke arrhythmias especially in patients with left ventricular dysfunction.

  - **Torsades de pointes:** Isoproterenol may be used as a temporizing procedure in patients with bradycardia dependent torsades de pointes before a temporary pacemaker can be inserted.

  - Isoproterenol should be given at the lowest dose possible. Because it enhances myocardial oxygen consumption, it can expand infarct size and cause complex ventricular and supraventricular arrhythmias.

## Labetalol (Normodyne): Pregnancy Category C

- **Indication:** Intravenous labetalol is indicated for the emergency treatment of hypertension. It does not carry indication for the treatment of cardiac arrhythmias.

- **Mechanism:** Labetalol is a nonspecific beta blocker with $\alpha_1$-, $\beta_1$- and $\beta_2$-adrenergic receptor blocking properties. In addition, it also has intrinsic sympathomimetic activity.

- **Dose:** For the treatment of hypertension, 10 mg is given IV push over 1 to 2 minutes. The dose is repeated or doubled every 10 minutes if needed to a maximum dose of 150 mg. Another option is to give an initial bolus followed by an infusion of 2 to 8 mg/minute.

## Lidocaine (Xylocaine HCL): Pregnancy Category B

- **Indication:** For acute suppression of VT or VF.
- **Mechanism of Action:** Lidocaine is Class IB antiarrhythmic agent. It blocks the sodium channel but has no effect on potassium channel. It does not prolong and may even shorten action potential duration and effective refractory period of the His-Purkinje system.
- **Dosing:**
  - In cardiac arrest, an initial bolus of 1.0 to 1.5 mg/kg is given. The higher dose is given only for ventricular fibrillation or pulseless VT after defibrillation and epinephrine has failed.
  - For refractory VT or VF, an additional bolus of 0.5 to 0.75 mg/kg is given IV over 3 to 5 minutes. The rate should not exceed 50 mg/minute. Lidocaine is distributed rapidly out of the plasma in <10 minutes. The initial dose therefore is only transiently therapeutic and additional boluses have to be given repeatedly every 5 to 10 minutes, as needed, for a maximum total loading dose of 3 mg/kg over 1 hour. The loading dose should be decreased in patients with heart failure.
  - The initial loading dose is followed by an IV infusion of 1 to 4 mg/minute to maintain therapeutic blood levels. Maintenance infusion should be adjusted to a lower rate in patients with heart failure and liver disease.
  - The volume of distribution does not reach steady state until after 8 to 10 hours or even longer, up to 24 hours in patients with liver disease, heart failure, or low output states.
- **Other things you should know about lidocaine:**
  - Lidocaine does not prolong action potential duration and therefore does not prolong the QT interval. The drug is useful in patients with normal or prolonged QT intervals or patients with monomorphic or polymorphic VT.
  - Is primarily indicated for patients with ischemic VT/VF and is the drug of choice for VT/VF associated with acute myocardial infarction.
  - Unlike most antiarrhythmic agents, lidocaine can be used in patients with impaired left ventricular function.
  - It is not effective in blocking the AV node and therefore is not useful in supraventricular arrhythmias. It may even enhance AV conduction, which can result in 1:1 AV conduction in atrial flutter.
  - Lidocaine as well as its metabolites undergoes degradation through the CYP 450 3A4 pathway. Continuous infusion of lidocaine at the same dose for 24 to 48 hours increases its half-life and generally leads to toxicity.
  - Symptoms of toxicity are usually from central nervous system involvement, which include seizures, dysarthria or slurred speech, muscle twitching, drowsiness, altered consciousness, or even coma.
  - Lidocaine should generally be discontinued 12 hours after the arrhythmia has been successfully suppressed unless there is an indication to infuse the medication for a longer period.
  - After the infusion is terminated, plasma levels slowly decline over several hours. If the medication is no longer needed, the medication can be discontinued outright without tapering the dose.
  - Therapeutic blood levels can be monitored, which ranges from 1.5 to 5 mcg/mL.

## Magnesium Sulfate: Pregnancy Category C

- **Indication:** Replacement therapy in the presence of magnesium deficiency. Also used in the treatment of torsade de pointes characterized by polymorphous VT with prolonged QT interval.
- **Mechanism of Action:** Severe magnesium deficiency can cause cardiac arrhythmias including ventricular fibrillation and sudden cardiac death. Hypomagnesemia also prevents the correction of potassium deficiency.
- **Dosing:**
  - **For refractory VF:** In emergent conditions where there is refractory VF associated with magnesium deficiency, dilute 1 to 2 g magnesium sulfate in 100 mL D₅W and inject IV over 1 to 2 minutes.
  - **For torsade:** Even in the absence of magnesium deficiency, give a loading dose of 1 to 2 g mixed with 50 to 100 mL D₅W injected IV over 5 to 60 minutes, depending on the urgency of administration. Follow with a continuous IV infusion of 0.5 to 1.0 g/hour.
  - **For magnesium deficiency:** Dilute 5 g in 1 L D₅W, 0.9% NaCl or lactated Ringers solution and given as a continuous infusion. Maximum concentration is 4 g in 250 mL given IV over 3 hours. Dose should not exceed a total of 30 to 40 g in adults and rate should not exceed 50 mg/minute.

## Metoprolol (Lopressor): Pregnancy Category C

- **Indication:** Metoprolol is indicated for reduction of mortality in acute myocardial infarction. It is also indicated for angina and hypertension. It is effective as an antiarrhythmic agent in supraventricular arrhythmias and reduces incidence of ventricular tachycardia/fibrillation in patients with acute myocardial infarction.

- **Mechanism of action:** Metoprolol is a cardioselective $\beta_1$-adrenergic blocking agent.
- **Dose:** The initial IV dose is 5 mg slowly over 5 minutes. May be repeated every 5 minutes if well tolerated for a total of three doses or 15 mg over 15 minutes. If maintenance oral dose is necessary and patient is postoperative or NPO, give IV piggyback 20 mg over 2 hours. This is equal to 50 mg of oral metoprolol. The IV dose is followed by an oral dose of 50 mg BID $\times$ 24 hours, then 100 mg BID.
- **Other things you should know about metoprolol:**
  - The most recent 2007 focused update of the American College of Cardiology/American Heart Association 2004 guidelines for the management of ST elevation MI raises doubt about the safety of IV metoprolol or similar beta blockers based on the results of a large clinical trial (Clopidogrel and Metoprolol in Myocardial Infarction). Although metoprolol IV has been shown to decrease reinfarction and ventricular fibrillation in this study, there were more episodes of cardiogenic shock. Thus, the use of metoprolol IV is reasonable only when hypertension is present and the patient does not have any of the following findings:
    - ☐ Signs of heart failure
    - ☐ Low output state
    - ☐ Increased risk for cardiogenic shock (age >70 years, systolic blood pressure <120 mm Hg, sinus tachycardia >100 beats per minute, or heart rate <60 beats per minute and increased time since onset of acute MI).
    - ☐ Contraindications to beta blockade (PR >0.24 second, second- or third-degree AV block, reactive airway disease or active asthma).
  - The long-term use of beta blockers remains a Class I recommendation when given orally within 24 hours to patients who do not have contraindications and are not high risk for hypotension or cardiogenic shock.
  - In patients with left ventricular dysfunction, oral beta blocker therapy is recommended but should be gradually titrated.

## Norepinephrine: Pregnancy Category C

- **Indication:** Cardiac arrest and hypotension
- **Mechanism of Action:** Norepinephrine is a sympathomimetic agent with both alpha and beta adrenergic activity.
- **Dosing:** The initial dose is 0.5 to 1 mcg/minute given IV titrated to 8 to 30 mcg/minute. The dose is adjusted according to the blood pressure.
- **Other things you should know about norepinephrine:**

---

- The solution should be given IV using a large vein. Extravasation may cause sloughing and necrosis because of its $\alpha$-adrenergic effect resulting in vasoconstriction. After extravasation occurs, the area should be immediately injected with 10 to 15 mL of saline containing 10 mg of phentolamine.

## Procainamide: Pregnancy Category C

- **Indication:** Effective for both supraventricular and ventricular arrhythmias. It is indicated for conversion of atrial flutter and atrial fibrillation to normal sinus rhythm, for control of ventricular rate in atrial fibrillation in the setting of WPW syndrome, and for stable monomorphic wide complex tachycardia that may be ventricular or supraventricular.
- **Mechanism of Action:** Procainamide is a type IA antiarrhythmic agent (Class I agents inhibit the fast inward sodium channel causing a decrease in the maximum depolarization rate during phase 0 of the action potential). It decreases automaticity by decreasing the slope of spontaneous (phase 4) depolarization. Procainamide also inhibits the potassium channel and therefore prolongs the duration of the action potential. Conduction velocity in the atrium, AV node, His-Purkinje system, and ventricles is prolonged. The drug is metabolized to N-acetylprocainamide (NAPA), which is also an effective antiarrhythmic agent but has Class III effects. Class III drugs prolong the action potential duration as well as refractoriness of cardiac tissues.
- **Dosing:**
  - Procainamide is given IV at an infusion rate of 20 mg/minute. The dose should not exceed 17 mg/kg. The infusion is given until the arrhythmia is suppressed or toxic complications from the drug is manifested such as widening of the QRS complex by 50% when compared with baseline, prolongation of the QT interval or hypotension occurs.
  - When more rapid infusion is needed, an alternative is to give intravenous boluses of ≤100 mg for 3 minutes every 5 minutes. The drug can also be given at a faster infusion rate of 50 mg/minute, to a total dose of 17 mg/kg during cardiac resuscitation.
  - Infusion is maintained at 1 to 4 mg/minute but should be reduced if there is renal dysfunction.
- **Other things you should know about procainamide:**
  - Is effective for both atrial and ventricular arrhythmias.
  - The drug should not be given to patients with prolonged QT interval.
  - Procainamide is negatively inotropic and is proarrhythmic and should not be given to patients with congestive heart failure or patients with systolic left ventricular dysfunction (ejection fraction ≤40%).

- Hypotension can be precipitated if the drug is injected too rapidly.
- Unlike quinidine, another type IA antiarrhythmic agent, procainamide does not increase digoxin levels.
- The drug is metabolized to NAPA, which is also an effective antiarrhythmic agent. When procainamide blood levels are checked, NAPA levels should be included. Therapeutic level of procainamide is 4 to 8 mcg/mL and for NAPA 7 to 15 mcg/mL.
- The drug is mainly excreted through the kidneys unchanged with a half-life of approximately 3 hours. Excretion is delayed when there is renal dysfunction or heart failure.
- Blood levels should be checked when there is renal dysfunction or maintenance infusion exceeds 2 mg/minute or infusion exceeds 48 hours.
- Can cause drug induced lupus when oral therapy is continued for prolonged periods.

## Propranolol (Inderal): Pregnancy Category C

- **Indication:** Propranolol has approved indications for hypertension, angina pectoris, acute myocardial infarction, and treatment of cardiac dysrhythmias including conversion of SVT to normal sinus rhythm.
- **Mechanism:** Propranolol is a nonselective beta blocker with $\beta_1$- and $\beta_2$-adrenergic blocking properties.
- **Dose:** Approximately 1 to 3 mg is initially given. IV administration should not exceed 1 mg/minute. Additional doses may be repeated after 2 minutes if needed. The total IV dose should not exceed 10 mg administered in three equal parts. The total dose can also be given IV piggyback over 10 to 15 minutes. The IV dose is followed by a maintenance oral dose of 180 to 320 mg daily in divided doses.
- **Other things you should know about propranolol:**
  - The elimination half-life of propranolol is 4 hours. After the initial dose, additional IV doses should not be given until after 4 hours after the last dose.
  - The drug is eliminated by hepatic metabolism.

## Sotalol: Pregnancy Category B

- **Indication:**
  - Sotalol is indicated in converting atrial fibrillation to normal sinus rhythm in patients with WPW syndrome when the duration of the atrial fibrillation is ≤48 hours.
  - It is also indicated for monomorphic ventricular tachycardia.

- **Mechanism of action:** Sotalol is a Class III antiarrhythmic agent. Similar to amiodarone, it prolongs action potential duration and increases refractoriness of atrial and ventricular myocardium. It also has nonselective beta blocking properties.
- **Dosing:** The dose is 1 to 1.5 mg/kg given IV at 10 mg/minute.
- **Other things you should know about sotalol:**
  - The intravenous preparation of sotalol is not available in the United States.
  - According to the American College of Cardiology/American Heart Association/European Society of Cardiology 2006 guidelines for the management of patients with atrial fibrillation, sotalol is not effective for conversion of atrial fibrillation to sinus rhythm but is effective for maintenance of sinus rhythm and is used for preventing recurrence of atrial fibrillation after the patient has converted to normal sinus rhythm.
  - In patients with monomorphic VT, sotalol should be given only when left ventricular systolic function is preserved.
  - Sotalol has beta blocking properties. It should not be given to patients who are already on beta blockers.
  - The intravenous infusion can cause bradycardia and hypotension. Sotalol is also proarrhythmic and can cause torsade de pointes.

## Vasopressin (Pitressin): Pregnancy Category C

- **Indication:** VT/VF. Intended as an alternative to epinephrine during cardiac resuscitation.
- **Mechanism of action:** Vasopressin is a non-adrenergic peripheral vasoconstrictor that is naturally present in the body. It is an antidiuretic hormone. The agent becomes a powerful peripheral vasoconstrictor when given in much higher doses than normally present in the body. It does not have beta adrenergic activity and directly stimulates non-adrenergic smooth muscle receptors. It mimics the positive effects but not the adverse effects of epinephrine and has a longer half-life of 10 to 20 minutes compared with epinephrine, which is 3 to 5 minutes.
- **Dosing:** A one-time bolus injection of 40 units given IV during cardiac resuscitation for VT/VF. This substitutes for epinephrine during resuscitation for cardiac arrest, although epinephrine can still be given in repeated doses if necessary after 10 to 20 minutes if vasopressin is not effective.
- **Other things you should know about vasopressin:**
  - Vasopressin is a powerful non-adrenergic vasoconstrictor given as a one-time dose of 40 units. It is

effective even in the presence of severe acidosis, which commonly occurs during cardiac resuscitation.

■ May be effective in asystole and pulseless electrical activity.

## Verapamil (Isoptin): Pregnancy Category C

■ **Indication:** Conversion of paroxysmal supraventricular tachycardia to normal sinus rhythm, control of ventricular rate in atrial flutter, or fibrillation or in patients with multifocal atrial tachycardia.

■ **Mechanism of action:** Verapamil is a nondihydropyridine calcium channel blocker that increases refractoriness of the AV node. It can also slow down the rate of the sinus node. It is a negative inotropic agent and can decrease myocardial contractility resulting in heart failure in patients with left ventricular dysfunction. It is also a peripheral vasodilator and can cause hypotension.

■ **Intravenous dose:** The drug should not be given to patient with left ventricular dysfunction. Give slowly IV 2.5 to 5 mg over 2 minutes, longer in elderly patients, under continuous electrocardiogram and blood pressure monitoring. If not effective, and no adverse event is noted, repeat with another dose of 5 to 10 mg every 15 to 30 minutes to a maximum dose of 20 mg. Another option is to give 5-mg boluses every 15 minutes to a maximum dose of 30 mg.

■ **Other things you should know about verapamil:**
  ■ Nondihydropyridine calcium channel blockers such as verapamil and diltiazem are very effective agents in converting PSVT to normal sinus rhythm. They are the next agents that should be used for conversion of PSVT to normal sinus rhythm if adenosine is not effective or is contraindicated.
  ■ Verapamil is a vasodilator and is negatively inotropic. It should not be given to patients with left ventricular dysfunction or patients with congestive heart failure.
  ■ Verapamil should be given only to paroxysmal supraventricular tachycardia with narrow complexes or supraventricular tachycardia with wide QRS complexes with normal left ventricular function. When there is wide complex tachycardia and the diagnosis of the tachycardia is uncertain, verapamil should not

be given. If the wide complex tachycardia turns out to be ventricular, the administration of verapamil may cause severe hypotension or even death.

■ Intravenous hydration and calcium chloride or calcium gluconate IV may be given to counteract the hypotensive effect of verapamil or diltiazem without diminishing its antiarrhythmic effect.

## Suggested Readings

2005 American Heart Association Guidelines for cardiopulmonary resuscitation and emergency cardiovascular care. Part 7.2: management of cardiac arrest. *Circulation.* 2005: 112;58–66.

Antman EM, Hand M, Armstrong PW, et al. 2007 focused update of the ACC/AHA 2004 guidelines for the management of patients with ST-elevation myocardial infarction. *J Am Coll Cardiol.* 2008;51:210–247.

Blomstrom-Lundqvist C, Scheinman MM, Aliot EM, et al. ACC/AHA/ESC guidelines for the management of patients with supraventricular arrhythmias—executive summary. A report of the American College of Cardiology/American Heart Association Task Force on Practice Guidelines and the European Society of Cardiology Committee for Practice Guidelines. *J Am Coll Cardiol.* 2003;42:1493–1531.

Fuster V, Ryden LE, Cannom DS, et al. ACC/AHA/ESC 2006 guidelines for the management of patients with atrial fibrillation—executive summary; a report of the American College of Cardiology/American Heart Association Task Force and the European Society of Cardiology Committee on Practice Guidelines and the European Society of Cardiology Committee for Practice Guidelines (Writing Committee to Revise the 2001 Guidelines for the Management of Patients with Atrial Fibrillation). *J Am Coll Cardiol.* 2006;48:854–906.

Hazinski MF, Cummins RO, Field JM, eds. *AHA 2002 Handbook of Emergency Cardiovascular Care.* 4th ed. Dallas: American Heart Association; 2002.

Micromedex Healthcare Series. Thomson Healthcare. http://www.thomsonhc.com. Accessed January 2008.

*Physicians' Desk Reference.* 62nd ed. Montvale: Thomson Healthcare Inc; 2008.

Zipes DP, Camm AJ, Borggrefe M, et al. ACC/AHA/ESC 2006 guidelines for management of patients with ventricular arrhythmias and the prevention of sudden cardiac death: a report of the American College of Cardiology/American Heart Association Task Force and the European Society of Cardiology Committee for Practice Guidelines (Writing Committee to Develop Guidelines for management of patients with ventricular arrhythmias and the prevention of sudden cardiac death). *J Am Coll Cardiol.* 2006,48:e247–e346.

Pages numbers in italics denote figures; those followed by a t denote tables.